Design and Development of Affordable Healthcare Technologies

Arindam Bit
National Institute of Technology Raipur, India

A volume in the Advances in Medical Technologies and Clinical Practice (AMTCP) Book Series

IGI Global
DISSEMINATOR OF KNOWLEDGE

Published in the United States of America by
IGI Global
Medical Information Science Reference (an imprint of IGI Global)
701 E. Chocolate Avenue
Hershey PA, USA 17033
Tel: 717-533-8845
Fax: 717-533-8661
E-mail: cust@igi-global.com
Web site: http://www.igi-global.com

Library of Congress Cataloging-in-Publication Data

Names: Bit, Arindam, 1985- editor.
Title: Design and development of affordable healthcare technologies / Arindam Bit, editor.
Description: Hershey, PA : Medical Information Science Reference, [2018] | Includes bibliographical references.
Identifiers: LCCN 2017032789| ISBN 9781522549697 (hardcover) | ISBN 9781522549703 (eBook)
Subjects: | MESH: Biomedical Technology--instrumentation | Equipment Design | Biomedical Engineering--instrumentation | Micro-Electrical-Mechanical Systems--instrumentation | Equipment and Supplies--ethics
Classification: LCC R857.M3 | NLM W 26 | DDC 610.28/4--dc23 LC record available at https://lccn.loc.gov/2017032789

This book is published in the IGI Global book series Advances in Medical Technologies and Clinical Practice (AMTCP) (ISSN: 2327-9354; eISSN: 2327-9370)

British Cataloguing in Publication Data
A Cataloguing in Publication record for this book is available from the British Library.

All work contributed to this book is new, previously-unpublished material. The views expressed in this book are those of the authors, but not necessarily of the publisher.

For electronic access to this publication, please contact: eresources@igi-global.com.

Advances in Medical Technologies and Clinical Practice (AMTCP) Book Series

Srikanta Patnaik
SOA University, India
Priti Das
S.C.B. Medical College, India

ISSN:2327-9354
EISSN:2327-9370

Mission

Medical technological innovation continues to provide avenues of research for faster and safer diagnosis and treatments for patients. Practitioners must stay up to date with these latest advancements to provide the best care for nursing and clinical practices.

The **Advances in Medical Technologies and Clinical Practice (AMTCP) Book Series** brings together the most recent research on the latest technology used in areas of nursing informatics, clinical technology, biomedicine, diagnostic technologies, and more. Researchers, students, and practitioners in this field will benefit from this fundamental coverage on the use of technology in clinical practices.

Coverage

- Medical Imaging
- Patient-Centered Care
- Clinical High-Performance Computing
- Medical informatics
- Neural Engineering
- Biomedical Applications
- Diagnostic Technologies
- Nursing Informatics
- Biomechanics
- Telemedicine

IGI Global is currently accepting manuscripts for publication within this series. To submit a proposal for a volume in this series, please contact our Acquisition Editors at Acquisitions@igi-global.com or visit: http://www.igi-global.com/publish/.

The Advances in Medical Technologies and Clinical Practice (AMTCP) Book Series (ISSN 2327-9354) is published by IGI Global, 701 E. Chocolate Avenue, Hershey, PA 17033-1240, USA, www.igi-global.com. This series is composed of titles available for purchase individually; each title is edited to be contextually exclusive from any other title within the series. For pricing and ordering information please visit http://www.igi-global.com/book-series/advances-medical-technologies-clinical-practice/73682. Postmaster: Send all address changes to above address.

Titles in this Series

For a list of additional titles in this series, please visit: www.igi-global.com/book-series

Multifunctional Nanocarriers for Contemporary Healthcare Applications
Md. Abul Barkat (K.R. Mangalam University, India) Harshita A.B. (K.R. Mangalam University, India) Sarwar Beg (Jubilant Generics, India) and Farhan J. Ahmad (Jamia Hamdard, India)
Medical Information Science Reference • copyright 2018 • 335pp • H/C (ISBN: 9781522547815) • US $265.00

Biomedical Signal and Image Processing in Patient Care
Maheshkumar H. Kolekar (Indian Institute of Technology Patna, India) and Vinod Kumar (Indian Institute of Technology Roorkee, India)
Medical Information Science Reference • copyright 2018 • 312pp • H/C (ISBN: 9781522528296) • US $265.00

Next-Generation Mobile and Pervasive Healthcare Solutions
Jose Machado (University of Minho, Portugal) António Abelha (University of Minho, Portugal) Manuel Filipe Santos (University of Minho, Portugal) and Filipe Portela (University of Minho, Portugal)
Medical Information Science Reference • copyright 2018 • 286pp • H/C (ISBN: 9781522528517) • US $245.00

Innovative Research in Thermal Imaging for Biology and Medicine
Ricardo Vardasca (University of Porto, Portugal) and Joaquim Gabriel Mendes (University of Porto, Portugal)
Medical Information Science Reference • copyright 2017 • 340pp • H/C (ISBN: 9781522520726) • US $210.00

Internet of Things and Advanced Application in Healthcare
Catarina I. Reis (Polytechnic Institute of Leiria, Portugal) and Marisa da Silva Maximiano (Polytechnic Institute of Leiria, Portugal)
Medical Information Science Reference • copyright 2017 • 349pp • H/C (ISBN: 9781522518204) • US $210.00

Integrating Biologically-Inspired Nanotechnology into Medical Practice
B.K. Nayak (K.M. Centre for Post Graduate Studies, India) Anima Nanda (Sathyabama University, India) and M. Amin Bhat (Sathyabama University, India)
Medical Information Science Reference • copyright 2017 • 394pp • H/C (ISBN: 9781522506102) • US $190.00

Recent Advances in Drug Delivery Technology
Raj K. Keservani (Rajiv Gandhi Proudyogiki Vishwavidyalaya, India) Anil K. Sharma (Delhi Institute of Pharmaceutical Sciences and Research, India) and Rajesh Kumar Kesharwani (National Institute of Technology, Warangal, India)
Medical Information Science Reference • copyright 2017 • 510pp • H/C (ISBN: 9781522507543) • US $215.00

IGI Global
DISSEMINATOR OF KNOWLEDGE

701 East Chocolate Avenue, Hershey, PA 17033, USA
Tel: 717-533-8845 x100 • Fax: 717-533-8661
E-Mail: cust@igi-global.com • www.igi-global.com

Table of Contents

Detailed Table of Contents

The rapid growth in information technology (IT) has reshaped traditional infrastructure in several application domains including education, business, and health. Access to patient information, specifically, is vital for effective functioning of a healthcare system; the unavailability of such medical information leads to management issues. IT is no longer perceived as just a supporting tool; it is a tactical necessity for establishing an integrated healthcare infrastructure. Developed nations benefit from the use of modern technology within healthcare to maximize life expectancy and decrease disease. This chapter presents an overview of healthcare conditions of south Asia region. A framework is presented that embeds IT within the healthcare system. The proposed framework has potential to not only restructure but also remove many errors that plague healthcare system. In addition, key problems within the healthcare sector of south Asian countries—Bangladesh, India, Pakistan, and Sri-Lanka—have been highlighted, and recommendations are proposed to overcome the challenges.

There are several classes of surgical instruments such as graspers, clamps, and occluders for blood vessels and other organs; retractors used to spread open skin, ribs, and other tissue; distractors, positioners, and stereotactic devices; mechanical cutters (scalpels, lancets, surgical scissors, etc.); dilators and specula for access to narrow passages or incisions; suction tips and tubes for removal of bodily fluids; sealing devices such as surgical staplers; irrigation and injection needles, tips, and tubes for introducing fluid; powered devices, such as drills, dermatomes; scopes and probes, including fiber optic endoscopes and tactile probes; carriers and appliers for optical, electronic, and mechanical devices; ultrasound tissue disruptors, cryotomes, and cutting laser guides; measurement devices, such as rulers and calipers; and many more. This chapter overviews surgical instruments for the operation theatre.

Rehabilitation is an area of focus by experts and researchers from different disciplines owing to the increase in number of various types of disabilities. This chapter covers information relating to causes and need for rehabilitation devices for differently abled people with motor, vision, or hearing impairment. The chapter begins with a brief on the disability population worldwide and in India, and progresses towards presenting available devices in global market and possible improvement that can be made to improve the functionality of the device and in turn improve the quality of life (QoL) of the users. Towards the end of the chapter, a reader can acquire the fundamental knowledge about the different types of disability, suitable aids, and working.

Occupational morbidities during manual material handling operations are routine at workplaces. This is a global burden contributing substantially to the economy. The multifactorial etiology for musculoskeletal disorders (MSDs) along with workplace stressors require multidisciplinary preventive effort. Biomechanics plays a pivotal role in occupational health research quarrying into the root cause analysis of posture, load handling, muscular loading, balance, and stability at work. Sophisticated instrumentation and experimental techniques assist in understanding the biomechanical mechanisms of MSDs and ergonomic principles, etc. Kinetic, kinematic, isotonic, isokinetic, as well as isometric experimental modes investigate body postures and muscular responses. Foundation of biomechanics instrumentation and injury mechanism would aid researchers alongside ergonomists in dealing with identification, assessment, and control of workplace risks through participatory ergonomics approach. Judicious utilization of this discipline would approach a long-term sustainable solution to protect health and safety of workers at the workplace.

The term control release means the release of the molecules from any reservoir in very precise and constant amounts and following zero-order or near-to-zero-order release kinetics. This type of formulation and device has a huge market over the medical world. The basic foundation of sustained release drug delivery system enhances the biopharmaceutical and pharmacodynamics pharmacokinetic properties of a drug in such a way that its usefulness is exploited, side-effects are reduced, and cure of the disease is attained easily. The international controlled-release drug delivery technology market has been divided on the basis of technology, application, release mechanism, and geography. This chapter describes these topics: metered dose inhalers, transdermal and ocular patches, drug eluting stents, activation-modulated drug delivery systems, polymer coating systems microelectromechanical technology, implants, micro reservoir partition controlled drug delivery systems, hydrophilic polymer matrix systems, targeted delivery, enzyme activated device.

The confluence of wireless body area network (WBAN) advancement has led to a great shift in the healthcare sector and has enormous potential to reduce long-term costs, social problems, workforce issues, and improve quality of healthcare service. Based on existing literature on WBANs, technologies, and standards, a WBAN is proposed to bridge the gap of information between patients and healthcare professional through sharing of high quality of information (QoI) whereby the latter can have real-time and historical view of patient's condition for effective and timely monitoring. This feature will also address the time and space restriction of healthcare service. Moreover, a best fit glucose prediction model considering various exogenous inputs based on autoregressive (ARX) model is proposed to perform data analytics in a WBAN system. The performance of the model is evaluated through performance metrics. Potential challenges and future research work are pointed out for further development of WBAN.

Implantable drug delivery devices have shown promise for drug administration for management of several diseases spanning chronic diseases to emergency medicine as they overcome the limitations of continuous monitoring by medical physician or paramedical professional. Micro-electro mechanical systems (MEMS) technologies are they key enabling technology platform that allow fabrication of miniature devices with precise control over drug dosing rates. Recently, many of these technologies are also finding applications in microfluidic chips applications. MEMS are composed of microvalves, microchannels, microsensors, and micropumps within a miniaturized control device. Among these, micropumps play a dynamic role in determining the extent of control over drug dispensation. In this chapter, principles and developments of MEMS-based drug delivery systems with micropumps are presented, which may allow future development of affordable technologies based on this principle.

Before starting semi-pilot/pilot production plants for biochemical metabolites production, it is essential to optimize the fermentation media. This chapter discusses the classical and advanced techniques of media optimization. The statistical approaches save experimental time for developing processing and improving quality. Recent years have seen the growth of integrated approaches of microbial cultures.

This chapter is an attempt to understand the effect of audio-visual stimulus with a humorous content on the cardiac electrophysiology. Electrocardiogram (ECG) signals were acquired from 11 female volunteers under the pre- and the post-stimulus conditions. Artificial neural network (ANN)-based classification of the ARMA model coefficients computed from the RR interval signals suggested significant variation in the autonomic nervous system activity. Analysis of the Gabor denoised ECG signals indicated a change in the electrical activity of the heart in the post-stimulus condition, which was confirmed by the ANN-based classification. Recurrence analysis of the RR interval suggested plausible differences of the cardiac activity amongst both the conditions. The audio-visual stimulus has resulted in significant alterations in the ANS and the cardiac physiology.

This chapter is aimed at identifying the variation in the cardiac electrophysiology due to the abuse of the cannabis products (bhang) in a non-invasive manner. ECG signals were acquired from 25 Indian women working in the paddy fields. Amongst them, 10 women regularly abused bhang and the rest 15 women never abused bhang. The ECG signals were preprocessed and subjected to wavelet packet decomposition (WPD) up to the level 3 using db04 wavelet. Ninety-six statistical features were extracted from the wavelet packet coefficients and analyzed using linear and non-linear statistical methods. The results suggested a variation in the cardiac electrophysiology due to the abuse of bhang. Artificial neural networks (ANNs), namely, radial basis function (RBF) and multilayer perceptron (MLP) were able to classify the ECG signals with an accuracy of $\geq$95%. This supported the hypothesis that abuse of bhang may alter the cardiac electrophysiology. The results of the study may be used to increase awareness among people to avoid the abuse of cannabis products.

Preface

Medical devices are major backbone of healthcare industries of modern ear. It covers wide spectrum of support to diagnose, interpret, intervention and therapeutic procedures for users. With the increase of diversified diseases, cross-sectional and highly interdisciplinary approaches are required to address solutions for severely affected diseased situations in light of advancement of medical sciences. This book preview few of the fascinating venture of highly multi-modal diagnostic systems for the detection and possible solution to a few critical diseases. The main objective of this book is to enlighten the readers with innovative and further simplified techniques for detection and tackle many critical diseases. This book also serves with wide domain of application of many diagnostic techniques like ECG and EEG for detecting and diagnosis of many diseases/habits and outcomes of certain physiological practices and treatment procedures. This book also enlightens the readers with the application of modern days computational technique as tools for integrating many multi-model expert systems.

This book contains 16 chapters. The Introduction covers an introductory phase of the entire spectrum of modern days laboratory and trial stages technologies which can play significant role in converging modern healthcare technology in affordable form. In order to illustrate the various band of spectrum of these technologies, the remaining 16 chapters are contributed by some of the most distinguished authors specializing in the field of healthcare technologies.

Chapter 1, "Healthcare Services in Developing Countries of the South-Asian Region: Present and Future Perspectives," illustrates the scenario of present healthcare sector in South-Asian region. The chapter also illustrates the prospective future development in healthcare sector in light to the fast-growing development of laboratory research in domain of healthcare sector.

Chapter 2, "Overview on Surgical Instruments for Operation Theatre," illustrates a comprehensive description of all modern days surgical instruments which are essential for operation theatre. It explains the working principle of all those instruments. It was followed by instruments used for rehabilitation.

Therefore, Chapter 3, "Devices for Rehabilitation," explains the working principles of advanced rehabilitation devices. Here, it brings the cross-talk between multi-disciplinary technology to address better solution for rehabilitation engineering.

Chapter 4, "Application of Biomechanics Instrumentation in Occupational Health Research," deals with the cross-talk of biomechanical principles and occupational problems and illustrates prospective solutions for occupational therapy. Until now, technology for delivery of targeted drug has not been discussed.

Therefore, Chapter 5, "Devices for Controlled Release Advancements and Effectiveness," illustrates the working principle of precise devices which perform drug-delivery in targeted organ of the body in a controlled rate.

Chapter 6, "Low Cost Body Areas Network for Monitoring of Diabetic Patient," illustrates an example of drug-delivery in human body. This chapter explains the working principle of various drug-delivery techniques to address the management of drug-delivery to patients with diabetes in correlation to continuous monitoring of various physiological parameters of the body relevant to diabetes.

Chapter 7, "Advances in MEMS and Micro-Scale Technologies for Application in Controlled Drug-Dosing Systems: MEMS-Based Drug Delivery System," explains the application of MEMS architecture to establish controlled drug-delivery unit. Once again, a cross-disciplinary approach has been adopted to address an advancement in healthcare unit.

Another dimension of advancement of drug-delivery and continuous effective diagnosis of diseased organ of human body in non-invasive manner has been illustrated in Chapter 8, "Optimization Techniques Application in Biochemical Engineering and Controlled Drug Delivery: Current Practices and Forthcoming Challenges". This chapter also illustrates the working principle of various optimization technique for the designing and development of drug-delivery unit.

Chapter 9, "Segmentation of Liver From Three-Dimensional Medical Imaging Dataset for Diagnosis and Treatment Planning of Liver Disorder," reveals the diagnostic technique of liver diseases and continuous evaluation of the treatment protocol using image processing tools and most modern advancement in technology. This chapter illustrates the efficiency of multi-modal technology for non-invasive diagnosis of liver anatomy.

Another example of multimodal technology advancement is in the form of rehabilitation devices. And it has been illustrated in Chapter 10, "Development of Text-to-Speech Scanner for Visually Impaired People". In this chapter, a projection has been made to elaborate various principles of multi-lingual character-speech scanner which are systemically evaluated for blind people. In this way the discontinuity in sensory paradigm of challenged people are addressed using modern healthcare toolkits. In another segment of this book, role of electrophysiological signals for intervention of various diseases has been represented in a systemic manner.

Chapter 11, "Analysis of ECG Signals to Investigate the Effect of a Humorous Audio-Visual Stimulus on Autonomic Nervous System and Heart of Females," illustrates the method of establishment of correlation between autonomic nervous system and heart-rate of female under the influence of emotional audio-video stimulus. It illustrates the technique of ECG signal analysis for interpretation of the autonomic and cardiac crosstalk. In further chapter, various techniques of ECG signal analysis are illustrated for interpretation of various diseases.

Chapter 12, "Wavelet Packet Analysis of ECG Signals to Understand the Effect of Cannabis Abuse on Cardiac Electrophysiology of Indian Women Working in Paddy Fields," illustrates wavelet analysis technique for processing of ECG signals of paddy field workers for intervention of cardiac physiological state under the influence of abuse due to cannabis.

In the following chapter, "Analysis of the Changes in the RR Interval Signals of Smokers Using Recurrence Analysis and ANN Classification," recurrence analysis is illustrated for determination of R-R interval of ECG signals of smokers. Further, R-R interval related features are classified by artificial neural network techniques. In this chapter, a glimpse of machine – learning algorithm for intervention of features of biosignals, mainly cardiological signals has been elaborated. Further, modern techniques of telemedicine are also employed for cardiological signals have been elaborated.

Chapter 14, "Remote Monitoring via EEG of Persons in Severe Depression," elaborates the telemedicine technology for analysis of EEG signal of patients suffering from severe depression. It elaborates the feasibility of continuous remote monitoring of big data and its rapid analysis.

Subsequent chapter, "Effect of Motivational Songs on the Autonomic Nervous System and the Heart of Indian Male Volunteers," illustrates the intervention of autonomic nervous system and its correlation with heart rate of individual under the influence of motivational songs. Entropy of EEG spectrum are evaluated, and features of EEG signal in relevance to motivational songs are extracted using advance machine learning algorithms. Lastly, the book is concluded with illustration on wide spectrum of machine-learning features in healthcare sector.

Chapter 16, "Application of Machine Learning Techniques in Disease Classification From Medical Images: Recent Practices and Future Challenges," illustrates the utility of various algorithms of machine learning for the intervention of diseases on the basis of feature extraction from medical images. However, along with the advancement in science and technology of soft computing techniques, the various aspects of limitation of machine learning techniques towards the robustness and enhancement of accuracy of the outcomes of feature selection is also discussed as a section of limitation and future challenges.

Introduction

AN OVERVIEW OF DESIGN AND DEVELOPMENT OF AFFORDABLE HEALTHCARE TECHNOLOGIES

Health plays a vital role in the life of an individual. Health can be described as the physical and mental ability to tolerate any changes that may occur in the environment. Each and every individual has a right to health: that means access to all medical services, devices, healthy conditions and environment.

Health care technologies can be described as organization established to meet the health needs of targeted population. According to World Health Organization (WHO), for a healthcare system to work properly, it requires sufficient financing and well trained team for implementation of healthcare policies.

Healthcare system varies with country to country depending on the population, economical, social and health policies of individual country. Developed countries will have good economy and will be able to make healthcare system available to their population. On the contrary, under developed countries still has to suffer to meet the basic health needs. The present situation of the healthcare system around the world is that the developed countries are thriving to improve the present system while some economically poor countries are still struggling to improve the facilities for basic health care. The main reasons why poor countries are unable to provide complete healthcare system to their population is the lack of sufficient medicines, trained professionals, inadequate fund and lack of coordination between public and private sector.

In this book, we have illustrated the healthcare technologies that can be provided at very affordable cost so that each and every individual will have access to it.

With the help of developing technologies, many devices can be developed to detect or treat various abnormalities. But, the question that arises is the cost of the device. If the device is too costly, then most of the population cannot afford that. So, here in this book, we have discussed some of the devices developed that are accessible to majority of the population.

Conventional drug delivery system is facing some problems such as incorrect dosing, drug permeability, toxicity and side effects. Mostly, drugs in use are hydrophobic and cannot dissolve in blood stream resulting in reduced pharmacological efficiency. To overcome these problems, local and targeted drug delivery systems are considered as alternatives. Localized drug delivery has many advantages over conventional methods like minimizing fluctuations in plasma concentration of drug, pharmacodynamics and lowering the dose-dependent toxicity. Some of the advanced drug delivery devices include Microelecromechanical systems (MEMS), microchip based drug delivery, magnetically controlled MEMS etc.

According to WHO, 36 million population are blind and 217 million population are having moderate to severe vision impairment. For a blind person, it is very difficult to learn language and lead normal.

Although many devices are available to convert speech to text, they are expensive and cannot be afforded by common people. To make those kind of devices affordable, device is made that captures the image, converts to text and then again gets converted into voice. This speech scanner device developed is not only affordable but also portable which makes easy for visually impaired persons to read the text material.

In some diseases like cancer, diagnosis is very difficult. the conventional method for cancer detection is biopsy which is very costly at the same time very painful procedure. So, the alternative method researchers have developed are diagnosis that are done using machines and imaging such as CAD(Computer Aided Diagnosis) in which diagnosis is done with the help of images.

Rehabilitation is any form of permanent or temporary inability, malfunction of body part of individual which effects the quality of living. Although many devices are available to correct the inabilities, most of them are highly expensive. In this chapter, we discuss about development of prosthesis and orthosis, so that they can reach most of the impaired populations.

The liver is one of the largest organ in the human body. The major activities of liver are metabolism of fat, carbohydrates, processing of blood plasma proteins, cholesterol etc. With the changes in the living habits and other condition of an individual, liver suffers from many kinds of abnormalities like Hepatitis, Cirrhosis, Fibrosis etc. Other major disease affecting liver is cancer. As Liver plays major role in maintaining and regulating many chemicals in the body, it is important to detect the condition of effected liver at early stages to control further damage. Although there are many devices for detection like MRI, CT scan, Ultrasound, etc., they are expensive and out of reach of common population. So there is huge demand for devices to detect liver disease at very low cost so that most of the population will be benefited.

Diabetes is a condition where blood glucose (blood sugar) levels of an individual increase. Though it does not seems to be very critical disease, if left untreated, diabetes can cause many complication like blindness, heart attacks, kidney failure and so on. Early diagnosis and simple changes in lifestyle of an individual can control the diabetes. Although there are many devices for diagnosis, researchers are mainly focusing on simple diagnosis tools including development of sensors which can accurately measure the blood sugar levels and can be handled by the individual itself at an affordable rate.

Even though there is an advancement in health care technology, still its use is limited all across the globe due to either lack of awareness, cost and complexity. Therefore, nowadays many attempts are made to have affordable and accessible health care technology with main focus on cost effectiveness and simplicity. The emerging health care technology represents evolution of cost effective and simple to operate health care systems with guaranteed increase in life expectancy.

A number of diagnostic tools were developed utilizing the advantage of miniaturization technology. MEMS is one of the versatile application of electronics. Patients get benefited from the development of microelectronics such as MEMS. Among the MEMS technology, micropumps are widely used in biomedical industries for drug delivery. A very detailed description of the various types of MEMS based micropumps along with their comparison is explained in this book.

Biomechanics contains the concepts of fluid and solid mechanics to study different problems of biology and mechanics of human organism by reacting to different types of external stimuli. This helps in diagnosis by establishing relation between phenomena of blood flow. In Chapter 7 various biomechanical instruments to carry out the biomechanical research are described.

Chapters 1-4 of this book presented topics on ECG based data, intending to give an advanced understanding of the topic, allowing readers to create their own ideas to design experiment based on ECG derived non-invasive data. There exists many literature having discussion on cardiovascular disease as common cause of death. ECG signals derived can be used to monitor all the cardiac activities. In Chapter 1, ECG data indicates that Cannabis Savita users are having significantly more variation in cardiac electrophysiology. The effect of Cannabis Savita based products mainly the bhang whose abusing results in the physiological variation of the heart, causing cardiovascular diseases. These variations can be analyzed using ECG signal feature extraction which reduces the dimensions of the original ECG data. The desired signal processing operations are carried out by various feature extraction methods and classification techniques among which the multi-parametric nature of ANN proves to be the easiest and accurate statistically significant feature analyzing technique. Also the effect of Tobacco consumption using ECG based data is presented in Chapter 4. The abuse of tobacco-based products such as Cigarette smoking has been reported to detriment the cardiac physiology by increasing the plasma catecholamine level and tachycardia effect. The baroreflex sensitivity is impaired due to smoking, thereby, increasing the blood pressure and the heart rate. The R-R interval variability or heart rate variability (HRV) signals are non-stationary signals and are analyzed via non-linear techniques like empirical mode decomposition and recurrence analysis which provides an easy and noninvasive means to analyse the ANS-based regulation of the cardiac physiology which were subjected to ANN classification. Chapter 2 tells about recording of ECG signals to do HRV analysis. As music plays an important role in the alteration of psychological state of emotion. The psychological processes like promoting sleep, reducing anxiety, and increasing brain activities are controlled by the functioning of ANS. The HRV analysis are achieved by studying the ANS functioning on cardiac activity which includes the beat-to-beat interval variation of the heart. HRV is studied by recording ECG signals and computing recurrence analysis which provides information about the temporal variation in a time series due to any stimulus or pathological condition. The HRV and the ECG (either original or wavelet processed) signal statistical parameters were used to classify the differences in both the pre- and the post-stimulus conditions of ANS activity and cardiac activities. Chapter 3 explains that the SA node is the collection of excitatory cells which are responsible for rhythmic contraction of the heart. The nerve innervations of the ANS is responsible to assess the emotions such as sadness, happiness, fear, disgust and neutral in humans. The audio-visual stimuli have also been exploited to evaluate the effect of the ANS activity and the mood states by monitoring the variation in the time duration of the consecutive 'R' peaks. The EEG signals about the electrical activities and the RRI time series describes the change in the heart rate, galvanic skin response and respiratory activities non-invasively.

Even though there is a wide development, still surgeries are always considered as the global health priority. As it plays important role to help those suffering from either emergency, complications or chronic disability through instrumental and manual means. In Chapter 6 effective explanation of close attention on the appropriate design, variety is presented which can help to enhance its use in modern health care. Recent robotic based surgery equipment's allow surgeons to have an effective interventional procedure in surgery. This robotic based surgery helps to have surgery using minimally invasive procedures. This Minimally Invasive Surgery (MIS) can help in reduction of cost with many others benefits for the patients and even surgeons. This robot based technology have revolutionized modern surgical instruments, but can be widely accepted only after having proper knowledge of its application and use.

CONCLUDING REMARKS

Modernization in the healthcare field can be expanded by revolutionizing the field of health care support technology by educating the user. The combination of MEMS technologies with the Internet-of-Things (IoT), wireless and digital data transmission forms a driving force for health technology. Further major impact in enhancing expertise in the medical technology field can be done by integrating computational biology with biomechanics field.

Also cardiac disease can be predicted by changes in the ECG signals. With this non-invasive technique, the growing complications with intake of Cannabis Savita and tobacco over cardiovascular disease has been studied effectively and further in-depth analysis can be also done to classify the exact changes occurring in the ECG signals. Also the effect of music on emotions by extracting RRIs from ECG signals to do recurrence, HRV analysis for understanding the ANS activity. The Recurrence analysis of the ANS activity and the electrophysiology of the heart suggested a difference in the dynamic nature of the pre- and the post-stimulus RRI time series and shows 100% classification accuracy using statistically significant features, obtained from the ARMA model coefficients. The classification of the statistically significant features shows >95% efficiency of the de-noised ECG signals using Gabor transform.

Research in manufacturing of surgical instruments need to be done, where hypotheses should be made on the graphical design of the instruments, usage on instruments to maintain accuracy, development of modern medical instruments based on the surgery to be done or to find suitable materials for manufacturing the instruments. This will help to have low cost and optimized surgery to reduce disease burden.

Science and technology has developed very rapidly over the decades. Especially in healthcare system, we can say that, almost each and every disease can be diagnosed and cured with the available devices and treatments. With this, we can attain 100% healthy population which is not the case. Coming to the reality, even though there are so many advanced equipments and devices in the healthcare system, almost all are very expensive and not in reach to common population. Even if there are some affordable devices, they are not reaching to the population, either due to lack of knowledge or ignorance. The main aspect of the non- availability of healthcare systems in underdeveloped countries is not only the lack of economic stability, but also illiteracy and lack of awareness by concerned government to approach each and every group of population. At the beginning of the book, we have discussed some healthcare devices for common diseases like diabetes, liver diseases, blindness, etc. that can be developed to make it affordable. The main challenge is not only to develop affordable devices but also to create awareness among the people with which the purpose will be fulfilled completely.

Arindam Bit
National Institute of Technology Raipur, India

Chapter 1
Healthcare Services in Developing Countries of the South Asian Region: Present and Future Perspectives

Hiba Shah
Mehran University of Engineering and Technology, Pakistan

Areej Fatemah Meghji
Mehran University of Engineering and Technology, Pakistan

Naeem A. Mahoto
Mehran University of Engineering and Technology, Pakistan

ABSTRACT

The rapid growth in information technology (IT) has reshaped traditional infrastructure in several application domains including education, business, and health. Access to patient information, specifically, is vital for effective functioning of a healthcare system; the unavailability of such medical information leads to management issues. IT is no longer perceived as just a supporting tool; it is a tactical necessity for establishing an integrated healthcare infrastructure. Developed nations benefit from the use of modern technology within healthcare to maximize life expectancy and decrease disease. This chapter presents an overview of healthcare conditions of south Asia region. A framework is presented that embeds IT within the healthcare system. The proposed framework has potential to not only restructure but also remove many errors that plague healthcare system. In addition, key problems within the healthcare sector of south Asian countries—Bangladesh, India, Pakistan, and Sri-Lanka—have been highlighted, and recommendations are proposed to overcome the challenges.

DOI: 10.4018/978-1-5225-4969-7.ch001

INTRODUCTION

Health is an essential need of human beings. A healthy person is an asset of the country. To ensure fine health, in such a complex and busy world, there is an increasing need of healthcare systems (Lindblad et al., 2017). Healthcare, as the word suggests, is caring for health; essentially this means meeting the basic medical needs of an individual or a population. It encompasses the prevention and cure of diseases by providing vaccines, ensuring sanitary conditions, adequate hospital facilities and educating the masses on awareness of diseases.

Healthcare systems can be seen as organizations specifically established to meet the needs of a certain targeted population. According to the World Health Organization (WHO), in order for healthcare systems to function well, they require a mechanism of steady financing; a workforce that is properly trained and sufficiently-paid; reliable information on which decisions can be based; and health facilities that are adequately maintained.

Policies of a country vary in relation to personal and population based health care goals. Similarly, access to healthcare varies across individuals, regions and countries, being highly influenced by not only economic and health policies of the region, but also social conditions. Developed nations have always laid great emphasis on high quality healthcare. Campaigns and policies promoting healthcare have influenced political outcomes. One such example is the Patient Protection and Affordable Care Act, nicknamed Obamacare (Rosenbaum, 2011).

We live in a world where digital innovation is at the forefront of transforming healthcare, where technology is advancing to provide better data, allowing more informed decisions (Weaver et al., 2016). Care providers are creating new ways to improve the quality and cost of patient care. Apart from this, cultural shifts, policy adjustments and due to recent technological advances, over the last decade, a more patient empowered approach is being adopted by many hospitals by prioritizing prevention. Use of Electronic Records, Telemedicine, Remote Monitoring and Wearable Technology has reshaped the healthcare infrastructure (Tomines et al., 2013; Mupela et al., 2011). Developed nations are benefiting from the use of technology within healthcare to maximize life expectancy and decrease disease (Kevin, 2016).

One problem with the use of technology in healthcare, however, is that many healthcare devices operate in silos (Eric, 2014). Over a third of healthcare organizations don't apply data from connected devices to other business processes; an issue that creates inefficiency, potential for data loss and mistakes in diagnosis. Effective healthcare depends on speed and accuracy. There thus emerges a need to somehow connect these devices and share their data over a centralized platform. In doing so, patients will no longer have to carry files with background medical information and treatments as they visit hospitals. More importantly their medical history will be accessible, without omissions, for a better diagnosis. The introduction and integration of technology, specifically the Internet of Things (IoT), in the health sector has the potential to overcome these issues.

The networked interconnection of everyday objects, which are often equipped with ubiquitous intelligence, may be a simple explanation for the term IoT. IoT provides the facility of integrating every object for the purpose of interaction via embedded systems, which leads to a highly distributed network of devices communicating with each other as well as human beings (Xia et al., 2012). IoT is redefining healthcare by introducing innovative ways that apps, devices and people interact when delivering healthcare solutions.

The use of technology in healthcare can mean different things to different people. For most people it means some form of connectivity that connects things and people across the healthcare ecosystem to acquire, aggregate and analyze data in order to glean actionable insights (Tan & Ong, 2002). The more common use cases in healthcare involve connecting people; consumers, clinicians and caregivers. Healthcare organizations have piloted many connected health projects merely aimed at improving consumer engagement. The ability to connect consumers and patients and affect their behavior will encourage them to make healthier decisions, which in turn will lead to better outcomes and lower healthcare costs (Fernandez & Pallis, 2014).

Nevertheless where developed nations are striving to elevate healthcare infrastructures, healthcare does not top the priority list in most developing nations. Healthcare in south Asian counties like Pakistan, Bangladesh, India and Sri-Lanka face a range of problems (Van et al., 2016). The infrastructure of healthcare in Pakistan, for instance, is extremely weak. It faces a range of problems, from mismanagement to the lack of professionalism, inadequacies of staff, insufficient equipment and medicines and lack of coordination between private and public sector hospitals (Arif, 2017). As diseases and fatalities in the country continue to increase, the status of healthcare system in Pakistan continues to stay stagnant, worsen and declined (Shehzad, 2005). Likewise, current state of healthcare services in Sri-Lanka is inadequate and insufficient (Van et al., 2016). India is also not an exception in healthcare services in comparison with its neighboring nations. Poor health conditions, infrastructure and lack of effective policies have been observed as major issues in India (Ma & Sood, 2008). This year, the highest budget has been allocated for health in the USA (Federal Budget, 2016). Similar trends were observed in other developed nations such as UK, Germany, Australia, Italy and Germany (OECD, 2015). A lack of interest of the government towards the healthcare system in Pakistan is clearly reflected in the annual budget allocation for healthcare (Pakistan Federal Budget, 2016). The similar trends have been observed in other south Asian nations: India, Bangladesh and Sri-Lanka (Van et al., 2016).

The emerging innovations of IT hold the key to reshape the healthcare paradigm. However, developing nations, especially south Asian region, lack from such human friendly technological solutions at broad level (World Report, 2017). Therefore, there is an ever-growing need for determining the gaps and key challenges that result in the poor health conditions in south Asian countries. The aim of this chapter is identifying the fundamental issues that result in the poor healthcare services of south Asian nations. Furthermore, chapter proposes recommendations to address the gap and a generic model (i.e., Framework) to rapidly resolve the several issues with technological solutions.

This chapter begins by presenting current conditions of the healthcare services, budget, policies and priorities of the developing countries of south Asia. It also includes similar statistics of developed countries to compare and identify gaps. After identification of gaps, recommendations have been made. Besides, a framework has been proposed in order to improve healthcare services, because there is an ever-growing need for a generic model that incorporates the various aspects in developing countries like Bangladesh, India, Pakistan and Sri-Lanka. Although the current healthcare systems in south Asian nations face a lot of problems, the introduction and centralized use of advanced IT in this sector can significantly help overcome many of the obstacles. The implementation of proposed model will reduce the human errors. The proposed framework may help to reshape the existing healthcare system to adopt technological solutions.

This chapter is organized as follows: Section *Background* indicates a brief outline of health priorities in developed and developing countries. Healthcare systems of several countries have been explored in *Overview of healthcare systems in different countries* section. The next section, *Health System comparison between developing and developed countries,* presents a comparison in health conditions based on factors such as health expenditure, health facilities, population, life expectancy, level of mismanagement and use of technology within developed and south Asian developing countries. The details of the different technologies and systems that are being used in healthcare around the globe are described in the *Emerging changes in healthcare system* section. The details of the suggested framework/model are described in *Proposed Framework* section to tackle previously highlighted problems. Further, *Applications of the Proposed Framework* and *Recommendations* are given, and finally the conclusion is presented in the *conclusion* section.

BACKGROUND

Healthcare system has evolved over the years, with many of the changes being influenced by technological advances. Routine procedures like surgical removal of a cataract, which required several hours of surgery and intensive care, over extensive time duration after the procedure, is now performed in 15 minutes on an outpatient basis (Vance, 2017). Patients suffering from kidney ailments have the facility of installing a dialysis machine at home (Garrick et al., 2012). Today, using high resolution cameras and smaller incisions allow faster healing while performing Laparoscopic surgery (Chambers et al., 2011).

Over the years a high emphasis has been paid on treating patients quickly and reducing the amount of time they spend in hospitals. Researchers have been trying to come up with innovative ways to use technology within healthcare to influence better treatment. Although steady improvement has been seen across the globe in Australia, England, Germany and United States of America, the healthcare system in developing countries, namely Bangladesh, India, Pakistan and Sri Lanka, continues to face many problems; weak infrastructure, poor outcomes to total health expenditure, poor use of technology and poor governance to name a few (Cline & Luiz, 2013). The public healthcare system, specifically, faces many problems as private hospitals are delivering better health services as compared to public hospitals (Irfan & Ijaz, 2011). A study by (Van et al.,2016), has shown that the total expenditure on health as percentage of Gross domestic Product (GDP) in developing countries is maximum 4%, whereas in Developed Countries it is 17% of the maximum GDP rate (The World Bank, 2016)

Studies have been carried out and frameworks have been proposed to improve healthcare in developing countries. For instance, (Leite et al., 2012), presented the concept of using mobile technologies in hospital systems in order to make them automated. Further, he suggested an architecture showing how the hospitals can be automatized, patient conditions monitored and their data extracted using sensors. (Leite et al.,2012), also suggested an architecture for implementing mobile technologies in hospital management in order to improve healthcare services.

According to (Mahoto et al., 2014), integration of wireless technologies in healthcare can improve the quality of service in hospitals. The authors suggested an innovative framework to improve hospital management by means of integrated wireless technology (WBAN). Sensors have been employed to collect healthcare data; furthermore, the collected data has been examined/analyzed by using data mining techniques for extracting meaningful knowledge. Moreover, this architecture can help in managing the hospital resources, and also for managing the required services.

OVERVIEW OF THE HEALTHCARE SYSTEM IN DIFFERENT COUNTRIES

Generally, healthcare system falls in two categories: 'public' and 'private' sectors. Both sectors run in parallel in many of countries of the world. Some countries provide free of charge medical care as public hospitals are funded, owned and run by the government; thus giving them the alternate name of government hospitals. On the other hand, private hospitals are funded privately or by any company and the patients themselves pay money for any kind of medical services.

In developing countries, the healthcare system is somewhat inadequate; especially, the quality of care is largely ignored (John, 2006). Some suggest that public healthcare systems are poor because of the economic condition of the government (Kurji et al., 2016). However, apart from the economic factor, public hospitals suffer from structural fragmentation, poor management caused by a lack of doctors and nurses, and poor infrastructure (Mills, 2014). With the overload to the doctors and staff due to shortage of human resources and the manual work, human error is common. In contrast, the services provided by the private hospitals are far better than public hospitals (Irfan & Ijaz, 2011). It is due to this and the dismal conditions in public hospitals, that people have started preferring private hospitals over their public counterparts (Jabnoun & Chaker, 2003)..

Although private hospitals offer efficient use of well-equipped instruments and resources, a patient cannot always afford the treatment costs of such an institution (Jahanzeb, 2017). It is estimated that every year 100 million people are pushed into poverty because they have to pay directly for health services (Anup, 2011). This makes obtaining good quality treatment extremely hard for people with financial constraints. In India, for instance, private hospitals as growing rapidly with better medical facilities, but unfortunately these are unaffordable for an average Indian due to poverty (Ma & Sood, 2008). It thus becomes even more important for public sector hospitals to provide adequate healthcare service. Unfortunately in developing countries, the total expenditure spent on health as percentage of GDP is under 4%, which is clearly insufficient. (The World Bank, 2016).

In countries like USA, England and Australia, health insurance is mandatory and is provided to citizens by the government (Robertson et al., 2014). Penalty may be fined who do not obtain health insurance (Michelle, 2014; Phil, 2015). Health insurance covers services including consultation to doctors, lab tests and hospitalization (Utkarsh, 2016).

A large share of health budget in the GDP is the prime reason for good healthcare system. For instance, health share in the budget of the USA is 17% of the GDP (OECD, 2017), which is remarkable. Due to such huge shares in budget, the developed world is able to provide competitive public health facilities, contrary to their counterpart world. Secondly, the availability of technology in developed countries results in effective procedures for treatment. Thirdly, awareness among people on how to use technology and understand their needs is essential in the success of the system. Finally, to add more to the effectiveness of the system, infrastructure plays an elementary role.

The use of Information Technology (IT) includes electronic patient registration, computerized medical records in hospitals, use of Internet for communication and information exchange. Additionally, for user identification they use medical cards, electronic scheduling systems for appointments, examinations and hospital admissions (Tomasi et al., 2004) and continuing research in medical science. Moreover, computerized protocols for diagnosis and treatment support are just a few examples.

HEALTH SYSTEM COMPARISON BETWEEN DEVELOPING AND DEVELOPED COUNTRIES

This section explores the differences in healthcare in terms of healthcare expenditure, population, healthcare facilities, level of mismanagement, life expectancy rate and use of technology within developed and developing nations.

Healthcare Expenditure

Health expenditure is the amount of money spent on health services and facilities. It generally includes public and private expenditures. Government as well as non-government donators spend in health systems as budget highly affects the quality and effectiveness of healthcare services.

In developed countries, the total expenditure spent on health is higher in numbers of GDP. This year highest budget for health sector has been allocated in the USA, which is 17.1% of GDP on health in fiscal year 2016 (The World Bank, 2016). Likewise, in other developed countries it is: UK - 9.8%, Australia - 9.3%, Germany - 11.1% (OECD, 2016). However, in developing countries the expenditure on health is under 4%, which clearly shows the priority of the government towards healthcare services. One example of developing country of south Asia is India, where the expenditure spent on health is just 4% in FY 2016. While the budget share of health in fiscal year 2016 of Pakistan remains lower, that is 2.8% of the GDP. Similarly, Sri Lanka - 3.2% and Bangladesh - 3.7% (Van et al., 2016). The drastic difference of spending on health between the developed and developing countries reflects in the difference in the effectiveness and technological adoption in their health systems.

Moreover, the provision of healthcare is not only the responsibility of the government, but also a basic right of the citizens. With rapid growth in the inhabitants of a country, explicit measures need to be taken to ensure adequate healthcare facilities. Sadly, the healthcare system in south Asian countries continues to steadily decline. Consider an example of the healthcare facilities in Pakistan. The healthcare system in Pakistan is plagued with numerous problems. One major problem is the lack of doctors, nurses and the poor infrastructure of hospitals especially in case of public hospitals (Sara, 2016; Arif, 2016). According to Pakistan Bureau of Statistics, the population of the country is approximately 196,744,376 and the number of medically trained professionals to cater to this population is 175,223 doctors and 90,276 nurses. This makes the ratio of one doctor for every 1000 people and one hospital bed for 1000 people, clearly showing the inadequacy of healthcare in Pakistan ("Public Hospitals", 2015).

In Sri Lanka, there are 631 hospitals, 80,581 hospital beds and 19,429 doctors (See Table 1) which is very less according to the population of Sri Lanka. Additionally the ratio of one doctor per 1000 people clearly shows shortage of health facilities (Fernando et al., 2012)

By contrast, in Germany and Australia, there are 4 doctors available for 1000 people in FY2015. The Australian government provides most of the funds to their public hospitals (Biggs, 2013). For a complete listing of healthcare statistics please refer to Table 1.

Population

The volume of health services should be sufficient in accordance with population. In the developed world, low birth rates result in lower populations and thus, there are adequate facilities to cater the needs of the country. The population growth rates of USA and Germany are 0.8% and 0.5%, respectively. Moreover,

Table 1. Healthcare statistics

Country	Year	Doctors	Nurses	Hospitals	Hospital Beds	No: of Doctors per 1000 People	No: of Beds per 1000 People
Pakistan	2015	175,223	90,276	1,142	118,041	1	1
	2014	167,759	86,183	1,113	118,378	1	1
	2013	160,289	82,119	1,207	107,537	1	1
Sri-Lanka	2015	19,429	32,272	631	80,581	1	3.8
	2014	17,903	38,451	622	80,105	1	3.9
	2013	11,204	26,429	624	78,243	1	3.8
India	2015	9,36,488	4,734,123	22,401	8,45,190	1	1
	2014	9,38861	3,589,003	19,817	6,28,708	1	1
	2013	9,88,922	3,431,000	16.713	4,12,160	1	1
Germany	2015	340,591	10683000	3,186	668,560	4.2	4
	2014	332,695	1064000	3,138	666337	4.11	4
	2013	325,407	1045000	3,183	667,560	4.04	4
Australia	2015	102,805	140,213	1,322	92,114	3.4	4
	2014	95,690	130,399	1,359	89,500	3.5	3.9
	2013	92,503	124,584	1,347	87,300	3.4	3.9

Source: (Pakistan Bureau of Statistics, 2013-2015: Ministry of Health, Nutrition and Indigenous Medicine: WHO,2013-2015: Australian Institute Of Health and welfare, 2013-2015: OECD, 2013-2015:).

populations of US and Germany are 327 million and 80 million, respectively (Mossialos et al., 2016). High birth rates lead to higher population and the dearth of facilities make the healthcare system ineffective. The population growth rates of Pakistan and India are 2.1% and 1.2%, respectively. The population stands approximately as: Pakistan - 192.8 million, India - 1.32 billion, Bangladesh - 162.9 million (Worldometers, 2016). The higher population in the developing countries adds a layer of complication due to high number of patients.

Level of Mismanagement

Mismanagement impacts healthcare service delivery. It makes small budgets, yet smaller in the developing world. Also, the level of mismanagement and corruption in south Asian countries continues to grow without any check and balance (Thampi, 2002). Such mega corruption includes the mismanagement of medicine, lack of medical utilities such as water supply, fans and other related material, absenteeism of the doctors and staff – a serious issue in the health sector (Kurji et al., 2016), poor condition of toilets and lack of cleanliness (Mahapatra, Srilatha, and Sridhar, 2001; Ma & sood, 2008). Although many countries have an established healthcare activity and staff monitoring system, countries in South Asia continue to face monitoring challenges. Countries like Afghanistan, India and Pakistan face a significant lack of monitoring mechanism (Ashfaq, 2016; Ma & Sood 2008).

An example of mismanagement in Afghanistan and Pakistan is clearly reflected in the fact that these are the only two countries in the world where Poliomyelitis remains an endemic. The eradication of Polio has long been on the priority list of the government of Pakistan. Even though Polio has been completely removed throughout the globe, Pakistan and Afghanistan still regularly report cases of Polio (Ashfaq, 2016). Lack of governance and accountability along with local groups opposing vaccination are jeopardizing efforts to rid the country of this disease. Even though the number of cases per year has been declining, both the countries lack firm commitment and managerial strategy needed to eradicate a disease that no longer exists in the rest of the world. (Ahmad, 2007), suggests that internal corruption and biased hiring of health officials is also a growing hindrance towards the eradication of Polio.

Apart from Pakistan, corruption and mismanagement continues to foster in other south Asian countries such as India, Sri Lanka and Bangladesh (World Report, 2017). India is considered as Asia's most corrupt country, particularly in case of healthcare sector and Education (Suparna, 2017). The impact of corruption has badly affected the lives of people as the people of India don't get any proper health facilities. Lack of medicine, equipment, instruments, inadequate services, and unqualified doctors continue to plague the healthcare system (Rumani, 2014). Particularly the government hospitals are in shabby conditions with no check and balance (Rumani, 2014).

Another example of mismanagement is the poor sanitation conditions observed in India as it does not provide clean water to citizens which causes many ailments such as diarrhea, typhoid, cholera (Tyagi et al., 2010; Kumar et al., 2011). To counter such mega corruption in developing countries of the south Asian region the government should implement strict rules and regulations, also better laws and action for the healthcare system must be taken against the corruption within the system.

Life Expectancy Rate

Another comparison parameter is "life expectancy", as it is shown in Figure 1 that in the developed countries the life expectancy of individuals is more than 80 years, whereas in south Asian countries, it is either in 60's or limited to 70's.

Figure 1. Life expectancy rate in developed and developing countries
Source: (WHO, 2013-2015).

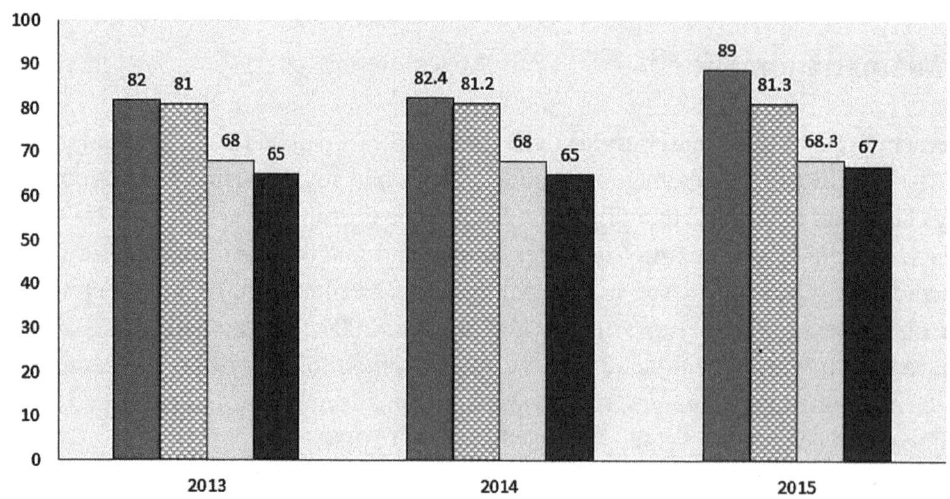

Use of Technology

Good technology tends to better the quality of services. In developed countries, high-tech machines are used in the hospitals such as the use of software applications in the hospitals in order to make it automated. Also, there is a wide use of Internet of things (IoT) based devices in the hospitals (Islam et al., 2015). An example of IoT is the wireless body area network (WBAN) sensors. It is a sensor that is attached to patients' body in order to capture the patient's condition or to examine patient's vital signs of human automatically (Mahoto et al., 2014). Another example of IoT based device used in hospitals is the use of beacons, NFC tags and RFID tags. The purpose of beacons is that it is attached to wall and it transmits the messages directly to smart phones or laptop, tablet PC. These technologies help in maintaining patient's records automatically and electronic health record, data collection through wireless sensors (Islam et al., 2015).

On the other hand, in developing countries, there is poor use of such technologies. Almost procedure is manual and paper-based, leading to human errors (Cline & Luiz, 2013). Therefore, high-tech mechanism is the necessity in the developing world. IT can be a panacea as it can help them contain absenteeism, manage human resources, control corruption, simplify high number of patients' record and centralize whole of the healthcare system (Cline & Luiz, 2013). The use of technology would be the fundamental development in improving the health related issues, which is lacking in south Asian countries.

It is concluded that the health system in developing countries of south Asia is not on the priority list as it faces a lot of challenges, such as:

- Poor governance
- Lack of resources and Equipment
- Weak infrastructure of hospitals
- Absenteeism of health workers
- Poor maintenance of health facilities
- Lack of technologies

Despite these challenges that the healthcare system in south Asian nations is not on the priority list, many programs have been introduced to improve the healthcare system. The government of Pakistan, for instance, has initiated the "National health insurance scheme", "programs on immunization", "lady health worker training initiative" and a program specifically to target polio called "polio eradication" across the country. But still the healthcare system is not encouraging (Hafeez et al., 2011; Ikram, 2016)

Developing countries' healthcare system is improving slowly and it is in progress since many years, most of countries have tried to improve the healthcare system but still a big change has not been seen, most of the problems and challenges have not as yet been resolved(Van et al., 2016). Therefore, it is the responsibility of government to pay more focus on the infrastructure of the healthcare system. Besides, number of health programs should be introduced and also the budget should be increased so that the system can be improved. Also there is a need of integrating information technology (IT) in health sector.

EMERGING CHANGES IN HEALTHCARE SYSTEM

Technology in healthcare has not only improved medical practices but also reduces time and provides better treatment. Today, the search of medical conditions has been observed in online user community. They not only look up treatments but also symptoms and preferred medicines (Hannan, 2010). Use of social media is also helping reach wider audiences and has been used to launch awareness campaigns and outreach programs (Ventola, 2014). Hand held devices are being used to record patient medical history as well as monitor ongoing treatments. Databases are being created to record and preserve results of lab tests, vital signs and patient history, all of which can be referred to as needed. Use of EMR (Electronic Medical Records) makes it convenient for both the doctor and the patient to access patient information (Sikhondze, & Erasmus, 2016). Consolidating these emerging databases, rich in medical history, provide the opportunity to better study diseases and trends to prevent breakthroughs even before they occur.

The following are some major breakthroughs of technological changes in healthcare system:

1. **Electronic Records:** The introduction of Electronic Medical records (EMR) has made it easier for healthcare facilities to store, use and disseminate patient information. This has resulted in a reduction of lost records. Information, instead of being held by individual specialists or doctors, is now being seamlessly shared, leading to a better system of healthcare (Hoerbst & Ammenwerth, 2010).

EMR systems are widely used in the developed countries and their healthcare sector have benefited from it. One example of EMR is "Electronic medical records adoption model (EMRAM)", used by hospitals in Canada, Europe and Australia, which shows the adoption of electronic medical record systems. Widespread adoption and remarkable growth of EMR systems has been seen in USA. On the other hand, the adoption of EMR systems in developing countries is very limited (Sikhondze, & Erasmus, 2016).

2. **Telemedicine:** Broadly defined as the use of telecommunication technology in the field of medicine. Using telemedicine, doctors are now able to use video, text and conferencing options to stay connected with patients and other doctors across the world (Nerlich, & Kretschmer, 1999; Williams et al., 2017). It has proved beneficial for treating patients in rural or devastated areas. Telemedicine provides the opportunity of not only treating patients without having to make them travel long distances but also of the physical need to remove them from their surroundings. The 24/7 availability of doctors allows medication to be prescribed using technology, and in special cases, as seen in Haiti, operate on patients using robotics (Perednia & Allen, 1995). Telemedicine services are in greater use in UK, Australia and USA (Scott et al., 2015). Telehealth solutions (Furht, 2007) specified the use of wireless body area network (WBAN) sensors in healthcare. The wearable health monitoring system (WHMS), is developed at the University of Alabama, which specifies the use of telemedicine system in order to monitor the health status of a user (Milenković et al., 2006). One major advantage brought about through telemedicine is that it has allowed healthcare to move out of the traditional setting and into daily environment of patients. This was accomplished through the use of i) Remote Monitoring and ii) Wearable Technology.
3. **Remote Monitoring:** Think of remote monitoring as a way to constantly connect a patient and a medical expert. It allows the patient to be evaluated all the time, from anywhere around the world, through a smartphone and/or certain devices. For instance, to monitor the glucose levels of a dia-

betic patient, glucose reading may be done through smartphone (e.g., wearable devices), which as a result may be monitored by medical expert remotely. One of the greatest benefits of remote monitoring is that it allows patients to heal in their own comfortable and known surroundings, with the assurance that medical expert is monitoring them. Using remote monitoring, patients are discharged from hospitals after a procedure earlier than ever. This reduces the cost of care for both, patient and hospital (Heidbuchel et al., 2015).

4. **Wearable Technology:** These are devices that monitor health and vital signs. They record data such as the exercise undertaken each day and things that are consumed, leading to more efficient plan of exercise routines and provisions for better diet. One such example of wearable technology is Fuelband, which tracks the user's body movement (Chris, 2017; Islam et al, 2015). The use of wireless communication has rid hospitals of the hassle of wide spread internet (Ethernet) cables and the fear of unplugging patient monitoring devices. This has indeed made drastic changes in the infrastructure of hospitals, allowing them to function effectively and provide better patient care (Igbokwe, 2004). A number of advanced wearable technologies have been introduced over the years in the system of healthcare, including devices which use human gestures to control user environments, Reemo being an example of such a device. Another example is Haloband, a wristband which is used as a heart tracker, designed specifically to track patient heart conditions. Some other wearable technologies include Syns Smart Band, iHealthBP, Phyode band and owlet (Islam et al., 2015).

With rise in internet-connected devices and the widespread adoption of technological advancements within healthcare, the Internet of Things (IoT) is another area quickly gaining a stronghold within healthcare. The use of IoT in healthcare may drastically reduce time and provide treatment to patients effectively.

5. **Internet of Things:** Use of Internet of Things (IoT) in healthcare is not new, but it has been gaining attention in recent years. IoT entails use of electronic devices, used to capture and/or monitor data. These devices are then connected to a cloud -private or public, which enables the automatic trigger of desired events.

Although numerous applications for IoT already exist in healthcare, this technology is still evolving (Rohokale et al., 2011). With huge amounts of data emerging from the healthcare sector, in form of fetal monitors, electrocardiograms, temperature monitors or blood cholesterol or glucose levels, one challenge for use of IoT will be the management of all the data it collects. Another challenge, which will also decide the future of IoT, will be the ability of healthcare organizations to convert that data into meaningful insights. Many devices have now started becoming connected as IoT takes hold within healthcare (Salunke & Nerkar, 2017). From handheld devices to health records to medical equipment, the industry is embracing the world of connected things. With a common language and a single platform for these devices to operate, the potential for IoT is limitless. For caregivers, the ability to easily monitor and manage patient health can save precious minutes every day. Without having to manually visit each patient, the expert can give a remote diagnosis and track medical assets, thus providing medical care more quickly and managing the healthcare environment more efficiently. Using sensors and wifi, the ability to locate the right department in the hospital, while retrieving essential information, becomes straightforward for both caregivers and patients. From patient heart monitors to temperature gauges, this real time data already exists in healthcare. Now, this data can be used to create a safer and more effective environment. Through a single application on a mobile device, patients and staff can securely manage IoT data. The use of IoT in healthcare allows for the automation of processes that have previously taken time and processes that have previously allowed human error.

PROPOSED FRAMEWORK

The computerized system of patients' record is a growing trend in the healthcare sector, as it collects tremendous amount of data, which is very difficult to manage on paper, thus a need for a framework (National database center) is paramount. It will not only help to reduce work-load of administrative staff but also to provide error-free system. This reduced error rate eventually may increase the efficiency of hospitals.

In many hospitals of south Asian nations, the patients' information is stored in thousands of folders all of which is paper-based thus arranging the entire data is cumbersome and time-consuming task (Tayade, & Karandikar, 2013) If all of these valuable data is computerized and stored electronically, then hospitals can be benefited. The Electronic retrieval of patient records will help to link many hospitals through data center. Figure 2 shows the proposed generic model of data center, which depicts how the patients' data can be electronically stored.

The framework strongly emphasizes the use of modern technology in the healthcare services and suggests that there should be a data center in hospitals throughout the country (i.e., especially south Asian region) where electronic health records are kept. Every hospital and medical expert should have access to that data to analyze previous history. The stored data should be shared among private and public hospitals of the country.

Figure 2. Generic model of data center: A proposed framework

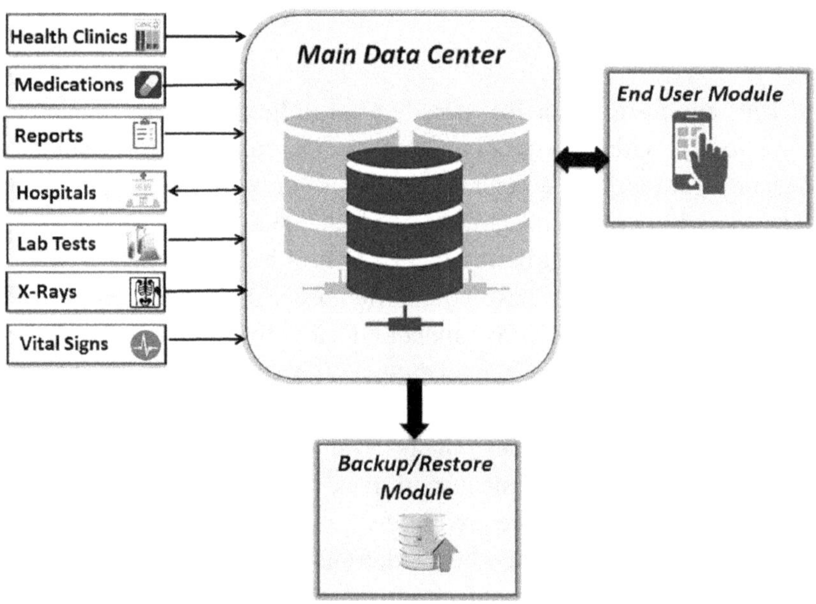

The data sources layer for the *Data Center* comprises of several means of input devices to enter information of patients into Data Center. The data sources layer are depicted in Figure 2 and are described below:

- **Health Clinics:** The data in the database will not be only regarding hospital checkups and admittance, but the data of the patient visiting a clinic will also be added. Clinical data including date of checkup, diagnosis, disease identified, medication history, medication prescribed as well as medical tests prescribed should be collected and stored in the data center.
- **Medications:** This parameter tells that what type of medications, the patients have taken and for what disease. The name of medicines, dosage of medicines and the frequency of using the medicine should also be stored in the data center.
- **Reports:** Reports comprises of medical data of the patient, such as laboratory tests reports, name and address of the lab, name of the doctor, name of patient, patient's phone number, name of the test performed, situation of the patient, X-ray reports, vital signs reports. These tests may be run either in separate laboratory or in the hospital lab. These valuable data can then be further used for the monitoring of the patient and the samples should be sent to the hospital or the laboratory for further analysis. This all data is essential for patient assessment and should be stored in the data center.
- **Hospitals:** Patient data from the public as well as private hospitals should also be included in the data center. It particularly comprises of complete record of a patients' name, address, identity Card, email, telephone number, the duration of patient in the hospital, medical treatment, disease of the patient, infection, patient's room number, hospital name, medical prescription, medications, and laboratory test reports.
- **Vital Signs:** Vital signs are the measurements providing physiological data of patients indicating any changes in body functions. These signs are used to detect risk situations at the earlier stage. It provides the data, which particularly indicates conditions of the person and help in health assessment and diagnosis. Few of the examples of vital signs are: blood pressure, heart rate, respiratory rate, body temperature, glucose and sugar level. These vital signs should be part of the data center, since these will help medical experts in diagnosis and treatment prescription.

Main Data Center

The Data Center is the essential component of the proposed framework. A key benefit of a central data center allows easy access to patient's information. The data may be stored on clouds (i.e., data storage on remote computers or server machines) as well as local and national level data storages. The 24/7 accesses to Data Center provide immediate information on patient medical history, current medical status as well as on-going treatments. The historical health related data may also be used for the research purposes to derive interesting knowledge and aware the public as well as take decisions for the betterment of healthcare procedures.

The public as well private hospitals may be given access to National Data Center in order to effective examine the patient's medical history and avoid unnecessary medical tests for the diagnosis. A mobile device and/or computer (*End User Module*) with certain application installed can be used to access the National Data Center over the Internet. Likewise, medical experts may monitor patient's medical records through their mobiles or computers. The sharing of data stored in National Data Center may ease government to retrieve information of its population based on several diseases, location-based statistics to effectively make policies and overcome severe diseases with better and proactive actions. Furthermore, government may ensure policies to keep private information secure from the reach of un-authorized users.

Backup/Restore Module

Another important component is the backup module; this module is responsible for archive. The word backup means copying of the original data so that it can be used to restore original contents of the data later after a data loss event.

For instance, if the main server is down due to power-supply interruption or Internet issues, the data will be saved in this module. The module will make data available all the time without the fear of data loss. As the issues related to server get resolved, the data is resolved.

End User Module

Through End User Module, the patients' can access their data through mobile device or computer having certain application installed. The hospitals and the Patients will have a mobile application. The application will help patients see the record through End user Module. On practical grounds, a patient can compare the sugar level taken currently with the data regarding sugar level in the past. This application will enable the patients to access all the previous data.

Applications of the Proposed Framework

The proposed framework would be much productive, in case, IoT and WBAN technologies are integrated to it. The framework already offers data source layer, which actually provides data to be stored in the Data Center. WBAN and Sensors can be used as continuous data sources to feed Data Center with real-time data of the patients.

The Figure 3 reports the scenario, in which sensory data of a patient with the help of WBAN can be stored in the Data Center. The implementation of IoT may provide the effective notification of the sever cases. For instance, whenever patients' glucose level values pass certain threshold values; automatic alarming may be notified to medical experts. Similarly, if the ECG of certain patient is alarming, the IoT devices may send these reports with alarming messages to Mobile devices or Emergency Unit to handle the situation urgently.

WBAN and IoT can be the essence of the proposed framework. The south Asian nations may get benefits from these technologies to rapidly overcome the healthcare challenges.

RECOMMENDATIONS

Due to the well-functioning and efficient health systems, the health facilities in developed countries keep on improving. However, in developing countries, particularly south Asian region, lack of proper health systems lead towards worsening health conditions.

Figure 3. WBAN and IoT integrated in proposed framework

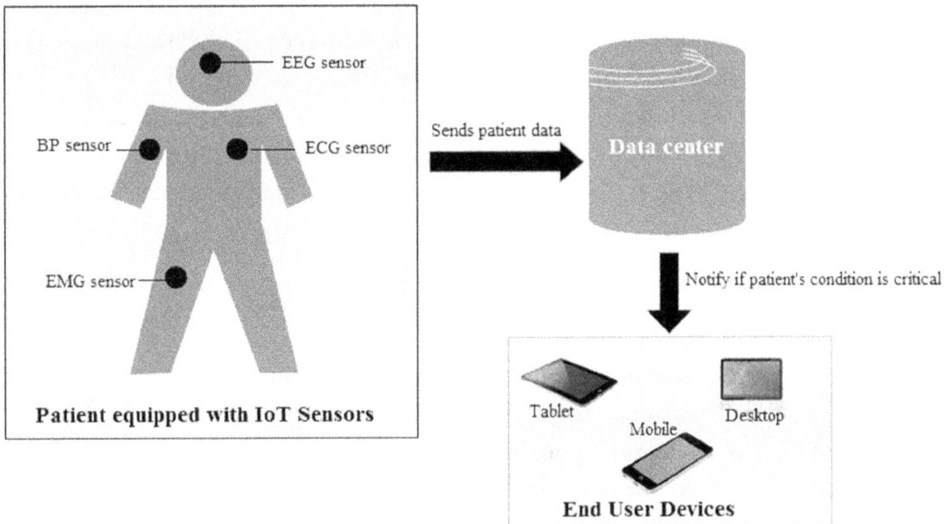

Table 2. Identified problems and proposed recommendations

Problem	Recommendation
Lack of Infrastructure	
Hospitals	Hospitals should be provided according to the population of the region.
Doctors	Sufficient doctors should be available, well trained and their punctuality be ensured.
Staff	Well-trained and efficient staff should be available in sufficient number.
Medicines	Medicine and equipment of the latest technology should be provided as per population ratio.
Lack of Coordination	
Public and Private Hospitals	A well-coordinated network between public and private hospitals should be maintained. The urban as well as countryside areas should remain in focused for healthcare units provision.
Central Database	Hospitals collect huge amounts of patient data. This data should be collected and stored at a National Level. A Centralized National Database can adequately tackle the carelessness of administrative staff as well as open channels for further Data Analysis.
Budget	Increase in healthcare budget is greatly needed for improving healthcare services.
Improper Sanitation	Level of sanitation in healthcare system is questionable from patient interaction to the usage of various instruments and their proper disposal. Proper sanitary measures should be taken including the safety of healthcare workers, patients and all other middle parties involved. This includes the use of gloves, masks, sterilization of equipment and clean water.
Improper Use of Technology	Use of Artificial Intelligence (AI) and Data Mining techniques can result in early detection of severe conditions or emergence of certain disease in specific regions. Internet of Things based devices and mobile phones are in common use. According to (kakria et al., 2015), usage of cellphone is increasing rapidly in developing countries. Almost 94% of the world population is the subscriber of cell phones and about 2.7 billion people are using the internet. These devices can be used in developing countries in order to provide better healthcare services. Wearable devices are playing a vital role in healthcare systems. Sensors can be installed in a patient's body according to the type of disease. This way, the patients can go home and the doctors can still monitor their health as those sensors are scanned and tracked in the hospital. Wearable devices can greatly enhance patient care in remote areas.
Lack of Joint Ventures	Memorandum of Understandings (MOUs) with International health services is very important for advancing and upgrading medical facilities, practices and technology. Signing the MOUs will get the hospitals in touch with latest practices and treatments. The hospital will learn new methods and will have alternatives to select best suitable for it. With the exposure of different hospitals, development will definitely take place in different areas of hospital related aspects.

As discussed in earlier sections, several steps can be taken to improve the condition of health system in the developing countries of south Asia. The proper utilization of budget, the eradication of corruption and the increased use of technology can greatly aid in reshaping the healthcare system. Table 2 reports the challenging problems of south Asian countries and their recommendations.

The Healthcare system of developing countries of south Asia, in particular, needs an overhaul, so that it may cater the current needs of the time. If all of these suggestions/recommendations are followed in letter and spirit, the healthcare system may witness a considerable improvement in south Asian nations.

CONCLUSION

This chapter reported the current healthcare conditions of the developing nations, in particular, south Asian countries: Bangladesh, India, Pakistan and Sri-Lanka. The mismanagement, lack of resources, equipment & infrastructure, lack of policies & priorities of government in south Asian developing countries result in errors and poor health conditions. The key issues that worsen the health related services have been determined, for instance, lack of infrastructure, co-ordination among healthcare units, insufficient budget, medical experts, lack of advanced technological solutions. To overcome the identified issues and challenges, recommendations have been proposed.

Furthermore, A Generic Model (i.e., Framework) of Data Center has been proposed for future perspectives, which emphasizes on the national level data storage to improve the healthcare services and procedures. The proposed data center may help to improve management processes and enhance quality of service. The National Data Center may also open doors towards research paradigm. The stored data may be used to extract interesting information that eventually provides insights in decision-making and policy-making. Centralized data will also reduce paper work, improve infrastructure and reduce errors and may help resolving current issues related to improper record keeping and poor health conditions due to unavailability of medical history of patients.

REFERENCES

Ahmad, K. (2007). Pakistan struggles to eradicate polio. *The Lancet Infectious Diseases*, *7*(4), 247. doi:10.1016/S1473-3099(07)70066-X PMID:17419137

Arif, M. (2016, January 4). Health cards will not end Pakistan's Healthcare nightmare. *DAWN*. Retrieved from http://www.dawn.com/news/1230294

Ashfaq, Y. (2016, January 12). Pakistan, Afghanistan need extra efforts to eradicate polio. *DAWN*. Retrieved from https://www.dawn.com/news/1232373

Australian Institute of Health and Welfare. (n.d.). Retrieved from http://www.aihw.gov.au/

Biggs, A. (2013). *Health in Australia: A quick guide*. Parliamentary Library.

Chambers, W. M., Bicsak, M., Lamparelli, M., & Dixon, A. R. (2011). Single-incision laparoscopic surgery (SILS) in complex colorectal surgery: A technique offering potential and not just cosmesis. *Colorectal Disease*, *13*(4), 393–398. doi:10.1111/j.1463-1318.2009.02158.x PMID:20002691

Cline, G. B., & Luiz, J. M. (2013). Information technology systems in public sector health facilities in developing countries: The case of South Africa. *BMC Medical Informatics and Decision Making*, *13*(1), 13. doi:10.1186/1472-6947-13-13 PMID:23347433

Fernandez, F., & Pallis, G. C. (2014, November). Opportunities and challenges of the Internet of Things for healthcare: Systems engineering perspective. In *Wireless Mobile Communication and Healthcare (Mobihealth), 2014 EAI 4th International Conference on* (pp. 263-266). IEEE.

Fernando, J. L. I. N., Wickramaratne, C. P., Dissanayake, R. S. B., Kolambage, S. H., Aminda, M. A. U., Cooray, N. H., ... Muthukudaarachchi, A. D. (2012). Studying current status of intensive care services in Sri Lanka. *International Journal of Critical Illness and Injury Science*, *2*(1), 11. doi:10.4103/2229-5151.94884 PMID:22624096

Furht, B. (2007). *Encyclopedia of Wireless and Mobile Communications-3 Volume Set*. Auerbach Publications. doi:10.1201/NOE1420043266

Garrick, R., Kliger, A., & Stefanchik, B. (2012). Patient and facility safety in hemodialysis: Opportunities and strategies to develop a culture of safety. *Clinical Journal of the American Society of Nephrology; CJASN*, *7*(4), 680–688. doi:10.2215/CJN.06530711 PMID:22282480

Hafeez, A., Mohamud, B. K., Shiekh, M. R., Shah, S. A. I., & Jooma, R. (2011). Lady health workers programme in Pakistan: Challenges, achievements and the way forward. *JPMA. The Journal of the Pakistan Medical Association*, *61*(3), 210. PMID:21465929

Hannan, A. (2010). Providing patients online access to their primary care computerised medical records: A case study of sharing and caring. *Journal of Innovation in Health Informatics*, *18*(1), 41–49. doi:10.14236/jhi.v18i1.752 PMID:20429977

Heidbuchel, H., Hindricks, G., Broadhurst, P., Van Erven, L., Fernandez-Lozano, I., Rivero-Ayerza, M., ... Beeton, I. (2015). EuroEco (European Health Economic Trial on Home Monitoring in ICD Patients): A provider perspective in five European countries on costs and net financial impact of follow-up with or without remote monitoring. *European Heart Journal*, *36*(3), 158–169. doi:10.1093/eurheartj/ehu339 PMID:25179766

Hoerbst, A., & Ammenwerth, E. (2010). Electronic health records. *Methods of Information in Medicine*, *49*(4), 320–336. doi:10.3414/ME10-01-0038 PMID:20603687

Howell. (2016). *5 Ways Technology is Transforming Developing Nations*. Available: http://epics.ieee.org/582-2/

Igbokwe, O. (2004). *Wireless technology and healthcare*. Academic Press.

Ikram, J. (2016, January 1). PM launches Health scheme for the poor. *DAWN*. Retrieved from https://www.dawn.com/news/1229970

Irfan, S. M., & Ijaz, A. (2011). Comparison of service quality between private and public hospitals: Empirical evidences from Pakistan. *Journal of Quality and Technology Management*, *7*(1), 1–22.

Islam, S. R., Kwak, D., Kabir, M. H., Hossain, M., & Kwak, K. S. (2015). The internet of things for health care: A comprehensive survey. *IEEE Access: Practical Innovations, Open Solutions, 3*, 678–708. doi:10.1109/ACCESS.2015.2437951

Jabnoun, N., & Chaker, M. (2003). Comparing the quality of private and public hospitals. *Managing Service Quality: An International Journal, 13*(4), 290–299. doi:10.1108/09604520310484707

Jahanzeb, E. (2017, April 7). Those who can't afford to live are left to die - my experiences as a doctor in karachi. *Dawn.* Retrieved from https://www.dawn.com/news/1325471

Kakria, P., Tripathi, N. K., & Kitipawang, P. (2015). A real-time health monitoring system for remote cardiac patients using smartphone and wearable sensors. *International Journal of Telemedicine and Applications*, 8.

Kumar, G. S., Kar, S. S., & Jain, A. (2011). Health and environmental sanitation in India: Issues for prioritizing control strategies. *Indian Journal of Occupational and Environmental Medicine, 15*(3), 93. doi:10.4103/0019-5278.93196 PMID:22412284

Kurji, Z., Premani, Z. S., & Mithani, Y. (2016). Analysis of the health care system of Pakistan: Lessons learnt and way forward. *Journal of Ayub Medical College, Abbottabad, 28*(3), 601–604. PMID:28712245

Leite, C. R. M., Sizilio, G. R., Ribeiro, A. G., Valentim, R. A., Neto, P. F., & Guerreiro, A. M. (2012). Mobile Technologies Applied to Hospital Automation. In *Advances and Applications in Mobile Computing*. InTech. doi:10.5772/36478

Lindblad, S., Ernestam, S., Van Citters, A. D., Lind, C., Morgan, T. S., & Nelson, E. C. (2017). Creating a culture of health: Evolving healthcare systems and patient engagement. *QJM: An International Journal of Medicine, 110*(3), 125–129. PMID:27803364

Ma, S., & Sood, N. (2008). *A comparison of the health systems in China and India* (Vol. 212). Rand Corporation.

Mahapatra, P., Srilatha, S., & Sridhar, P. (2001). A Patient Satisfaction Survey in Public Hospitals. *Journal Academy of Hospital Administration, 13*(2).

Mahoto, N. A., Shaikh, F. K., & Chowdhry, B. S. (2014). Innovative Architecture to Enhance Quality of Service for Laboratory Management Information Systems. *Laboratory Management Information Systems: Current Requirements and Future Perspectives: Current Requirements and Future Perspectives, 237.*

Michelle, A. (2014, March 24). FAQ: What are the penalties for not getting Health insurance? *PBS Newshour.* Retrieved from http://www.pbs.org/newshour/updates/faq-penalties-getting-health-insurance/

Milenković, A., Otto, C., & Jovanov, E. (2006). Wireless sensor networks for personal health monitoring: Issues and an implementation. *Computer Communications, 29*(13), 2521–2533. doi:10.1016/j.comcom.2006.02.011

Mills, A. (2014). Health care systems in low-and middle-income countries. *The New England Journal of Medicine, 370*(6), 552–557. doi:10.1056/NEJMra1110897 PMID:24499213

Ministry of Finance. (n.d.). Retrieved from http://www.finance.gov.pk/

Ministry of Health. (n.d.). *Nutrition and Indigenous Online*. Retrieved from http://www.health.gov.lk/moh_final/english/

Mossialos, E., Wenzl, M., Osborn, R., & Anderson, C. (2016). *2015 International Profiles of Health Care Systems*. The Commonwealth Fund. doi:10.15868ocialsector.25100

Mupela, E. N., Mustarde, P., & Jones, H. L. (2011). Telemedicine in primary health: The virtual doctor project Zambia. *Philosophy, Ethics, and Humanities in Medicine; PEHM*, *6*(1), 9. doi:10.1186/1747-5341-6-9 PMID:21569490

Nerlich, M., & Kretschmer, R. (Eds.). (1999). *The impact of telemedicine on health care management* (Vol. 64). IOS Press.

OECD. (2015). Retrieved from https://www.oecd.org/health/health-systems/Focus-Health-Spending-2015.pdf

OECD. (2016). Retrieved from http://www.oecd.org/

OECD. (2017). *Doctors (indicator)*. OECD. doi: 10.1787/4355e1ec-en

OECD Online. (n.d.). Retrieved from http://www.oecd.org/

Pakistan Bureau of Statistics. (n.d.). Retrieved from http://www.pbs.gov.pk/

Pakistan Federal budget spending for fiscal years 2016-2017. (n.d.). Retrieved from https://en.dailypakistan.com.pk/headline/live-finance-minister-unveils-budget-for-2016-2017/

Perednia, D. A., & Allen, A. (1995). Telemedicine technology and clinical applications. *Journal of the American Medical Association*, *273*(6), 483–488. doi:10.1001/jama.1995.03520300057037 PMID:7837367

Phil, G. (2015, July 21). 7.5 million Americans paid fine for having no health insurance in 2014. *PBS Newshour.* Retrieved from http://www.pbs.org/newshour/rundown/7-5-million-americans-paid-fine-health-insurance-2014/

Public hospitals become part of problem rather than solution. (2015, August 31). *International the news.* Retrieved from https://www.thenews.com.pk/print/59580-public-hospitals-become-part-of-problem-rather-than-solution

Robertson, R., Gregory, S., & Jabbal, J. (2014). *The social care and health systems of nine countries.* The King's Fund.

Rohokale, V. M., Prasad, N. R., & Prasad, R. (2011, February). A cooperative Internet of Things (IoT) for rural healthcare monitoring and control. In *Wireless Communication, Vehicular Technology, Information Theory and Aerospace & Electronic Systems Technology (Wireless VITAE), 2011 2nd International Conference on* (pp. 1-6). IEEE.

Rosenbaum, S. (2011). The Patient Protection and Affordable Care Act: Implications for public health policy and practice. *Public Health Reports*, *126*(1), 130 135. doi:10.1177/003335491112600118 PMID:21337939

Rumani, S. P. (2014). *Impact of Corruption in India's Healthcare Sector*. Retrieved from https://www.mapsofindia.com/my-india/india/impact-of-corruption-in-indias-healthcare-sector

Sahu, U. (2016). *8 Major Differences Between Healthcare In The US And India*. Available: http://www.huffingtonpost.in/utkarsh-sahu/a-tale-of-two-nations-ind_b_9261892.html

Salunke, P., & Nerkar, R. (2017). IoT Driven Healthcare System for Remote Monitoring of Patients. *Journal for Modern Trends in Science and Technology*, *3*(06), 100–103.

Sara, M. (2016, June 27). Pakistan's Healthcare crisis. *DAWN*. Retrieved from https://www.dawn.com/news/1267410

Scott, R. E., Mars, M., Scott, R. E., & Mars, M. (2015). Telehealth in the developing world: Current status and future prospects. *Smart Homecare Technology and TeleHealth*, *3*, 25–37. doi:10.2147/SHTT.S75184

Shah. (2011). *Health Care Around the World*. Available: http://www.globalissues.org/article/774/health-care-around-the-world

Shehzad, S. (2005). *Alternative Resource Mobilization Strategies for Pakistan's Health Care*. Sustainable Development Policy Institute.

Smith, C. (2017). *Nike FuelBand: The rise and fall of the wearable that started it all*. Retrieved from https://www.wareable.com/nike/not-so-happy-birthday-nike-fuelband-2351

Suparna, G. (2017). *Study Finds India Is Asia's Most Corrupt Country, While Japan Comes In Last*. Retrieved from https://www.forbes.com/sites/suparnagoswami/2017/03/08/study-finds-india-is-asias-most-corrupt-country-while-japan-comes-in-last/#7fea8d931201

Tan, L. T. H., & Ong, K. L. (2002). The impact of medical technology on healthcare today. *Hong Kong Journal of Emergency Medicine*, *9*(4), 231–236. doi:10.1177/102490790200900410

Tayade, M. C., & Karandikar, P. M. (2013). Role of data mining techniques in healthcare sector in India. *Sch J App Med Sci*, *1*(3), 158–160.

Thampi, G. K. (2002). *Corruption in South Asia: Insights and benchmarks from citizen feedback surveys in five countries*. Transparency International.

The World Bank. (2016). Retrieved from http://www.worldbank.org/

Thompson, V. (2017). *Cataract surgery*. Available: http://www.allaboutvision.com/conditions/cataract-surgery.htm

Tomasi, E., Facchini, L. A., & Maia, M. D. F. S. (2004). Health information technology in primary health care in developing countries: A literature review. *Bulletin of the World Health Organization*, *82*(11), 867–874. PMID:15640923

Tomines, A., Readhead, H., Readhead, A., & Teutsch, S. (2013). Applications of electronic health information in public health: Uses, opportunities & barriers. *EGEMS (Washington, DC)*, *1*(2), 5. doi:10.13063/2327-9214.1019 PMID:25848571

Tyagi, A., Hutton, G., & Sen, S. (2010). *The economic impacts of inadequate sanitation in India: Inadequate sanitation costs India Rs. 2.4 trillion (US $53.8 billion)*. Academic Press.

USA FY16 Federal Budget Spending Estimates for Fiscal Years 2015 – 2020. (n.d.). Retrieved from http://www.usgovernmentspending.com/health_care_budget_2016_1.html

van Weel, C., Kassai, R., Qidwai, W., Kumar, R., Bala, K., Gupta, P. P., ... Howe, A. (2016). Primary healthcare policy implementation in South Asia. *BMJ Global Health*, *1*(2), e000057. doi:10.1136/bmjgh-2016-000057 PMID:28588938

Ventola, C. L. (2014). Social media and health care professionals: Benefits, risks, and best practices. *P&T*, *39*(7), 491. PMID:25083128

Weaver, C. A., Ball, M. J., Kim, G. R., & Kiel, J. M. (2016). *Healthcare information management systems*. Cham: Springer International Publishing. doi:10.1007/978-3-319-20765-0

WHO. (n.d.). Retrieved from http://www.who.int/en/

Wicklund, E. (2014). *"Silo" one of healthcare's biggest flaws*. Available: http://www.healthcareitnews.com/news/silo-one-healthcares-biggest-flaws

Williams, O. E., Elghenzai, S., Subbe, C., Wyatt, J. C., & Williams, J. (2017). The use of telemedicine to enhance secondary care: Some lessons from the front line. *Future Hospital Journal*, *4*(2), 109–114.

World Report. (n.d.). Retrieved from https://www.hrw.org/world-report/2017

Worldometers. (n.d.). Retrieved from http://www.worldometers.info/world-population/pakistan-population/

Xia, F., Yang, L. T., Wang, L., & Vinel, A. (2012). Internet of things. *International Journal of Communication Systems*, *25*(9), 1101–1102. doi:10.1002/dac.2417

ADDITIONAL READING

Akram, M., & Khan, F. J. (2007). *Health care services and government spending in Pakistan (No. 22184)*. East Asian Bureau of Economic Research.

Hassanalieragh, M., Page, A., Soyata, T., Sharma, G., Aktas, M., Mateos, G., . . . Andreescu, S. (2015, June). Health monitoring and management using Internet-of-Things (IoT) sensing with cloud-based processing: Opportunities and challenges. In *Services Computing (SCC), 2015 IEEE International Conference on* (pp. 285-292). IEEE.

Rechel, B., Buchan, J., & McKee, M. (2009). The impact of health facilities on healthcare workers' well-being and performance. *International Journal of Nursing Studies*, *46*(7), 1025–1034. doi:10.1016/j.ijnurstu.2008.12.008 PMID:19166997

Shaikh, B., Rabbani, F., Safi, N., & Dawar, Z. (2010). Contracting of primary health care services in Pakistan: Is up-scaling a pragmatic thinking. *JPMA. The Journal of the Pakistan Medical Association*, *60*(5), 387. PMID:20527614

Shaikh, S. B., Ejaz, E. I., Achakzai, A. D., & Shafiq, S. Y. (2013). Political and economic unfairness in health system of Pakistan: A hope with the recent reforms. *Journal of Ayub Medical College, Abbottabad*, *25*(1-2), 198–203. PMID:25098095

KEY TERMS AND DEFINITIONS

Data Center: A data center is a network of computers, specifically designed for storing large amount of data.

EMR (Electronic Medical Record): A process of collecting medical record, it comprises of patients' medical history which is stored electronically.

GDP: GDP stands for "gross domestic product"; it is a way to measure the country's economy.

IoT (Internet of Things): The IoT is the inter-networking of electronic devices, used for capturing and monitoring the data connected to a cloud. The purpose of IoT is to make smart objects, which make use of physical devices to gather and monitor the data and trigger the events automatically.

Telemedicine: The two-way communication that makes use of the telecommunication technologies to diagnose the patient remotely.

Chapter 2
Overview of Surgical Instruments for the Operation Theatre

Sandip Bag
JIS College of Engineering, India

ABSTRACT

There are several classes of surgical instruments such as graspers, clamps, and occluders for blood vessels and other organs; retractors used to spread open skin, ribs, and other tissue; distractors, positioners, and stereotactic devices; mechanical cutters (scalpels, lancets, surgical scissors, etc.); dilators and specula for access to narrow passages or incisions; suction tips and tubes for removal of bodily fluids; sealing devices such as surgical staplers; irrigation and injection needles, tips, and tubes for introducing fluid; powered devices, such as drills, dermatomes; scopes and probes, including fiber optic endoscopes and tactile probes; carriers and appliers for optical, electronic, and mechanical devices; ultrasound tissue disruptors, cryotomes, and cutting laser guides; measurement devices, such as rulers and calipers; and many more. This chapter overviews surgical instruments for the operation theatre.

INTRODUCTION

According to "Medical Dictionary" Surgery is defined as the "branch of medicine that is concerned with the conditions that are amenable to, or require operative procedures." During an operation or surgical procedure, a trained surgeon uses various tools to manipulate the body's tissues and organs. While some surgical tools such as scalpels and suturing needles are used for most operative procedures, others are more specialized and may be used only within a certain branch of surgery such as orthopaedics or neurosurgery.

A surgical instrument is a specially designed tool or device for performing a surgery or operation for specific actions of carrying out desired effects such as modifying biological tissue, or to provide access for viewing it. Over the years, many different kinds of surgical instruments and tools have been invented and utilized. Some surgical instruments are designed for general use in surgery, while others

DOI: 10.4018/978-1-5225-4969-7.ch002

are designed for specific surgery. Accordingly, the nomenclature of surgical instruments follows certain patterns, such as a description of the action it performs (for example, scalpel, hemostat), the name of its inventor(s) (for example, the Kocher forceps) ("Meriam Webster", n.d.), or a compound scientific name related to the kind of surgery (for example, a tracheotome is a tool used to perform a tracheotomy).

The expression surgical instrumentation is somewhat interchangeably used with surgical instruments (Nimitz, 2010) but its meaning in medical jargon is really the activity of providing assistance to a surgeon with the proper handling of surgical instruments during an operation, by a specialized professional, usually a surgical technologist or sometimes a nurse or radiographer (Kirup, 2006).

Due to the advancements of the medical science a number of surgeries are growing every year with the application of modern surgical instruments having cutting edge of medical technology. New techniques and procedures mean that new instruments and devices must be developed.

HISTORY

Surgical instruments have been designed and manufactured since the era of pre-history (Bonfils-Roberts, 1972). Rough trephines for performing round craniotomies were discovered in neolithic sites in many places. It is believed that they were used by shamans to release evil spirits and alleviate headaches and head traumas caused by war-inflicted wounds.

In the Antiquity, surgeons and physicians in Greece and Rome developed many ingenious instruments manufactured from bronze, iron and silver, such as scalpels, lancets, curettes, tweezers, speculae, trephines, forceps, probes, dilators, tubes, surgical knifes, etc. They are still very well preserved in several medical museums around the world. Most of these instruments continued to be used in medieval times, albeit with a better manufacturing technique ("General Instrument Sourcebook", 2006).

In the Renaissance and post-Renaissance era, new instruments were again invented and designed, in order to accompany the increased audacity of surgeons. Amputation sets originated in this period, due to the increased severity of war-inflicted wounds by shot, grapnel and cannon.

However, it was only with the discovery of anesthesia and surgical asepsis that new surgical instruments were invented to allow the penetration of the inner sanctum, or the previously forbidden body cavities, namely the skull, the thorax and the abdomen. A veritable explosion of new tools occurred with the hundreds of new surgical procedures which were developed in the 19th century and first decades of the 20th century. New materiais, such as stainless steel, chrome, titanium and vanadium were available for the manufacturing of these instruments. Precision instruments for microsurgery in neurosurgery, ophthalmology and otology were possible and, in the second half of the 20th century, energy-based instruments were first developed, such as electrocauteries, ultrasound and electric scalpels, surgical tools for endoscopic surgery, and finally, surgical robots.

TYPES OF SURGICAL INSTRUMENTS

There are several classes of surgical instruments such as Graspers, Clamps and occluders for blood vessels and other organs, Retractors used to spread open skin, ribs and other tissue, Distractors, positioners and stereotactic devices, Mechanical cutters (scalpels, lancets, surgical scissors etc.), Dilators and specula for access to narrow passages or incisions, Suction tips and tubes for removal of bodily fluids, Sealing devices such as surgical staplers, Irrigation and injection needles, tips and tubes for introducing fluid, Powered devices, such as drills, dermatomes, Scopes and probes, including fiber optic endoscopes and tactile probes, Carriers and appliers for optical, electronic and mechanical devices, Ultrasound tissue disruptors, cryotomes and cutting laser guides, Measurement devices, such as rulers and calipers and many more (Heller, 2016).

Surgical instruments can be generally divided into five classes by function. These classes are:

1. **Cutting Instruments and Dissecting:** Scalpels, scissors, saws.
2. **Grasping or Holding Instruments:** Smooth [anatomical] and toothed [surgical] forceps, towel clamps, vascular clamps, and organ holders.
3. **Haemostatic Instruments:** Kocher's and Billroth's clamps, hemostatic "mosquito" forceps, atraumatic hemostatic forceps, Deschamp's needle, Höpfner's hemostatic forceps.
4. **Retractors:** Farabef's C-shaped laminar hook, blunt-toothed hook, sharp-toothed hook, grooved probe, tamp forceps.
5. **Tissue Unifying Instruments and Materials:** Needle holders, surgical needles, staplers, clips, adhesive tapes.

BASIC SURGICAL INSTRUMENTS

Surgical instruments are specially designed tools that assist health care professionals to carry out specific actions during an operation. Most instruments crafted from the early 19th century on are made from durable stainless steel. Some are designed for general use and others for specific procedures. There are many surgical instruments available for almost any specialization in medicine. There are precision instruments used in microsurgery, ophthalmology and otology. Most surgical instruments can be classified into these 4 basic types:

- **Cutting and Dissecting:** These instruments usually have sharp edges or tips to cut through skin, tissue and suture material. Surgeons need to cut and dissect tissue to explore irregular growths and to remove dangerous or damaged tissue. These instruments have single or double razor-sharp edges or blades. Nurses and or personnel need to be very careful to avoid injuries, and regularly inspect these instruments before using, for re-sharpening or replacement (Kirkup, 2006). Cutting and dissecting instruments are used for cutting, incising, scraping, punching and puncturing. This type of instruments includes scissors (Figure 1), scalpels, chisels, elevators, curettes, punches, drills and needles.

Surgical Scalpels

A scalpel, or lancet, is a small and extremely sharp bladed fine edge cutting instrument used for surgery, anatomical dissection, and various arts and crafts (called a hobby knife) (KMedic, 2008). Scalpels are available in both single-use disposable or re-usable i.e. stainless steel varieties, and in a range of sizes. Re-usable scalpels can have permanently attached blades that can be sharpened or, more commonly, removable single-use blades. Disposable scalpels usually have a plastic handle with an extensible blade (like a utility knife) and are used once, and then the entire instrument is discarded. Scalpel blades are

Figure 1. Iris scissors

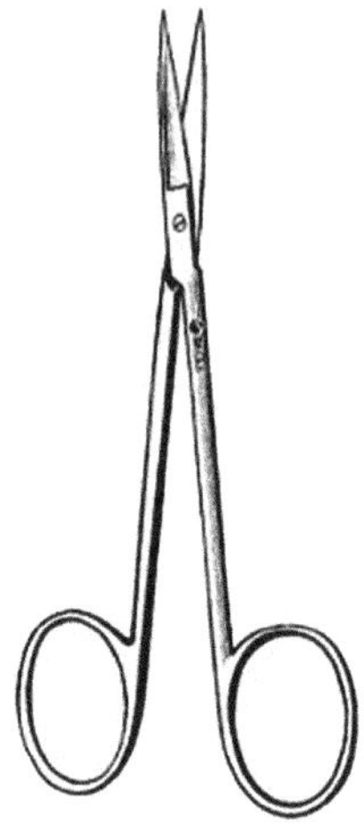

usually individually packed in sterile pouches but are also offered non-sterile. Double-edged scalpels are referred to as "lancets". The scalpel is most commonly used to make the initial incision that opens the body for surgery (Figure 2).

Scalpel blades are usually made of hardened and tempered steel, stainless steel, or high carbon steel; in addition, titanium, ceramic, diamond and even obsidian knives are not uncommon. For example, when performing surgery under MRI guidance, steel blades are unusable (the blades would be drawn

Figure 2. Different types of scalpel blades with handle

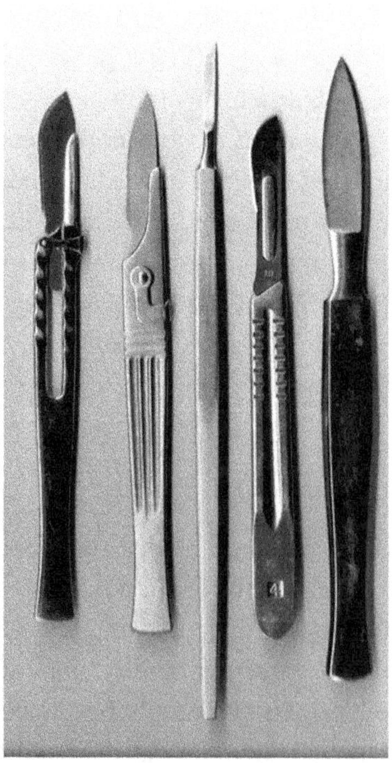

to the magnets, or may cause image artifacts). Historically, the preferred material for surgical scalpels was silver, on account of its antimicrobial properties (although the mechanics were not understood at the time). Scalpel blades are also offered by select manufacturers with a zirconium nitride-coated edge to improve sharpness and edge retention. Others manufacture blades that are polymer-coated to enhance lubricity during a cut. Alternatives to scalpels in surgical applications include electrocautery and lasers.

Surgical scalpels consist of two parts, a blade and a handle. The handles are often reusable (Figure 3 and 4), with the blades being replaceable. In medical applications, each blade is only used once (even if just for a single, small cut).

The handle is also known as a "B.P. handle", named after Charles Russell Bard and Morgan Parker, founders of the Bard-Parker Company. Morgan Parker patented the 2-piece scalpel design in 1915 and Bard-Parker developed a method of cold sterilization that would not dull the blades, as did the heat-based method that was previously used.

The handle of medical scalpels comes in two basic types. The first is a flat handle used in the #3 and #4 handles. The #7 handle is more like a long writing pen, rounded at the front and flat at the back. A #4 handle is larger than #3. Blades are manufactured with a corresponding fitment size so that they fit on only one size handle.

Gripping of Medical Scalpel

Gripping of medical scalpel has immense importance as initial cutting of any surgery is made my scalpel. There are two types of scalpel grips are there which includes Palmer grip and Pencil grip.

Palmar Grip

Also called the "dinner knife" grip. The handle is held with the second through fourth fingers and secured along the base of the thumb, with the index finger extended along the top rear of the blade and the thumb along the side of the handle (Figure 5). This grip is best for initial incisions and larger cuts.

Pencil Grip

Best used for more accurate cuts with smaller blades (e.g. #15) and the #7 handle. The scalpel is held with the tips of the first and second fingers and the tip of the thumb with the handle resting on the fleshy base of the index finger and thumb (Figure 6). Care should be taken not to allow the handle to rest too far along the index finger as this promotes an unstable grip and cramped fingers.

Figure 3. Reusable handle

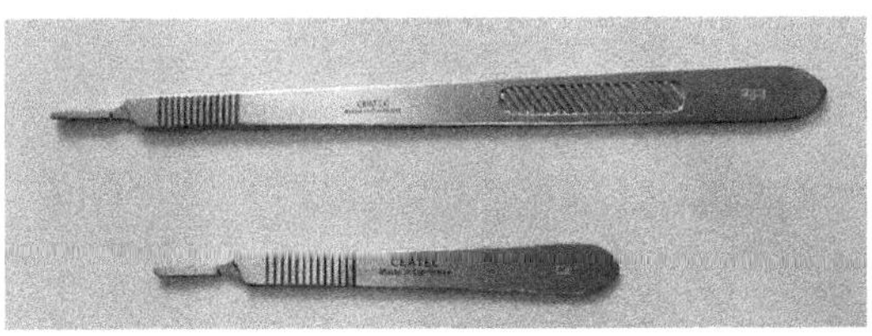

Figure 4. Disposable scalpels

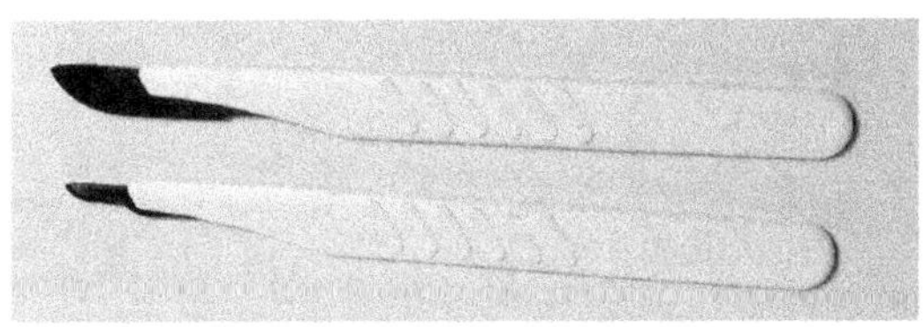

Figure 5. Palmar grip

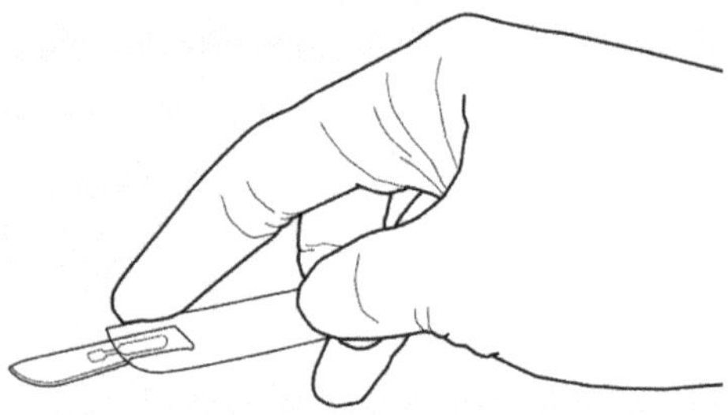

Figure 6. Pencil grip

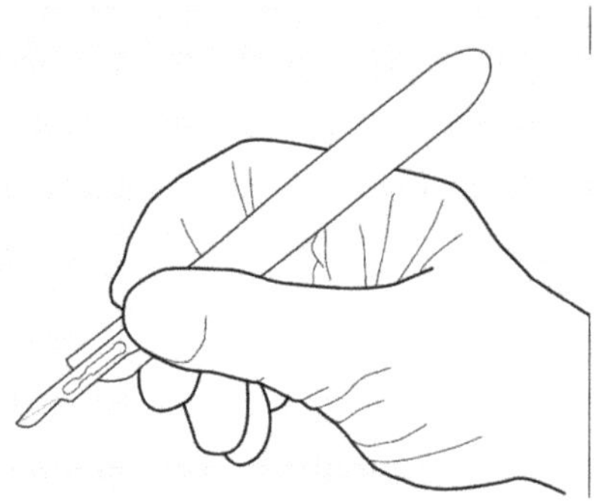

Graphic Design and Arts and Crafts Blades

Graphical and model-making scalpels tend to have round handles, with textured grips (either knurled metal or soft plastic) (Figure 7). These are often called by the name of the most well-known manufacturer of graphic arts blades, X-Acto knives. The blade is usually flat and straight, allowing it to be run easily against a straightedge to produce straight cuts.

There are many kinds of graphic arts blades; the most common around the graphic design studio is the #11 blade which is very similar to a #11 surgical blade (q.v.). Other blade shapes are used for wood carving, cutting leather and heavy fabric etc.

Ancient Scalpels

- Obsidian scalpels older than 2100 BC have been found in a Bronze Age settlement in Turkey. Skulls from the same time and place show signs of brain surgery.
- Indian surgeon Susruta used various scalpels to perform surgery in 8th century B.C.
- Ancient Egyptians made incisions for embalming with scalpels of sharpened obsidian, a material that is still in use.
- The first medical writings of ancient Greeks indicate they were commonly using tools identical to today's scalpels around 500 BC.
- Ancient Romans used more than 150 different surgical instruments, including scalpels.
- Indian Ayurvedic medicine mentions the use of sharp bamboo splinters.

Figure 7. Round handle scalpel

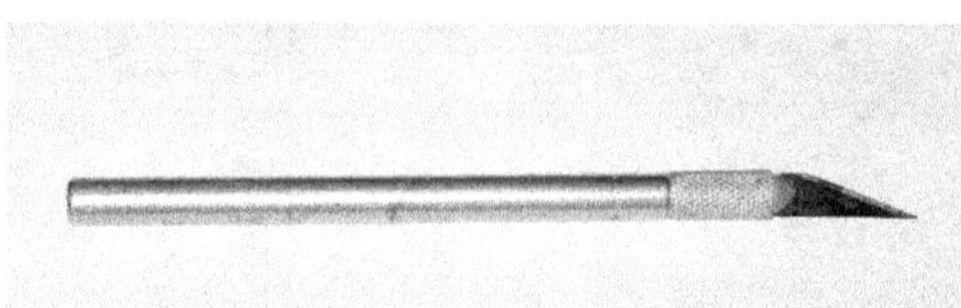

Safety Scalpels

Safety scalpels are becoming increasingly popular as their prices come down and also on account of legislation such as the Needle Stick Prevention Act. There are essentially two kinds of disposable safety scalpels offered by various manufacturers. They can be either classified as retractable blade or retractable sheath type. The retractable blade version made by companies such as OX Med Tech, DeRoyal, Jai Surgicals, and Swann Morton are more intuitive to use due to their similarities to a standard box-cutter. Retractable sheath versions have much stronger ergonomic feel for the doctors and are made by companies such as Aditya Dispomed, Aspen Surgical and Southmedic. A few companies have also started to offer a safety scalpel with a reusable metal handle. In such models, the blade is usually protected in a cartridge. Such systems usually require a custom handle and the price of blades and cartridges is considerably more than for conventional surgical blades.

However, CDC studies shows that up to 87% of active medical devices are not activated. Safety scalpels are active devices and therefore the risk of not activating is still significant. There is a study that indicated there were actually four times more injuries with safety scalpels than reusable scalpels.

Blade Removers

There are various scalpel blade removers on the market that allows users to safely remove blades from the handle, instead of dangerously using fingers or forceps. In the medical field, when taking into account activation rates, the combination of a single-handed scalpel blade remover with a passing tray or a neutral zone was as safe and up to five times safer than a safety scalpel. Companies like Qlicksmart offers a single-handed scalpel blade remover that complies with regulatory requirements such as US Occupational Safety and Health Administration Standards.

Safety

The usage of both safety scalpels and a single-handed blade remover, combined with a hands-free passing technique, are potentially effective in reducing scalpel blade injuries. It is up to employers and scalpel users to consider and use safer and more effective scalpel safety measures when feasible.

Scissors

Scissors are used to cut tissue or other materials during operative procedures, and come in a range of sizes and types. All scissors are classified as either sharp or blunt and straight or curved. Mayo scissors may be used to cut sutures and heavy body tissues, while smaller varieties, such as Metzenbaum scissors, are employed in cutting delicate materials. Blunt scissors are used to cut sutures and dressings.

Surgical scissors, also known as “forceps” in some countries outside of the United States, are surgical instruments usually used for cutting. They include bandage scissors, dissecting scissors, iris scissors, operating scissors, stitch scissors, tenotomy scissors, Metzenbaum scissors, plastic surgery scissors, and Mayo scissors. Surgical scissors are usually made of very hard stainless steel for ongoing toughness. Some scissors have tungsten carbide reinforcements along their cutting edges. The hardness of this material allows the manufacturers to create sharper edges, which allows for easier and smoother cuts and keeps the scissors sharp for longer.

Types of Surgical Scissors

There are two types of scissors used in surgeries.

- Ring scissors look much like standard utility scissors with two finger loops.
- Spring forceps are small scissors used mostly in eye surgery or microsurgery. The handles end in flat springs connected with a pivot joint. The cutting action is achieved by pressing the handles together. As the pressure is released, the spring action opens the jaws.

Scissors are available in various configurations like

- Blunt/blunt blades
- Blunt/sharp blades
- Sharp/sharp blades

Metzenbaum scissors are surgical scissors designed for cutting delicate tissue and blunt dissection (Figure 8). The scissors come in variable lengths and have a relatively long shank-to-blade ratio. They are constructed of stainless steel and may have tungsten carbide cutting surface inserts. Blades can be curved or straight. The blade tips are usually blunt. This is most common in organ operations. It is also used in heart operations.

Mayo scissors are a type of surgical scissor, often used in the cutting of fascia (Figure 9).

Bandage scissors, or bandage forceps, are angled tip scissors, with a blunt tip on the bottom blade, which helps in cutting bandages without gouging the skin (Figure 10). Bandage scissors were invented by Henry A. Kimmel in 1961 to prevent injury when removing a tight bandage. They are very popular in any health care facility because they are designed to safely lift bandages away from skin for easy cutting. The bottom blade of the scissor is longer and goes easily under the bandages. The blunt tip design of the scissor prevents accidental injury while making bandage removal very easy, smooth, and quick.

- **Clamping and Occluding:** Are used in many surgical procedures for compressing blood vessels or hollow organs, to prevent their contents from leaking. Occlude means to close or shut. Therefore, these instruments are also used to control bleeding. They are either straight, curved or angled, and have a variety of inner jaw patterns (Figure 11). Hemostats and mosquito forceps are some examples of these types of instruments.

Figure 8. Metzenbaum scissors

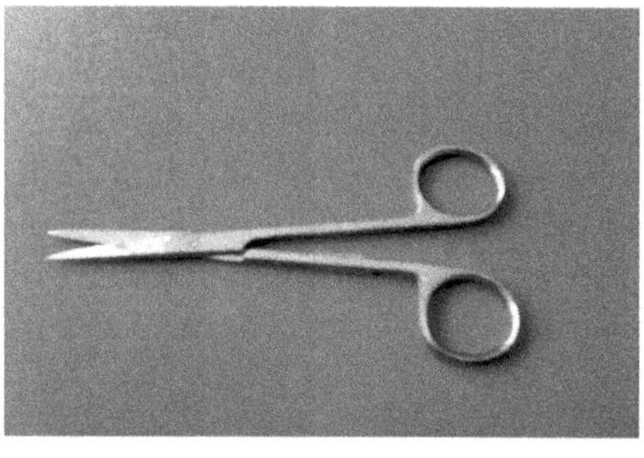

Figure 9. Mayo scissors

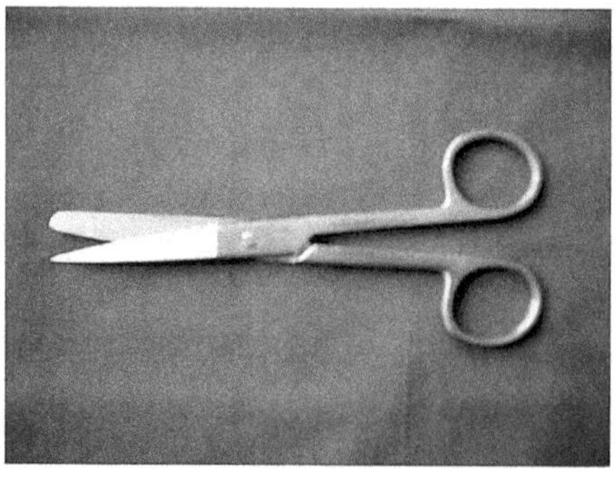

Figure 10. Bandage scissors

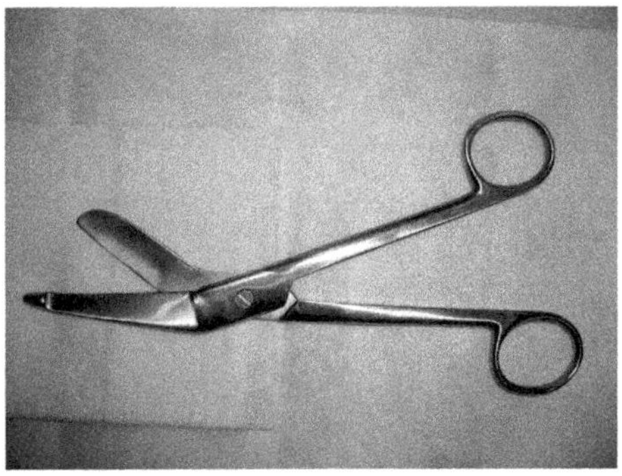

Figure 11. Clamping instrument

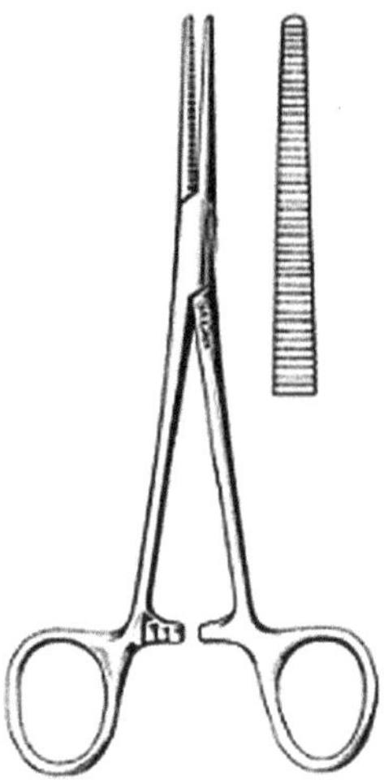

Clamp

A clamp is a fastening device used to hold or secure objects tightly together to prevent movement or separation through the application of inward pressure. In the United Kingdom and Australia, the term cramp is often used instead when the tool is for temporary use for positioning components during construction and woodworking; thus a G cramp or a sash cramp but a wheel clamp or a surgical clamp.

There are many types of clamps available for many different purposes (Figure 12). Some are temporary, as used to position components while fixing them together, others are intended to be permanent. In the field of animal husbandry, using a clamp to attach an animal to a stationary object is known as "rounded clamping." A physical clamp of this type is also used to refer to an obscure investment banking term; notably "fund clamps." Anything that performs the action of clamping may be called a clamp, so this gives rise to a wide variety of terms across many fields.

A hacmostat is used to clamp the blood vessels or tag sutures (Figure 13). Its jaws may be straight or curved. Other names are crile, snap or stat.

Figure 12. Surgical clamp

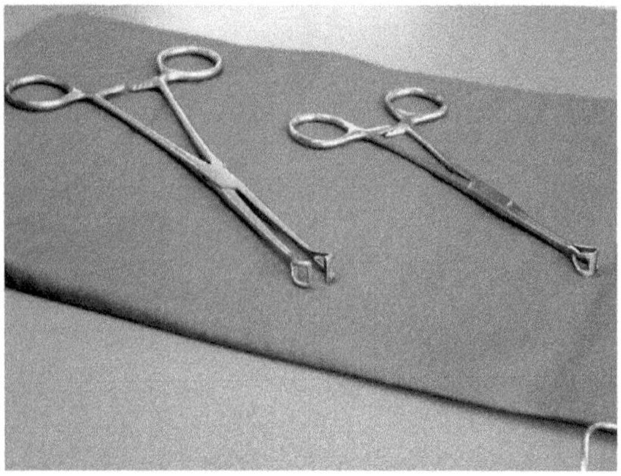

Figure 13. Haemostat

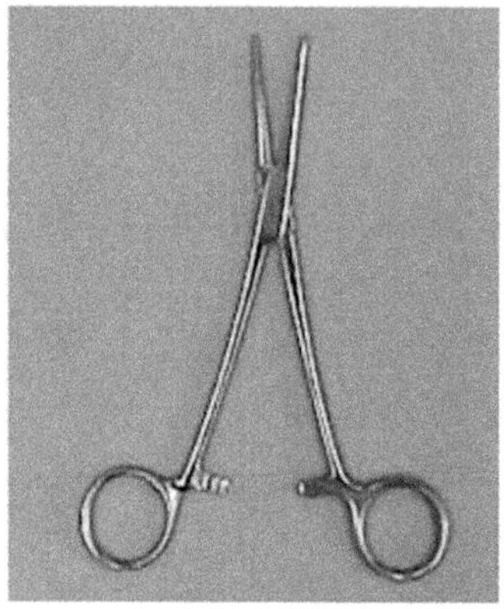

A mosquito is used to clamp small blood vessels. Its jaws may be straight or curved (Figure 14).

Kelly is used to clamp larger vessels and tissue. Available in short and long sizes. Other nanames include Rochester Pean (Figure 15).

A burlisher is used to clamp deep blood vessels (Figure 16). Burlishers have two closed finger rings. Burlishers with an open finger ring are called tonsil hemostats. Other names are Schnidt tonsil forcep, Adson forcep.

Figure 14. Hemostat, mosquito (left to right)

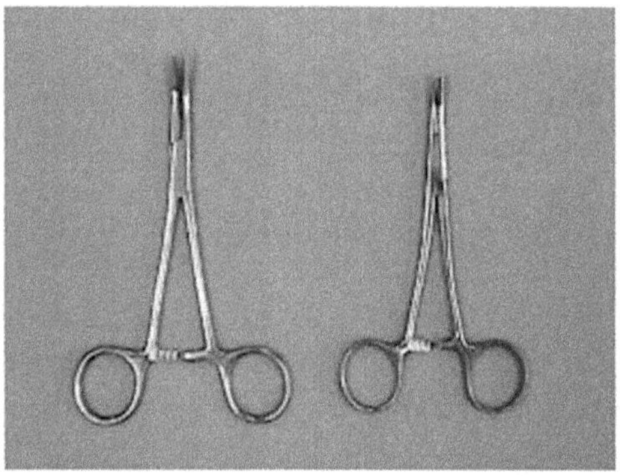

Figure 15. Kelly, hemostat, mosquito (left to right)

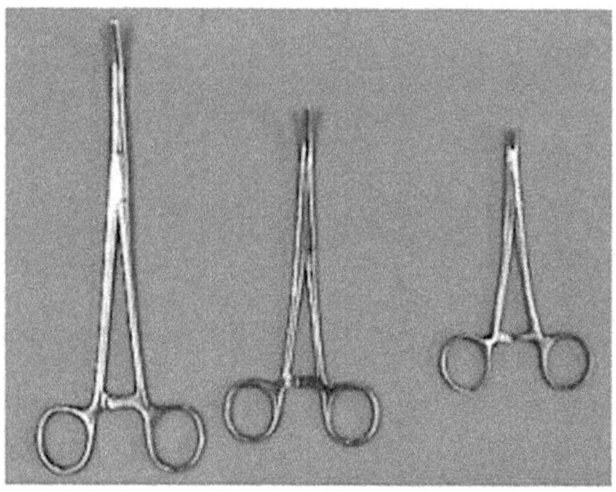

Figure 16. Burlisher

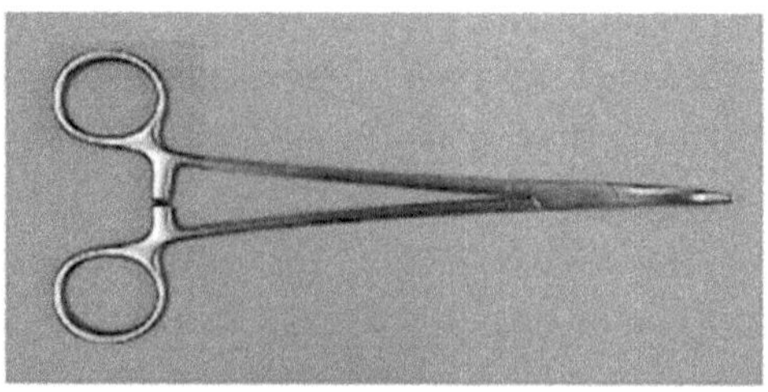

A right angle is used to clamp hard-to-reach vessels and to place sutures behind or around a vessel (Figure 17). A right angle with a suture attached is called a "tie on a passer." Other names: Mixter.

A hemoclip applier with hemoclips applies metal clips onto blood vessels and ducts which will remain occluded (Figure 18).

- **Retracting and Exposing:** These surgical instruments are used to hold back, or retract organs and tissue so the surgeon has access to the operative area. They spread open the skin, ribs and other tissue; and are also used separate the edges of a surgical incision. Some retracting and exposing instruments are "self-retaining," meaning they stay open on their own. Others manual styles need to be held open by hand.

Retracting and exposing instruments are used to hold back or retract organs or tissue to gain exposure to the operative site (Figure 19). They are either "self-retaining" (stay open on their own) or "manual" (held by hand).

Figure 17. Right angle

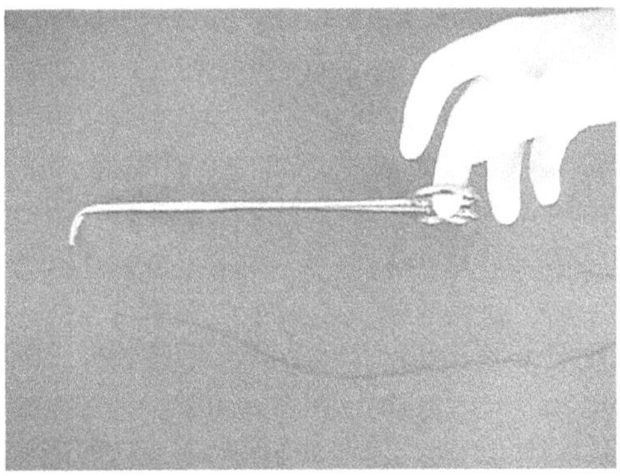

Figure 18. Hemoclip applier with hemoclips

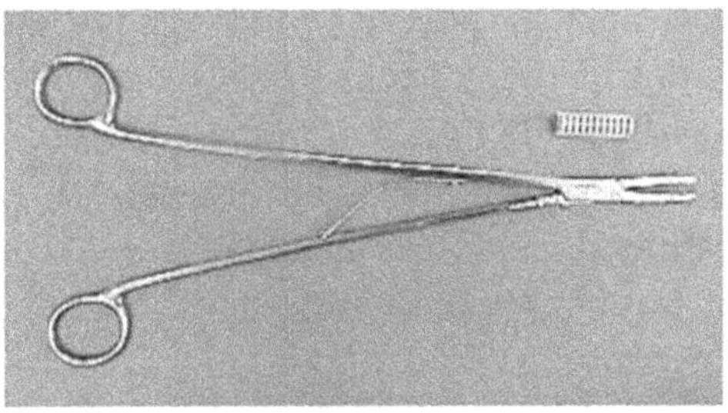

Figure 19. Volkman retractor

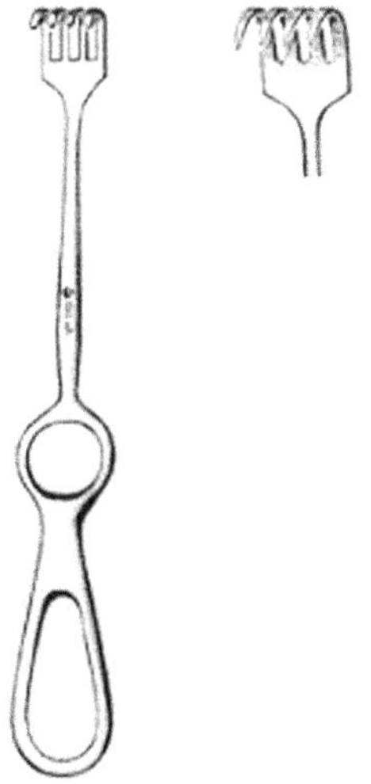

Retractors

Surgeons use surgical retractors to pull back, hold open or move tissues during surgery. Two types of retractors are used: self-retaining and hand-held. While self-retaining retractors lock into place, the hand-held variety must be held in place by an assistant during a procedure. The design of retractors reflects their function; surgeons use lung retractors, rib spreaders and skin retractors, among others (Figure 20). The design of retractors is similar to scissors--a hinged instrument, but with prongs or ridges on the ends for grabbing.

The two are each available in many shapes, sizes, and styles. The general term *retractor* usually describes a simple handheld steel tool possessing a curved, hooked, or angled blade fitted with a comfortable handle, that when in place maintains the desired position of a given region of tissue.

A retractor is a surgical instrument with which a surgeon can either actively separate the edges of a surgical incision or wound, or can hold back underlying organs and tissues, so that body parts under the incision may be accessed. The two are each available in many shapes, sizes, and styles. The general term retractor usually describes a simple handheld steel tool possessing a curved, hooked, or angled blade fitted with a comfortable handle, that when in place maintains the desired position of a given region of tissue. These simple retractors may be handheld, clamped in situ, or suspended at the end of a robotic arm. Retractors can also be self retaining and not need to be held once inserted by having two or more opposing blades or hooks which are separated via spring, ratchet, worm gear or some other method and pull on opposite sides of a wound. The term retractor is also used to describe the distinct, hand-cranked devices such as rib spreaders (also known as thoracic retractors, or distractors) with which surgeons may forcefully drive tissues apart to obtain the exposure. For specialized situations such as spinal surgery retractors have been fitted both with suction and with fiberoptic lights to keep a surgical wound dry and illuminated.

Surgical retractors probably originate with very basic tool use in the Stone Age (KMedic, 2008). Branches or antlers of various shapes were used to dig and extract food from the ground. As the use of tools evolved, a variety of instruments came about to substitute for the use of hooked or grasping fingers in the butchering of meat or dissection of bodies. The use of metals in tool making was of great importance. A variety of Roman metal instruments of the hook and retractor family have been found by

Figure 20. Different types of retractors

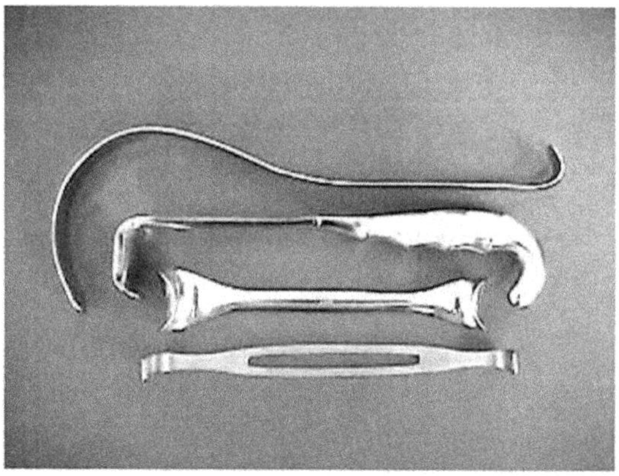

archeologists. These instruments would generally be called hooks if the end was as narrow as the handle of the instrument. If the end was broad, it would be called a retractor. Also arising from this group of tools were other related tools for displacing (elevators and spatulas) and scooping (spoons and curettes).

In 4th century CE, Indian physician Susruta used surgical tools such as retractors. In a description of the procedure of tonsillectomy from the 7th century CE, Paul of Aegina documents the use of a tongue spatula to keep the tongue out of the way while a form of tonsil hook is used to bring the tonsil forward for excision (Kmedic, 2008).

Jan Mikulicz-Radecki's invention of a hinged rib spreading retractor in 1904 prompted a flurry of development of retractors in the early 20th century, culminating in 1936 in our modern device based on the design of Enrique Finochietto (Bonfils-Robert, 1972).

A Deaver retractor (manual) is used to retract deep abdominal or chest incisions. Available in various widths (Figure 21).

A Richardson retractor (manual) is used to retract deep abdominal or chest incisions (Figure 22).

An Army-Navy retractor (manual) is used to retract shallow or superficial incisions (Figure 23).

A goulet (manual) is used to retract shallow or superficial incisions (Figure 24).

A malleable or ribbon retractor (manual) is used to retract deep wounds (Figure 25)

Figure 21. Deaver retractor

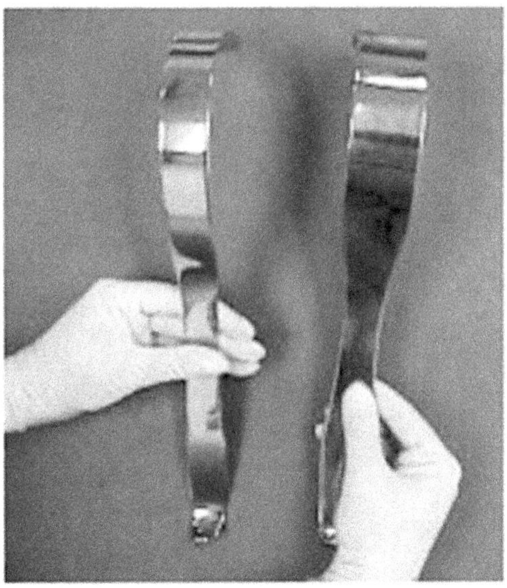

Figure 22. Richardson retractor

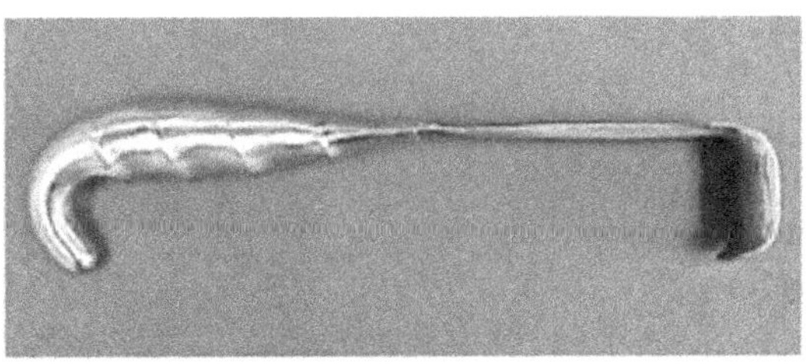

Figure 23. Army Navy retractor

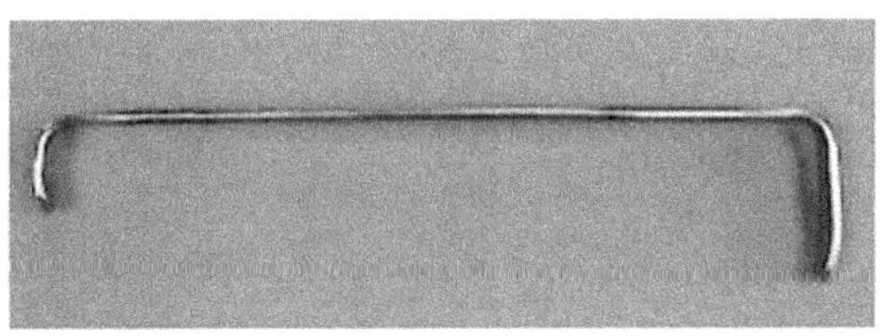

Figure 24. Goulet

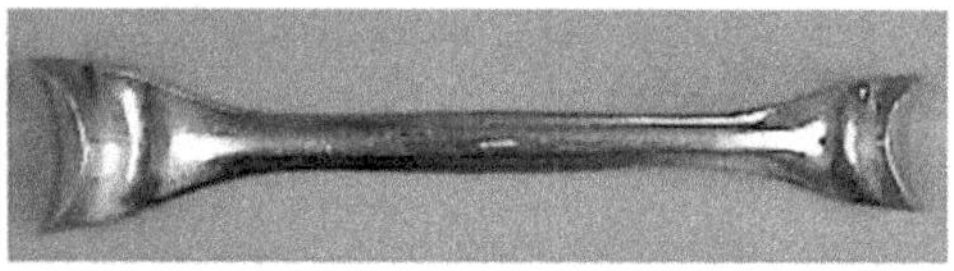

Figure 25. Malleable or ribbon retractor

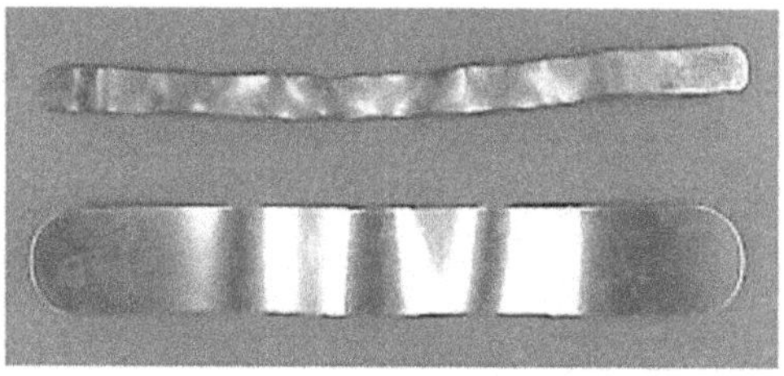

A Weitlaner retractor (self-retaining) is used to retract shallow incisions (Figure 26).

A Gelpi retractor (self-retaining) is used to retract shallow incisions (Figure 27).

A Balfour with bladder blade (self-retaining) is used to retract wound edges during deep abdominal procedures (Figure 28).

Figure 26. Weitlaner retractor

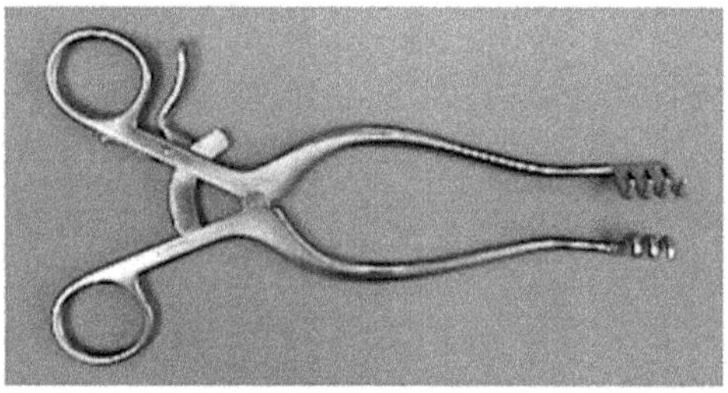

Figure 27. Gelpi reactor

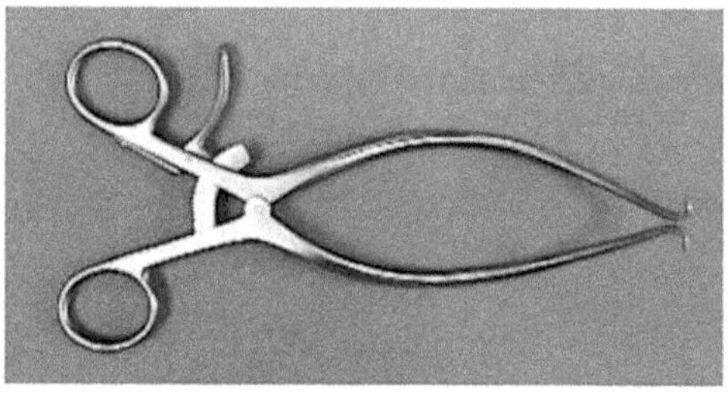

Figure 28. Balfour

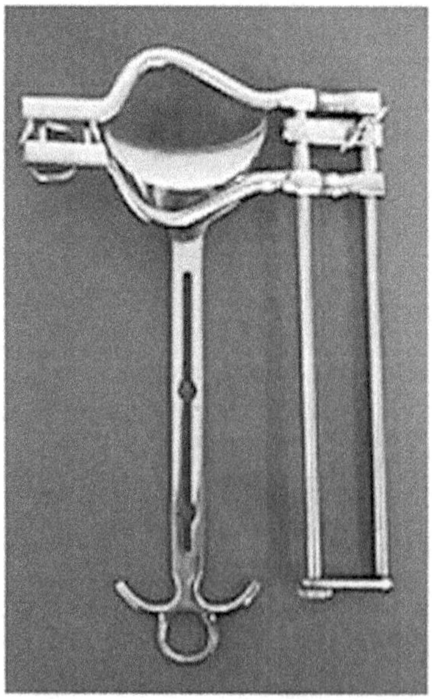

Grasping and Holding

These instruments, as their name suggests, are used to grasp and hold tissue or blood vessels that may be in the way during a surgical procedure. Medical assistants must make sure these instruments are working correctly, and that their locking mechanisms are lubricated for easy opening and closing, particularly after cleaning and reprocessing. Forceps are a very good example of these types of instruments.

In addition to these major categories, there are other narrow instrument classifications –such as viewing (specula, endoscopes), dilators/probes, suturing (needle holders), aspirating (suction tubes), and accessories (mallets, etc.) (Figure 29).

An Allis is used to grasp tissue (Figure 30). Available in short and long sizes. A "Judd-Allis" holds intestinal tissue; a "heavy allis" holds breast tissue.

A Babcock is used to grasp delicate tissue (intestine, fallopian tube, and ovary) (Figure 31). Available in short and long sizes.

A Kocher is used to grasp heavy tissue (Figure 32). It may also be used as a clamp. The jaws may be straight or curved. Other names: Ochsner.

A Foerster sponge stick is used to grasp sponges (Figure 33 and Figure 34) Other names: sponge forceps.

Figure 29. Different types of Grasping instruments

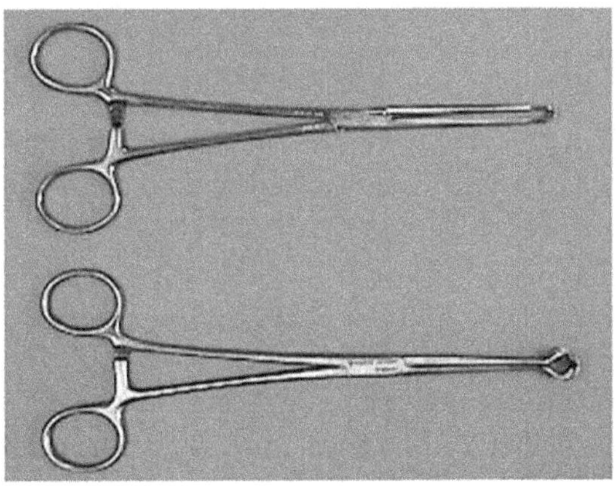

Figure 30. Allis tissue forceps

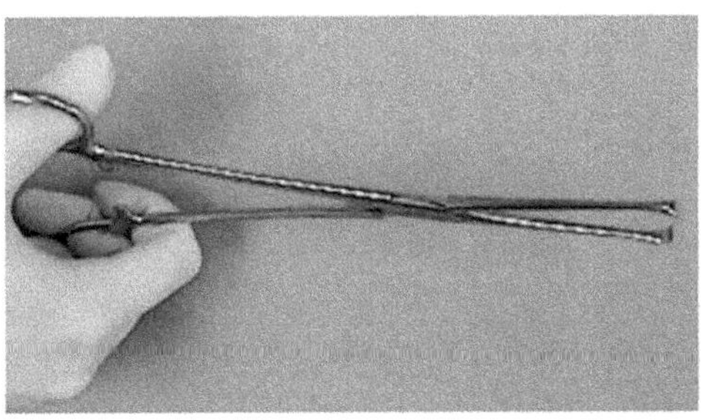

Figure 31. Babcock

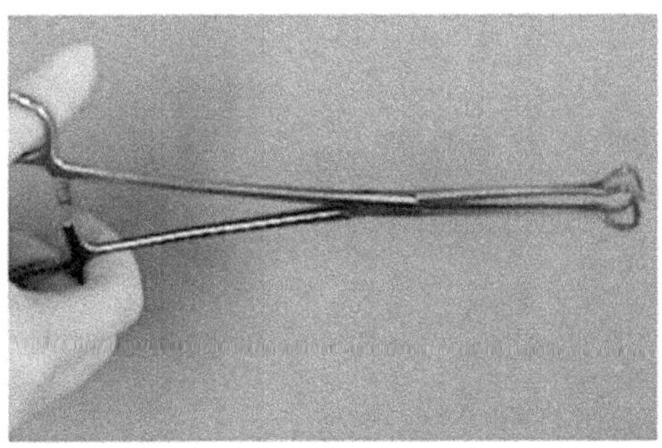

Figure 32. Kocher

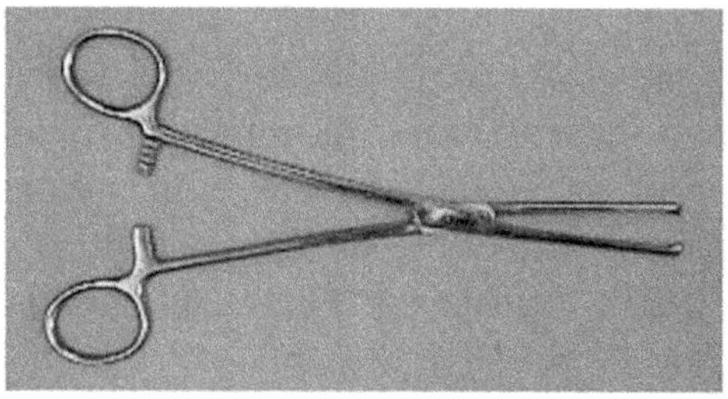

Figure 33. Foerster sponge stick

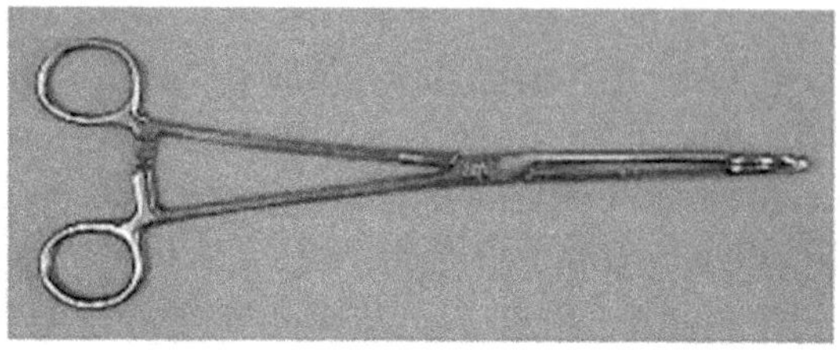

Figure 34. Sponge sticks holding a 4 X 4 and probang

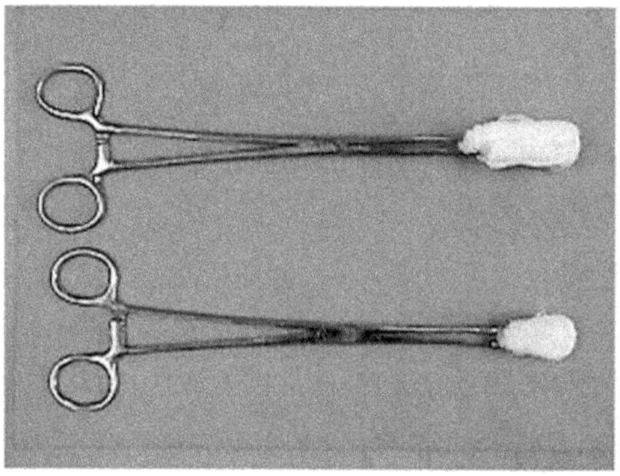

A dissector is used to hold a peanut (Figure 35). Ex: Dissector holding a peanut (Figure 36).

A Backhaus towel clip is used to hold towels and drapes in place (Figure 37 and Figure 38). Other name: towel clip.

Forceps

Forceps are a handheld, hinged instrument used for grasping and holding objects. Forceps are used when fingers are too large to grasp small objects or when many objects need to be held at one time while the hands are used to perform a task. The term 'forceps' is used almost exclusively within the medical field. Outside medicine, people usually refer to forceps as tweezers, tongs, pliers, clips or clamps.

Surgeons use forceps during surgical procedures to hold onto or manipulate tissues and to clamp blood vessels. Surgical forceps are hinged instruments, similar in design to scissors, but with tong-like or flat

Figure 35. Dissector

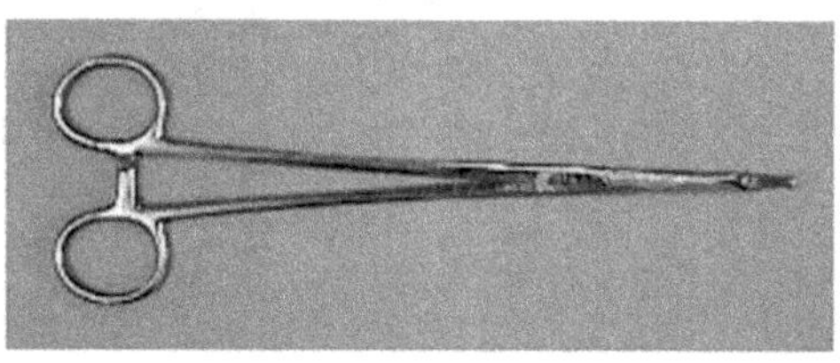

Figure 36. Dissector holding a peanut

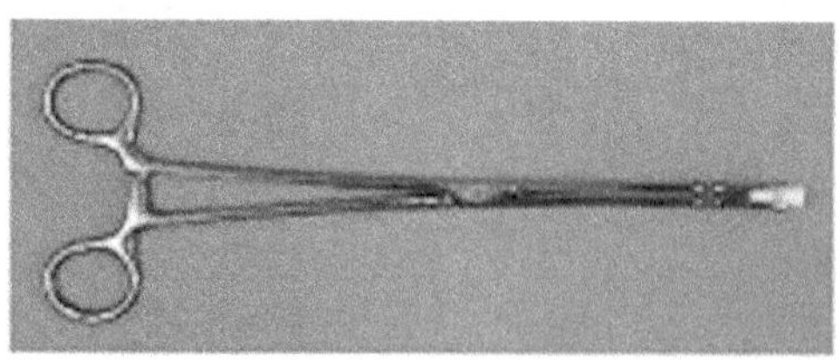

Figure 37. Backhaus towel clip

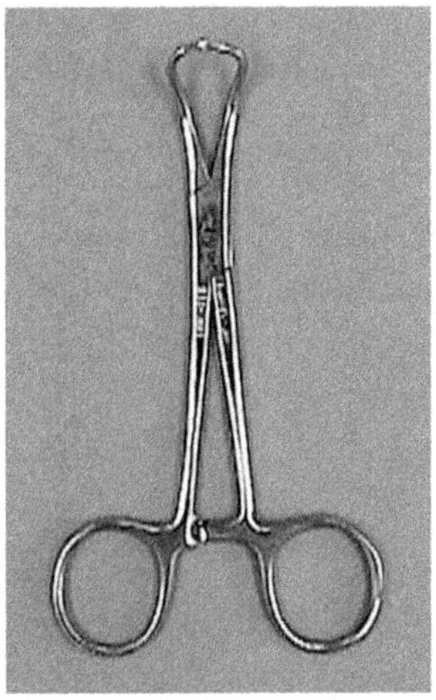

Figure 38. Large and small towel clips

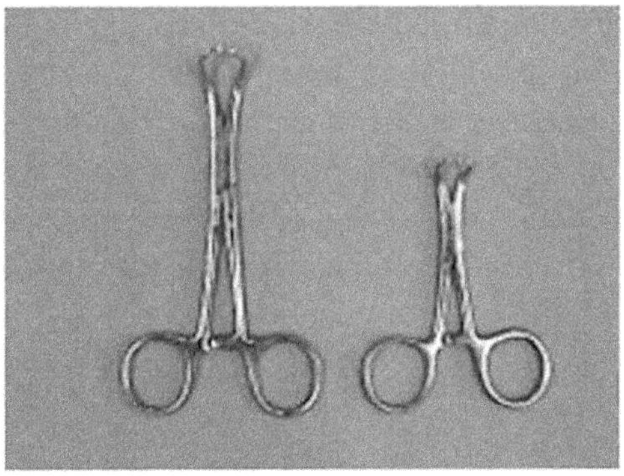

tips that are used to hold, clamp or move tissues during surgery. Forceps come in three varieties: tissue/ dressing forceps, intestinal forceps and hemostats (used to clamp blood vessels). Forceps, like scissors, may be classified as curved or straight and may or may not have small "teeth" at the tips.

Mechanically, forceps employ the principle of the lever to grasp and apply pressure.

Depending on their function, basic surgical forceps can be categorized into the following groups Viz:

1. **Non Disposable Forceps:** They should withstand various kinds of physical and chemical effects of body fluids, secretions, cleaning agents, and sterilization methods.
2. **Disposable Forceps:** They are usually made of lower quality materials or plastics which are disposed after use.

Surgical forceps are commonly made of high-grade carbon steel, which ensures they can withstand repeated sterilization in high-temperature autoclaves Some are made of other high-quality stainless steel, Chromium and Vanadium alloys to ensure durability of edges, and restlessness. Lower quality steel is used in forceps made for other uses. Some forceps Disposable, intended to be used once and then discarded, are made of plastic. The invention of surgical forceps is attributed to Stephen Hales.

There are two basic types of forceps: non-locking (often called 'thumb forceps' or 'pick-ups') and locking, though these two types come in dozens of specialized forms for various uses. Non-locking forceps also come in two basic forms: hinged at one end, away from the grasping end (colloquially such forceps are called tweezers) and hinged in the middle, rather like scissors. Locking forceps are almost always hinged in the middle, though some forms place the hinge very close to the grasping end. Locking forceps use various means to lock the grasping surfaces in a closed position to facilitate manipulation or to independently clamp, grasp or hold an object.

Thumb Forceps

Thumb forceps are commonly held between the thumb and two or three fingers of one hand, with the top end resting on the first dorsal interosseous muscle at the base of the thumb and index finger. Spring tension at one end holds the grasping ends apart until pressure is applied. This allows one to quickly and easily grasp small objects or tissue to move and release it or to grasp and hold tissue with easily variable pressure. Thumb forceps are used to hold tissue in place when applying sutures, to gently move tissues out of the way during exploratory surgery and to move dressings or draping without using the hands or fingers (Figure 39). Thumb forceps can have smooth tips, cross-hatched tips or serrated tips (often called 'mouse's teeth'). Common arrangements of teeth are 1×2 (two teeth on one side meshing with a single tooth on the other), 7×7 and 9×9. Serrated forceps are used on tissue; counter-intuitively, teeth will damage tissue less than a smooth surface because one can grasp with less overall pressure. Smooth or cross-hatched forceps are used to move dressings, remove sutures and similar tasks.

Locking Forceps

Locking forceps, sometimes called clamps, are used to grasp and hold objects or tissue. When they are used to compress an artery to forestall bleeding they are called hemostats. Another form of locking forceps is the needle holder, used to guide a suturing needle through tissue. Many locking forceps use finger loops to facilitate handling (see illustration, below, of Kelly Forceps). The finger loops are usually grasped by the thumb and middle or ring fingers, while the index finger helps guide the instrument.

The most common locking mechanism is a series of interlocking teeth located near the finger loops. As the forceps are closed, the teeth engage and keep the instrument's grasping surfaces from separating. A simple shift of the fingers is all that is needed to dis-engage the teeth and allow the grasping ends to move apart. Forceps are also used for surgery.

Figure 39. Blunt-nosed thumb forceps with serrated tips for increased grip

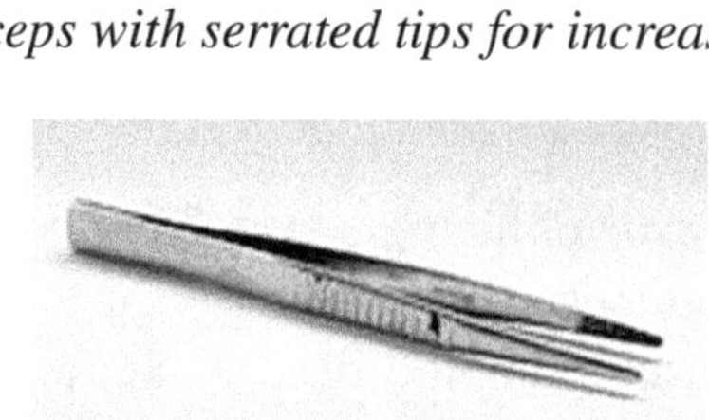

Kelly Forceps

Kelly forceps are a type of hemostat usually made of stainless steel. They resemble a pair of scissors with the blade replaced by a blunted grip. They also feature a locking mechanism to allow them to act as clamps. Kelly forceps may be floor grade (regular use) and as such not used for surgery (Figure 40). They may also be sterilized and used in operations, in both human and veterinary medicine. They may be either curved or straight. In surgery, they may be used for occluding blood vessels, manipulating [tissues], or for assorted other purposes. They are named for Howard Atwood Kelly, M.D., first professor of obstetrics and gynecology at Johns Hopkins. The "Mosquito" variant of the tool is more delicate and has smaller, finer tips. Other varieties with similar, if more specialized, uses are Allis clamps, Babcocks, Kochers, Carmalts, and tonsils; all but the last bear the names of the surgeons who designed them.

Pick ups, thumb forceps and tissue forceps are available in various lengths, with or without teeth, and smooth or serrated jaws (Figure 41).

Russian tissue forceps are used to grasp tissue (Figure 42).

Adson pick ups are either smooth: used to grasp delicate tissue; or with teeth: used to grasp the skin (Figure 43). Other names: Dura forceps.

Long smooth pick-ups are called dressing forceps. Short smooth pick-ups are used to grasp delicate tissue (Figure 44).

DeBakey forceps are used to grasp delicate tissue, particularly in cardiovascular surgery (Figure 45). DeBakey forceps

Thumb forceps are used to grasp tough tissue (fascia, breast) (Figure 46). Forceps may either have many teeth or a single tooth. Single tooth forceps are also called "rat tooth forceps.

Figure 40. Kelly forceps, shown closed and open

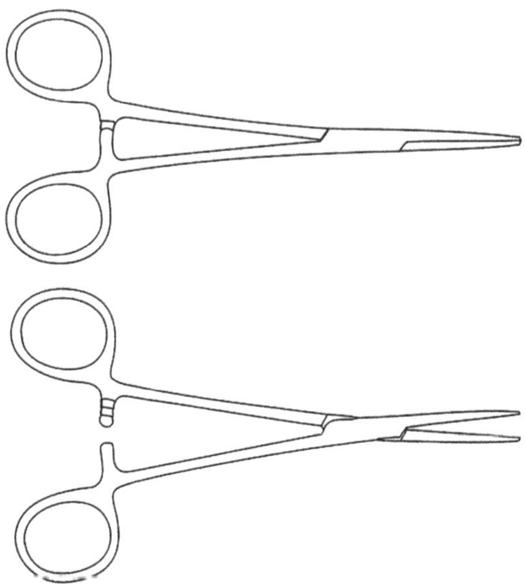

Figure 41. Different types of forceps

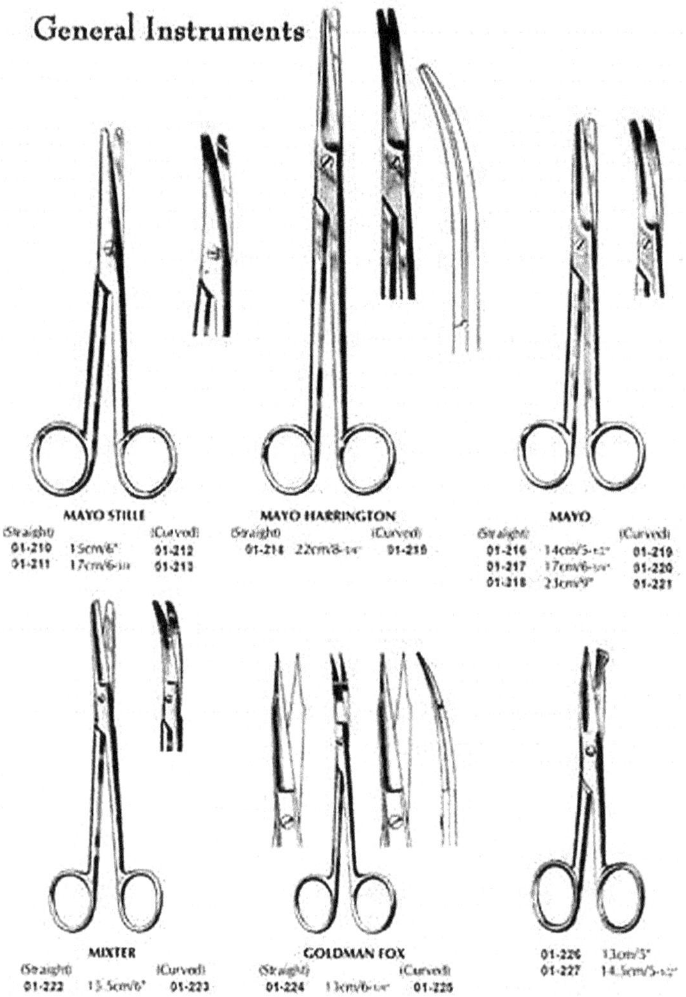

Figure 42. Russian tissue forceps

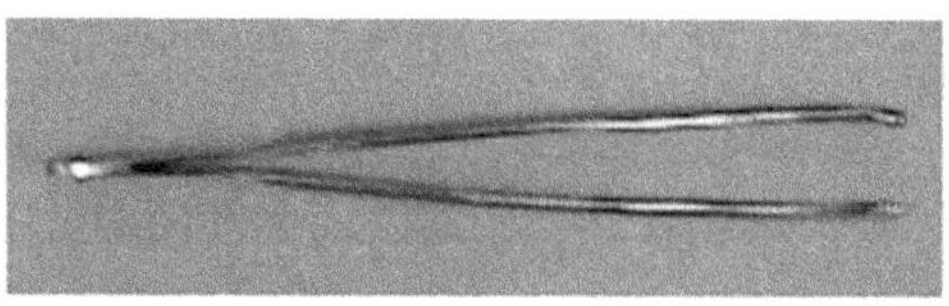

Suction Instruments

In medicine, devices are sometimes necessary to create suction. Suction may be used to clear the airway of blood, saliva, vomit, or other secretions so that a patient may breathe. Suctioning can prevent pulmonary aspiration, which can lead to lung infections. In pulmonary hygiene, suction is used to remove fluids from the airways to facilitate breathing and prevent growth of microorganisms (Allen, 1996).

Figure 43. Adson pick ups

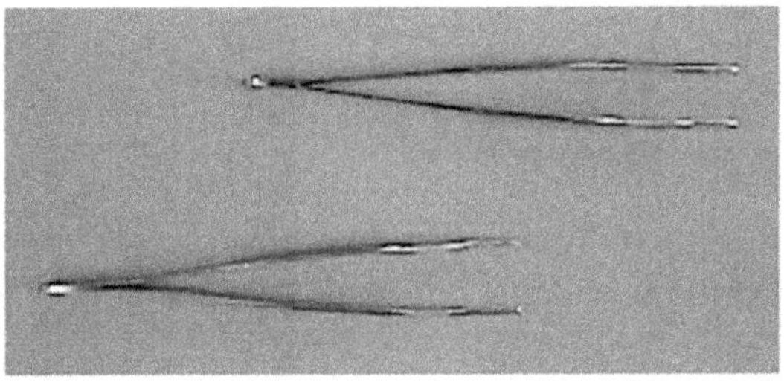

Figure 44. Smooth forceps

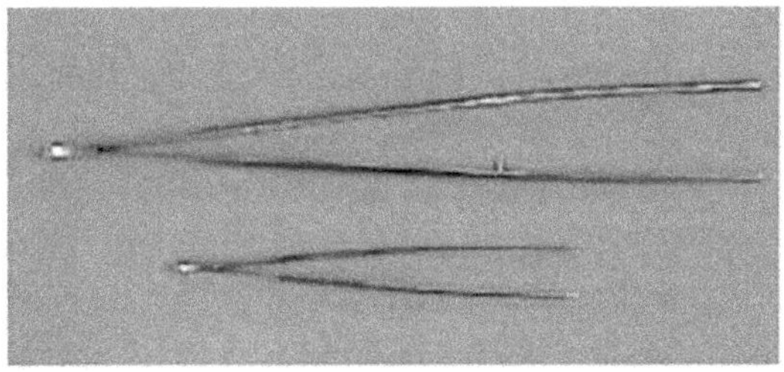

Figure 45. DeBakey forceps

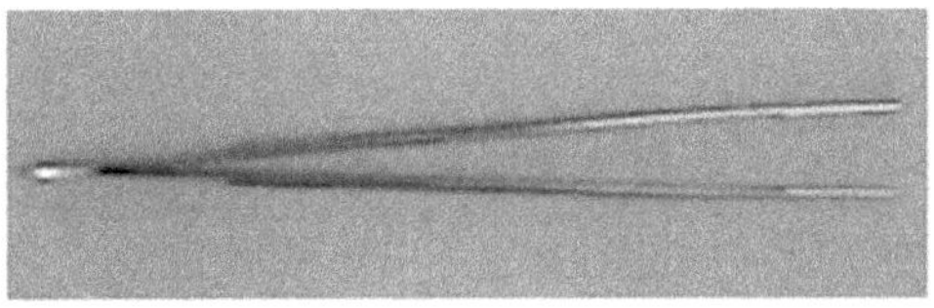

Figure 46. Single tooth forceps, many teeth forceps

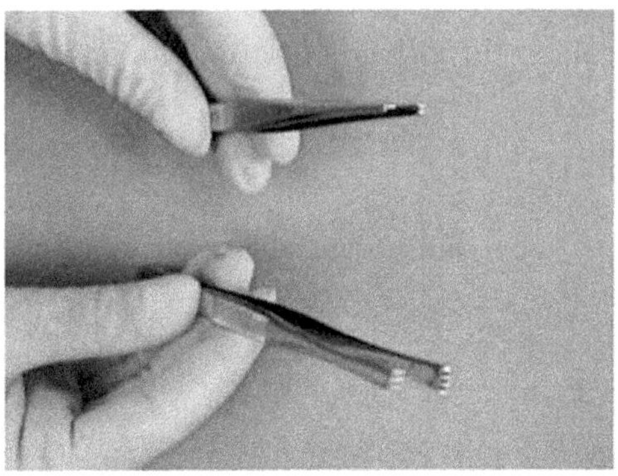

In surgery suction can be used to remove blood from the area being operated on to allow surgeons to view and work on the area. Suction may also be used to remove blood that has built up within the skull after an intracranial hemorrhage (Valadka, 2004).

Suction devices may be mechanical hand pumps or battery or electrically operated mechanisms. The plastic, rigid Yankauer suction tip is one type of tip attached to a suction unit. Another is the plastic, nonrigid French or whistle tip catheter (Pollak, 2011).

Drain

A surgical drain is a tube used to remove pus, blood or other fluids from a wound (Durai et al, 2009). They are commonly placed by surgeons or interventional radiologists. Drains inserted after surgery do not result in faster wound healing or prevent infection, but are sometimes necessary to drain body fluid which may accumulate and in itself becomes a focus of infection or retained blood complications (Carter, 1993; Pollak, 2011).

Types of Drains

Surgical drains can be broadly classified into:

- **Jackson-Pratt Drain:** Consists of a perforated round or flat tube connected to a negative pressure collection device. The collection device is typically a bulb with a drainage port which can be opened to remove fluid or air. After compressing the bulb to remove fluid or air, negative pressure is created as the bulb returns to its normal shape (Rayatt et al, 2005).
- **Blake Drain:** A round silicone tube with channels that carry fluid to a negative pressure collection device. Drainage is thought to be achieved by capillary action, allowing fluid to travel through the open grooves into a closed cross section, which contains the fluid and allows it to be suctioned through the tube (Tsuda et al, 2003).
- **Penrose Drain:** A soft rubber tube
- **Negative Pressure Wound Therapy:** Involves the use of enclosed foam and a suction device attached; this is one of the newer types of wound healing/drain devices which promotes faster tissue granulation, often used for large surgical/trauma/non-healing wounds.
- **Redivac Drain:** (Bharathan et al, 2009).
- **Pigtail Drain:** Has an exterior screw to release the internal "pigtail" before it can be removed
- **Davol**
- **Chest Tube:** Is a flexible plastic tube that is inserted through the chest wall and into the pleural space or mediastinum
- **Wound manager.**

There are many types of drains, tubes and catheters used in surgery. These next few pages will outline many of these and their major uses.

- Catheters are used for evacuating or injecting fluids. Catheters are sized on a French scale according to the diameter of the lumen. The smallest diameter on this scale is 3 French.
- Drains and tubes are devices used to drain fluid from the body when excessive drainage is expected. A drain or tube is often placed in a separate small incision site known as a stab wound, close to the operative site (Allen et al, 1996).

Foley catheters are commonly used as an indwelling catheter to drain the bladder. It has an inflatable balloon near the tip which holds the catheter in place. There are 2 (Figure 47) and 3 way Foleys (Figure 48). The 3 way Foley has an inlet for irrigation.

A rectal tube is used to expel flatus from the rectum. The opening at the end of the tubing differentiates it from the Robinson catheter. The clear rectal tube is disposable (Figure 49).

Figure 47. A 2 way Foley

Figure 48. A 3 way Foley

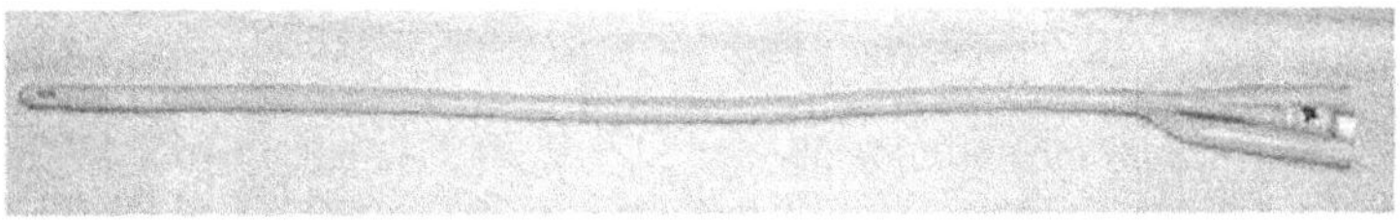

Figure 49. Two types of rectal tubes

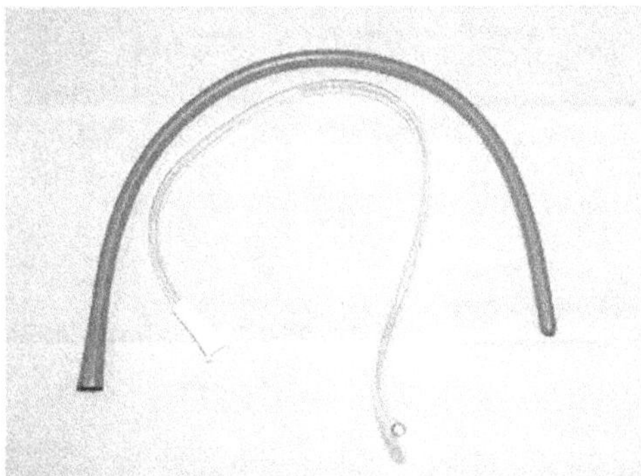

Thoracic catheters are used to drain blood and other fluids from the thoracic cavity (Figure 50).

The trocar catheter with a large trocar needle is used for a closed thoracostomy (Figure 51).

The thoracic or trocar catheter is usually connected to a disposable chest drainage collection unit (Figure 52).

Feeding tubes are used to feed a premature infant (Figure 53).

A Penrose drain, made of soft, pliable rubber, is used to drain incisions (Figure 54).

Surgical Staple

Surgical staples are specialized staples used in surgery in place of sutures to close skin wounds, connect or remove parts of the bowels or lungs (Zeebregts, Heijmen, Dungen, Schilfgaarde, 2003; Konstantinov,

Figure 50. A thoracic catheter

Figure 51. A trocar catheter with trocar inserted

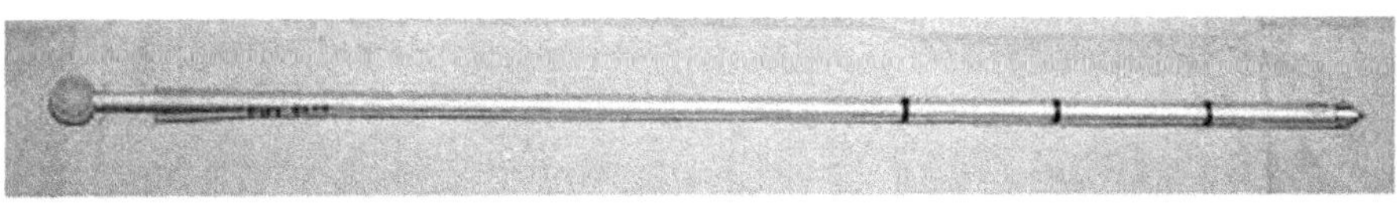

Figure 52. A thoracic catheter

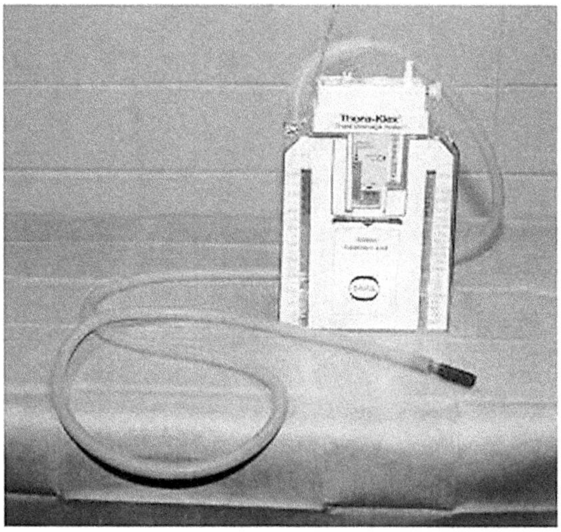

Figure 53. A feeding tube

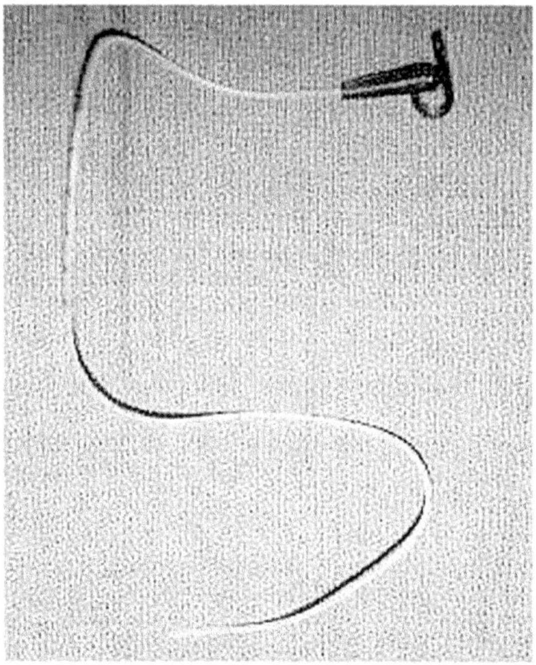

Figure 54. A Penrose drain

2004). A more recent development, from the 1990s, uses clips instead of staples for some applications; this does not require the staple to penetrate.

Stapling is much faster than suturing by hand, and also more accurate and consistent (Brundage, Jurkovich, Hoyt, Patel, Ross, Marburger, Stoner, Ivatury, Ku, Rutherford, Maier, 20001). Staples are primarily used in bowel and lung surgery, because staple lines are more consistent and therefore less likely to leak blood, air or bowel contents. Still, several randomized controlled trials have shown no significant difference in bowel leakage after anastomoses performed either manually with suture by experienced surgeons, or after mechanical anastomoses with staples. In skin closure, dermal adhesives (skin glues) are also an increasingly common alternative (Hsu, Chen, Haung, Lee, Lee, 2004).

Types and Applications

The first commercial staplers were made of stainless steel with titanium staples loaded into reloadable staple cartridges. Modern surgical staplers are either disposable and made of plastic, or reusable and made of stainless steel (Stefano, Manelli, Gasidlo, Rinaldo, Luigi, Zonta, 1990). Both types are generally loaded using disposable cartridges. The staple line may be straight, curved or circular. Circular staplers are used for end-to-end anastomosis after bowel resection or, somewhat more controversially, in esophagogastric surgery (Shiffrin, Schwierz, Wassilijew, Caggianos, 2007). The instruments may be used in either open or laparoscopic surgery, different instruments are used for each application. Laparoscopic staplers are longer, thinner, and may be articulated to allow for access from a restricted number of trocar ports.

Some staplers incorporate a knife, to complete excision and anastomosis in a single operation. Staplers are used to close both internal and skin wounds. Skin staples are usually applied using a disposable stapler, and removed with a specialized staple remover. Staplers are also used in vertical banded gastroplasty surgery (popularly known as "stomach stapling") (Shifrin, Moore, Bell, Kolvenbach, Daniline, 2007)(Figure 55).

Vascular stapler for reducing warm ischemia in organ transplantation. With this model each stapler end can be mounted on donor and recipient by independent surgical teams without care for reciprocal orientation, being the maximal possible vascular axis torsion ≤30°. Activating guide-wire is connected just immediately before firing.

Figure 55. Surgical stapler

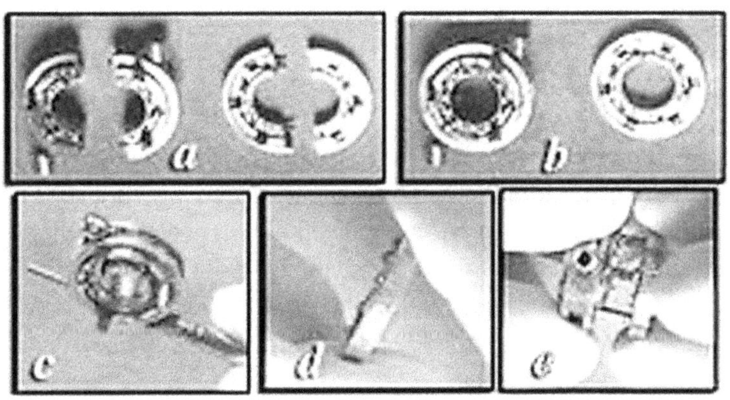

While devices for circular end-to-end anastomosis of digestive tract are widely used, in spite of intensive research circular staplers for vascular anastomosis never had yet significant impact on standard hand (Carrel) suture technique (Teoh, Bird, 1987). Apart from the different modality of coupling of vascular (everted) in respect to digestive (inverted) stumps, the main basic reason could be that, particularly for small vessels, the manuality and precision required just for positioning on vascular stumps and actioning any device cannot be significantly inferior to that required to carry out the standard hand suture, then making of little utility the use of any device. An exception to that however could be organ transplantation where these two phases, i.e.device positioning at the vascular stumps and device actioning, can be carried out in different time, by different surgical team, in safe conditions when the time required does not influence donor organ preservation, i.e. at the back table in cold ischemia condition for the donor organ and after native organ removal in the recipient. This is finalized to make as brief as possible the donor organ dangerous warm ischemia phase that can be contained in the couple of minutes or less necessary just to connect the device's ends and actioning the stapler (Wickens, 2014).

Although most surgical staples are made of titanium, stainless steel is more often used in some skin staples and clips. Titanium produces less reaction with the immune system and, being non-ferrous, does not interfere significantly with MRI scanners, although some imaging artifacts may result. Synthetic absorbable (bioabsorbable) staples are also now becoming available, based on polyglycolic acid, as with many synthetic absorbable sutures.

Titanium staples are not suspected of causing nickel reactions because nickel is rarely if ever used in titanium alloys.

Periodontal Probe

A periodontal probe is an instrument in dentistry commonly used in the dental armamentarium. It is usually long, thin, and blunted at the end. The primary purpose of a periodontal probe is to measure pocket depths around a tooth in order to establish the state of health of the periodontium. There are markings inscribed onto the head of the instrument for accuracy and readability.

There are many different types of periodontal probes, and each has its own manner of indicating measurements on the tip of the instrument. For example, the Michigan O probe has markings at 3 mm, 6 mm and 8 mm and the Williams probe has circumferential lines at 1 mm, 2 mm, 3 mm, 5 mm, 7 mm, 8 mm, 9 mm, and 10 mm. The PCP12 probe with Marquis markings has alternating shades every 3 mm. Unlike the previous two mentioned, the Naber's probe is curved and is used for measuring into the furcation area between the roots of a tooth.

Use

Proper use of the periodontal probe is necessary to maintain accuracy. The tip of the instrument is placed with light pressure of 10-20 grams into the gingival sulcus, which is an area of potential space between a tooth and the surrounding tissue. It is important to keep the periodontal probe parallel to the contours of the root of the tooth and to insert the probe down to the base of the pocket (Figure 56). This results in obscuring a section of the periodontal probe's tip. The first marking visible above the pocket indicates the measurement of the pocket depth. It has been found that the average, healthy pocket depth is around

Figure 56. Michigan O probe with Williams markings (left) and Naber's probe with shades alternating every 3 mm (right)

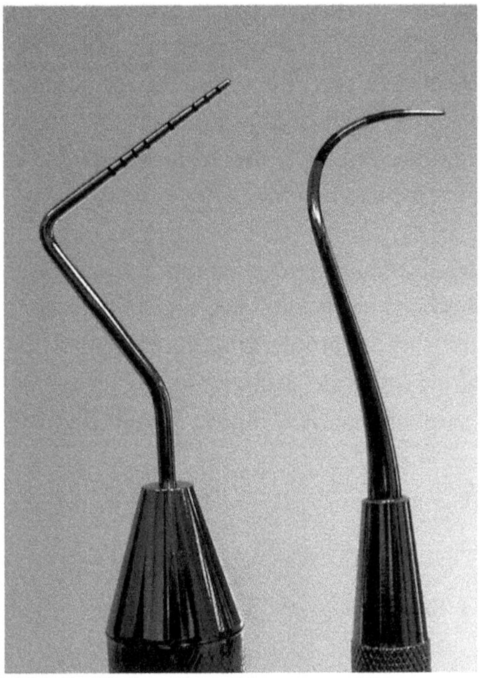

3 mm with no bleeding upon probing. Depths greater than 3 mm can be associated with "attachment loss" of the tooth to the surrounding alveolar bone, which is a characteristic found in periodontitis. Pocket depths greater than 3 mm can also be a sign of gingival hyperplasia.

The periodontal probe can also be used to measure other dental instruments, tooth preparations during restorative procedures, gingival recession, attached gingiva, and oral lesions or pathologies. Bleeding on probing (BoP), even with a gentle touch, can also occur in this situation. It is due to the periodontal probe damaging the increased blood vessels in the capillary plexus of the lamina propria, which are close to the surface because of the ulceration of the junctional epithelium (JE). The presence of bleeding is one of the first clinical signs of active periodontal disease in uncomplicated cases and should be recorded per individual tooth and tooth surface in the patient record. However, in patients who smoke, the gingival tissue rarely bleeds because of unknown factors that do not seem related to dental biofilm and calculus formation.

Surgical Suture

Surgical suture is a medical device used to hold body tissues together after an injury or surgery. Application generally involves using a needle with an attached length of thread. A number of different shapes, sizes, and thread materials have been developed over its millennia of history. Surgeons, physicians, dentists, podiatrists, eye doctors, registered nurses and other trained nursing personnel, medics, and clinical pharmacists typically engage in suturing. Surgical knots are used to secure the sutures.

Needles

Eyed or reusable needles are needles with holes called eyes which are supplied separate from their suture thread. The suture must be threaded on site, as is done when sewing at home. The advantage of this is that any thread and needle combination is possible to suit the job at hand. Swaged, or atraumatic, needles with sutures comprise a pre-packed eyeless needle attached to a specific length of suture thread. The suture manufacturer swages the suture thread to the eyeless atraumatic needle at the factory. The chief advantage of this is that the doctor or the nurse does not have to spend time threading the suture on the needle, which may be difficult for very fine needles and sutures. Also, the suture end of a swaged needle is narrower than the needle body, eliminating drag from the thread attachment site. In eyed needles, the thread protrudes from the needle body on both sides, and at best causes drag. When passing through friable tissues, the eye needle and suture combination may thus traumatise tissues more than a swaged needle, hence the designation of the latter as "atraumatic".

There are several shapes of surgical needles (Figure 57 and Figure 58). These include:

- Straight
- 1/4 circle
- 3/8 circle
- 1/2 circle. Subtypes of this needle shape include, from larger to smaller size, CT, CT-1, CT-2 and CT-3.
- 5/8 circle
- compound curve
- half curved (also known as ski)
- half curved at both ends of a straight segment (also known as canoe)

The ski and canoe needle design allows curved needles to be straight enough to be used in laparoscopic surgery, where instruments are inserted into the abdominal cavity through narrow cannulas.

Needles may also be classified by their point geometry; examples include:

Figure 57. Eyed surgical needles which form 3/8th of a circle, in different sizes

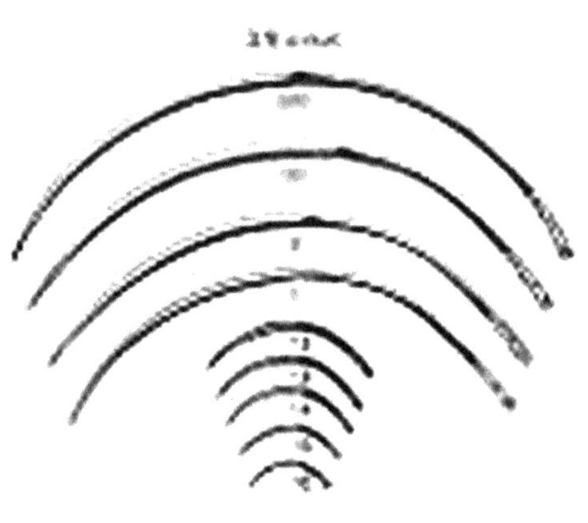

Figure 58. Eyed surgical needles which are semi-circular, in different sizes

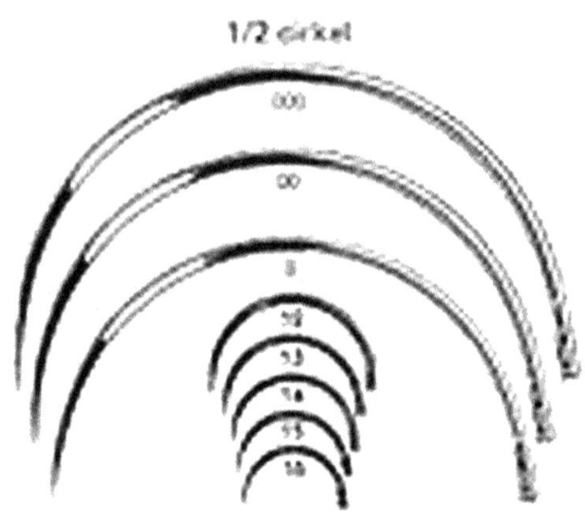

- Taper (needle body is round and tapers smoothly to a point)
- Cutting (needle body is triangular and has a sharpened cutting edge on the inside curve)
- Reverse cutting (cutting edge on the outside)
- Trocar point or tapercut (needle body is round and tapered, but ends in a small triangular cutting point)
- Blunt points for sewing friable tissues
- Side cutting or spatula points (flat on top and bottom with a cutting edge along the front to one side) for eye surgery

Finally, atraumatic needles may be permanently swaged to the suture or may be designed to come off the suture with a sharp straight tug. These "pop-offs" are commonly used for interrupted sutures, where each suture is only passed once and then tied.

Sutures can withstand different amounts of force based on their size; this is quantified by the U.S.P. Needle Pull Specifications.

Thread

Suture thread is made from numerous materials. The original sutures were made from biological materials, such as catgut suture and silk. Most modern sutures are synthetic, including the absorbables polyglycolic acid, polylactic acid, Monocryl and polydioxanone as well as the non-absorbables nylon, polyester, PVDF and polypropylene. The FDA first approved triclosan-coated sutures in 2002; they have been shown to reduce the chances of wound infection. Sutures come in very specific sizes and may be either absorbable (naturally biodegradable in the body) or non-absorbable. Sutures must be strong enough to hold tissue securely but flexible enough to be knotted. They must be hypoallergenic and avoid the "wick effect" that would allow fluids and thus infection to penetrate the body along the suture tract.

Mayo-Hegar needle holders are used to hold needles when suturing (Figure 59 and Figure 60). They may also be placed in the sewing category.

Figure 59. Needle holders (short, medium and long)

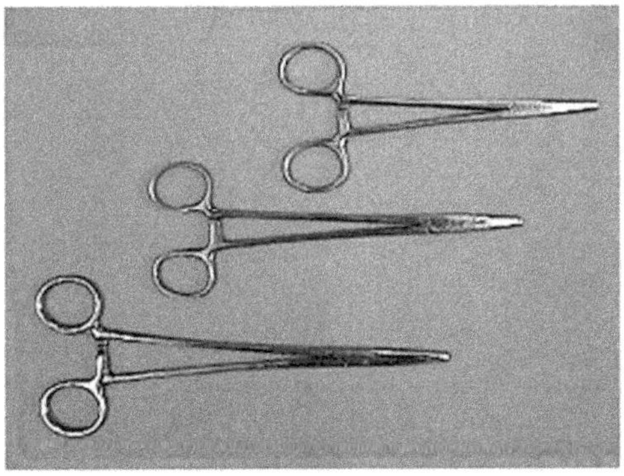

Figure 60. Needle holder with suture

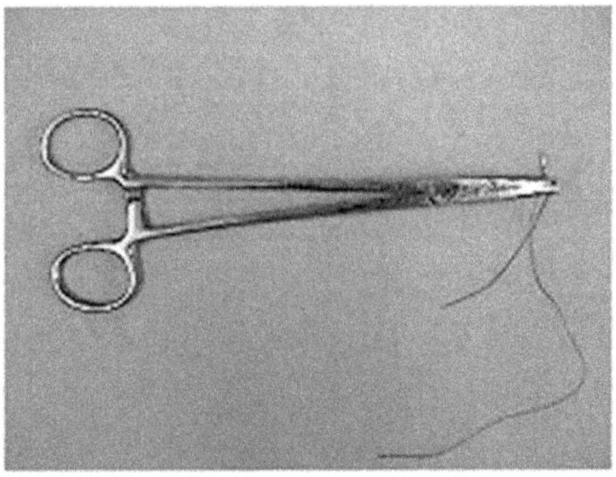

Modern Surgical Instruments

Apart from basic surgical instruments, some special instruments are required in cardiovascular surgery, neurosurgery and other purposes. Some of the modern instruments includes Bronchus Clamps, Bulldog Clamp, Dilators, Needles (Specially designed), Punches, Rongeurs, Special Scissors, Tissue forceps, Tourniquets, Tunnelers, Valvulotomes, Vein Passers, Vein strippers, Vessel clips & appliers and Wire Twisters for cardiaovascular surgey (Figure 61).

Neurosurgery, or neurological surgery, is the medical specialty concerned with the prevention, diagnosis, surgical treatment, and rehabilitation of disorders which affect any portion of the nervous system including the brain, spinal cord, peripheral nerves, and extra-cranial cerebrovascular system (Preul, 2005; Kroh, 2015).There are numerous types of neurological instruments are there for diagnosis, treatment and surgery. But the commonly used tools in neurosurgery are critically designed includes bipolar forceps, Dissectors and Rongeurs, various drill bits, wire and pin instruments, specially designed Elevators and Impactors, Retractors (Hand held and self-retaining), Spreaders etc (Figure 62 and Figure 63).

Figure 61. Cardiovascular instruments

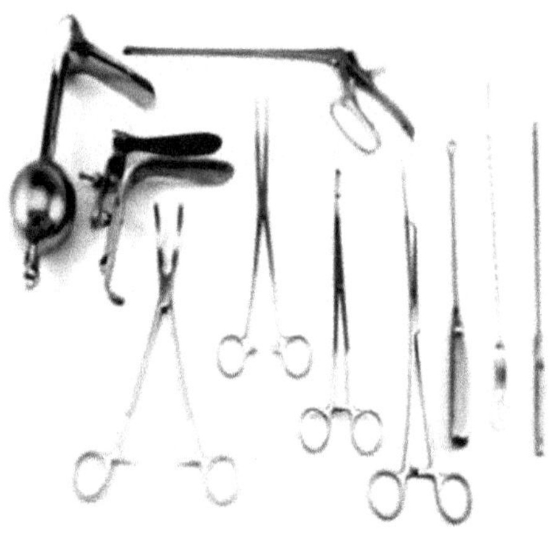

Figure 62. Instruments for neurosurgery

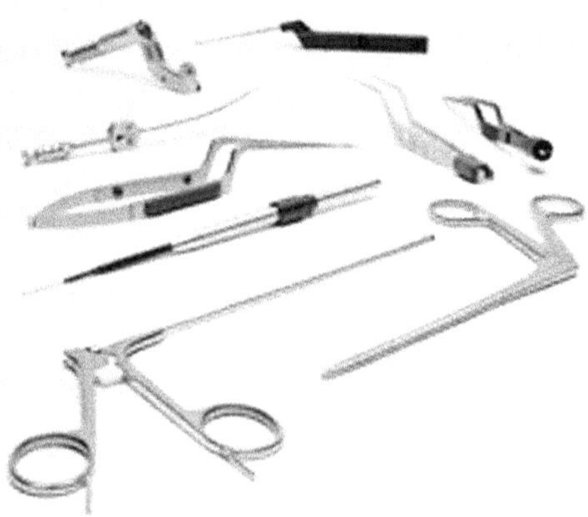

Figure 63. Neuroendoscopic instrument

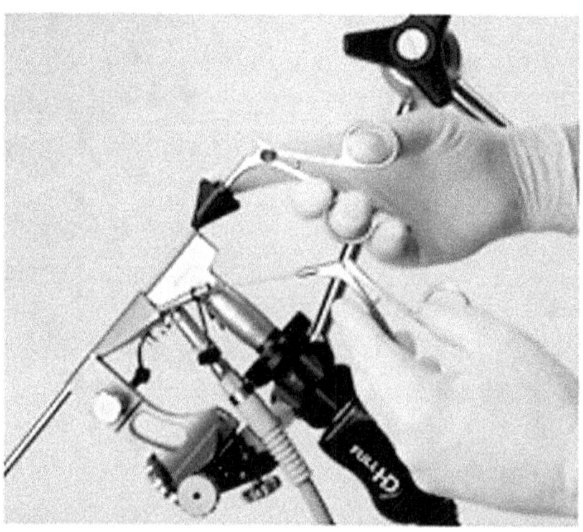

Instruments for Robotic Surgery

Robotic surgery is one of the most promising techniques in modern days for minimally invasive surgery (Gerthardus, 2003; Zangnolo, Garbi, Achilare, Minig, 2017). During the surgery the miniaturized instruments are mounted on three separate robotic arms, allowing the surgeon maximum range of motion and precision. The surgeon controls these instruments and the camera from a console located in the operating room. Placing his fingers into the master controls, he is able to operate all four arms of the robot that literally places him inside the patient, giving him a better, more detailed 3-D view of the operating site than the human eye can provide (Figure 64). Every movement he makes with the master controls is replicated precisely by the robot. When necessary, the surgeon can even change the scale of the robot's movements: If he selects a three-to-one scale, the tip of the robot's arm will move just one inch for every three inches the surgeon's hand moves. And because of the console's design, the surgeon's eyes and hands are always perfectly aligned with his view of the surgical site, minimizing surgeon fatigue.

The ultimate effect is to give the surgeon unprecedented control in a minimally invasive environment. Utilizing this advanced technology, our surgeons are able to perform a growing number of complex urological, gynecological, cardiothoracic and general surgical procedures (Finkelstein, Eckerserger, Sardi, Taneja, Lepor, Djavan, 2010). Since these procedures can now be performed through very small incisions, our patients experience a number of benefits compared to open surgery, including less trauma on the body, minimal scarring, and faster recovery time.

The patient-side cart has three robotic arms and an optional fourth arm. One arm holds the endoscope, while the other arms hold interchangeable surgical instruments.

CONCLUSION

A wide range of surgical instruments are available in the market. So, surgeons must know the applications and limitations of these instruments. Junior surgeons usually select instruments according to the advice

Figure 64. Surgical robotic arm

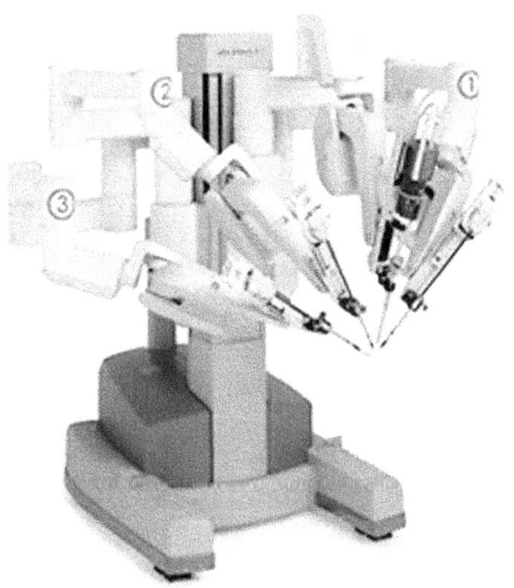

and habits of their surgical mentors. Personal experience modifies, and often limits, the selection of instruments eventually used by the advanced surgeon. Cutting instruments for surgery include scalpels, scissors, and instruments that use electrosurgery or other energy sources (eg, ultrasound, laser). For scalpels, the size of blade and handle chosen depend upon the task. The needle-holder's purpose is to firmly hold a curved surgical needle as it is passed through tissue, to easily release the needle, and then to easily regrasp the needle. Ideally, the needle-holder should be designed to grasp the needle firmly without flattening or bending it or damaging the suture material. Surgical forceps serve as an extension of the surgeon's thumb and index finger and enable grasping of small structures in limited spaces. The design of all forceps is very similar, with differences limited to length, width, and type of surface that grips the tissue. A variety of specialized clamps has been designed to accomplish the surgical purpose. All retractors have the same basic function of providing exposure of the surgical field. Knowledge and appropriate selection of retractors can simplify a procedure. Conversely, inadequate exposure can create difficulties in an otherwise easy operation. A number of new medical surgeries are growing up with new medical instruments in which medical robots are new addition as surgical instruments.

REFERENCES

Allen, G. S., & Coates, N. E. (1996). Pulmonary contusion: A collective review. *The American Surgeon*, *62*(11), 895–900. PMID:8895709

Allen, G. S., & Coates, N. E. (1996). Pulmonary contusion: A collective review. *The American Surgeon*, *62*(11), 895–900. PMID:8895709

Bharathan, R., Dexter, S., & Hanson, M. (2009). Laparoscopic retrieval of retained Redivac drain fragment. *Journal of Obstetrics & Gynaecology*, *29*(3), 263–264. doi:10.1080/01443610902754000 PMID:19358050

Bonfils-Roberts, E. (1972). The Rib Spreader: A Chapter in the History of Thoracic Surgery. Chest, 61(5), 469–474.

Bonfils-Roberts, E. (2008). The Rib Spreader: A Chapter in the History of Thoracic Surgery. *Chest*, *61*(5), 469–474. doi:10.1378/chest.61.5.469 PMID:4558402

Brundage, Jurkovich, Hoyt, Patel, Ross, Marburger, … Maier. (2001). Stapled versus Sutured Gastrointestinal Anastomoses in the Trauma Patient: A Multicenter Trial. *The Journal of Trauma Injury Infection and Critical Care*, *51*(6), 1054–1061.

Carter, P. (1993). Perforation of the bowel by suction drains. *British Journal of Surgery*, *80*, 129. PMID:8428277

Durai, R., Mownah, A., & Ng, P. C. (2009). Use of drains in surgery: A review. *Journal of Perioperative Practice*, *19*(6), 180–186. doi:10.1177/175045890901900603 PMID:19591322

Finkelstein, J., Eckersberger, E., Sadri, H., Taneja, S. S., Lepor, H., & Djavan, B. (2010). Open Versus Laparoscopic Versus Robot-Assisted Laparoscopic Prostatectomy: The European and US Experience. *Reviews in Urology*, *12*(1), 35–43. PMID:20428292

Gerhardus, D. (2003). Robot-assisted surgery: The future is here. *Journal of Healthcare Management, 48*(4), 242–251. doi:10.1097/00115514-200307000-00008 PMID:12908224

Haciibrahimoglu, G., Solak, O., Olcmen, A., Bedirhan, M. A., Solmazer, N., & Gurses, A. (2004, February). Management of Traumatic Diaphragmatic Rupture. *Surgery Today, 34*(2), 111–114. doi:10.100700595-003-2662-8 PMID:14745609

Hsu, H.-H., Chen, J.-S., Huang, P.-M., Lee, J.-M., & Lee, Y.-C. (2004, June). Comparison of manual and mechanical cervical esophagogastric anastomosis after esophageal resection for squamous cell carcinoma: A prospective randomized controlled trial. *European Journal of Cardio-Thoracic Surgery, 25*(6), 1097–1101. doi:10.1016/j.ejcts.2004.02.026 PMID:15145015

John, K. (2006). *The Evolution of Surgical Instruments – An Illustrated History from Ancient Times to the Twentieth Century*. Norman Publishing.

Kocher's Forceps. (2016). In *Merriam-Webster Medical Dictionary*. Retrieved from merriam-webster.com

Konstantinov, I. E. (2004). Circular vascular stapling in coronary surgery. *The Annals of Thoracic Surgery, 78*(1), 369–373. doi:10.1016/j.athoracsur.2003.11.050 PMID:15223474

Kroh, M. (2015). *Essentials of robotic surgery*. Cham: Springer. doi:10.1007/978-3-319-09564-6

Laparoscopic graspers. (n.d.). Retrieved from Laparoscopic.md

Manelli, Gastaldo, Rinaldo, Luigi, & Zonta. (1990). A new vascular stapler for pulmonary artery anastomosis in experimental single lung transplantation. *Proceedings of the 4th Annual Meeting of The Association for Cardio-Thoracic Surgery*.

Michelle, H. (2016). *Clinical Medical Assisting: A professional*. Field Smart Approach to the Workplace.

Nimitz, R. (2010). *Surgical Instrumentation: an Interactive Approach*. Saunders.

Ochsner, J. (1999). The surgical knife. *Bulletin of the American College of Surgeons, 84*(2), 27–37. PMID:10350986

Pollak, A. N. (Ed.). (2011). Airway Management. Emergency Care and Transportation of the Sick and Injured. Jones and Bartlett Publishers.

Preul, M, C. (2005). History of brain tumor surgery. *Neurosurgical Focus, 18*(4), 1. doi:10.3171/foc.2005.18.4.1 PMID:15844868

Rayatt, S. S., Dancey, A. L., & Jaffe, W. (2005). Soft fluted silicone drains: A prospective, randomized, patient-controlled study. *Plastic and Reconstructive Surgery, 115*(6), 1605–1608. doi:10.1097/01.PRS.0000160696.19137.37 PMID:15861064

Richterich, J. P., Heigl, A., Muff, B., Luchsinger, S., & Gutzwiller, J. P. (2008). Endo-SPONGE: A new endoscopic treatment option in colonoscopy. *Gastrointestinal Endoscopy, 68*(5), 1019–1022. doi:10.1016/j.gie.2008.02.038 PMID:18534581

Shiffrin, E., Schwierz, E., Wassiljew, S., & Caggianos, C. (2007). Evaluation of an aortic stapler for an open aortic anastomosis. *The Journal of Cardiovascular Surgery, 48*(5), 659–665. PMID:17989637

Shifrin, E. G., Moore, W. S., Bell, P. R. F., Kolvenbach, R., & Daniline, E. I. (2007). Intravascular Stapler for "Open Aortic Surgery: Preliminary Results". *European Journal of Vascular and Endovascular Surgery, 33*(4), 408–411. doi:10.1016/j.ejvs.2006.10.019 PMID:17137806

Teoh, M. K., & Bird, D. A. (1987). Removal of skin staples in an emergency. *Annals of the Royal College of Surgeons of England, 69*, 222–224. PMID:3314634

Tsuda, Y., Takemura, T., Shimamura, Y., & Iwasa, S. (2003). Usefulness of silicone Blake drains after cardiac surgery (in Japanese). *Kyobu Geka, 56*, 1017–1019. PMID:14608925

Valadka, A. B. (2004). Injury to the cranium. In E. J. Moore, D. V. Feliciano, & K. L. Mattox (Eds.), *Trauma* (pp. 385–406). New York: McGraw-Hill, Medical Pub. Division.

Wickens, A. , P. (2014). *A History of the Brain: From Stone Age surgery to modern neuroscience*. Psychology Press.

Zanagnolo, V., Garbi, A., Achilarre, M. T., & Minig, L. (2017). Robot-assisted surgery in Gynecologic cancers. *Journal of Minimally Invasive Gynecology, 24*(3), 379–396. doi:10.1016/j.jmig.2017.01.006 PMID:28104497

Zeebregts, C. J., Heijmen, R. H., van den Dungen, J. J., & van Schilfgaarde, R. (2003). Non-suture methods of vascular anastomosis. *British Journal of Surgery, 90*(3), 261–271. doi:10.1002/bjs.4063 PMID:12594661

Chapter 3
Devices for Rehabilitation

Jessee Moirangthem
North Eastern Hill University, India

Sateesh Reddy Avutu
North Eastern Hill University, India

Meena Gupta
North Eastern Hill University, India

Dinesh Bhatia
North Eastern Hill University, India

ABSTRACT

Rehabilitation is an area of focus by experts and researchers from different disciplines owing to the increase in number of various types of disabilities. This chapter covers information relating to causes and need for rehabilitation devices for differently abled people with motor, vision, or hearing impairment. The chapter begins with a brief on the disability population worldwide and in India, and progresses towards presenting available devices in global market and possible improvement that can be made to improve the functionality of the device and in turn improve the quality of life (QoL) of the users. Towards the end of the chapter, a reader can acquire the fundamental knowledge about the different types of disability, suitable aids, and working.

REHABILITATION ENGINEERING

Disability Data

Many people in the world live with some form of disability. It may either be a temporary or permanent impairment leading to difficulties in quality of living. According to the World Health Organization (WHO), the estimated figure of people with disability increased from 10% as reported from 1970s to 15% of the world's population as reviewed in 2011 factsheet of disability and health (Table 1). As estimated by World Health Survey and Global Burden of Disease that 110-190 million people globally suffer from serious form of disabilities with significant difficulties in functioning (Table 2). The growth in

DOI: 10.4018/978-1-5225-4969-7.ch003

Table 1. Percentage of disabled population to total population, India

Residence		Persons (In Millions)	Males (In Millions)	Females (In Millions)
Total	2011	2.21	2.41	2.01
	2001	2.13	2.37	1.87
Rural	2011	2.24	2.43	2.03
	2001	2.21	2.47	1.93
Urban	2011	2.17	2.34	1.98
	2001	1.93	2.12	1.71

Table 2. Percentage of disabled population by type of disability, India: 2011

Type of Disability	Persons (In Millions)	Males (In Millions)	Females (In Millions)
Sight	18.8	17.6	20.2
Hearing	18.9	17.9	20.2
Speech	7.5	7.5	7.4
Motor/Movement	20.3	22.5	17.5
Mental retardation	5.6	5.8	5.4
Mental illness	2.7	2.8	2.6
Any other	18.4	18.2	18.6
Multiple disorder	7.9	7.8	8.1
Total	**100**	**100**	**100**

the number of people with disabilities is due to varied reasons such as increase in the number of ageing population, chronic diseases, health conditions, environment and other factors.

According to the Census of India 2011, "Data on Disability", information on eight types of disability namely sight, hearing, speech, motor, mental retardation, mental illness, any other and multiple disability was collected (Table 3). The report showed that the percentages of disabled population were more in rural areas as compared to urban areas and more in males in comparison to females. Also, the percentages of disabled population in each division showed a significant increase in 2011 figures as compared to 2001 records (Table 1).

Rehabilitation Engineering and Its Goal

Any form of disability cannot be fully restored but measures and efforts can be put in to improve the conditions. Rehabilitation engineering and assistive device/technology are terms which are often used interchangeably. However, there is difference between the two. In 1982, James Reswick, a pioneer in the field of rehabilitation engineering defined it as "the application of science and technology to ameliorate the handicaps of individuals with disabilities" while, assistive technology is product of rehabilitation

Table 3. Definitional changes from 2001-11

Type of Disability	Definition
Sight	• In 2001, one eyed persons were treated as disabled. • In 2011, one eyed persons have not been treated as disabled in seeing. Enumerators were asked to apply a simple test to ascertain blurred vision.
Hearing	• In 2001, persons having problem in hearing through one ear although the other ear is functioning normally was considered having hearing disability. Persons using hearing aid have not been treated as disabled. • In 2011, persons using hearing aid have been treated as disabled while persons with hearing problem only on one ear were not considered as having hearing disability.
Speech	Definition was made clearer in Census 2011 to record persons with speech disability. For instance, "persons who speak in single words and are not able to speak in sentences" was specifically mentioned to be treated as disabled.
Motor/Movement	Specific mention of the following was made in the definition for Census 2011: 1. Paralytic persons 2. Those who crawl 3. Those who are able to walk with the help of aid 4. Have acute and permanent problems of joints/muscles 5. Have stiffness or tightness in movement or have loose, involuntary movements or tremors of the body or have fragile bones 6. Have difficulty balancing and coordinating body movement 7. Have loss of sensation in body due to paralysis, Leprosy etc. 8. Have deformity of body like hunch back or are dwarf.
Mental Retardation	• In 2001, Mental Retardation was covered under the category of mental disability. • In 2011, It was introduced as a new category.
Mental Illness	• In 2001, Mental Illness was covered under the category of mental disability. • In 2011, It was introduced as a new category.
Any other	New category introduced at Census 2011 to ensure complete coverage. This option enabled respondents to report those disabilities which are not listed in the question. In such cases, where informant was not sure about the type of disability this option of reporting disability as 'Any Other' was available to her/him.
Multiple Disability	New category introduced at Census 2011. The question has been designed to record as many as three types of disabilities from which the individual was reported to be suffering.

*Courtesy for Table 1, Table 2 and Table 3: "C-Series, Table C-20, Census of India 2011, Data on Disability", Office of the Registrar General and Census Commissioner, India. Website: http://censusindia.gov.in, accessed on 4th October 2016

engineering (Bronzino, 2014). For a better understanding, let us take an example of a person with one side of the leg amputee below the knee is using a prosthetic leg to aid him in locomotion. The process involved from designing to developing the prosthetic leg is known as rehabilitation engineering and the product obtained i.e., the prosthetic leg is known as an assistive device.

The area of rehabilitation is quite vast and extensive (John, 2006). It can range from correction in any deformity to replacing a whole part of the body with an aim to improve the quality of life of an individual from the current deprived condition. Major practices of rehabilitation and the assistive devices involved will be discussed in the following sections of this chapter.

When a person has some or the other forms of disability, one or more of the following functions are deprived:

1. A person may not be able to perform activities of daily living (ADL) independently and all such activities require support and assistance of another individual or caretaker. This may not only be embarrassing but at times bring about depression or disturb the mental balance of the patient.

2. Some form of disability may compensate a person with his ability to move around. They may require a minimal assistance of a walking stick or a walker for mobility or using a wheelchair in severe cases.
3. In some conditions, a person might be able to perform activities of daily living but are not functionally independent i.e., they may not be able to cook, clean, etc.
4. Disability may at times result in a person being less socially interactive or totally avoiding social participation. This may lead to social exclusion, stress and loneliness.
5. Goal setting is an important aspect in rehabilitation management, as it will help channel the plan and expedite the process of rehabilitation. In any rehabilitation process, a bi-directional goal is required for effective rehabilitation, one from the giver's end and the other from the receiver's end. With a SMART goal working in a two-way process, rehabilitation will be a sure success. Goals in rehabilitation engineering require plan and interventions to address as solutions for the above discussed functionalities.

MODERN DAY PROSTHETICS AND ORTHOTICS DEVICES

Definition of Prosthetic and Orthotic

Prosthetics and orthotics are two frequently used terms in rehabilitation. Prosthetic refers to "replacement" of a missing body part while orthotics refers to "correction" of some deformity, While prosthetics aims at replacing and restoring the functionality of a missing body part, orthotics aims at correcting, aligning and supporting, preventing deformities or to improve the function of a moving body part. "Prosthetic" or "prosthesis" and "orthotic" or "orthosis" are terms often use interchangeably. However, it is not to be confused. The "sis" is the noun form and "tic" is the adjective form of the words. Also, while prosthetic can be an external or internal artificial part, orthotic only refers to an artificial external device.

Prosthetic and orthotic have existed even before the advent of technology. Since then it has undergone transformation improving in aspects of function, strength, compatibility and aesthetic concerns. Prosthetic as stated earlier is replacement of an amputee or missing body part (Robitaille, 2010). If a person with an amputee limb is replaced with an artificial limb for the missing part then it is referred to as prosthetic. While, if a splint or brace is used to limit the movement of a sprained wrist, it is referred to as orthosis.

Need for Prosthesis and Orthosis

Limb deficient people not only faces problem in physical ability and appearance but also causes psychological damage and slowly diminishes their existence in the society. The society has a great influence on the existence of people with disability. People's attitude and reaction towards a disabled has its impact on the physical, psychological and social being of the individual. This makes survival either tough or lively.

Absence of a limb or part of a limb not only raises the concern of appearance but also the loss of function of that part. Until another part can replace the function of the lost part, need for restoring the lost function still lingers. The use of the word prosthesis often brings in mind replacement in the limbs. However, the application of prosthetic is not only limited to the limbs. Prosthesis represents an artificial part. Apart from prosthetic limbs, artificial parts of heart and breast implants are also a part of the prosthetic family. Detailed information regarding these will be discussed in section 2.3.

Orthosis refers to artificial device which is used to correct or support or prevent or assist deformities. While prosthesis can be used both external and internal, orthosis is external assist or can be referred to as assistive device like prosthesis, on the use of the word orthosis, limb orthosis often pops up. Apart from limb orthosis, trunk orthosis is another area of application of orthosis referring to areas of neck and spine section 2.4 discusses different types of orthosis.

The long lying goal of using prosthetic is to totally replicate the function of the missing body part. However, the human body is a unique system with unique design. It functions due to interconnection between different sub-systems. Replicating such a system completely is a difficult task. However, due to advances in technology, it is slowly overcoming this barrier. Only concerns for function do not wrap the envelope of prosthetics. Design, comfort and cosmetic concerns also arise. It is important to consider these aspects as it is the wearer who should be benefited by the prosthesis. While the design and comfort will keep in check the function and physical benefit, the aesthetic value will re-instill the social existence of the user (Whitelock, 2006). Also, the use of prosthesis should not result in other physical side-effects. Orthotic on the other hand is the field which explores different techniques to correct or prevent deformities. This will not only result in a better alignment of body parts but also improve the functions lost due to the deformities.

Prosthesis

Before the advent of technology, prosthetics were developed only to replace the missing part. However, with the advent and advancement of technology the goal of prosthetic now is not only to replace the missing part but also to replicate the function of that part. Even if medical science has explained the mechanics involved with the movement of each body part, replicating the exact function is a big challenge as the human system is a complicated complex system. Advances in prosthetics are discussed in the proceeding topics.

Limb Prosthesis

Regaining the ability to walk or perform activities is the prime goal in any prosthesis for rehabilitation. From being a passive device, prosthetic technology has advanced in using active elements such as the bio-signals for developing motorized prosthesis. The major consideration in developing prosthesis is to make use of the residual limb for the function and attachment of the prosthesis. Frequent use of prosthesis helps in delivering rehabilitation to amputees. However, due to the poor cosmetic appearance and lack of functionalities in the traditionally developed prosthesis, amputees hardly use it. In recent years, use of prosthesis by amputee is gaining popularity due to advancement in technology which delivers multiple functions and also, improved cosmetic appearance has made amputee to frequently use it making their everyday life better.

All signals for initiating and controlling movement processing occurs in the brain and follows the motor pathway (through sensory and motor neuronal pathway). These signals are made use in for initiating and controlling movement in advanced prosthesis. Signals are stronger underneath the skin and skull which can be obtained by implanting electrodes (Reinkensmeyer, 2016). However, these are invasive procedures and also may include the risk of material rejection of the implanted electrode. A safer method is by using intracranial electroencephalography (iEEG) which involves placing the electrodes on the surface of the brain to record electrical activity. This in turn initiates the functioning of the prosthesis. Another widely used non-invasive method is the use of EMG signals. EMG is signals obtained from the muscle. One such application of EMG as a driving force for prosthesis is the myoelectric arm. In this, EMG signal from voluntarily contracted muscles within a person's residual limb is used to control movements of the prosthesis. Movement supported by myoelectric arm includes elbow flexion/extension, wrist pronation/supination and opening/closing of fingers. Some of the developed myoelectric arm:

- **Michelangelo Hand:** It features a thumb that electronically moves into position and can perform multiple grip functions.
- **Bebionic 3:** It is a multi-articulating myoelectric hand and features 14 grip patterns. It has optimized weight distribution which makes the hand feel lighter in weight and is available in 9 different skin shades.
- **i-Limb:** The i-limb features five (5) individually powered digits and fully articulated joints. It features key grips with precision and can be used for activities which needs power.
- **Boston Arm:** It is Psychic robot limb moved just by thinking. Movement of hand will be created using motor fixed in the elbow position. The sensory electrodes are fixed at the wearer's arm. The motor will respond according to the tiny electrical charge signal captured by electrodes.

Another method approached for prosthesis is targeted muscle reinnervation (TMR). In cases following amputation, the peripheral nerves are still active in carrying signals between the brain and the peripheral nerves for motor control. TMR makes use of these peripheral nerves in order to redirect these signals to other muscles to control prosthesis. Through surgical procedures, the nerves in the residual arm are attached to some other healthy muscle in the body such as the chest muscle. When the patient tries to move, the redirected signal causes contraction of the chest muscle. Electrodes in the chest muscle sense the electrical activity and transfer the signal to the prosthesis and control it. The TMR provides control of prosthesis using signal which is originally used to control the hand unlike traditional myo electrically controlled prosthesis which uses another group of muscle not intended for the activity to control the prosthesis. Till date, this method has been used for amputees with shoulder disarticulation but, it is being tested for possibilities in applications in other amputation levels.

Figure 1. Michelangelo hand

Source: http://www.ottobockus.com/prosthetics/upper-limb-prosthetics/solutionoverview/michelangelo-prosthetic-hand/ on 11th June 2017.

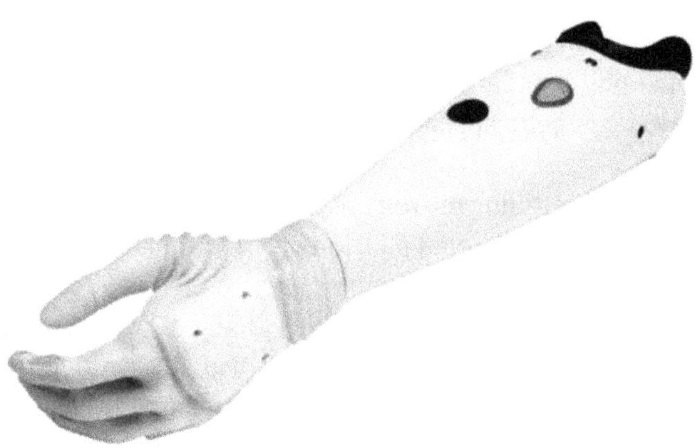

Figure 2. Bebionic 3
Source: http://bebionic.com on 11th June 2017.

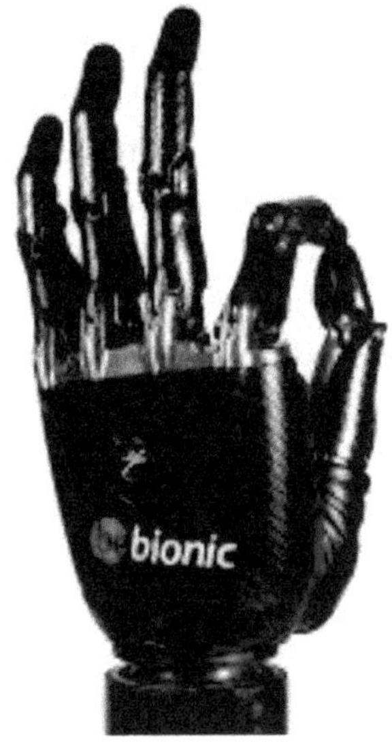

Figure 3. i-limb
Source: http://www.touchbionics.com on 11th June 2017.

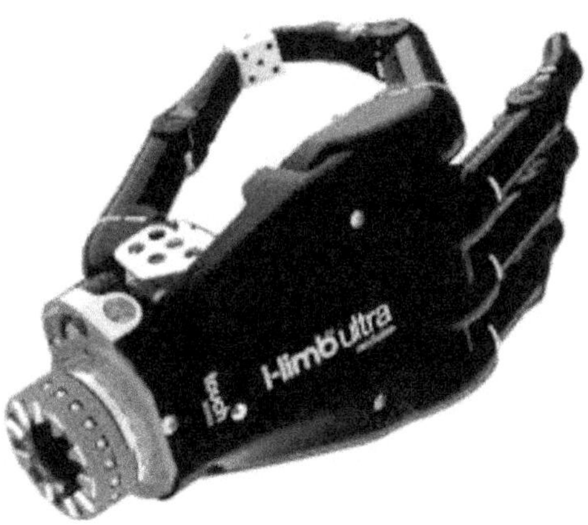

Figure 4. Boston arm
Source: http://www.liberatingtech.com/products/elbows/LTI_Boston_Digital_Arm_Systems_for_Adults.asp on 11th June 2017.

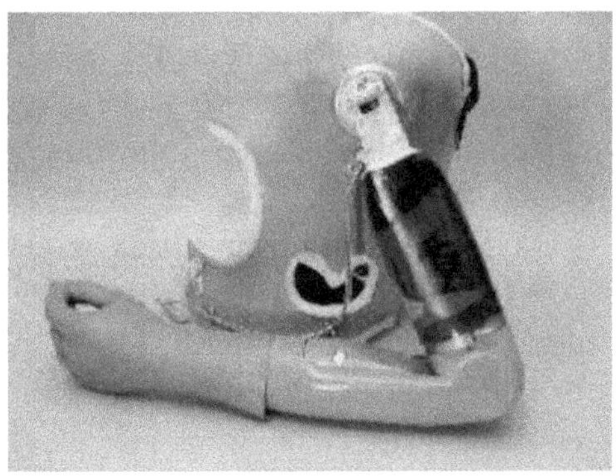

Orthosis

Orthosis is a corrective measure which in turn increases the efficacy and protecting the body in long run by:

- **Resisting Motion:** For cases in which a joint or a part of the body has sustained injury and owing to which forced or use of that part can lead to greater injury, orthosis is advised to those patients. This not only resists the motion of that part but due to the restricted motion aids in the process of healing.

- **Assisting Motion:** When the movement is hindered due to deformity, orthosis provides support and assists in performing action. For example, a patient with limb length deformity will possess a different gait pattern. To correct this, he may be given a foot orthosis wherein the sole of one side of the footwear is thicker than the other side to equalise the difference in length.
- **Transferring the Force:** Force plays an important role in biomechanics and motion. Rightful origin of force is required for performing an action such as running water searching for a route to continue its flow, in case of deformities, the force also searches for alternative pathways to generate the force in order to perform the action. Such prolong practice will lead to damage in other parts of the body. Use of orthosis enables transferring the force to a valid point of origin or for work to prevent any induced damage added to the existing deformity.
- **Proper Leverage:** There are many activities which we carry out in daily life which requires following the rules of the lever system. This gives efficient mechanical advantage and lesser force required to carry out the work. Lifting of weights, balancing, walking, carrying loads on back, etc. are some of the activities which require proper leverage. For patients with deformities following proper rules of the lever system is difficult. Use of orthosis as assist enables them in performing actions with proper leverage preventing adverse injuries.

Limb Orthosis

The limb or appendages are important parts of the body as they are the key to performing activities of daily living (ADL) and locomotion. While the lower limb is the weight bearing portion, the upper limb is responsible for carrying out activities. Simple form of orthosis used by people from all walks of life is braces, splints and straps (elastic). These orthosis are used in injuries such as sprain and aids in resisting, restricting motion and enhancing the process of healing.

The lower limb being the weight bearing portion is prone to injuries. Also, deformities in lower limb make locomotion difficult. The following are the different forms of lower limb orthosis that exists:-

- **FO (Foot Orthosis):** Heel pads, metatarsal pads, insoles, soles, footwear
- **AFO (Ankle-Foot Orthosis):** AFO devices are used to solve the major complicated issues associated with the foot slap during load response and toe-drag during swing. AFO can be designed with or without articulated joint with various motion control elements like springs, dampers, series elastic actuator and four-bar mechanism.
- **KAFO (Knee-Ankle-Foot Orthosis):** AFO plus knee control (locked or hinged). Locked KAFOs and KAFO with a posterior off-set knee joint are the different types available in the market.
- **HKAFO (Hip-Knee-Ankle-Foot Orthosis):** Extension of KAFO by adding a pelvic band.

Trunk Orthosis

The human body excluding the appendages is referred to as the trunk. When talks about orthosis are done, trunk orthosis is often neglected while concentrating on limb orthosis. The trunk holds all vital organs and this is necessary for functioning of the human system in the format it is designed for. Trunk orthosis comprises of orthosis application to the skull, neck and spinal portion, cervical, lumbosacral, thora columbo sacralare are the regions for which orthosis is prescribed. These regions are vital for

Figure 5. Foot orthosis
Source: http://www.medicalexpo.com/prod/orthomerica/product-80482-639596.htmlon 11th June 2017.

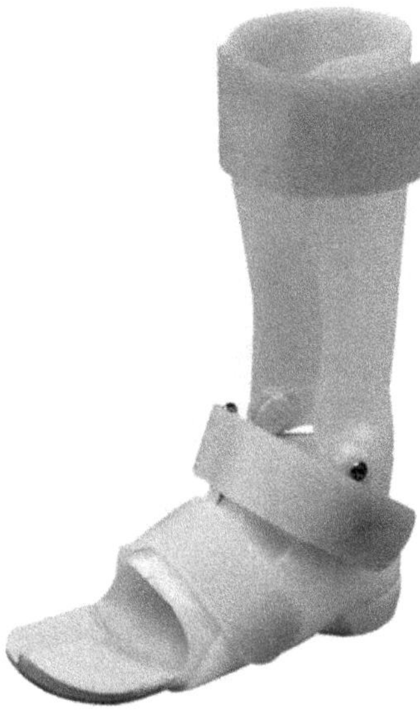

Figure 6. Types of knee-ankle-foot orthosis
Source: http://www.artificiallimbcenter.com/knee-ankle-foot-orthosis.htmlon 11th June 2017.

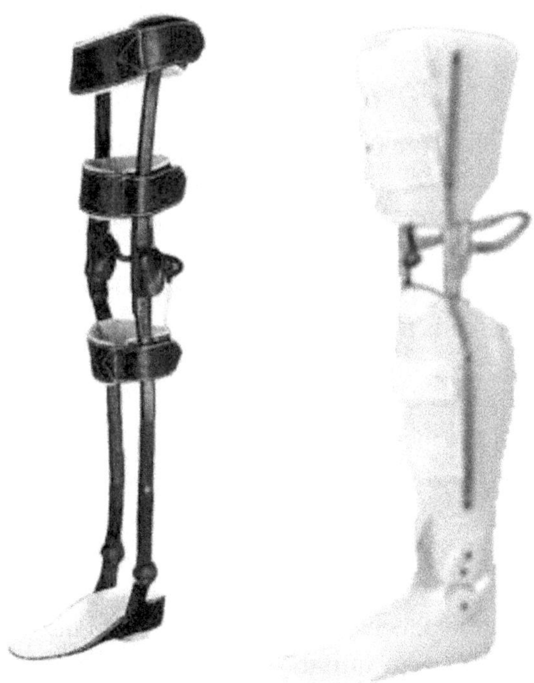

Figure 7. Hip-knee-ankle-foot orthosis
Source: http://www.artificiallimbcenter.com/knee-ankle-foot-orthosis.htmlon 11th June 2017.

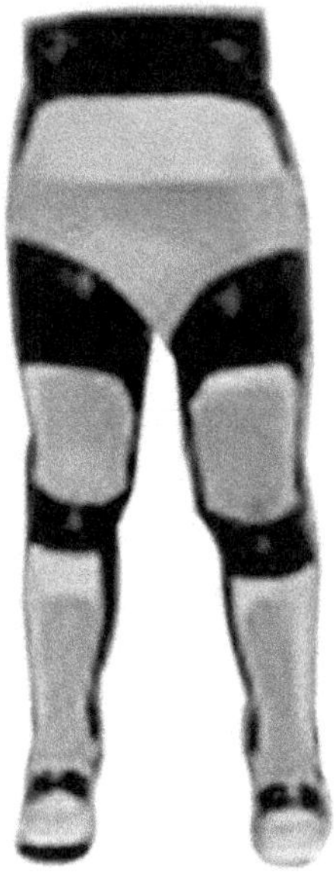

posture and weight distribution on the lower limbs. Compared to orthosis advised for patients in other regions, orthosis in these regions are more rigid to restrict movement and maintain posture.

Exoskeleton

Skeleton is the support system of the human body. "Exo" means external and skeleton is the internal framework. Exoskeleton is an external framework which is often a robotic mechanical suit worn by human being. It is a type of advanced orthosis used in conditions where a patient cannot use his upper or lower extremities or both (Ali, 2014).It can be considered as a type of mobile machine which moves as the wearer moves. It provides additional strength and support to the wearer. Apart from its role as orthosis, a whole body exoskeleton is used in by people with dangerous or tiring jobs. Some examples exoskeletons are:

- **Rex:** It is self balancing, hands-free robotic device for rehabilitation. It will provide the power to move Rex and a user of up to 100Kg. The main benefit for patient is, he/she can get full range of movement in legs.
- **HAL 5:** Designed to help the disabled and elderly. It is used to support movement and to lift weights.
- **Ekso Suit:** Used by paralyzed patients for standing, walking and climbing stairs. I consist of pair of powered robotics legs. The users turn themselves into Ekso suit placing their feet on the foot-plates and securing straps around their legs, hips, and torso. The Ekso Suit transfers their weight to the ground, and they uses two arm braces to keep themselves from falling over.

Figure 8. 01. Linear actuators 02. Carbon fibre pelvis 03. Onboard microprocessors 04. Length adjustment 05. Holding straps 06. Wide foot plates 07. Rechargeable batteries 08. Carbon fibre cuffs.
Source: http://www.rexbionics.com/product-information/ on 11th June 2017.

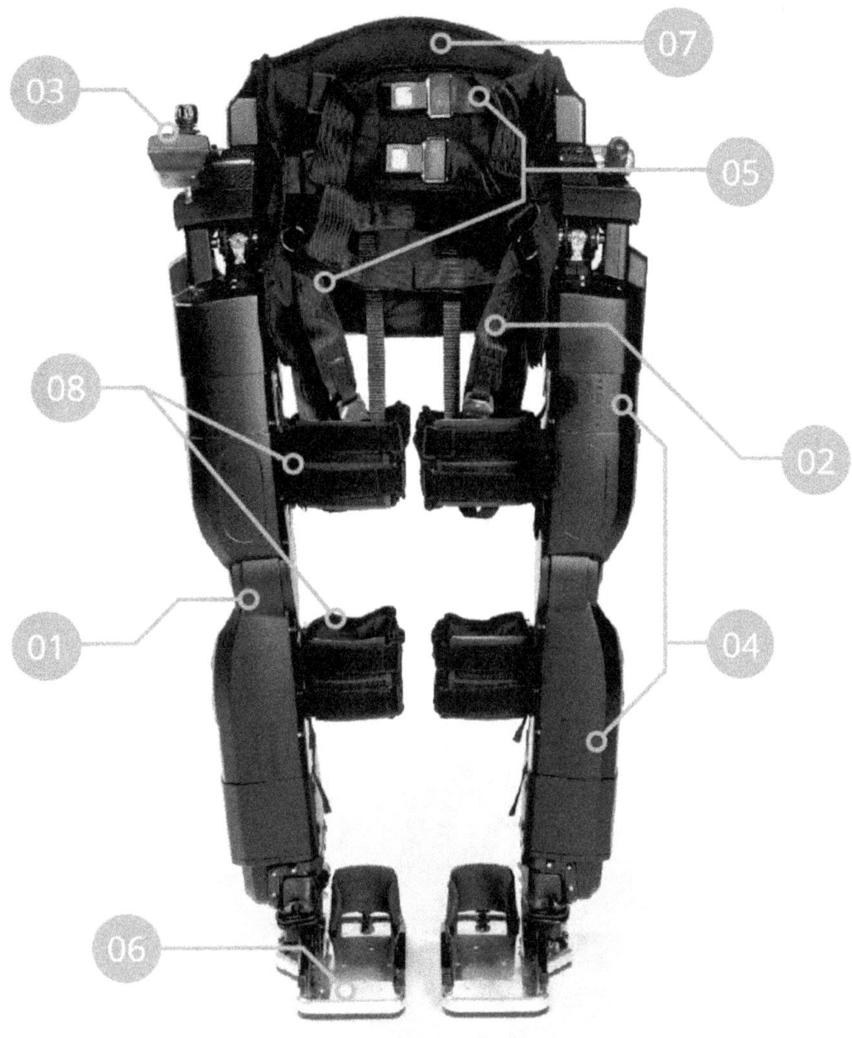

- **Berkeley Lower Extremity Exoskeleton (BLEEX):** Lower extremity exoskeletons seek to supplement the intelligence and sensory systems of a human with significant strength and endurance of a pair of wearable robotic legs that supports a payload.

Components and Working of Exoskeleton

The basic components of an exoskeleton are: (i) the skeleton (made of light weight metals like aluminium, nickel, titanium and hard plastics); (ii) micro computers (for controlling movement of various motors for joint movement and signal relays; (iii) power supply (powered by an internal combustion engine,

Figure 9. Hal 5
Source: http://cdn.walk-again.com/wp-content/uploads/hal_overview_700.jpg on 11th June 2017.

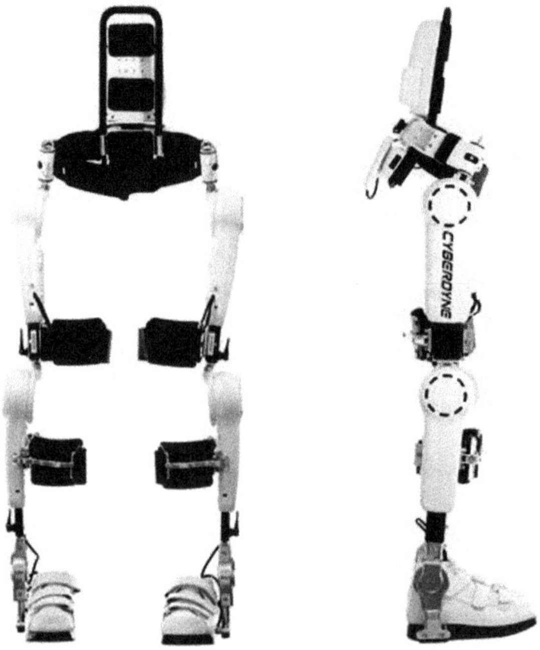

Figure 10. Ekso suit
Source: http://josefmicanekdesign.com/ekso-suit-helps-the-paralyzed-walk-again/ on 11th June 2017.

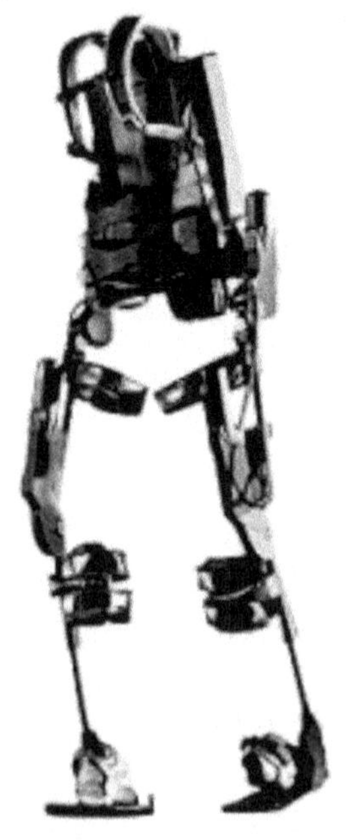

Figure 11. BLEEX
Source: http://bleex.me.berkeley.edu/research/exoskeleton/bleex/ on 11th June 2017.

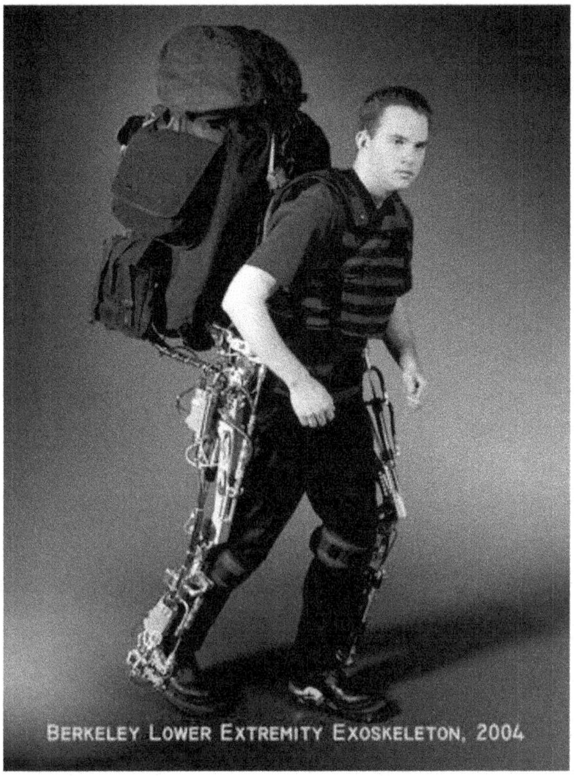

batteries or potentially fuel cells); (iv) multi-speed motors (for adjusting and performing as required); (v) control pad (enables the user to select various modes of movement); (vi) sensors (for sensing and recognizing movements such as grasping, holding, lifting etc. with precision)

Exoskeleton functions like the musculoskeletal system involving the signals of brain for movement. When a person attempts to move, the signal from the muscles are picked up from the skin or beneath (implanted) by the bioelectric sensors. These signals are used to control and activate the motor suit for the movement of the exoskeleton along with the muscle movement of the wearer aiding the wearer to move and perform activities. This is called 'voluntary control system' that provides movement interpreting the wearer's intention from the bio signals in advance of the actual movement.

Applications of Exoskeleton

The use of exoskeleton is not only limited for use in conditions of mobility issues. Exoskeleton is used in fields of:

- **Medical:** Assist the disabled and elderly to move from one place to another and in their daily tasks. It can also be used to help paralytic patients to stand, walk and even climb stairs and to amplify muscle strength for people with muscular dystrophy and other neuromuscular disabilities.

- **Military:** It has potential use in the military as an aid to increase endurance, speed, and strength, particularly that of wounded soldiers that would otherwise be helpless. It can be used to protect soldiers from enemy fire by repelling bullets. This increases the efficiency of soldiers. It can be used for mission in places where vehicles can't access.
- **Rescue:** It can be used in any physically demanding job such as disaster rescue or construction, rescue operations in hazardous or hard-to-access environments.
- **Entertainment:** It is used in activities which demands extreme and dangerous performance while ensuring the safety of the performer such as performing superhuman stunts without risking the person's life and is used as a preventive measure in extreme sports.

Jaipur Foot

In 1968, Jaipur foot was first developed and carried forward by Bhagwan Mahaveer Viklang Sahayata Samiti, India for societal betterment in 1975. Jaipur Foot is a renowned one for its facilitation in changing lives of many physically challenged people worldwide. The development of the Jaipur Foot proved to be a remarkable triumph in the history of prosthetic foot (Coupland RM, 1991). It is an artificial limb which replaces the missing extremity. According to one research by Dr. Goutam Reddy from Massachusetts Institute of Technology it is low cost, durable, water proof and can be used without shoes. Jaipur Foot, named after the place where it was designed, is flexible along multiple axes, which allows natural movement of the foot. The Jaipur Foot technology is based on traditional craft using small local production methods. It has already helped over 900,000 amputees in developing and landmine-affected countries (Sethi PK 1972). The limb is so efficient that a person can walk like a normal person and sit in a crossed leg position. It helps them to go back to their jobs and earn for their families. In a world where prosthetics is a complicated and expensive industry, there is an operation of impressive scope that offers hope to the some of the most impoverished citizens of India and maybe even the world. It offers these handicapped citizens a chance to return to their livelihoods and pursue their dreams.

Figure 12. Jaipur foot
Sources: http://hdimagegallery.net/jaipur+foot+history 1st August 2017.

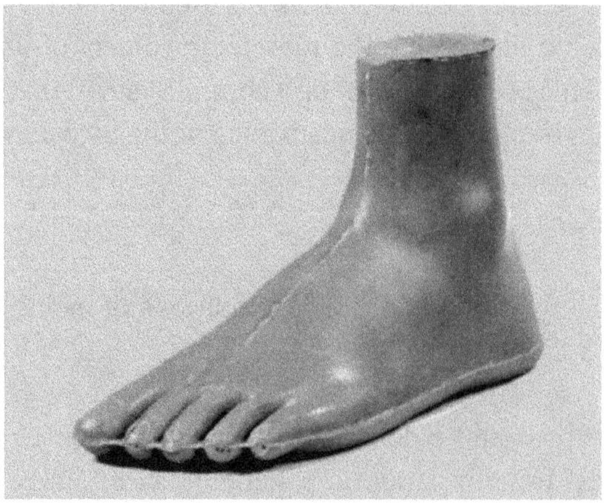

Working Method of Jaipur Foot

The Jaipur foot was designed according to the socio-culture needs of handicapped people of India keeping in view cost factor, ease of use and product quality. Due to its unique property it permits squatting, sitting in crossed leg position, walking on uneven surface, even in wet muddy field. It has proved to be a 'universal design' and can interface with prosthetic technology used around the globe. It is distinguished from other prosthesis because it have central keel which permits mobility in all planes despite having non articulation.

Devices for Mobility

Overview of Robotic Aids for Mobility

Over the past few decades, technology has advanced immensely serving as a boon to rehabilitation and assistive technology. Not only has it helped in developing devices with sophisticated functionalities, but also enhancing its aesthetic value. This gives the user of assistive devices a positive mental attitude towards the use of the device thus aiding in the rehabilitation process.

Apart from the basic need of food, cloth and shelter, the other needs of an individual are independence in carrying out his/her own activities and independence in movement. However, owing to unfortunate events, this independence may be compensated partially or totally. Engineering science and technology proves as a boon in such conditions. It has helped traditional techniques in rehabilitation become automatic and closely tailor-made as possible to suit a wide scale of patient conditions.

Basic everyday activities or often referred to as activities of daily living (ADL) include eating, cleaning, dressing, brushing, reading, etc. Performing such activities requires free movement of the body and its parts. In case of patient suffering from motor disabilities, such movements are often largely compensated. Often rehabilitation practices through occupational therapy and physical therapy serves as a helping hand in training for performing such activities. Additionally, assistive aids such as grabbers, feeders, wheelchair, etc., provide assistance in helping perform activities better.

From activities such as brushing to moving about in vicinity or beyond that, technology has come up with solutions to help people with motor disability to help them perform activities. Feeders and grabbers for people with compensated freedom of movement in the upper limb are available. This makes them hold things and transfer food without spilling or dropping all over and boosting their confidence to perform activities.

The generations of wheelchair has also advanced from manual wheelchairs to powered wheelchairs. Sophisticated features such as voice-controlled, EOG-controlled, EEG-controlled, joystick controlled wheelchairs are also available in market and research (Bourke, 2001). The design and materials used have also transformed to give best comfort and suit patient conditions. Motorized tricycle, scooters, modified licensed vehicles, walkers with brakes and many such innovative introductions are made for a better social involvement of person with challenges in mobility.

Manual and Attendant Propelled Wheelchair

Chair with wheels was invented in the 5th century. Since then, ithas undergone continuous modifications in design and technology associated with it. A basic manual wheelchair incorporates a seat, foot rests, four wheels (2 caster wheels at the front, 2 large wheels at the back).The two large wheels usually have hand rims (metal or plastic) to aid in propulsion by the patient. Push handles at the top of the back for manual propulsion by second person assisting the device user. A wheelchair acts as an assist to people for whom walking is difficult or impossible due to illness, injury or disability.

Traditional wheelchairs are manually propelled or attendant propelled. It requires physical effort for propulsion in both the cases. In case of manually propelled wheelchairs, the two hind wheels are made large enough to allow the user for proper biceps elevation and alignment for propulsion. This alignment is necessary to avoid any upper extremity problems, possibility of stroke and loading in the hand. In any wheelchair, the back-hip alignment, knee-foot alignment is always maintained at 90° to maintain a proper posture in order to avoid additional problems. Cushions are fitted at seat to prevent pressure sores from long sitting hours and also at back for rest. In an attendant propelled wheelchair, included for safety. Push handle bracket are fitted at the top of the back of the wheelchair. This allows easy propulsion of the wheelchair.

There are different types of wheelchairs based on the utility, duration and patient conditions. For example, wheelchairs used in hospitals, brief outings, airports etc., are not quite comfortable but serves the purpose as it is used for a short duration of time. However, wheelchairs used at home or work (in few cases) are quite different from the above mentioned as they are ergonomically designed for longer use time and also to suit the comfort and work environment and conditions. All wheelchairs can be customized for user's need such as seat dimensions, height, seat angle, footrests, leg rests, front caster, and backrests etc. Wheelchair designs are based on factors such as intended use, abilities of the user, resources available, existing products, durability, function, aesthetics and comfort.

Special Purpose Wheelchair

Moving forward from traditional wheelchairs, there are other types of wheelchair which are designed for special purposes (Gomi, 1998). There are wheelchairs for different types of sports, recreational activities, racing wheelchairs, wheelchairs for staircase ascend or descend with the introduction of Paralympics

Figure 13. Types of wheelchair
Source: http://www.wheelchairsmanufacturers.com/ on 11th June 2017.

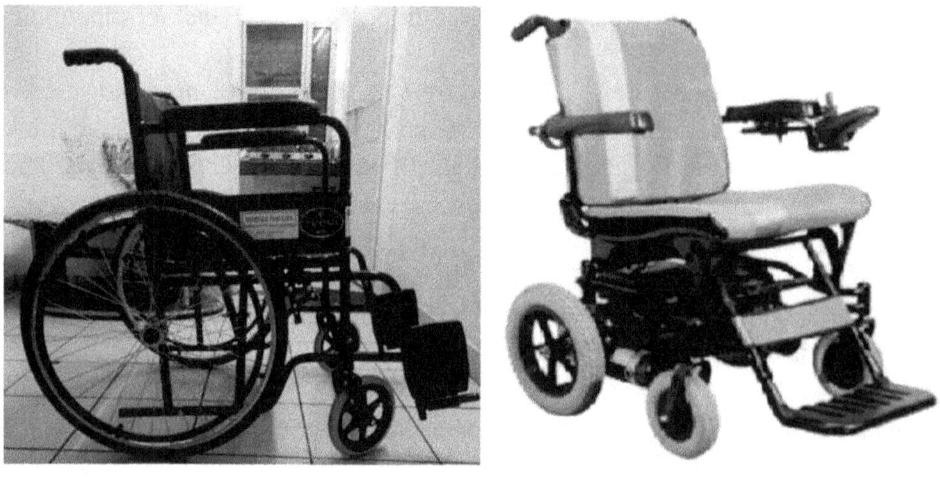

and growing interests in sport activities by people with motor disabilities, wheelchairs have undergone a drastic evolution to serve the purpose. However, such wheelchairs are for recreational use and not for use in daily life and long run.

Not all environments are made friendly for people on four wheels. There are steps and irregular terrain everywhere and also presence of slides is less common compared to flights. Therefore, there are wheelchairs modified for use for staircase to ascend and descend. However, these wheelchairs are costly and not commercially available but mostly on a trial stage.

There are other types of wheelchairs for staircase ascend and descend (Chaichanasiri, 2011). However, these are not specially designed for the purpose. Instead spokes are attached as appendage on the hind portion of the wheelchair between the hind wheels.

Automated and Powered Wheelchair

Manually and attendant propelled wheelchair which requires physical effort are tiresome for long duration use. Also, it may sometimes lead to other physical and functional problems both for the attendant and the user. To remove these difficulties, implementation of technologies for developing automated and powered wheelchair is available and research for improvements are taking place. This has transformed wheelchair into a "will-chair".

In automated and powered wheelchair, there is no manual physical effort involved. The rotation of the wheels which in turn is responsible for the movement of the wheelchair is done with the help of motors. The motor is the source for movement of the wheelchair. Power source for the functioning of the motor is provided using battery. The motor and power source assembly is such that it produces enough power to carry the load of the wheelchair and the user sitting on it and move carrying the total load. The direction and velocity for movement is controlled by an interface between the user and the wheelchair. Another important component of an automated wheelchair is the controller.

The basic components of an automated and powered wheelchair are as follows:

- **Input Device:** A joystick is the most standard way of controlling a powered wheelchair. It is mounted on either side of the wheelchair. Some alternative ways to control a motorized wheelchair are: (i) mini joystick: These are smaller than the normal joystick used in the wheelchairs and require less force to operate, a pressure as low as 18g; (ii) touchpad: It is similar to what you find in computer for controlling its cursor. The touchpad is based on touch but not pressure. Touchpad can be configured for the user such that touching a specific spot with respect to the centre will move in a configured direction or just dragging the finger on touchpad in the desired direction; (iii) sip and puff controls: These are controlled by sucking and blowing to a mouthpiece. The sip and puff can be programmed such that it will have mode to operate other controls. It requires some practice for the user to get good at driving the wheelchair. The system can also determine the strength of sip and puff besides just distinguishing them.
- **Controller:** The controller acts as the intermediate between the user and input device i.e. joystick or other forms of input device discussed above. It includes the electronics and software that is required to modify the signal from the input device, which is then converted to output and passed to the wheelchair for control. In other words the function of a controller is to translate various commands from the input and monitor performance and provide feedback to the user.

- **Power Controller:** Its function is control the electrical power delivered to the motors which controls the wheelchair speed.
- **Motor:** The basic function is to generate driving torque and to provide steering control for the wheelchair. The wheelchairs commonly make use of permanent magnet direct current motors with brushes. Most permanent magnet motors have conversion efficiency in the range of 60-80%.
- **Drive Trains:** They provide transmission of motor's torque for driving the wheel and to provide required speed versus torque reduction. The drive trains can convert high motor speed to low speed with increase in the torque. It's done with efficiency of 50-70%.
- **Battery:** The powered wheelchairs basically use rechargeable deep-cycle batteries rated 12-80 amperes-per-hour. The batteries can be wet-cell or dry-cell batteries. Majority of the manufactures use gel-cell based batteries over wet-cell due to its low maintenance and other environmental concerns.

Advantages of Wheelchair

Wheelchairs have given mobility life to people with motor disability. This has provided them with a feel for independence to a certain extent. Use of wheelchair gives them better performance in daily life. Movement in rough terrain happens at ease. Wheelchair provides benefit in most of the aspects of its utility except that it is costly.

Devices for Visually Impaired

Visual System

Visual system is the part of higher function of brain that is central nervous system (CNS). It gives ability to the organism to process the visual details. Visual system also detects and interprets information from visual light to build a representation of the surrounding environment. Visual system comprises (Hersh, 2008) of many parts such as eyes specially retina, optic nerve, optic chiasma, optic tract, genticulate body and visual cortex.

Function of Visual System

During the mechanism of work cornea and lens refract light into a small image and shine it on the retina. The retina transfers this image into rod and cone cell of the eyes. Optic nerve which is the part of cranial nerve carries these electric pluses through optic canal and reached to the optic chisma (Toh, 2008). The structure of eyes involve many parts such as eyes specially retina, optic nerve, optic chiasma, optic tract, genticulate body and visual cortex.

- **Eye:** It provide organisms vision, it have ability to process visual field as well as enabling many photo response function as that are dependent of vision. The main function of eye is to detect light. In eyes retina consists of a large number of photo receptor cells which contains particular protein molecules called opsins. In humans, two types of opsins are involved in conscious vision: rod opsins and cone opsins. It transmits a signal to the cell through a signal transduction pathway, resulting in hyper-polarization of the photoreceptor.

- **Optic Nerve:** It is a part of cranial nerve, it paired nerve that transmits visual information from the retina to the brain. It is derived from optic stalks during developmental period of life and composed of retinal ganglion cell axons and glial cell. In human body optic nerve extends from the optic disc to the optic chisma and continues as optic track (Vilensky, 2015, Selhorst, 2009). Optic nerve is the part of cranial nervous system because it derived from an out pouching of the diencephalon (Optic stalks) during embryonic development.
- **Optic Chiasma:** The optic nerve of both the eyes where meets and cross each other that point is called optic chisma (Turner, 2010). It situated at the base of hypothalamus of the brain.. At this point the information coming from both eyes is combined and then splits according to the visual field. The corresponding halves of the field of view (right and left) are sent to the left and right halves of the brain, respectively, to be processed(Nolte, 2002)
- **Optic Tract:** Optic tractis a part of the visual system in the brain. It is a continuation of the optic nerve that relays information from the optic chiasm to the ipsilateral lateral geniculate nucleus (LGN), pretectal nuclei, and superior colliculus (Britannica, 2011).
- **Visual Cortex:** It passes the visual information through the visual hierarchy, the complexity of the neural representation increases. It receives the impulses sent to it from the eye that contain what the image.

Types of Visual Impairment

Visual impairment is defined as decreased ability to see to a degree that causes problems not fixable by usual means, such as glasses. Some also include those who have a decreased ability to see because they do not have access to glasses or contact lenses. Visual impairment is often defined as a best corrected visual acuity of worse than either 20/40 or 20/60. According to world health organization the visual impairment (Sinha, 2015) or visual acuity can be defined as in many forms such as given below (Maberley, 2006).

- **Low Visual Acuity:** Vision between 20/70 and 20/400 with the best possible correction in visual field of 20 degree or less than 20 degree.
- **Mild Blindness:** Visual acuity worse than 20/400 with the best possible correction, or visual field of 20 degree or less.
- **Blindness:** Visual acuity of 20/200 or worse with best possible correction in visual field 20 degrees or less.

Causes of Visual Impairment

Types of impairment are different for different causes of visual impairment.

- **Visual Impairment in Glaucoma:** In glaucoma normal fluid pressure increases as compared to normal pressure inside the eye. In glaucoma peripheries seem to be normal.
- **Age Related Macular Degeneration (AMD):** In this type of visual impairment central area of the eye becomes woolly or cottony opacity obsures the central part of the vision. The peripheries may be normally seen. In usually blurs the sharp, central vision that is needed for closely viewed activities like reading sewing and driving. Patients have no pain in the visual impairment.

- **Cataract:** There is general clouding of the vision. In this condition whole eye lens is affected the blurring or vision may be diffuse until it is totally lost.
- **Diabetic Retinopathy:** Diabetes leads to damage of the smaller arties and blood vessels at the back of the eyes over the retina. Diabetic retinopathy is the most common diabetic eye disease and a leading cause of blindness in adults. Usually vision impairment in diabetics begins as black spots or floating shapes that appear in the field of vision. Slowly compete vision may be lost if left unchecked.
- **Near Sightedness:** Myopia or near sightedness or short sightedness means a person can see nearby objects clearly but distant objects appears blurred. High myopia may lead to vision impairment.
- **Retinitis Pigmentosa:** This is genetic condition which initially manifests as night blindness. As the disease progress there may be a tunneling of vision with loss of peripheral vision followed by the compete blindness.

Cortical and Retinal Implant

Cortical and retinal implants are used to enhance vision or substitute parts of organ system function. Cortical implant consists of a chip or cable implanted in the visual cortex in the brain and the useful vision is enabled through camera or glasses. In case of retinal implants, the chip containing about 3500 solar cells with its own stimulating electrodes in about 2mm in diameter is implanted. The cells convert light energy into pulses to stimulate the remaining functioning part of the retina. There are two approaches for implant:

Epiretinal approach: In this, the electrode array is implanted on the surface of the retina to stimulate the overlying cells of the retina (ganglion cells).

Subretinal approach: In this, the implant is made behind the retina between the photoreceptor layer and the retinal pigment epithelium, directly stimulating retinal cells and relying on the normal processing of the inner and middle retinal layers.

Mobility Aids

Mobility for the visually impaired or blind has been a hindrance as most of the designs in the environments were not done taking such groups into consideration. Although designs are being implement in few places and transport system. However, it cannot ease up the movement problem faced by the group. Assistance acts as a boon in such cases. White cane is widely used by blind and visually impaired to aid them in mobility. An improvised version is use of ultrasound technology in white cane of the user to help them identify the presence of object on their route and traverse avoiding it.

Ultrasound is a sound wave ranging in the frequency of 15-20 kHz. Most objects in nature reflect ultrasound. This is used in developing the improvised white cane with ultrasound technology. In this, the hand held portion of the cane has control buttons that emits ultrasonic waves on a press. Around the tip of the cane, ultrasound transmitter and receiver are present. The transmitter transmits the sound waves which upon hitting an object (if any) reflect the waves and the user receives indication on object in the form of light vibrations. This has helped in making the group of users more independent with regards to movement.

Devices for Hearing Impaired

Auditory Pathway

Auditory system is a sensory system which is meant for sense of hearing. It includes both sensory and auditory parts of the sensory system.In auditory pathway cochlear nerve fibers synapse into the dorsal and ventral cochlear nuclei. Cochlear nuclei contain second order neurons so the auditory pathway is bilateral in nature (Harlow 1946). In auditory pathways fibers decussate remains ipsilateral that the pathway ascends in the lateral leminscus and then in the brachium of the caudal collicus from which neurons send their axons through the internal capsule to cerebral cortex surrounding the sylvian sulcus.

In auditory pathway cochlear nuclei receives input from the ipsilateral cochlear nerve. Similarly dorsal nucleus of trapezoid body receives input from right and left ears. Cochlear nucleus works as sound localization, for example it detecting phase and intensity different between the two ears. After detecting the sound location it sends the output to cranial nerves V and VII for reflex contraction of tensor tympani and stapedius muscle to dampen loud sound. In auditory pathway nucleus is the main source of efferent axons which tune the spinal organ for frequency discrimination.

Functional Hearing Assessment

A hearing test provides an evaluation of the sensitivity of a person's sense of hearing. The hearing test is performed by audiologist by using instrument called audiometer. It determines a person hearing sensitivity at different frequencies. Before hearing assessment ear examination is required prior to hearing test. In this examination the ear of the patient are usually examined with an otoscope to make sure they are free of wax that the eardrum is intact, ear are not infected and the middle ear is free of fluid (Johnson 1993). There are many genetic dis-order, ageing problems, exposure to noise, environmental pollution, birth complication and side effects of medication that results the hearing loss and hearing impartment.

Type of Hearing Tests

- **Pure Tone Audiometry:** It is the most oldest and common method of hearing testing. It measure the air and bone conduction thresholds for each ear in a set of eight standard frequency from 250Hz to 8000Hz (Yusuf Kemal Kemaloglu 2005). This test is performed in sound booth using a pair of headphones connected to an external audiometer and the result of this test is ploted in form of audiogram diagram form at the tested frequency.
- **Web and Rinne Test:** This test helps to determine the kind of hearing loss is present in the patient. In this examination of hearing test vibrating tuning fork is placed behind the ear near to the mastoid process. When patient can no longer feel/hear the vibration (Yueh, 2003) the tuning fork is held in front of the ear; the patient should once more be able to hear a ringing sound. If patient so not perform this test mean there is conductive hearing loss in the ear. In that condition patient is then asked if the sound is localized ion the centre of the head. If again there is conductive hearing loss it should be louder in the affected ear and if there is only sensor neural hearing loss it will be quieter in the affected ear.

- **Physiological Tests:** Auditory brainstem response testing, oto acoustic emission audiometry and tympanometry comes under the physiological test. These tests are mainly performed to describe neurological or mechanical functioning of the auditory system but these test do not involve person being tested.
- **Behaviour Test:** It required participation of the individual being tested. Most common behaviour test involve pure tones which generate sound by machine. These machine generated sounds are very controlled for their pitch and loudness. All natural sounds, especially speech, contain a combination of different frequencies (pitch) of varying intensity (loudness). During pure tone testing, audiologists are trying to find an individual's threshold at various frequencies. Threshold is the intensity level where a sound can just be detected. There is not an exact one-to-one correspondence between auditory thresholds and what an individual can do with her or his hearing, but pure tone testing is important to use as a starting point for predictions and to use as the basis for hearing aid fitting.

Auditory Augmentation and Substitution

Hearing impairment may be mild or profound. In case of mild impairment, auditory augmentation is provided for rehabilitation of the impairment while auditory substitution is required in case of profound impairment.

Hearing aid is a type of auditory augmentation. A hearing aid is an electronic device which amplifies the incoming sound for perception. The different components that are assembled together form a hearing aid are described below.

- **Microphone:** A microphone serves the function of the external ear of receiving sound. The received sound is then converted into electrical impulses and sent to the amplifier.
- **Amplifier:** The amplifier increases the intensity of the electrical impulses generated by the microphone.
- **Receiver:** The receiver's role is to convert the amplified electrical signals to sound with greater intensity than the perceived sound. It then delivers the sound to the inner portion of the ear.
- **Battery:** Battery serves as a source of power for the operation of the device.

Hearing aids are available in different styles to suit the requirement and choice of an individual. The components are held in a small case making the hearing aid highly portable and hardly visible. The different styles indicate the location for placement of the hearing aid. Hearing aids are mostly digital or of programmable type.

- **Behind-the-Ear (BTE):** BTE hearing aids is placed behind the ear and has a hook shaped plastic moulded extension from the case which is used for fit in concha. The sound travels from the case and is delivered into the ear through the mold. It is used for mild to profound hearing loss and can used by all ages. However, BTE is visible and might be an embarrassment to the user. Hence, other styles are preferred in many cases.
- **In-the-Ear (ITE):** An ITE hearing aid completely fits in the orifice of the outer ear. The components are held in a hard plastic case for a proper casing. Due to its small size, the ITE has problems

Figure 14. BTE
Source: http://www.alimco.in/content/854_1_BehindTheEarHearingAidDigital.aspx on 11th June 2017.

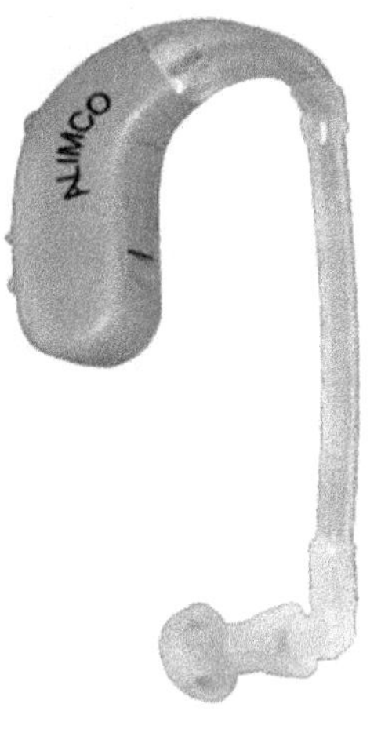

for fit and also damages can occur due to earwax or fluids. It is not worn by children as the casing needs to be replaced as the ear grows. It is used for mild to severe hearing loss.

- **In-the-Canal (ITC):** It is a customized hearing aid in which the case is developed for perfect fit depending on the size and shape of the ear canal. It is used for mild to moderately severe hearing loss.
- **Completely-in-Canal (CIC):** CIC is another custom-fit hearing aid and concealed in the ear canal. It is smaller in size as compared to other hearing aids and is not comfortable for repeated removal and adjustment. It is also prone for damage by earwax and fluids.

When hearing impairment is profound, auditory augmentation is of vain. The subject needs to have auditory substitution i.e., an artificial auditory pathway is required. Cochlear implant is a form of auditory substitution. It consists of 4 main parts: microphone; speech processor; transmitter-receiver and implanted electrode array. The microphone is employed for collecting sound from the environment and feeding it to the speech processor. The speech processor has the necessary volume adjust. Its primary role is to convert the incoming sound into matching intensity of electrical signals. This signal is then sent to the parts present inner in the ear via the transmitter-receiver assembly. The transmitter-receiver as the name suggests does the function of transmitting the electrical signal from the external portion of the

Figure 15. ITE
Source: http://www.alimco.in/content/854_1_BehindTheEarHearingAidDigital.aspx on 11th June 2017.

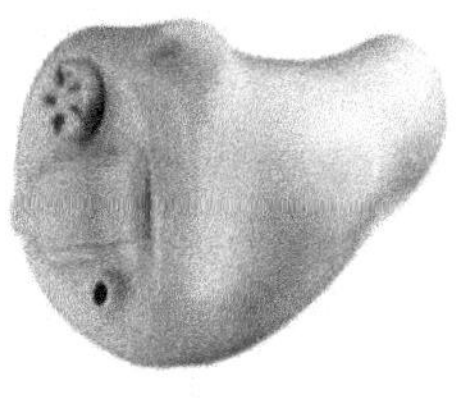

Figure 16. ITC
Source: http://www.alimco.in/content/854_1_BehindTheEarHearingAidDigital.aspx on 11th June 2017.

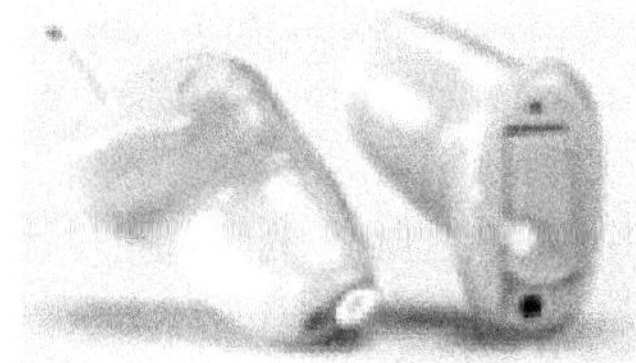

implant components to the internal portion. This can occur in two ways: transcutaneous or percutaneous. The electrode array is a wire consisting of multiple electrodes placed in the scala tympani. It stimulates the hair cells with the electrical signal received from the receiver.

Tactile Sensors

A tactile sensor is a device that measures information arising from physical interaction with its environment (A. S. Hsieh, 1995). Tactile sensors are generally modeled after the biological sense of cutaneous touch which is capable of detecting stimuli resulting from mechanical stimulation, temperature, and pain. Tactile sensors are used in robotics, computer hardware and security systems. A common application of tactile sensors is in touchscreen devices on mobile phones and computing. Tactile sensors may be of different types including piezo-resistive, piezoelectric, capacitive and elasto-resistive sensors (Cutkosky, M. R.1989).

Applications of Tactile Sensors

Tactile sensors are nowadays employed in everyday life having innumerable applications such as lighting lamps which dim or lighten up by touching the base or the elevator button. They have several applications in the field of rehabilitation and assistive devices for disabled. Sensors are quite small in appearance but they have high sensitivities which suit several medical applications. They are designed keeping in view having minor effect on what parameter is being measured; thereby making the sensor smaller that often improves their sensitivity and introduces other advantages (A. M. Wing 1993). Tactile sensors can be used to test the performance of all types of applications. For example, these sensors have been used in the manufacturing of automobiles (brakes, clutches, door seals, gasket), battery lamination, bolted joints, fuel cells etc. Nowadays tactile sensors are much familiar in field of rehabilitation such as soft silicone tactile sensor for measuring pressure while gait training in stroke or hemiparetic patients, alternative tactile sensors for perceptron neural networks by applying the contact evaluation according to the algorithm, pressure sensor for detecting normal force on human weight nearing joints and biological inspired tactile sensors for finger pressure measurements.

Computer Brain Interfacing (BCI)

Research on brain computer interfacing (BCIs) began in the 1970s at the University of California, Los Angeles (UCLA) under a grant from the National Science Foundation (Adjouadi M. A 2000). The papers published after this research also mark the first appearance of the expression brain–computer interface in scientific literature. Computer interfacing is a process of shared boundary across which two or more separate components of computer system exchange information. The exchange can be between software, computer hardware, peripheral devices, humans and combinations of these. Some computer hardware devices, such as a touchscreen, can send and receive data through the interface, while others such as a mouse or microphone may only provide an interface to send data to a given system. A brain computer interface (BCI), sometimes called a mind-machine interface (MMI), direct neural interface (DNI), or brain–machine interface (BMI), is a direct communication pathway between an enhanced or wired brain and an external device (Evarts EV.1966). BCIs are often directed at researching, mapping, assisting, augmenting, or repairing human cognitive or sensory-motor functions.

Figure 17. BCI
Sources: https://en.wikipedia.org/wiki/Brain%E2%80%93computer_interface (on 1st August 2017).

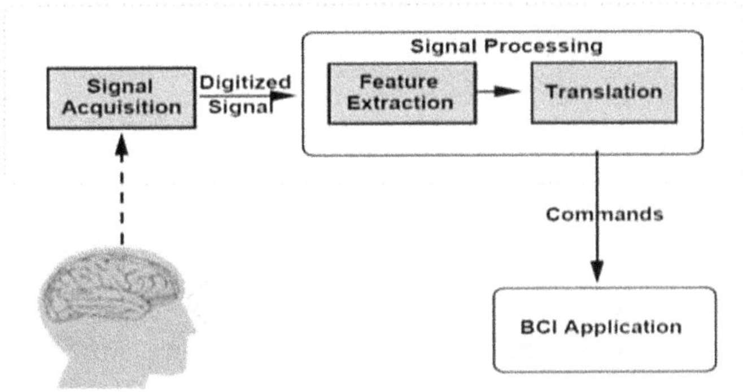

Basic block diagram of a BCI system incorporating signal detection, processing and deployment

The history of brain–computer interfaces (BCIs) starts with Hans Berger's discovery of the electrical activity of the human brain and the development of electroencephalography (EEG). In 1924, Berger was the first person to record human brain activity by means of EEG. Berger was able to identify oscillatory activity, such as Berger's wave or the alpha wave (8–13 Hz), by analysing EEG traces. It is a direct communication pathway between an enhanced or wired brain and an external device. BCIs are often directed at researching, mapping, assisting, augmenting, or repairing human cognitive or sensory-motor functions.

Cost Analysis of Affordable Devices for Rehabilitation

Cost-effectiveness and cost-benefit studies are conducted at a level that involves more than just a local program (such as an individual's state strengthening project). Sometimes they also involve following up over a long period of time, to look at the long-term impact of interventions. They are often used by policy analysts and legislators to make broad policy decisions, so they might look at a large federal program, or compare several smaller pilot programs that take different approaches to solving the same societal problems. People often use the terms interchangeably, but there are important differences between them.

Cost Effective Analysis Helps Us in Following Aspects

- Cost analyses can provide estimates of what a program's costs and benefits are likely to be, before it is implemented.
- Cost analyses may improve understanding of program operation, and tell what levels of intervention are most cost-effective.
- Cost analyses may reveal unexpected costs.
- Whether or not the outlined program is having a significant net effect on the desired outcomes.
- Whether the least expensive alternative is always the best alternative.

ADVANTAGES OF USING COST ANALYSES

- Promotes fiscal accountability in programs.
- Helps set priorities when resources are limited
- Can be extremely powerful and persuasive to legislators, policy makers, and other funders.

DISADVANTAGES OF USING COST ANALYSES

- Requires a great deal of technical skill and knowledge
- Market costs (what people actually pay for something) don't always reflect "real" social costs
- Sometimes there are multiple competing goals, so we need to weight them or prioritize them in some way.
- Sometimes costs and monetary values are considered less important than other, more intangible values or program outcomes
- The best-known cost-benefit studies have looked at long-term outcomes, but most program evaluations don't have the time or resources to conduct long-term follow-up studies.

CONCLUSION

In this chapter, the importance of Rehabilitation Engineering was well explained in section – 1, based on the census data 2011 provided by the Government of India and World Health Organization. Section – 2 explains about the trends in development of prostatic and orthotic devices and how, the technology can be used to improve the current devices in the market. Devices for mobility and its development were explained in section – 3. Devices for visual impairment and hearing impairment and its uses are explained in section 4 and 5 respectively.

REFERENCES

Ades & Brookhart. (1949). The central auditory pathway. *Neurophysiology*, *13*(1), 1–2. PMID:15415767

Ali, H. (2014). *Bionic Exoskeleton: History, Development and the Future.* Paper presented at the IOSR Journal of Mechanical and Civil Engineering (IOSR-JMCE), International Conference on Advances in Engineering & Technology.

Barreto, A. B., Scargle, S. D., & Adjouadi, M. A. (2000). practical EMG-based human–computer interface for users with motor disabilities. *Journal of Rehabilitation Research and Development*, *37*, 53–63. PMID:10847572

Beebe, D. J., Hsieh, A. S., Denton, D. D., & Radwin, R. G. (1995). A Silicon Force Sensor for Robotics and Medicine. *Sensors and Actuators. A, Physical*, *50*(1-2), 55–65. doi:10.1016/0924-4247(96)80085-9

Bourke, T. (2001). *Development of a robotic wheelchair.* University or Wollongong.

Bronzino, J. D., & Peterson, D. R. (2014). *Biomedical engineering fundamentals*. CRC press.

Chaichanasiri, E., & Puangumpan, T. (2011). *A prototype of a stair-climbing system for a wheelchair*. Paper presented at the The Second TSME International Conference on Mechanical Engineering.

Coupland, R. M., & Koever, A. (1991). Injuries from antipersonnel mines: The experience of the International Committee of the Red Cross. *BMJ (Clinical Research Ed.)*, *330*(6816), 1509–1512. doi:10.1136/bmj.303.6816.1509 PMID:1838290

Cutkosky, M. R., & Kao, I. (1989). Computing and controlling the compliance of a robotic hand. *IEEE Transactions on Robotics and Automation*, *5*(2), 151–165. doi:10.1109/70.88036

Evarts, E. V. (1966). Pyramidal tract activity associated with a conditioned hand movement in the monkey. *Journal of Neurophysiology*, *29*(6), 1011–1027. doi:10.1152/jn.1966.29.6.1011 PMID:4961643

Flanagan, J. R., & Wing, A. M. (1993). Modulation of Grip Force with Load Force during point-to-point arm movements. *Experimental Brain Research*, *95*(1), 131–143. doi:10.1007/BF00229662 PMID:8405245

Gomi, T., & Griffith, A. (1998). Developing intelligent wheelchairs for the handicapped. *Assistive Technology and Artificial Intelligence*, 150-178.

Hersh, M. A., & Johnson, M. A. (2008). Disability and assistive technology systems. *Assistive technology for visually impaired and blind people*, 1-50.

John, G. W. (2006). Encyclopedia of Medical Devices and Instrumentation, 6 Volume Set. Wiley-Interscience.

Johnson,, C.D., & Almen. (1993). Revison based on Functional Listening Evaluation: Curr. *Neurophysiology*, *21*(5), 45–78.

Maberley, D., Hollands, H., Chuo, J., Tam, G., Konkal, J., Roesch, M., ... Bassett, K. (2006). The prevalence of low vision and blindness in Canada. *Eye (London, England)*, *20*(3), 341–346. doi:10.1038j.eye.6701879 PMID:15905873

Nolte, J., & Sundsten, J. (2002). *The human brain: an introduction to its functional anatomy* (Vol. 5). Mosby St. Louis.

Reinkensmeyer, D. J., & Dietz, V. (2016). *Neurorehabilitation technology*. Springer. doi:10.1007/978-3-319-28603-7

Robitaille, S. (2010). *The Illustrated Guide to Assistive Technology and Devices*. Academic Press.

Selhorst, J. B., & Chen, Y. (2009). *The optic nerve*. Paper presented at the Seminars in neurology.

Sethi, P. K. (1972). A rubber foot for amputees in underdeveloped countries. *The Journal of Bone and Joint Surgery. British Volume*, *54-B*, 177–178.

Toh, K. L. (2008). Basic science review on circadian rhythm biology and circadian sleep disorders. *Annals of the Academy of Medicine, Singapore*, *37*(8), 662–668. PMID:18797559

Turner, H. R. (2010). *Science in medieval Islam: an illustrated introduction*. University of Texas Press.

Vilensky, J. A., Robertson, W., & Suarez-Quian, C. A. (2015). *The Clinical Anatomy of the Cranial Nerves: The Nerves of" On Old Olympus Towering Top*. John Wiley & Sons. doi:10.1002/9781118491959

Whitelock, J., & Melrose, J. (2006). *Wiley Encyclopaedia of Biomedical Engineering*. Wiley.

World Health Organization. (2008). *Change the definition of blindness.* Retrieved from http://www. who. int/blindness/ChangetheDefinitionofBlindness. pdf

Yueh, B., Shapiro, N., MacLean, C. H., & Shekelle, P. G. (2003). Screening and management of adult hearing loss in primary care: Scientific review. *Journal of the American Medical Association*, *289*(15), 1976–1985. doi:10.1001/jama.289.15.1976 PMID:12697801

Yusuf, K. K., Bulent, G., & Selda, G. (2005). Pure tone audiometery in children. *International Journal of Pediatric Otorhinolaryngology*, *69*(2), 209–214. doi:10.1016/j.ijporl.2004.08.018 PMID:15656954

Chapter 4
Application of Biomechanics Instrumentation in Occupational Health Research

Sanjay M. Kotadiya
National Institute of Occupational Health, India

Joydeep Majumder
National Institute of Occupational Health, India

Sunil Kumar
National Institute of Occupational Health, India

ABSTRACT

Occupational morbidities during manual material handling operations are routine at workplaces. This is a global burden contributing substantially to the economy. The multifactorial etiology for musculoskeletal disorders (MSDs) along with workplace stressors require multidisciplinary preventive effort. Biomechanics plays a pivotal role in occupational health research quarrying into the root cause analysis of posture, load handling, muscular loading, balance, and stability at work. Sophisticated instrumentation and experimental techniques assist in understanding the biomechanical mechanisms of MSDs and ergonomic principles, etc. Kinetic, kinematic, isotonic, isokinetic, as well as isometric experimental modes investigate body postures and muscular responses. Foundation of biomechanics instrumentation and injury mechanism would aid researchers alongside ergonomists in dealing with identification, assessment, and control of workplace risks through participatory ergonomics approach. Judicious utilization of this discipline would approach a long-term sustainable solution to protect health and safety of workers at the workplace.

BACKGROUND

Biomechanics is the study of the mechanics of a living body, especially of the forces exerted by muscles and gravity on skeletal structure. This discipline is most common in sport science, where the laws of mechanics are applied in order to gain a categorical understanding of athletic performance through mathematical modeling, computer simulation and measurement. In this era of advanced research regime,

DOI: 10.4018/978-1-5225-4969-7.ch004

applied subfields of biomechanics including kinesiology, gait analysis, musculoskeletal biomechanics, ergonomics, human factors engineering and occupational biomechanics have been extended beyond sport biomechanics.

Biomechanics is meticulously close to engineering discipline; as often traditional engineering sciences are used to analyze biological systems (Aström & Murray, 2010). In this advanced research arena, biomechanics has turned on the computerization of the technologies. It would be imperative to mention that this discipline incorporates an integrated series of analysis techniques during a single experimental work simulation. Computational biology approaches in biomechanics and biomedical engineering also open up avenues for the importance of integrating the disciplines of engineering with medical technology and clinical expertise. Such integration is ought to have a major impact on health care in the near future. Researchers focus on two general areas of biomechanics- kinematics and kinetics. In kinematics, human motion during an activity is only monitored; while in kinetic studies, motion along with forces and torques involved in the activity is taken in to account.

Occupational biomechanics emerged as a sub-discipline within the general field of biomechanics that studies the physical interactions of workers with their tools, machines, and materials to improve the working condition, enhance worker performance while minimizing the risk of musculoskeletal disorders/injuries (MSDs). Since, occupational health deals with performance of a worker, sustainable livelihood factors such as anthropometric measurements, individual risk factors (age, gender, inherited genetic characteristic), workplace risk factors (methods, materials, machines, environment, and physical stressors), psychological factors, economic concerns and return to work issues are considered during biomechanics study. Occupational biomechanics research thus provides intellectual inputs as a subsidiary discipline during the development of important ergonomics guidelines.

Musculoskeletal Disorders are one of the major causes of variety of morbidity, and have a significant influence on health and quality of life. It imposes an enormous burden of cost on the healthcare system (Jenkins et al., 2016). Especially work-related MSDs are the commonest source of morbidity among workers in range of occupation, resulting in physical impairment and disability to psychological stress. MSD is considered as a primary contributor to the global burden of non-communicable diseases and the reported global prevalence ranges from 14-42% (Sharma, 2012). In the American workplace too, work related musculoskeletal disorders account for one of the largest category of claims in workers' compensation (Bhattacharya, 2014). Studies in various other countries revealed that the prevalence of MSDs in Malaysia (~21%) (Veerapen et al., 2007), Israel (35%) (Sharma, 2012), India (26%) (Yashobant & Rajkumar, 2014) is substantial and alarming. An ICMR Task Force Study in three centres of India reported a prevalence of 7-11.5% (Sharma, 2012), with functional limitation to 85% people with nearly 10% absenteeism.

Given the multifactorial etiology for MSD and its association with individual and workplace risk factors, their reduction and prevention will require a multidisciplinary effort. The science of ergonomics, biomechanics, epidemiology and medicine together better understand the interdependence of MSD, as well as long-term sustainable solution. Biomechanical intervention may determine safety or solution to these problems. Most work related injuries can be viewed as biomechanical damage to a tissue or organ.

Thus biomechanical hazards may be single or repetitive movements and forces imposing stress on the body with a potential to cause or contribute to injury or disease affecting the musculoskeletal or neurological systems. To identify these hazards and develop effective control measures, it is important to understand the principles of biomechanics as well as relevant physics, engineering and behavioural science concepts. Biomechanics principle helps in machine control and workplace design in occupational setups. Its fundamental principles explore mechanisms of occupational injuries, its interventions and implementation (Van Der Beek et al., 2017; Herman et al., 2009). Applying biomechanics in various industries and work situations helps in prevention and reduction of musculoskeletal injuries in the workplace.

These disciplines vary largely in their contribution to work-related MSD prevention research, ranging from classic injury surveillance and etiological studies to detailed laboratory studies and animal models exploring injury mechanisms, and studies evaluating

BIOMECHANICS IN OCCUPATIONAL HEALTH RESEARCH

In regards to occupational health research, better posture, optimal load handling, muscular loading, balance and stability gets priority when biomechanics studies are planned. Occupational research laboratories use sophisticated biomedical instrumentation and experimental techniques to understand the biomechanical mechanisms of musculoskeletal disorders, ergonomic principles etc. (Nag et al., 2013, Singh et al., 2015). Such research utilizes force platforms to study ground reaction forces and infrared videography to capture the trajectories of markers attached to the workers' body to study 3D motion. Electromyography (EMG) is further studied to understand the muscle activation. Integrating kinematics, kinetics and EMG techniques during a simulative work experiment makes it feasible to investigate the workers' body movements as well as muscular responses to the external forces, simultaneously (Nag et al., 2013). Therefore, both kinematics and kinetic studies along with EMG become essential in occupational biomechanics.

Gait analysis is the study of human motion, using the eye and the brain of observers, augmented by instrumentation for measuring body movements, body mechanics, and the activity of the muscles. Gait analysis has been found to be an efficient clinical tool used in diagnostics and treatment of pathological gait. It provides an objective and quantifiable assessment before and after intervention that aim to improve a worker's gait ability. Further to understand the kinematics, motion capture system digitally records and analyze the movement of a worker performing a particulate task.

This use of kinetics, however, does not result in information for individual muscles but muscle groups. To detect the activity and contribution of individual muscles to movement, it is necessary to investigate the electrical activity of muscles. It investigates the activation time of muscles and magnitude of their activation-thereby assessing their contribution to gait. Further, in occupational health research., it becomes important to look in the time zone of an activity i.e., intermittent or endurance type of work regime, along with the force required to perform it. There, the EMG assist in understanding the indefatigability of the muscles and henceforth the design of optimal time of work can be suggested to avoid overloading of the muscles. Deviations from normal kinematic, kinetic, or EMG patterns are used to diagnose specific postural abnormalities, predict the outcome of investigations, or determine the effectiveness of training programmes.

Further ahead, testing of the maximum allowable human strength (involving a group of muscles) became very essential for designing an equipment, as well as plan a proper work rest schedule. Isometric strength testing in simulative work situation provides the maximum voluntary strength from which limits can be set. In the next stage, improving the performance by training is a most effective tool. Computer-controlled exercise and testing machines are another example of how biomechanics contributes to strength and conditioning. Isokinetic muscle strength exercise, conditions the muscles towards cascade elevation of strength in terms of endurance sustainability.

Many industries nowadays consider poor muscular strength as a potential pre-employment risk factor for workers (Dale et al., 2014). It is strongly felt that quantification of muscular capability can predict susceptibility to many work related disorders. Consequently, health professionals in industries require objective tools to determine whether prospective employees possess the muscular strength necessary to safely meet the demands of the positions at the very pre-employment stage. Muscle strength testing and conditioning provides objective, reproducible measures that can be correlated with the physical demands of different jobs. Such pre-employment testing enables the concerned to assess whether job applicants will become true assets to their workforce or add on to risks of injuries, absenteeism, poor productivity, low morale as well as susceptible to diseases.

FUTURE RESEARCH DIRECTIONS: BIOMECHANICS INSTRUMENTATION

Literature categorically iterates that biomechanical studies complement epidemiological studies to comprehend the complex process between exposures and physical risk factors that result in sprain, strain, injuries or occupational diseases (Keyserling, 2000). Research in biomechanics is dependent on subject knowledge, expertise, instrumentation, data analysis and interpretation. In the recent years, sophisticated instrumentation integrating various dimensions of biomechanics principle has enabled generation of large amount of flawless data. Particularly in occupational health research, the biomechanics studies during actual work activity is grueling. Therefore, classical biomechanics instrumentation assimilating multiple dimensions of movement, balance, muscular activity and strength together gives quality information in less extensive experimentation process during laboratory based simulation studies (Keyserling, 2000; Chao, 2003; Marin et al., 2017). This ultimately assists in excavating out a solution to the occupational problem being researched. Some of the instrumentation are enumerated which caters the research in occupational biomechanics.

Force Platform

Force platforms or force plates are instruments used to measure the ground reaction forces and moments generated by a body while standing, walking, running and jumping. Force plates contribute to research on stability, gait and other parameters of biomechanics. Original workplaces are arduous for measurement of such parameters on sophisticated instrumentation are difficult to be used in such working conditions. Therefore, simulated experimentation especially in occupational health research is the viable option.

It measures the three-dimensional components of the single equivalent force applied to the surface and its point of application, usually called the centre of pressure (CoP), as well as the vertical moment of force (Robertson et al., 2004). It helps to demonstrate relationships between force, acceleration, velocity, and displacement. It is used individually or arranged in a walkway format to collect multiple footfalls. A complete standard system typically consists of a force plate, an amplifier, a computer or data acquisition system, mounting hardware, and interconnecting cables. Force plate with sensors attached to it gives an electrical output proportional to the force applied on the plate called piezoelectric phenomenon. Forces that cause human movement normally act on our hands or feet and exert strain on our entire musculo-skeletal system. For example, when a worker carries a load on the head in a construction site, he would have to maneuvre his own body weight and balance; in addition to the balance and stability of the load being carried. Simulating such conditions in laboratory using force platform would provide a detailed view of balance and stability during work by measuring ground reaction forces and CoP.

A load on the plate distorts each pedestal, depending on the direction and location of the placement of load on it. A piezoelectric or strain gauze transducer attached to each pedestal measures the occurring distortion. With the known force plate geometry and pedestal locations, the forces and moments acting on the plate are determined. The strain gauges at each corner deform with loading, causing a change in resistance which is measured by the change in voltage over the strain gauge. On contact with the platform, three forces and three moment components are measured. Fx, Fy, and Fz are the force components acting along the axes of an orthogonal x, y & z coordinates (Fx and Fy are horizontal components, and Fz is vertical force component). Mx, My and Mz are the three moment components, which are rotations around the corresponding x, y and z axes.

While simulating a walking or running activity at constant speed, horizontal force is not required. The front foot pushes forward on the ground, resulting in an impulse equal and opposite to the impulse generated when the back foot pushes backwards. While in the standing or stationary holding mode with both feet on a force plate, the vertical direction register $F = Mg$ (where, 'M' is mass of the individual and 'g' is gravitational force). During bending on knees for lifting or lowering of load, the centre of mass is lowered. Initially the force decreases and then increases before settling back to Mg (Wardoyo et al., 2016). However, while in upright standing position the whole body centre of mass continuously moves. But, the CoP underneath the feet is adjusted, maintaining the centre of mass within the feet. Thus, CoP motion plot (stabilogram) is used to assess the performer's standing/ seating balance during work.

Calibration of force platforms is an essential step before the data acquisition. These platforms are usually calibrated by applying a range of pre-quantified static loads that is the sensors are loaded with a range of known calibration weights at specified moment arms. However static loads can be applied only in one direction, which is a disadvantage. This is because actual forces exerted on force platforms are dynamic in nature and actuated multiple directions. Therefore, researchers while using sophisticated instrumentation go for manufacturer supplied calibration parameters to convert the voltages measured by the transducers into force and moment measurements. It is generally recommended to calibrate these instrumentations at least once in a year. However, it may be noted that recalibration intervals for sensors and measurement equipment may vary depending on the specific application and usage.

Motion Capture System

Quantifying human motion during an activity facilitate the understanding of pattern of work profile at workplace, angular deviation of the skeleton structure beyond normal as well as treatment and rehabilitation on injury. Conventionally biomechanical analysis systems used to capture brief snapshots of the mechanics of movement (Winter, 2009). In the recent era, with latest developments in wearable sensing technologies, biomechanical research has eased out permitting continuous monitoring and analysis (Wong et al., 2015).

Motion capture started as a photogrammetric analysis tool in biomechanics research around five decades back and expanded into education, training, and research as the technology advanced. Since the 20th century, with newer technology, the performer is worn markers near each joint to identify the motion by the positions or angles between the markers. Acoustic, inertial, LED, magnetic or reflective markers, or combinations of these, are tracked, optimally at least twice the frequency rate of the desired motion. The spatial resolution and temporal resolution is considered typically, as motion blur causes almost the same problems as low resolution. Modern systems extract the silhouette of the performer from the infrared motion camera images. Requisite joint angles are then calculated by fitting in a mathematic model into the silhouette.

Motion capture technology consists of motion capture cameras, other hardware and software. It is used in occupational health research to identify and prevent injuries, improve performance as well as aid ergonomists to build better products and increase production efficiency.

There are various types of motion capture systems:

1. **Optical-Passive:** Retroreflective markers tracked by infrared cameras.
2. **Optical-Active:** LED markers connected by wires to the motion capture suit with a battery or charger pack worn by the performer.
3. **Video/Markerless:** Markers are not required to be worn and instead relies on software to track the performers' movement.
4. **Inertial:** Cameras are not required except as a localization tool. Inertial sensors are worn on the performer's body at selective locations and the data from the sensors is transmitted wirelessly to a computer.

Data acquisition is performed by an infrared optoelectronic system and the analysis is based on the detection and three-dimensional construction of the silhouette from passive markers positioned on anatomical landmarks of the body. The labelling of the markers attached to the defined locations of the body is very important for identification of the correct two-point angular deviation within the software. These softwares generally carry out data acquisition and further elaboration of the trial, as well as interpretation of data in fidelity with conventional protocols like Davis protocol, SAFLo protocol etc. (Ferrari et al., 2008). Therefore, when an experiment is designed on the conventional protocols registered within the software, exact anatomical locations on three-dimensional coordinates needs to be recognized and linked to the corresponding real point on the performer. However, self-made protocols can also be used for the elaboration of a simulated work profile and interpreted.

Having said that any postural activity can be simulated, the precision and repeatability of data is dependent on the system calibration. Different systems have distinctive process of calibration. In general, these systems come with active wand, that calibrates both optical and video cameras while accounting for sensor edge distortion at the same time, to ensure synchronized overlay across entire volume. Calibration is performed using a rigid wand on which three markers are mounted and is swept through the volume of interest, in a dynamic acquisition, for simultaneous calibration of intrinsic parameters, and relative position, of the video cameras. Within the experimental overlay, the global frame of reference is determined by a three-axes calibration grid, placed on the ground.

Electromyography (EMG)

EMG is a technique of recording the electrical activity produced by skeletal muscles performed using an instrument called an electromyography to produce a record called an electromyogram. An electromyograph detects the electric potential generated by muscle cells when these cells are electrically or neurologically activated. EMG sensors and systems have been extensively researched and developed over a number of years incorporating the latest design principles and technologies for movement analysis and biofeedback. Understanding the electrical activity of the muscles provides a categorical view of the muscular overloading, limits of load, performers' capacity and sustainability and most importantly the indefatigability of the muscles leading to peripheral or central fatigue (Cifrek et al., 2009). This technology in addition to medical perspective is used in symmetry studies during gait, timing data in biomechanics, work profiling and fatigue, work environment and tool design, work performance and productivity oriented protocol as well as precisely in rehabilitation schema.

Electrical Characteristics of Muscles

When a muscle contracts, electrical activity is generated within the muscle which may be measured using electrodes placed on the surface of the skin. This electrical signal is usually in the order of up to 3,000 micro volts. Measured EMG potentials range between less than 50 μV and up to 20 to 30 mV, depending on the muscle under observation (Phinyomark et al., 2011).

Typical repetition rate of muscle motor unit firing is about 7-20 Hz, depending on the size of the muscle, previous axonal damage and other factors (Lee & Lee, 2008). Damage to motor units can be expected at ranges between 450 and 780 mV. EMG activity is linearly related to the amount of muscle contraction as well as the number of contracted muscles. This implies that stronger the muscle contraction and greater the number of activated muscles, the higher the recorded voltage amplitude.

Intramuscular and Surface EMG

Electromyography of specified muscle can be done in two ways: intramuscular and surface. Intramuscular EMG is a superior technique for the diagnostic examination of voluntary motor activity of the deeper muscles. This technique also comprehends the needle insertional activity. However, this technique is painful, the muscle may feel a little sore up for some post examination days. Depending on the purpose of experimentation particularly in case of measurement of electrical activity of a muscle during a simulative work process, surface EMG is a versatile, state of the art beneficial technique, which is reliable, accurate and easy to use. Its painless, non-invasive and can collect quality signals if the skin surface is prepared well. Therefore, especially for the occupational health research, where workers' posture remains dynamic, surface EMG is a judicious option to collect electrical signal for analysis. Surface EMG can be recorded by a pair of electrodes. More than one electrode is needed because EMG recordings display the potential difference (voltage difference) between two separate electrodes.

Placement of EMG electrodes over muscle groups of interest require a substantial level of anatomic knowledge to be able to get valid and reliable signals of high quality. EMG signal is collected in a bipolar technique i.e., the voltage difference between recording site and reference site. The EMG reference channels is placed on the bony body parts such as metacarpal, elbow, hip or collar bones. The shorter the size of connecting cables, lesser the electrical noise picked up from surrounding power sources.

Maximal Voluntary Contraction

One basic function of EMG is to see how well a muscle can be activated. The most common way that can be determined is by performing a maximal voluntary contraction (MVC) of the muscle that is being tested (Castelein et al., 2015). Several analytical methods for determining muscle activation are commonly used depending on the application. Most studies commonly use the maximal voluntary contraction as a means of analyzing peak force and force generated by target muscles. Researchers suggest that EMG data should be recorded alongside the peak EMG measure when assessing core exercises (Hibbs et al., 2011).

As said earlier, EMG can also be used for indicating the amount of fatigue in a muscle. In such cases, changes in the EMG signal is witnessed which signifies muscle fatigue like, an increase in the mean absolute value of the signal, increase in the amplitude and duration of the muscle action potential and an overall shift to lower frequencies. Monitoring the variability during different frequency changes is the most common way of using EMG to determine levels of fatigue. The lower conduction velocities enable the slower motor neurons to remain active (Cifrek et al., 2009).

EMG Signal Processing

Rectification is the translation of the raw EMG signal to a single polarity frequency. The purpose of rectifying a signal is to ensure the raw signal does not average zero. Half-length rectification deletes the EMG signal below the baseline. In doing so, the average of the data is no longer zero therefore it can be used in statistical analyses. The only difference between the two types of rectification is that full-wave rectification takes the absolute value of the signal array of data points.

It is imperative to note that occupational circumstances at workplace would be typically dynamic in nature. The movement, speed and angle of physical body deviation would resist accumulation of quality EMG data. Therefore, a portable instrument for any simulated laboratory experiment would be most effective for occupational health research. Further portable EMG machine synchronized with wireless position measurement systems to accurately study the amount of muscle activation for different activities such as lifting the arm up or during gait, would be the ideal one. Generally, the new generation devices include powerful software for the elaboration protocol creation by means of an innovative object interface that convert the biomechanics analysis language in a graphical way. In these systems, the user can develop quick and efficient customized analysis protocols. The real time data transmission between the system and the workstation occurs with Wi-Fi net using an access point. The software facilitates acquisition, display, processing, and reporting of electromyographic signals.

Mechanomyography (MMG)

In addition to the general technique of recording of electrical activity of muscles using EMG, the MMG is also used as an alternative to the EMG for monitoring the muscular activity. It is said to produce higher signal-to-noise ratio than the surface EMG and thus can be used to monitor muscle activity from deeper muscles without using invasive measurement techniques. It is a promising research area into prosthetic research and assistive technologies. The mechanomyogram is the mechanical signal from the surface of a muscle, on contraction, wherein the muscle shape causes a large peak in the MMG.

INTEGRATING MULTIPLE DIMENSIONS OF BIOMECHANICS

For the workers, posture at work, workplace design constraints and housekeeping management are important domain at workplace. Biomechanics tools aid in workplace design research, ensuring the safety at workplace as well as optimal posture of the worker for productivity at endurance. The measurements for the above three instrumentation systems (force platform, motion capture and EMG) can be either studied in isolation, or combined kinetic and/or kinematics to understand the principles of locomotion. If a worker makes a standing jump from a force plate, the data from the plate alone is sufficient to calculate acceleration, work and power output. Simultaneous video measurements of leg joint angles and force plate output can allow the determination of torque, work and power at each joint using a method called inverse dynamics. It also allows to perform advanced elaboration of the EMG signals, allowing to state for the muscular exertion as well as muscle fatigue. A customized analysis protocols integrating these dimensions would be a comprehensive advanced multimodal report.

ISOKINETIC SYSTEM

Another important facet of biomechanics study is the human strength quantification particularly for a group of muscles. This has a tremendous impact in the occupational health research in pre-employment screening, physical load handling limits, manual material handling, work rest schedule as well as safe work protocol for injury prevention. Research on human strength is done on three modes: isokinetic, isotonic and isometric mode.

Isokinetic Mode

The maximum dynamic capability throughout the range-of-motion is determined. It is an effective mode to comprehend the localization of pain, weakness and determine the dynamic physical capacity. It is also the most efficient method to improve strength, power in endurance as well as rehabilitation after an injury. The focal point for the experimentation is the dynamometer which functions on eccentric-concentric mode. Hence depending on the size (length) of the attachment/lever the resultant is quantified in torque (Nm).

Isotonic Mode

This mode is used to facilitate neuromuscular coupling improvement with functional isotonic concentric/eccentric resistance coupled with user defined velocity. During concentric contraction, the muscle tension is enhanced due to increment in resistance and remain the same with shortening of muscle. In eccentric mode, the muscle lengthens on account of grater resistance than the force generated by the muscle.

Isometric Mode

This mode of experimentation is typically used for quantification of maximum strength during a voluntary muscular exertion. While the dynamic mode sets the requisite motion for optimal strength and rehabilitation, isometric mode is a static function restricting the length of the muscle to be altered. Apparently the desirable posture during an activity is taken and the subject applies his/her maximum strength on the lever, precisely exerting the maximum voluntary contraction. The universally accepted protocol for short duration or intermittent experimentation is 5 second wherein 2 second is for strength build up and 3 second for retaining the maximum strength (Tiwari et al., 2010). For endurance exercise, 1 minute tests are applied; peak strength time, decremental plateau and sustainability of strength is noted.

Load cells of tension-tension type, tension-compression type are used. With the technological advancement, integrated instrumentation with the ability to experiment strength in isokinetic, isotonic and isometric mode are available. One such laboratory based integrated system is Humac Norm Testing and Rehabilitation system to cater the comprehensive experimentation of human strength at workplace.

CASE STUDY-I

A study was carried out to comprehend the balance and stability among young male workers while performing manual materials handling tasks. The excerpts from the study is presented below as a case study involving the principles and instrumentation in biomechanics.

Manual load handling continues to be a concern in everyday activities, particularly in the occupational set ups (Nag et al., 2014). Loss of balance associated with different forms of manual materials handling (MMH) tasks is a crucial factor causing workplace accident and injury. MMH tasks include the lifting, lowering, pushing, pulling, carrying, twisting and turning of materials (Kotadiya et al., 2013). Construction workers, food grain handlers, agricultural workers and labourers in manufacturing industries have frequently been engaged in lifting and other forms of MMH tasks (Deros et al. 2010; Maiti, 2008). With the premise that MMH tasks have potential consequences on postural balance and stability, there is a need to consider the effects of load positioning and magnitude on stability.

Postural control requires the ability for balancing the body in space through the visual, vestibular, and somatosensory systems and makes an appropriate musculoskeletal response to perturbations (Nashner, 2014; Paillard, 2012). The maintenance of an upright posture is a vital motor function and postural control is essential for the maintenance of posture and task performance (Ku et al., 2012). In humans, when the centre of gravity falls outside the base of support, the body has the ability to sense a threat to stability and in such instances, relevant muscles are activated to prevent falling (Ritzmann et al., 2017). Postural control strategies used are dependent on the assessment and control of many variables by the CNS. The strategies used to maintain balance differ according to an individual's goal, the environmental context and the task performed (Horak et al., 2008). Thus identifying a method of load handling which is relatively more stable can prevent falls and injury risks. Changes in postural responses can be identified through the use of EMG by measuring onset latencies, response amplitudes or postural strategies (Visser et al., 2008). Muscle fatigue affects postural control by increasing postural sway (Mello et al., 2007). Thus postural imbalance can be indicated through study of centre of pressure and electromyographic measurements. The simulated laboratory study was carried out with the hypothesis that muscle activity and centre of pressure displacements may be influenced by the changes in methods of MMH tasks and increase in grades of load.

The experimental set up included two large format multi-component piezoelectric force platforms (Kistler, USA) for measuring the ground reaction forces and 16-channel portable and Wi-Fi enabled pocket EMG machine (BTS Bioengineering, Italy) to measure muscular activities during MMH task. The electromyographic recording of neck, shoulder, spinal and leg muscles were examined. Primary MMH tasks viz. lifting-lowering, twisting-turning and holding activities were simulated. The simulated activities with the equipment set up are shown in Figure 1. The sEMG signals of muscles were captured by SMART capture software (BTS Bioengineering, Italy) and analyzed off-line using MYOLAB software (BTS Bioengineering, Italy) Piezoelectric force platform was used for measurement of three forces along the three orthogonal axes (F_x, F_y, and F_z) and three moments around the three axes — M_x, M_y, and M_z, thus ascertaining centre of pressure displacement parameters such as mediolateral CoP (ML CoP),

Figure 1. A volunteer performing MMH tasks on force platform during simulated experimentation set up

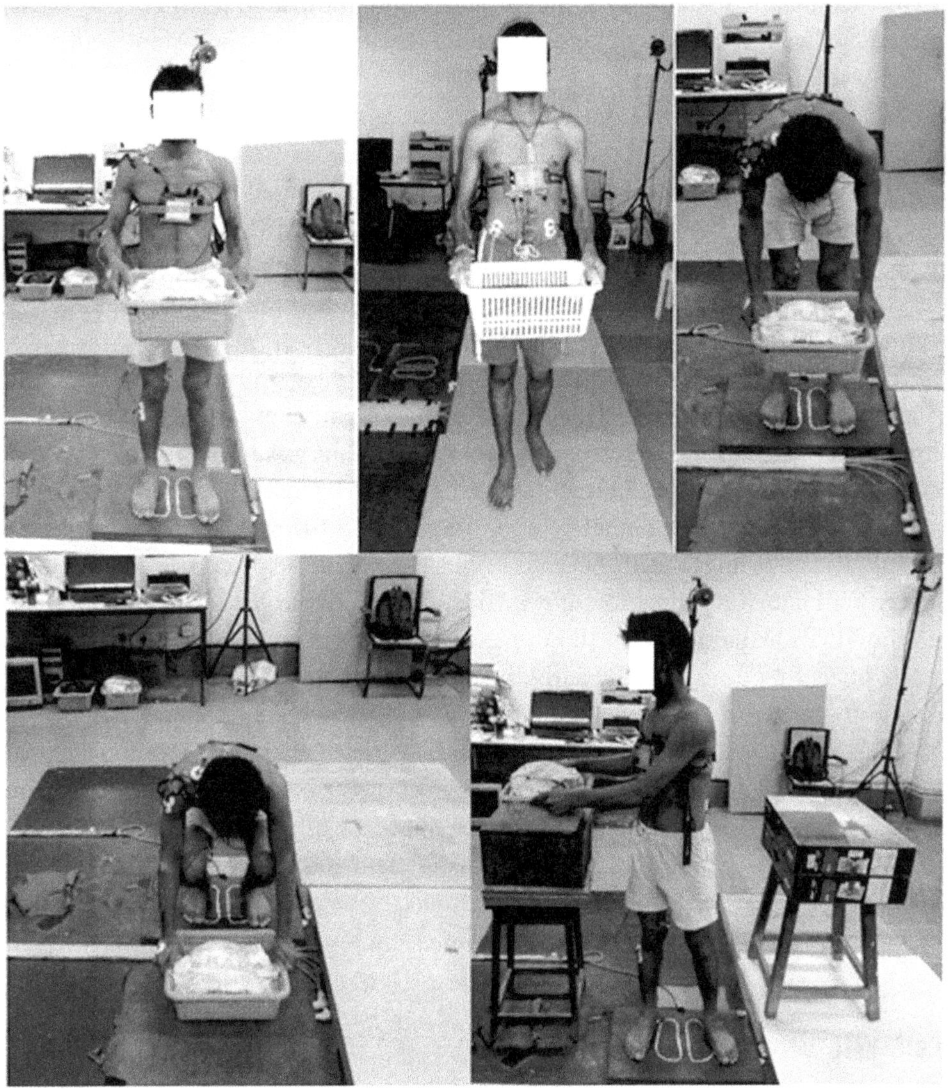

anterio-posterior CoP (AP CoP), radius of the stabilogram and speed of CoP displacement. Postural stability effects were evaluated using SWAY software.

In a designed research protocol, static loads of three different grades (4 kg, 8 kg and 12 kg) were lifted and lowered by the volunteers as a combined activity from ground to knee, waist and chest height at each three grades of load. The twisting-turning and holding activity was performed at iliocristale height. Both lifting-lowering and twisting-turning MMH task were performed for each three grades of load at standard frequency for continuous 10 min of sEMG recording. Holding activity was monitored while performing to hold each particular load for maximum voluntary duration.

Results revealed that the RMS values of muscles increased with increase in load from 4 to 8 to 12 kg. However, the trend was insignificant may be due to rest pause given between each trail. When the load was increased to thrice of the initial value (4 kg to 12 kg) significant influence was found on upper extremity muscles. Similar trend was not observed when load increased to twice of the initial value. Study also explained that increase in level (height) of handling the load from knee to waist to chest for each three grades of load, the RMS values of deltoid, rectus femoris and semitendinosus hamstring muscle also increased.

It was noted that median frequency (MDF) values significantly dropped as load level increased. Further, increase in load holding time demonstrated in decreased MDF values of the muscles. The decreasing trend of MDF values starts earlier with higher magnitude load as compared to lower one indicates muscles became fatigued earlier with higher grade of load suggesting any MMH holding activity in endurance would manifest in fatiguing nature of muscles. The response pattern showed that overloading of muscles leading to fatigue and/or injuries can be avoided by selection of appropriate magnitude of load with rest pause i.e. ergonomically designed work-rest schedule.

Interaction of multiple conditions and type of task performed has significant influence on stabilometric parameters included in the study. ML CoP and AP CoP have significant influences on all the MMH tasks with each three grades of load. The relative displacement of CoP was found higher in anterio-posterior direction as compared to medio-lateral direction during all MMH tasks. Carrying and holding tasks did not influence the CoP displacement parameters significantly. Twisting-turning task because of its nature of movement significantly influenced the anterio-posterior CoP displacement. Conversely, as lifting has been done from the forward direction, it significantly influenced the medio-lateral displacement of CoP. As both the MMH task influenced stabilometric parameters in characteristic manner, it indicated relative postural instability during MMH activities.

The study summarized that any MMH activity that involves frequent manipulation of load combined with change of handling level in endurance would manifest in the fatiguing nature of muscles and ultimately result in possibility of injuries. However, proper rest pause between work bouts would alleviate the possibility of injuries to some extent as well as enhance work performance. MMH tasks are also influenced the stabilometric parameters in characteristic manner, indicating relative postural instability during MMH activities. The incorporation of ergonomic principles of work-rest schedule design and limits of safe handling of weights would save the workers in long run.

CASE STUDY-II

Another study was carried out to quantify the human hand finger grasping and force exertion while doing manual drilling and screw-driving activities. The excerpts from the study is presented below as a case.

Forceful grasping, force exertion and prolonged activities, in combination, are common in day-to-day work life. Determination of hand-arm-shoulder force would elucidate the muscular capabilities of workers as well as provide an acceptable limit of operational force, restricting fatigue and consecutive injury at workplaces. Compared to hand-operated controls fixed in a static/dynamic machine, tools with one handle e.g., screw-drivers, drills etc. are usually held and moved in a power grip, requiring more of hand and shoulder muscle movement and less finger muscle movement/motion. In addition, wide-ranging straight translation motions and rotational motions are executed by hand-arm-shoulder system with less precision, but more force (Strasser, 2007). The determination of human strength capabilities is an important consideration in the development of ergonomic guidelines for pre-employment screening of workers performing manual materials handling jobs (NIOSH, 1981). Hand grip torque for the preferred hand in isometric mode among Indian agricultural workers varied between 2-19 Nm (Gite et al. 2009). Depending on the intensity and repetitiveness of the operation, the acceptable limit of force varies providing a safe force limit, restricting fatigue at workplace.

A test setup of screw-drivers and drilling equipment were fabricated and attached with CSMI Humac Norm Isokinetic and rehabilitation system as shown in Figure 2. Two screw-driver handles of dimensions (10 cm X 12 cm; 8 cm X 10 cm) & one drill handle with handgrip breadth 110 mm is fabricated and considered for the study.

Isometric strength testing of the preferred hand in concentric as well as eccentric movement is being recorded at 0 Nm torque and (+35^{0}) (-25^{0}) virtual range of motion. Isokinetic strength testing is being carried out at 500 Nm torque and (+35^{0}) (-25^{0}) actual range of motion. Volunteers were tested for isometric, isokinetic exercises for short duration (7 Sec) as well as long duration (60 Sec) maximum voluntary force exertion. Physical assessment of muscular strength in both isometric and isokinetic modes provide the maximum capability of the muscles at work.

For isometric pulling and pushing operation, the torque generated depreciated with time. Further, torque generated by the volunteers in pulling operation was found higher (24.3±1.4 Nm) than that in the pushing mode (20.7±1.3 Nm), length of the lever being 0.3 m. This may be due to the distribution of the force in horizontal plane as well as on the direction of gravity during pushing mode (Figure 3).

Comparison with short and long duration experimentation show that the torque generated and held in pulling mode in 7 second experimentation was higher (18.2%) than in 60 second experimentation. For isometric experimentation with screw-drivers (8X10 cm and 10X12 cm grip), the strength generated by 8X10 cm grip is less than that of the 10X12 cm grip. Also, the strength depreciated with time for both the two prototypes (Figure 4).

Such study determines the hand-arm-shoulder force elucidating the muscular capabilities of workers. It is an important consideration in the development of ergonomic guidelines for pre-employment screening of workers performing manual materials handling jobs as well as provide an acceptable limit of operational force, restricting fatigue and consecutive injury at workplaces.

Figure 2. A test setup of screw-driver attached with dynamometer of HUMAC Norm System during laboratory experimentation

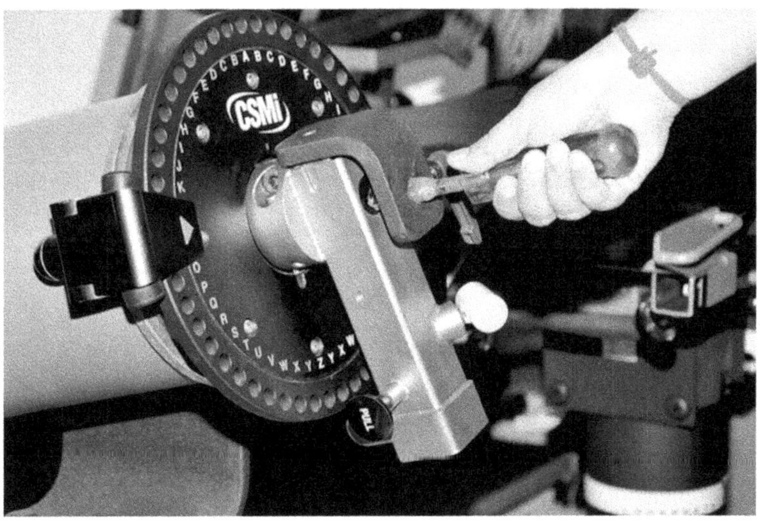

Figure 3. Pulling and pushing action during simulated drilling in three trials

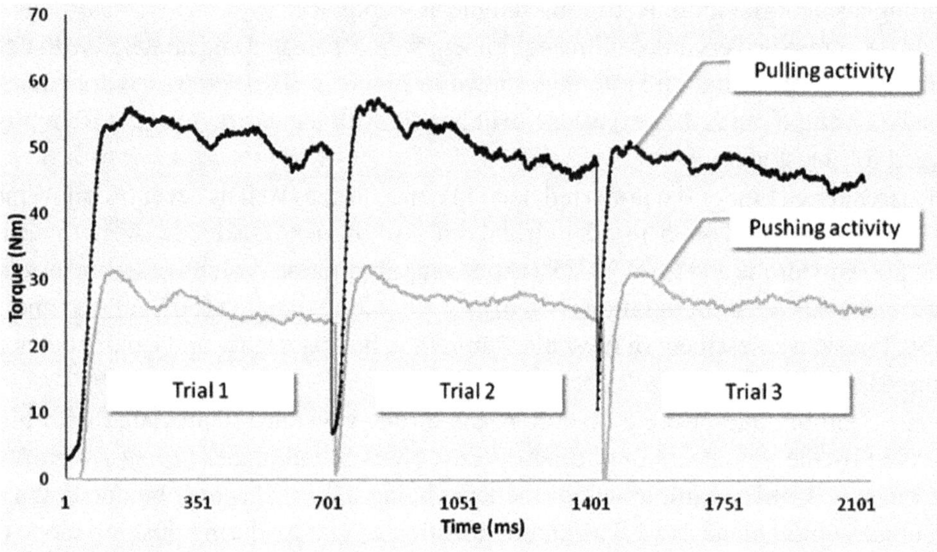

Figure 4. Concentric torque generated by two different screwdriver grips

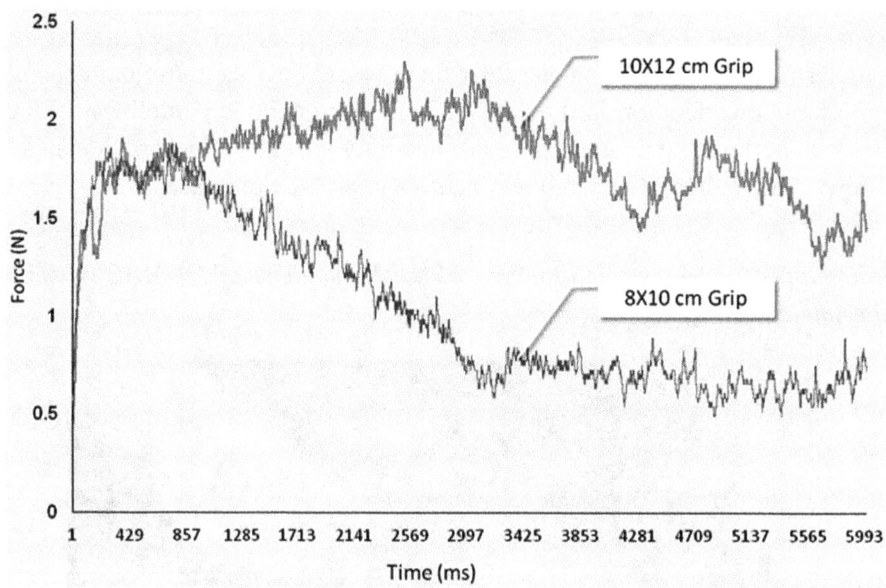

CONCLUSION

Confiscating the occupational health hazards at workplace is impossible in entirety, rather can be controlled. Engineering and administrative controls can substantively counter the probability of inadvertent incidents at workplace. However, the human component particularly the load limits, posture, duration of work i.e., the physical stress in causation of injuries, loss of productivity, absenteeism can be taken care of by biomechanics principles in close association with ergonomic inputs. This chapter has attempted to provide an overview of biomechanical hazards at workplace, with a focus on biomechanics instrumentation. In addressing the issues. Instrumentation in this field are complex, and need knowledge and expertise to gather data, analyze and interpret the results. Biomechanics research can aid in determining the cause of injury, helps to prevent future injuries by determining the safest method for performing a particular task. The goal towards increasing the productivity and decreasing the probability of accidents/injuries through judicious utilization of human resources can be achieved. Deep understanding of biomechanics can play a leading role in the design of work and workplaces that are injury free.

Having said that, acquiring the basic knowledge of biomechanics and mechanism of injury, occupational health professionals in combination with ergonomists can address the identification, assessment, evaluation and control of risks associated with manual efforts at workplaces. Participatory ergonomics can be helpful to develop and evaluate effective control measures in complex vulnerable situations at the work front.

REFERENCES

Aström, K. J., & Murray, R. M. (2010). *Feedback systems: An introduction for scientists and engineers*. Princeton, NJ: Princeton university press.

Bhattacharya, A. (2014). Costs of occupational musculoskeletal disorders (MSDs) in the United States. *International Journal of Industrial Ergonomics*, *44*(3), 448–454. doi:10.1016/j.ergon.2014.01.008

Castelein, B., Cagnie, B., Parlevliet, T., Danneels, L., & Cools, A. (2015). Optimal normalization tests for muscle activation of the levator scapulae, pectoralis minor, and rhomboid major: An electromyography study using maximum voluntary isometric contractions. *Archives of Physical Medicine and Rehabilitation*, *96*(10), 1820–1827. doi:10.1016/j.apmr.2015.06.004 PMID:26119465

Chao, E. Y. (2003). Graphic-based musculoskeletal model for biomechanical analyses and animation. *Medical Engineering & Physics*, *25*(3), 201–212. doi:10.1016/S1350-4533(02)00181-9 PMID:12589718

Cifrek, M., Medved, V., Tonković, S., & Ostojić, S. (2009). Surface EMG based muscle fatigue evaluation in biomechanics. *Clinical Biomechanics (Bristol, Avon)*, *24*(4), 327–340. doi:10.1016/j.clinbiomech.2009.01.010 PMID:19285766

Dale, A. M., Addison, L., Lester, J., Kaskutas, V., & Evanoff, B. (2014). Weak grip strength does not predict upper extremity musculoskeletal symptoms or injuries among new workers. *Journal of Occupational Rehabilitation*, *24*(2), 325–331. doi:10.100710926-013-9460-y PMID:23857165

Deros, B., Daruis, B., & Ismail, A. (2010). Work-related musculoskeletal disorders among workers' performing manual material handling work in an automotive manufacturing company. *American Journal of Applied Sciences*, *7*(8), 1087–1092. doi:10.3844/ajassp.2010.1087.1092

Ferrari, A., Benedetti, M. G., Pavan, E., Frigo, C., Bettinelli, D., Rabuffetti, M., ... Leardini, A. (2008). Quantitative comparison of five current protocols in gait analysis. *Gait & Posture*, *28*(2), 207–216. doi:10.1016/j.gaitpost.2007.11.009 PMID:18206374

Gite, L. P., Majumder, J., Mehta, C. R., & Khadatkar, A. (2009). *Anthropometric and strength data of Indian agricultural workers for Farm equipment design*. Bhopal, India: Central Institute of Agricultural Engineering.

Herman, D. C., Onate, J. A., Weinhold, P. S., Guskiewicz, K. M., Garrett, W. E., Yu, B., & Padua, D. A. (2009). The effects of feedback with and without strength training on lower extremity biomechanics. *The American Journal of Sports Medicine*, *37*(7), 1301–1308. doi:10.1177/0363546509332253 PMID:19299530

Hibbs, A. E., Thompson, K. G., French, D. N., Hodgson, D., & Spears, I. R. (2011). Peak and average rectified EMG measures: Which method of data reduction should be used for assessing core training exercises? *Journal of Electromyography and Kinesiology*, *21*(1), 102–111. doi:10.1016/j.jelekin.2010.06.001 PMID:20655245

Jenkins, N., Smith, G., Stewart, S., & Kamphuis, C. (2016). Pre-employment physical capacity testing as a predictor for musculoskeletal injury in paramedics: A review of the literature. *Work (Reading, Mass.)*, *55*(3), 565–575. doi:10.3233/WOR-162422 PMID:27792024

Keyserling, W. M. (2000). Workplace risk factors and occupational musculoskeletal disorders, Part 2: A review of biomechanical and psychophysical research on risk factors associated with upper extremity disorders. *AIHAJ-American Industrial Hygiene Association*, *61*(2), 231–243. doi:10.1080/15298660008984532 PMID:10782195

Kotadiya, S., Majumder, J., & Nag, A. (2013). *Muscular loading during manual material handling tasks*. National Institute of Occupational health, Annual Report 2012-13. Ahmedabad, India.

Ku, P. X., Osman, N. A., Yusof, A., & Abas, W. W. (2012). Biomechanical evaluation of the relationship between postural control and body mass index. *Journal of Biomechanics*, *45*(9), 1638–1642. doi:10.1016/j.jbiomech.2012.03.029 PMID:22507349

Lee, Y., & Lee, M. (2008). SMS application using EMG signal of clenching teeth for e-health communication. *Telemedicine Journal and e-Health*, *14*(6), 593–597. doi:10.1089/tmj.2007.0098 PMID:18729760

Maiti, R. (2008). Workload assessment in building construction related activities in India. *Applied Ergonomics*, *39*(6), 754–765. doi:10.1016/j.apergo.2007.11.010 PMID:18206852

Marin, J., Blanco, T., & Marin, J. J. (2017). Research Lines to Improve Access to Health Instrumentation Design. *Procedia Computer Science*, *113*, 641–646. doi:10.1016/j.procs.2017.08.323

Mello, R., Oliveir, L., & Nada, J. (2007). Anticipation mechanism in body sway control and effect of muscle fatigue. *Journal of Electromyography and Kinesiology*, *17*(6), 739–746. doi:10.1016/j.jelekin.2006.08.011 PMID:17142060

Nag, P., Nag, A., Vyas, H., & Shah, P. (2014). Occupation, participation, inclusion, work role postural control in different load handling tasks. *Work (Reading, Mass.)*, *49*(4), 577–584. PMID:24004795

Nag, P. K., Vyas, H., Nag, A., & Pal, S. (2013). Postural stability of sitting women. *International Journal of Occupational Safety and Ergonomics, 19*(4), 583–595. doi:10.1080/10803548.2013.11077022 PMID:24321637

Nashner, L. M. (2014). Practical biomechanics and physiology of balance. In *Balance Function Assessment and Management* (pp. 431–449). San Diego, CA: Plural Publishing.

NIOSH. (1981). *Work practices guide for manual load lifting*. Cincinnati, OH: National Institute for Occupational Safety and Health.

Paillard, T. (2012). Effects of general and local fatigue on postural control: A review. *Neuroscience and Biobehavioral Reviews, 36*(1), 162–176. doi:10.1016/j.neubiorev.2011.05.009 PMID:21645543

Phinyomark, A., Phukpattaranont, P., & Limsakul, C. (2011). A review of control methods for electric power wheelchairs based on electromyography signals with special emphasis on pattern recognition. *IETE Technical Review, 28*(4), 316–326. doi:10.4103/0256-4602.83552

Ritzmann, R., Gollhofer, A., & Freyler, K. (2017). Posture and Locomotion. In *Sensory Motor and Behavioral Research in Space* (pp. 1–35). Cham, Switzerland: Springer. doi:10.1007/978-3-319-68201-3_1

Robertson, G., Caldwell, G., Hamill, J., Kamen, G., & Whittlesey, S. (2004). *Research methods in biomechanics, 2E*. Champaign, IL: Human Kinetics.

Sharma, R. (Ed.). (2012). Epidemiology of Musculoskeletal Conditions in India. New Delhi, India: Indian Council of Medical Research (ICMR).

Singh, R. P., Batish, A. G., & Singh, T. P. (2015). *Ergonomic Investigations of Asymmetrical Manual Lifting Tasks on Indian Male Workers* (Doctoral dissertation).

Strasser, H. (2007). *Assessment of the ergonomic quality of handheld tools and computer input devices*. Amsterdam: IOS Press.

Tiwari, P. S., Gite, L. P., Majumder, J., Pharade, S. C., & Singh, V. V. (2010). Push/pull strength of agricultural workers in Central India. *International Journal of Industrial Ergonomics, 40*(1), 1–7. doi:10.1016/j.ergon.2009.10.001

Van Der Beek, A. J., Dennerlein, J. T., Huysmans, M. A., Mathiassen, S. E., Burdorf, A., Van Mechelen, W., ... Van Der Molen, H. F. (2017). A research framework for the development and implementation of interventions preventing work-related musculoskeletal disorders. *Scandinavian Journal of Work, Environment & Health, 43*(6), 526–539. PMID:28945263

Veerapen, K., Wigley, R. D., & Valkenburg, H. (2007). Musculoskeletal pain in Malaysia: A COPCORD survey. *The Journal of Rheumatology, 34*(1), 207–213. PMID:17216688

Visser, J. E., Carpenter, M. G., van der Kooij, H., & Bloem, B. R. (2008). The clinical utility of posturography. *Clinical Neurophysiology, 119*(11), 2424–2436. doi:10.1016/j.clinph.2008.07.220 PMID:18789756

Wardoyo, S., Hutajulu, P. T., & Togibasa, O. (2016). A Development of Force Plate for Biomechanics Analysis of Standing and Walking. *Journal of Physics: Conference Series*, *739*(1), 012118. doi:10.1088/1742-6596/739/1/012118

Winter, D. A. (2009). *Biomechanics and Motor Control of Human Movement*. Hoboken, NJ: Wiley. doi:10.1002/9780470549148

Wong, C., Zhang, Z. Q., Lo, B., & Yang, G. Z. (2015). Wearable sensing for solid biomechanics: A review. *IEEE Sensors Journal*, *15*(5), 2747–2760.

Yasobant, S., & Rajkumar, P. (2014). Work-related musculoskeletal disorders among health care professionals: A cross-sectional assessment of risk factors in a tertiary hospital, India. *Indian Journal of Occupational and Environmental Medicine*, *18*(2), 75–81. doi:10.4103/0019-5278.146896 PMID:25568602

Chapter 5
Devices for Controlled Release Advancements and Effectiveness

Arvind Kumar Singh Chandel
Central Salt and Marine Chemicals Research Institute, India

ABSTRACT

The term control release means the release of the molecules from any reservoir in very precise and constant amounts and following zero-order or near-to-zero-order release kinetics. This type of formulation and device has a huge market over the medical world. The basic foundation of sustained release drug delivery system enhances the biopharmaceutical and pharmacodynamics pharmacokinetic properties of a drug in such a way that its usefulness is exploited, side-effects are reduced, and cure of the disease is attained easily. The international controlled-release drug delivery technology market has been divided on the basis of technology, application, release mechanism, and geography. This chapter describes these topics: metered dose inhalers, transdermal and ocular patches, drug eluting stents, activation-modulated drug delivery systems, polymer coating systems microelectromechanical technology, implants, micro reservoir partition controlled drug delivery systems, hydrophilic polymer matrix systems, targeted delivery, enzyme activated device.

1. INTRODUCTION

The conventional drug delivery systems and devices having numerous problems such as incorrect dosing, limited drug solubility, limited drug permeability, poor drug distribution, overdose, short circulating time, poor selectivity, more side effects, toxicity and unfavourable pharmacodynamics/pharmacokinetics. Over these problems, the considerable research has directed in the last twenty years toward the development of advanced devices and more efficient drug delivery systems. (Jiang, W., Kim, B.Y., Rutka, J.T. and Chan, W.C., 2007; Ferrari, M. and Torchilin, V., 2008; Hoffman, A.S., 2008).

Almost 90% of drugs are hydrophobic which is currently in use, which unable to dissolve in the blood stream, and this phenomenon reduces drugs pharmacological efficiency. Such type of drug hav-

DOI: 10.4018/978-1-5225-4969-7.ch005

ing the challenging route of delivery (Murthy, C.D., Sunkara, G. and Young, D., 2007; Wolinsky, J.B., Colson, Y.L. and Grinstaff, M.W., 2012). The other hand, some therapeutics and bioactive agents such as enzymes, proteins, nucleic acids, and genes administered through intravenous or oral routes can be easily degraded, and loss their activity by various factors gastric HCL and first pass metabolism and that molecules are unable to show pharmacodynamics (Mainardes, R.M. and Silva, L.P., 2004; Kwon, G.S. and Okano, T.,1996; Brocchini, S., James, K., Tangpasuthadol, V. and Kohn, J.,1998). The Local and targeted drug delivery systems are considered a favourable alternative to systemic routes and conventional drug delivery system to address many of these challenges (Wolinsky, J.B., Colson, Y.L. and Grinstaff, M.W., 2012; Mainardes, R.M. and Silva, L.P.,2004; Kwon, G.S. and Okano, T., 1996; Brocchini, S., James, K., Tangpasuthadol, V. and Kohn, J., 1998; Florence, A.T. and Siepmann, J., 2009). Local and targeted drug delivery at the earlier stages of development were made of biodegradable implants based on various biomaterials such as, silk, chitosan, collagen, fibrin hyaluronic acid, and poly(glycolic acid), poly(methyl methacrylate) (PMMA), poly(lactic acid) (PLA), (PLGA) matrices, hydroxyapatite (HAP), ceramics and injectable calcium phosphate cements. They have been used for the delivery of bioactive agents in bone repair or tissue engineering (Florence, 2009). the effectiveness of drug therapy depends on the accessibility of the therapeutics concentrations at the site of affected body part. Localised drug Controlled and drug delivery systems deliver spatial and temporal control of drug release and provide significant advantages over burst release, and other drawbacks of conventional delivery systems by reducing fluctuations in plasma concentrations of drug, pharmacodynamics and lowering the dose-dependent toxicity. The Ideal conditions for a controlled, localised drug delivery system include, the ability to both deliver the drug to a target tissue and at a rate that matches the desired concentration at the target site. For various disease applications, the delivery of therapeutic concentrations on an on-demand basis would be of tremendous benefit (Pirmoradi, F.N., Jackson, J.K., Burt, H.M. and Chiao, M., 2011). To date, a huge number of localised controlled release systems for drug delivery have been developed, most of which are based on polymers with different physical or chemical characteristics (Narasimhan, B. and Langer, R, 1997). The release of the drug that is triggered by various external factors such as pH or temperature, osmotic pressure, radiation, vibration magnetic etc. (ma, S., Nijdam, A.J., Sinha, P.M., Walczak, R.J., Liu, X., Cheng, M.M. and Ferrari, M., 2006). These are the passively controlled drug delivery systems that are mostly rely on to deliver the drug payload slowly over a certain period of time and offer limited dosing flexibility and poor control over onset of release and release lifetime. Besides, difficulties in accomplishing controlled release of drugs using biodegradable polymers have been reported, including uncontrolled burst release of drugs in the first days of implantation, followed by non-zero order release kinetics (Wood, K.C., Zacharia, N.S., Schmidt, D.J., Wrightman, S.N., Andaya, B.J. and Hammond, P.T., 2008; Sharma, S., Nijdam, A.J., Sinha, P.M., Walczak, R.J., Liu, X., Cheng, M.M. and Ferrari, M., 2006). Some studies show that polymeric drug delivery systems that are responsive to external stimuli such as electric fields (Kost, J. and Langer, R., 2012) or magnetic fields8 have the advantage of providing on-demand drug release compared to passive degradation-based polymeric delivery system (Choi, B., Loh, X.J., Tan, A., Loh, C.K., Ye, E., Joo, M.K. and Jeong, B., 2015; Santini, J.T., Cima, M.J. and Langer, R., 1999). Other triggerable materials that are sensitive to visible light, near-infrared light, and ultrasound have been proposed for drug delivery (Narasimhan et al, 1997). These drug delivery systems can actively control the time of release but the control of delivery rate remains a major challenge. Furthermore, other issues (e.g. the presence of enzymes that increase the polymer degradation rate) may affect the functionality of polymeric systems. Microelectromechanical Systems (MEMS) technology offers the potential to develop drug delivery devices with accurate control of drug release which are typically suitable for implantation. Miniature reservoirs loaded with drug and sealed with thin film material have been introduced by Santini et al. (1999).

Considerable developments have been made in the field of drug delivery technology over the last two decades, subsequent in many inventions in the field of drug delivery and medicine (Choi, 2015). However, important classes of drugs have yet to benefit from these technological successes. One of the major necessities for implantable and other smart drug delivery devices is controlled release of therapeutic agents, especially biological molecules, as a delivery over a prolonged period of time. The aim here is to accomplish a continuous drug release profile consistent with zero-order kinetics where the concentration of the drug in blood remains constant throughout the delivery period (Santini, 1999). The Injected drugs have first-order kinetics, with initial high concentration in blood (above the therapeutic range), followed by an exponential decrease. Toxicity occurs when the peak concentration is above the therapeutic range, although efficacy of the drug diminishes as the drug concentration falls below this range. Consequently, the therapeutic advantages of continuous release of the drug by implantable delivery devices are important decreased adverse reactions by reducing the peak levels, expectable and extended duration of action, reduced inconvenience of frequent dosing, and so improved patient compliance (Narasimhan et al, 1997). Different technologies have been established to achieve this goal. However, they suffer from major disadvantages. Degradable polymer implants shows an initial 'burst effect' prior to sustained release and are typically not as effective in controlling release rates of small molecules (Wood et al, 2008). Implantable devices with percutaneous components such as ambulatory peritoneal dialysis, catheters, intravenous catheters, and orthopaedic implants are often associated with different failure modes. Infection, marsupialization, permigration, and avulsion are common occurrences (Sharma et al, 2006). Osmotic pumps lack the capabilities of electronic integration for achieving higher levels of functionality (i.e. pre-programming and remote activation) and are limited with respect to the type of drug they can deliver. Silicon microfabrication technology can permit the creation of drug delivery devices that possess a combination of structural, electronic, and mechanical features that may overcome some of these challenges (Narasimhan et al, 1997; Sharma et al, 2006; Wood et al, 2006; Kost et al, 2012; Choi et al, 2015).

2. PULMONARY DRUG DELIVERY

Research in the area of pulmonary drug delivery has gathered momentum in the last several years, with increased interest in using the lung as a means of delivering drugs systemically. Advances in device technology have led to the development of more efficient delivery systems capable of delivering larger doses and finer particles into the lung. As more efficient pulmonary delivery devices and sophisticated formulations become available, physicians and health professionals will have a choice of a wide variety of device and formulation combinations that will target specific cells or regions of the lung, avoid the lung's clearance mechanisms and be retained within the lung for longer periods (Labiris, N.R. and Dolovich, M.B, 2003).

The pulmonary drug delivery has in lime light since the last several years, with increased attention in using the lung for the delivering site of therapeutics systemically. Advances in device technology have led to the development of more efficient delivery systems capable of delivering high doses and finer particles into the lung. As more efficient pulmonary delivery devices and sophisticated formulations become accessible, physicians and health professionals will have a choice of a wide variety of device and formulation combinations that will target specific cells receptors or areas of the lung, avoid the lung's clearance mechanisms and be retained within the lung for longer periods (Barnes, P.J., Rodger, I.W. and Thomson, N.C. 1998; Ekroos, H., 2008).

2.1 Pulmonary Delivery Devices

The lungs are a route of drug administration since several centuries. The beginning of inhaled therapies can be outlined back 4000 years ago to India; people use to smoke the powdered leaves of the Atropa belladonna plant to use as suppressing the cough problem. In the 19th centuries, the asthmatic patients smoked asthma cigarettes that contain stramonium powder mixed with tobacco to treat the symptoms of their disease. The development of recent inhalation devices can divide into three different groups are Nebulizers Pressurized metered dose Compact inhalers and Dry powder inhalers, the modification of the nebulizer and the development of two types of compact portable devices, the metered-dose inhaler (MDI) and the dry powder inhaler (DPI) (Ekroos, H., 2008; Stockmann, C., Roberts, J.K., Yellepeddi, V.K. and Sherwin, C.M., 2015).

2.1.1 Nebulizers

The nebulizers are used for many years to treat asthma and other respiratory related diseases. Nebulizer are basically two types, jet and ultrasonic nebulizers. The jet nebulizer functions on the basis of Bernoulli principle by which compressed gas (air or oxygen) passes through a narrow orifice creating an area of low pressure at the outlet of the adjacent liquid feed tube. This results in drug solution being drawn up from the fluid reservoir and shattered into droplets in the gas stream. The ultrasonic nebulizer uses a piezoelectric crystal vibrating at a high frequency (usually 1–3 MHz) to generate a fountain of liquid in the nebulizer chamber; the higher the frequency, produces the smaller the droplets. (Preedy, E.C. and Prokopovich, P., 2013).

The deposition characteristics and efficacy of an aerosol in lungs depend mainly on the size the particle. Usually, the smaller the particle, the more chance of peripheral penetration and retention. Though, for very fine particles size below 0.5 μm in diameter not easily precipitated and were exhaled. The Task Group In 1966 concerned on Lung Dynamics, mainly with the toxic of inhalation of environmental pollutants, proposed a model for deposition of particles in the lungs system, and concluded that the, particles size >10 μm in diameter are most probable to deposit in the mouth and throat, and for those of 5–10 μm diameter a transition from mouth to airway deposition take place, and particles lesser than 5 μm in diameter deposit more frequently in the inferior airways and are appropriate for various pharmaceutical aerosols (Kwatra, S., Taneja, G. and Nasa, N., 2012).

2.1.2 Metered-Dose Inhalers

The Metered-dose inhalers was a revolutionary invention because of this overcame the problems of the hand-bulb nebulizer, the aerosol is majorly in use in the as the portable outpatient inhalation device today. The Metered-dose inhalers emit a drug aerosol driven force given by various propellants, such as chlorofluorocarbons and now days hydrofluoroalkanes through a nozzle at high velocity (>30 m s-1).

Figure 1. A diagrammatic representation of metered dose inhaler

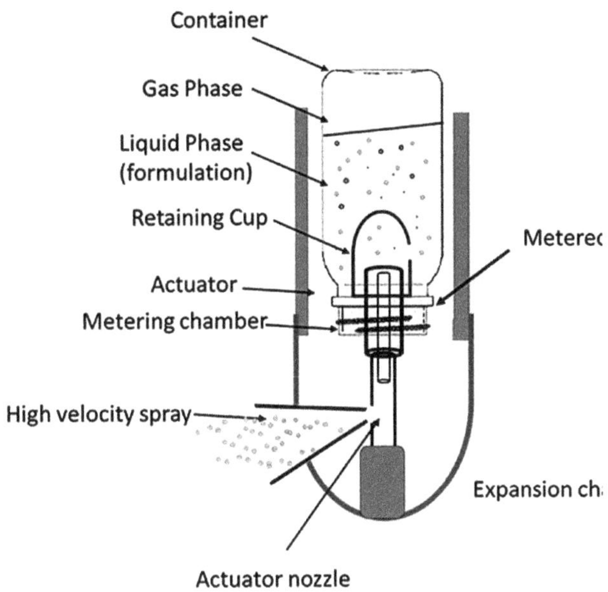

Metered-dose inhalers deliver only a small fraction of the drug dose to the lung. Typically, only 10–20% of the emitted dose is deposited in the lung (Jewett, W.R. and Williams III, R.C, 2011). The high velocity and large particle size of the spray cause almost 50–80% of the drug aerosol to impact in the oropharyngeal region (Jewett et al, 2011). Hand–mouth discoordination is another obstacle in the optimal use of the Metered-dose inhalers. Crompton and colleagues (Weinstein, L.A., Richards, F.M., Laun, D.A. and Middleton Jr, D.T., 1999). The delivery efficiency of an MDI depend on a patient's breathing pattern, inspiratory flow rate and hand–mouth co-ordination.

2.1.3 Dry Powder Inhalers

Dry powder inhalers eliminate the difficulties associated with the MDI. Wide attention in this delivery system has emanated from the urgency to eliminate CFC-containing MDIs. There is a wide variety of Dry powder inhalers devices in the current market, from single-dose devices loaded by the patient (e.g. Aerolizer, Rotahaler) to multiunit dose devices delivered in a blister pack (e.g. Diskhaler), multiple unit doses wrapped in blisters on a strip which transports through the inhaler (e.g. Diskus) or reservoir- type (bulk powder) systems (e.g. Turbuhaler). Lung deposition varies among the different Dry powder inhalers. Approximately 12–40% of the discharged dose is delivered to the lungs with 20–25% of the drug being retained within the device (Weinstein et al, 1999). Poor drug deposition with Dry powder inhalers can be ascribed to inefficient deaggregation of the fine drug particles from coarser carrier lactose particles or drug pellets. Slow IFR, high humidity and rapid, large changes in temperature are known to effect drug deaggregation and hence the efficiency of pulmonary drug delivery with dry powder inhalers (Vaghefi et al, 1999). With most Dry powder inhalers, drug delivery to the lungs is augmented by fast inhalation. For example, Borgstrom and colleagues (Vaghefi et al, 1999) demonstrated that improves the IFR from 35 min-1 to 60 min-1 through the Turbuhaler™ improved the total lung dose of terbutaline from 14.8% of nominal dose to 27.7%.

2.2 Inhaled Drug Formulations

Different drugs formulation plays a significant role in producing an effective inhalable medication it must be competently delivered into the lungs, to the appropriate site of action and remain in the lungs until the desired pharmacological effect occurs at the targeted site (Weinstein et al, 2001).

2.2.1 Lactose Carrier Systems

Lactose carrier required when the drug particles are requisite for deposition in the lung, the surface electric forces associated with the drug particles exceed the gravitational force acting upon them, subsequent in the growth cohesive poor flow rate powders that are hindering the formulation process (Jewett et al, 2001). Poor flow rate problem can be overcome with a diluent, and the drug is blended with a coarse carrier system (30–100 mm), such as lactose or other compatible carrier. Present market having dry powder inhalers contain either the pure drug alone or mixed with a bulk carrier, usually lactose (a-lactose monohydrate). Lactose is one of the permissible as carriers by the Food and Drug Administration. Lactose has good safety and compatibility profile and improves the flow properties of the various formulation necessary for reproducible filling and promoting dosing precision.

2.2.2 Liposomes

The sustained release from of a therapeutic aerosol can prolong the retention of an administered drug in the air passage or alveolar region, decrease the risk of adverse effects by subsiding its absorption rate systemically and increase patient compliance by minimising dosing frequency. A sustained- release formulation must escape the clearance mechanisms of the lung, by the mucociliary escalator of the conducting air passage and macrophages in the alveolar region. The liposomes, as a pulmonary drug delivery carrier, have been studied for several years and used as a means of transporting phospholipids to the alveolar surface for treatment of infant respiratory distress syndrome. Recently, researchers have been considered as a vehicle for sustained release dosages form in the treatment of respiratory disease, gene therapy and as a technique of delivering therapeutic molecule to the alveolar surface for the treatment of systemic diseases conditions (Thomas, D.A., Myers, M.A., Wichert, B., Schreier, H. and Gonzalez-Rothi, R.J., 1991).

Liposomes can be formed by the variety of phospholipids from various natural sources that are similar to endogenous to the lungs and that having either no charge or negative or positive charges on the surface (Thomas et al, 1991). They contain an aqueous part entrapped by one or more bilayers of natural or synthetic lipids with or without cholesterol moiety. They possess either as a single lipid bilayer sphere (unilamellar) or as a multilayer vesicle (multilamellar). They were having the capacity of encapsulating a variety of therapeutic agents with a wide range of lipophilicities. Hydrophobic drugs, such as corticosteroids, intercalate in the lipid bilayers, while others interact with the bilayer interface. Hydrophilic drugs, such as 5- fluorouracil partition in the aqueous spaces. Drugs with moderate solubility are poorly retained in liposomes. However, when the drugs are weak bases or weak acids the pH and chemical composition of the internal aqueous compartments can be manipulated as per need so that the drug concentrates in the interior part of the liposomes, resulting in a high degree of retention can be achieve (Thomas et al, 1991).

2.2.3 Large Porous Particles

MDI and DPI delivery systems. These particles can be prepared by of using polymeric or nonpolymeric excipients, by solvent evaporation as well as spray-drying techniques (Jewett et al, 2001). Pulmospheres™ are made of by phosphatidylcholine, the primary component of human lung surfactant. The formulation process is in a two-step.In the primary step, an oil-in-water emulsion is prepared by using oils, such as perfluoroctyl ethane or perflubron (Jewett, 2001). The oil phase serves as a 'blowing agent' all through the spray drying step, retarding shrinkage of drop lets while concurrently creating pores on the particle surface. The second step is the spray drying of the emulsion. Traditional medicinal powders consist of particles with a mass density of 1 ± 0.5 g cm-3 and mean geometric diameters of < 5 mm to exploit peripheral deposition. Pulmospheres™ are lighter and larger than the typical dry powder particles with a mass density of around 0.4 g cm-3 and geometric diameter of >5 mm. By virtue of their hollow and porous features, Pulmospheres™ give rise to smaller aerodynamic diameters than their geometric diameter. Because of their low mass and, density large size, the particles can aerosolize more competently (less aggregation) than smaller nonporous particles, resulting in more respirable fractions of the product. Cromolyn Pulmospheres™ have a respirable fraction (< 5 mm) of 68% compared with 24% with micronized cromolyn particles (Intal) Jewett et al, 2001; Weinstein et al, 1999). An increase in respirable fraction results in an increase in peripheral deposition and thus a lower the dose requirement to attain the same therapeutic effect. A decrease in oropharyngeal deposition of Pulmospheres™ also decreases the risk of local side-effects.

3. MAGNETICALLY CONTROLLED MEMS DEVICE FOR DRUG DELIVERY

A new kind of aerosol formulation is the large porous hollow particles, named Pulmospheres. They have very low particle densities, excellent dispersibility and also can be used in both MiMDI and DPI delivery systems (Pirmoradi, F.N., Jackson, J.K., Burt, H.M. and Chiao, M., 2011). These particles can be prepared by of using polymeric or nonpolymeric excipients, by solvent evaporation as well as spray-drying techniques. Pulmospheres™ are made of by phosphatidylcholine, the primary component of human lung surfactant. The formulation process is in a two-step.In the initial step, an oil-in-water emulsion is prepared by using oils, such as perfluorooctyl ethane or perflubron (Primoradi et al, 2011). The blowing agent (oil) all through the spray drying step, reducing shrinkage of droplets while concurrently creating pores on the particle surface. The second phase is the spray drying of the emulsion. Traditional medicinal powders consist of particles with a mass density of 1 ± 0.5 g cm-3 and mean geometric diameters of < 5 mm to exploit peripheral deposition. Pulmospheres™ are lighter and larger than the typical dry powder particles with a mass density of around 0.4 g cm-3 and geometric diameter of >5 mm. Under their hollow and porous features, Pulmospheres™ give rise to smaller aerodynamic diameters than their geometric diameter. Because of their low mass and, large density size, the particles can aerosolize more competently (less aggregation) than smaller nonporous particles, resulting in more respirable fractions of the product. Cromolyn Pulmospheres™ have a respirable fraction (< 5 mm) of 68% compared with 24% of micronized cromolyn particles (Intal) (Li, Y., Shawgo, R.S., Tyler, B., Henderson, P.T., Vogel, J.S., Rosenberg, A., Storm, P.B., Langer, R., Brem, H. and Cima, M.J., 2004). An increase in t respirable

Figure 2. A diagrammatic representation of Micro-Electro Mechanical Systems

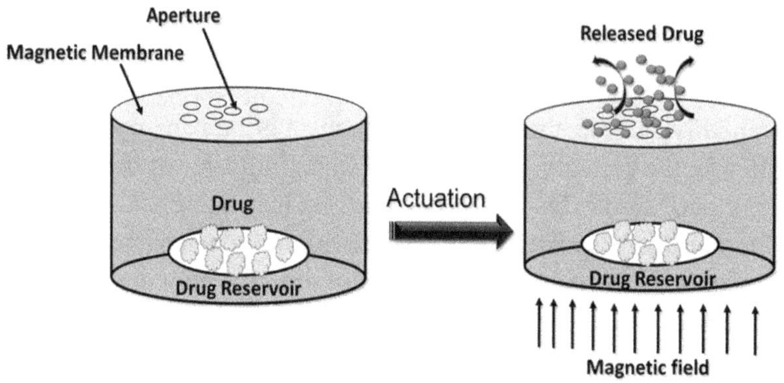

fraction results in an increase in peripheral deposition and thus a lower the dose required to attain the same therapeutic effect. A decrease in oropharyngeal deposition of Pulmospheres™ also reduces the risk of local side-effects (Li et al, 2004; Primoradi et al, 2011).

3.1 Working Principle

The device consists of a reservoir that contains drug and sealed with an elastic magnetic membrane with a laser-drilled aperture (100 100 mm^2). During actuation, the force generated by an external magnetic field causes the membrane to deform and build up pressure inside the reservoir to push the drug out, analogous to squeezing water out of a flexible bottle. The amount and timing of drug delivery can be controlled by adjusting different actuation parameters such as the number of actuation and the strength of the external magnetic field. On-demand actuation of the device by application of a magnetic field determines the time of drug release (Li et al, 2004; Primoradi et al, 2011).

4. REDOX RESPONSIVE CONTROLLED DELIVERY SYSTEM

Redox conditions present a promising stimuli for controlled delivery applications owing to the significantly different redox states between extracellular and intracellular spaces. It is well-known that the glutathione (GSH) level in intracellular spaces is 100–1000-fold higher than that in blood circulation and extracellular milieu. Therefore, these polymeric therapeutic Nano carriers are stable in blood circulation and extracellular milieu, however, when they accumulate in targeted sites and internalised by cells, these polymeric Nano systems will be disassembled and release their cargo. To date, a series of redox-responsive Nano systems including redox-responsive copolymers, Nano capsules, branched polymers, biodegradable polymers and redox-responsive poly (amino acid)s have been developed (Giri, S., Trewyn, B.G., Stellmaker, M.P. and Lin, V.S.Y., 2005).

The criterion for redox-responsive polymeric systems is that the polymers can respond to reduction or oxidation stimuli. Therefore, redox-responsive systems can typically be divided into reduction-responsive systems and oxidation responsive systems. Herein, we will mainly focus on redox polymeric systems that can potentially respond to redox stimuli from biological systems. The fundamental principle for designing these redox-responsive polymeric nanosystems is the incorporation of redox-responsive units such as disulphide, diselenide or ditellurium bonds into these polymers. These bonds embedded in polymers will break when the polymers are internalised by cells. This will lead to the disassembly of the polymeric Nano systems in intracellular spaces, releasing the biologically active agents. Taking advantage of the redox-responsiveness, different redox-responsive therapeutic systems can be elegantly fabricated for the potential delivery of cargo on demand (Giri et al, 2005; Luo, Z., Cai, K., Hu, Y., Zhao, L., Liu, P., Duan, L. and Yang, W., 2011).

4.1 Types of Redox-Responsive Polymeric Nano therapeutic Systems

4.1.1 Redox-Responsive Copolymers

Given advantages such as good biocompatibility, water dispersibility and designability of structures, the encapsulation of hydrophobic drugs into copolymers with both hydrophobic and hydrophilic segments has extensively explored for therapeutic agent delivery. Due to their amphiphilicity, copolymers will self-assemble into different nanostructures with different morphologies and sizes based on the types of hydrophobic and hydrophilic segments adopted and the ratio of hydrophobic and hydrophilic segments. By incorporation of dynamic linkages such as disulphide bonds into these copolymers, redox-responsive polymeric Nano carriers can be fabricated. Alginate sodium is the sodium salt of alginic acid; an anionic natural polysaccharide distributed widely in the cell walls of brown seaweed, which is composed of homopolymeric blocks of (1-4)-linked glycoside. Alginate sodium has been demonstrated to be food- and skin-safe and has widely used across a range of industries, including textile printing, food and pharmaceuticals. In a recent report, Li and colleagues fabricated redox-responsive polymeric Nano carriers for controlled delivery of DOX. The redox-responsive polymeric Nano carriers were fabricated in a facile manner via covalent linking of the carboxyl groups of alginate and the amino groups of cystamine using an EDC/NHS reaction. The chemotherapeutic agent (DOX) was readily loaded into the redox-responsive nano gels through electrostatic interactions between the anionic alginate and cationic DOX. The DOX-loaded polymeric carriers could be quickly internalised by CAL-72 cells, leading to higher DOX intracellular accumulation and enhanced cell killing effects. Moreover, because the DOX was concentrated in the polymeric Nano carriers, the side effects of DOX to normal tissues could thus be avoided or at least reduced through the EPR effect or functionalization with targeting agents. Therefore, the DOX could be effectively internalised by cells and released from the carriers into the cytoplasm, owing to the high GSH concentration in intracellular spaces (Giri et al, 2005; Lou et al (A), 2011; Mura, S., Nicolas, J. and Couvreur, P., 2013; Luo, Z. Cai, K., Hu, Y., Zhao, L., Liu, P., Duan, L. and Yang, W., (B), 2011).

4.2 Redox-Responsive Polymeric Nano Capsules

Polymeric Nano capsules, or hollow polymer capsules of nanometre size, have recently attracted significant research attention for potential biomedical applications because of their large hollow space for encapsulation of guest molecules and multifunctional potential via surface design.196 Much research effort has been devoted to fabricating many polymeric Nano capsules through the template-directed layer by layer strategy, template free super molecular assembly, or the recently developed template-directed mussel-inspired strategy. Among these, the template-free super molecular assembly approach has attracted much attention recently, and many polymeric Nano capsules with different compositions and responsive behaviours such as electricity, CO_2 and redox responsiveness have emerged. For Nano capsules to be desirable for drug delivery applications, they should fulfil the following requirements: excellent biocompatibility, simple preparation, facile surface functionalization, low cost and responsiveness. In a recent report, Kim and colleagues designed redox-responsive polymeric Nano capsules through a template-free strategy that relied on the host–guest interactions between cucurbit uril (CB) and polyamines.201 Moreover, many other functional agents such as targeting ligands and imaging probes could be facilely incorporated into these polymer Nano capsules by linking them with polyamines. In this work, both redox responsive and non-redox-responsive polymeric Nano capsules could be facilely prepared via covalent linkage of CB with redox responsive (containing disulphide bonds) or non-redox-responsive Lou et al (A), 2011; Mura, S., Nicolas, J. and Couvreur, P., 2013; Luo, Z. Cai, K., Hu, Y., Zhao, L., Liu, P., Duan, L. and Yang, W., (B), 2011; Du, J. and O'Reilly, R.K., 2009).

4.3 Redox-Responsive Biodegradable Polymers

The biodegradability of biomaterials is very important for their biomedical applications. In particular, biodegradable drug delivery carriers can avoid the accumulation and toxicity of materials in living organisms. Over the past few decades, various biodegradable polymers including many polysaccharides (e.g. chitosan, starch, dextran and hyaluronic acid) and synthetic degradable polymers (e.g. polylactic acid (PLA), polycaprolactone (PCL) and polycarbonate) have been considered as candidates for drug delivery. Through the incorporation of stimuli-responsive linkages into these biodegradable polymers, drug delivery carriers with both responsiveness and biodegradability could be fabricated. Zhu et al. recently reported the preparation of polymeric drug delivery nanocarriers via a ''one-pot'' strategy, and examined the redox-responsive properties of these polymeric carriers. An amphiphilic triblock copolymer was synthesised via polycondensation of the hydroxyl group of PEG with the carboxyl group of DL-thiomalic acid to obtain poly(oligo(ethylene glycol) thiomalicate) (POEGTMA) with multiple pendant mercapto groups, and then its terminal hydroxyl groups further served as initiators for the ring-opening polymerization of 3-caprolactone. An amphiphilic copolymer, denoted PCL-*b*-POEGTMA-*b*-PCL, could thus be obtained. Due to the existence of biodegradable hydrophobic segments (PCL), the amphiphilic triblock copolymer could be readily self-assembled into spherical nanoparticles with a size of about 45 nm. After the therapeutic drug (PTX) had been loaded into these micelles, the size of the micelles increased to about 65 nm according to the TEM images. The increase in the size of the micelles could likely be ascribed to the loading of PTX, which would increase the hydrophobic nature of the micellar core. Moreover, the amphiphilic copolymer still kept its structure in dimethyl formamide (DMF), which could dissolve both the hydrophobic and the hydrophilic segments of the copolymers. The above results suggested that these micelles were perfectly cross-linked by disulphide bonds (Giri et al, 2005; Lou et al (A), 2011; Mura, S., Nicolas, J. and Couvreur, P., 2013; Luo, Z. Cai, K., Hu, Y., Zhao, L., Liu, P., Duan, L. and Yang, W., (B), 2011).

5. NON-GASSING ELECTRO-OSMOTIC PUMPS

A new conducting polymer electrodes for non-gassing electroosmotic pumps are developed. The work describes the application of a redox-conducting poly(hydroquinone/benzoquinone) electrode which was synthesised by cationic polymerization of benzoquinone and containing parotic ceramic frit membranes. Laboratory made electro-osmotic pump was tested with developed polymer electrodes by varying different membrane thickness, applied voltage and flow-opposing (stall) pressure. As expected, with decrease in membrane thickness, flow rate was observed to increase, and the maximum flux per unit applied voltage was ~30.3 μL.min−1.cm−2 .V−1. The maximum stall pressure (at zero flow rate) was~10.0 kPa at 3.0 V with a membrane of 1.5 mm thick; stall pressure increased with increase in applied voltage. The maximum value of thermodynamic efficiency obtained was 0.16%. The pump could be operated continuously at 1.5 V and 3.0 V with flow rates of 4.0 ± 1.0 and 14.0 ± 1.0 μL.min−1, respectively. Obtained performance results vindicate the novel attempt of developing conducting polymer for applications in microfluidic devices, such as insulin pumps used for diabetes management (Sachan, V.K., Singh, A.K., Jahan, K., Kumbar, S.G., Nagarale, R.K. and Bhattacharya, P.K., 2014).

6. STRETCH RESPONSIVE SKIN PATCH

The strain-triggered, device has been developed for drug delivery. The stimuli-responsive delivery system based on mechanical force provides the easy and straightforward way to spatiotemporally controlled delivery. Wearable, tensile strain triggered device and micro gel depots can be used as triggered drug-delivery device. By applying a tensile strain to the elastomer film, the release of drug from the micro depots is promoted due to the enlarged surface area for diffusion and Poisson's ratio-induced compression on the micro depots. Here, both pulsatile and sustained release can be achieved. Our work demonstrated that the tensile strain, applied to the stretchable device, facilitated the release of therapeutics from micro depots for anticancer and antibacterial treatments. Moreover, polymeric microneedles were further integrated with the stretch-responsive device for transcutaneous delivery of insulin and regulation of blood glucose levels of chemically induced type 1 diabetic mice (i, J., Yao, S., Ye, Y., Cui, Z., Yu, J., Ghosh, T.K., Zhu, Y. and Gu, Z., 2015).

Figure 3. A diagrammatic representation of stretch responsive patch

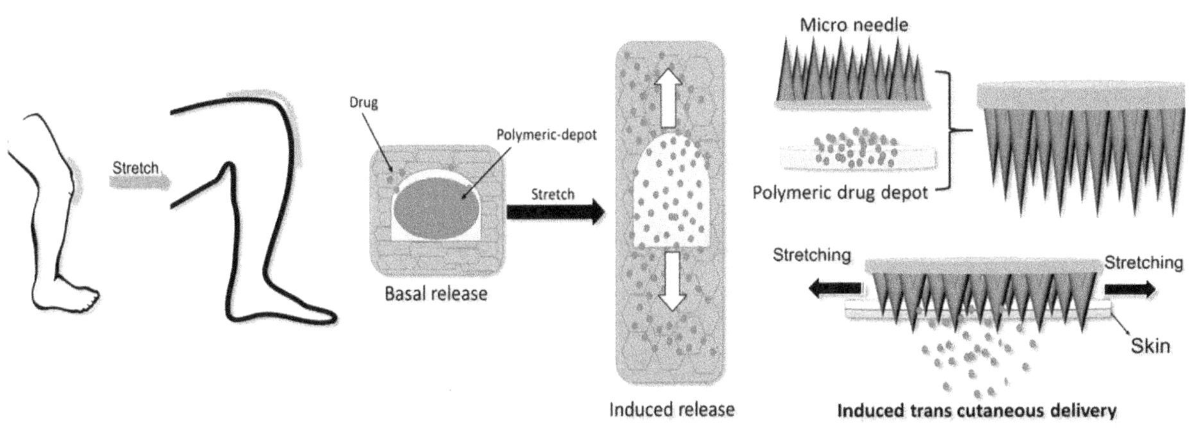

7. NASAL DRUG DELIVERY DEVICES

Nasal delivery is the logical alternative for topical treatment in the nasal route and paranasal sinuses including allergic and non-allergic rhinitis and sinusitis. The nose is considered an alternative route for needle-free vaccination and systemic drug delivery, especially when rapid absorption and effect are desired. Additionally, nasal delivery helps to improve bioavailability, faster absorption, control drug degradation, and adverse events in the gastrointestinal tract and avoid the first-pass metabolism. Conversely, in the case of nasal delivery devices and mechanisms, it is important to protect the lungs from the hazardous exposures, not to serve as a delivery route. The complex nasal geometry with cyclic physiological changes provide proficient filtration and conditioning of inspired air, enhance olfaction, and optimise gas exchange and fluid retention during exhalation. Though, this potential hurdles these functional features inflict on efficient nasal drug delivery are often ignored. The advantages and limitations of emerging nasal drug delivery devices and dispersion technologies are reviewed with the focus on their clinical performance. The importance and limitations of the in vitro testing in the FDA for nasal spray pumps and pressurised aerosols (metered-dose inhalers) with local action are discussed. However, the clinical utility of nasal studies and computer simulations of nasal airflow and compared with computational fluid dynamics software are considered. New emerging delivery technologies with the emphasis on Bi-Directional™ delivery, a novel concept for nasal delivery can be adapted for different dispersion technologies (Kozlovskaya, L., Abou-Kaoud, M. and Stepensky, D., 2014; Djupesland, P.G., 2013).

8. MULTI-PULSE DRUG DELIVERY

Controlled-release drug delivery systems have many applications in the treatment of hormone deficiencies and chronic pain. The biodegradable device providing multiple dose drug delivery can be advantageous for long-term treatment giving pulsatile drug release. The biodegradable polymeric microchips have been fabricated releasing four pulses of radiolabelled dextran, human growth hormone or heparin. Heparin released over 142 days retained 96 ± 12% of its bioactivity. The microchips were 1.2 cm in diameter, 480–560 µm thick and had 36 reservoirs each filled with a different therapeutics. The devices were fabricated using poly (L-lactic acid) and poly(D, L-lactic-co-glycolic acid) membranes of various molecular masses which cover the reservoirs. A drug delivery system with the potential to release pulses of different therapeutics at different intervals after implantation by using different molecular weights or materials for the membrane can be implemented (Grayson, A.C.R., Choi, I.S., Tyler, B.M., Wang, P.P., Brem, H., Cima, M.J. and Langer, R., 2003).

9. CARTRIDGE-BASED DRUG DELIVERY DEVICE

A liquid drug delivery device is made to order to be adhered to the skin by the skin-contacting surface having an adhesive coating. A cartridge serves as the reservoir for the therapeutics and can be incorporated in a covering which is connected to the base member in such a way that the longitudinal axis of the cartridge is disposed parallels to the skin surface. A delivery needle with the interior of the cartridge penetrates to the skin when the housing snaps downward relative to the base member. This action causes actuation of a citric acid or sodium bicarbonate gas generator generating gas to move a piston within the cartridge which compresses drug compartment. The compression causes a stopper to be penetrated by a channel in communication with the needle, releasing the drug from the compartment through the needle in subcutaneous tissue (Tsals, I., Gross, J. and Lavi, G., 199).

10. THERMAL VAPORIZING DEVICE FOR DRUG DELIVERY

A drug delivery device for delivery of various therapeutics to the lungs includes a tubular housing having a mouthpiece, a middle section and the heat source. The middle section has a chamber of inert inorganic particulates having therapeutics adsorbed as a coating. The heat source, the chamber of inert inorganic particulates in the middle section and the mouthpiece are connected through the interior to the distal end section to outside air. When suction is applied to the mouthpiece, air is drawn to the heat source by suction and is heated. The heated air is drawn into the chamber of the middle section to volatilize and desorb the drug from the inert particles. The volatilized and desorbed drug is then drawn from the chamber of the middle section into the mouthpiece and then into the mouth and lungs of the user (Kottayil, S., Crooks, P., Riggs, D. and Murty, R., Kottayil S. George and Crooks, 2001).

11. IMPLANTABLE MEDICAL DEVICE HAVING PROTRUDING SURFACE STRUCTURES

The implantable device, such as a stent, covered stent, or synthetic stent graft can be used for the drug delivery. The protruding structures are formed on the surface of the device. This structures having central depression region are surrounded by the lip. It can be in the variety of shapes, like circular, ovular shapes, or can form grooves. The structures can be used to engage a cover. Glue is also added to the protruding structures to help secure the cover. The protruding structures many times contains a therapeutic substance for release in situ. This structures can be formed by using a laser discharge to create a hole on the surface of the stent following directing a pressurised stream of grit at the surface (Wu, S.Z., Harish, S., Sanders-Millare, D. and Guruwaiya, J.A., 2001).

12. ELECTRONIC INSULIN PUMPS

The Insulin pumps are automatic computerised devices that are continuously deliver insulin according to need into the adipose layer below the skin by way of a soft flexible tube. The Insulin pumps are popular among those who require multiple routine injections of insulin. Safe and fruitful use of a pump requires appropriate education and training, their cost can be comparatively high. Insulin pumps are not characteristically used by those who are new to insulin, but can be an effective option once you have a minute more experience (Barnard, K.D., Lloyd, C.E. and Skinner, T.C., 2007). Figure 4 representing automatic insulin delivery pump.

Figure 4. A diagrammatic representation of insulin delivery pump

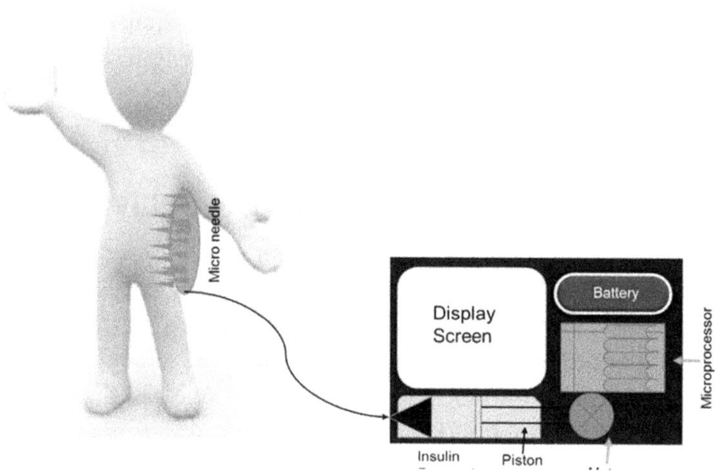

Table 1. List of insulin pens

Company	Brand Name	Insulin Type	Dose Delivery	Total Capacity	Details
Eli Lilly	HUMAPEN LUXURA HD	Humalog	Half-unit increments, up to 30 units at a time	300 units	Reusable
Eli Lilly	HUMALOG KWIKPEN	Humalog U-100/U-200/Mix 75/25/Mix 50/50	One-unit increments, up to 60 units at a time	300 units. 600 unit	Disposable
Eli Lilly	HUMULIN KWIKPEN	Humulin N Humulin 70/30	One-unit increments, up to 60 units at a time	300 units	Disposable
Novo Nordisk	NOVOLOG FLEXPEN	NovoLog NovoLog Mix 70/30	One-unit increments, up to 60 units at a time	300 units	Disposable
Novo Nordisk	FLEXTOUCH	Levemir	One-unit increments, up to 80 units at a Time. For Tresiba U-200, two-unit Increments, up to 160 units at a time.	300 units. For Tresiba U-200: 600 units	Disposable
Novo Nordisk	NOVOPEN ECHO	NovoLog PenFill Cartridges	Half-unit increments (starting at 0.5 units), up to 30 units at a time	300 units	Disposable Memory function shows units of last dose
Owen Mumford	AUTOPEN CLASSIC	Humalog	Comes in a one-unit increment version (with up to 21 units at a time) and a two-unit increment version (with up to 42 units at a time)	300 units	Reusable
Sanofi	APIDRA SOLOSTAR	Apidra	One-unit increments, up to 80 units at a time	300 units	Disposable
Sanofi	LANTUS SOLOSTAR	Lantus	One-unit increments, up to 80 units	300 units	Disposable
Sanofi	TOUJEO SOLOSTAR	Toujeo	One-unit increments, up to 80 units at a time	450 units	Disposable.

12. STENTS

The stents are typically metal mesh tubes inserted during PCI, a technique that widens the blocked artery by temporarily inserting and inflating a minute balloon. Stents help avoid the artery from becoming blocked again (restenosis). Even with stents, arteries can occasionally become blocked yet again. Drug-eluting stents can make this less likely to occur. Stents can be classified into two categories: bare-metal stents and drug-eluting stents (Htay, T. and Liu, M.W., 2005).

12.1 Drug-Eluting or Bare-Metal Stents for Coronary Artery Disease

The stent development is significant achievement in the field of the obstructive coronary artery disease treatment since the introduction of balloon angioplasty. However, hyperplasia occurring inside the stent leading to in-stent restenosis is the main complication in the long-term achievement of percutaneous coronary intervention (PCI). The modern introduction of drug-eluting stents (DES) contributes the main invention to interventional cardiology. Various large randomised clinical trials using DES have exposed a notable reduction in angiographic restenosis and target vessel revascularization when compared with bare metal stents (Htay et al, 2005).

The Drug-eluting stents (DES) are a typical metallic coronary stent with a polymer or co-polymer coating and an antiproliferative drug, such as paclitaxel which allows drug elution into the coronary endothelium for weeks to months after stent implantation. Drug-eluting stents, however, requires extended treatment with blood viscosity decreased to prevent the stents from closing because of blood clotting. This makes them less compliance for people with bleeding problems or those who will need any type of surgery after within a year the stent implant. Here's data to help you talk to your doctor approximately whether a drug-eluting stent is right for you (Htay et al, 2005; Bønaa, K.H., Mannsverk, J., Wiseth, R., Aaberge, L., Myreng, Y., Nygård, O., Nilsen, D.W., Kløw, N.E., Uchto, M., Trovik, T. and Bendz, B., 2016).

12.2 Bare-Metal Stents

There are no spacial coating on the Bare-metal stents. They serve as scaffolding to strengthener of blood vessels after they're stretched with angioplasty. As the artery heals, the tissue grows nearby the stent, holding it in place. But, sometimes an overgrowth of the scar tissue in the inner lining of the artery develops the risk of the re-blockage. The drug-eluting stents are coated with drug loaded polymer that is released controlled manner (eluted) to help inhibit the growth of scar tissue in the inner artery lining. This supports the artery maintains opened, and smooth ensuring normal blood flow. The drug-eluting stents can be used successfully by people having heart problems with, anticipating the need for more-invasive treatments, such as bypass surgery. The Drug-eluting stents help prevent the recurrence of disease symptoms, such as chest pain. This also reduces the need for repeat angioplasty procedures, which carry the risk of complications such as heart attack and stroke Htay et al, 2005; Bønaa et al,2016; Maisel, W.H. and Laskey, W.K., 2007).

Figure 5. A diagrammatic representation of drug eluting stent

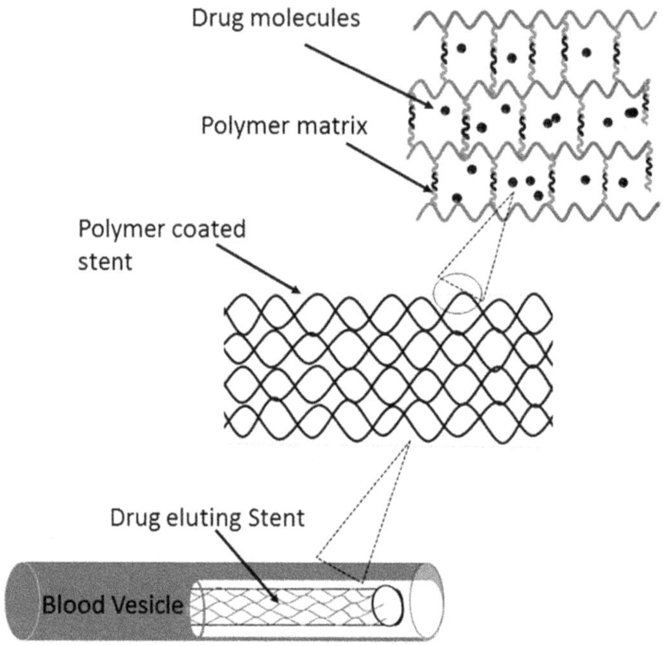

12.2.1 Bare-Metal Stents and Angioplasty

This type of stents may work adequately, but they may causes higher rate of restenosis than the drug-eluting stents. If anyone need some type of surgery that's not related to your heart (such as a stomach or hernia operation) soon after your stent placement, or if anyone having bleeding disorder, they may do well with a bare-metal stent.

12.2.2 Angioplasty and Drug-Eluting Stents

The Drug-eluting stents are very safer and effective in maximum conditions. These stents work well and have a lesser rate of restenosis than the bare-metal stents. For best effectiveness, you must take your medications as prescribed by the physician.

12.2.3 Angioplasty and Drug-Eluting Absorbable Stents

The latest option is a drug-eluting, fully absorbable stent that was recently approved by the FDA to treat coronary artery disease. The stent is intended to dissolve and be absorbed by the body over time. Long-term effects aren't yet known.

12.3 Commercially Available Drug-Eluting Stents

The commercial sirolimus-eluting Cypher™ stent (Cordis Corp, a Johnson and Johnson Company, Miami, FL, USA) was approved by Food and Drug Administration in April 2003. It is coated with a nonerodable polymer layer of 5 µm–10 µm thickness, which is integrated with sirolimus (140 µg sirolimus/cm2 of stent). An additional topcoat is sited on it as a diffusion barrier, which delivers the vehicle for controlled release of the API. It is designed as such that around 80% of the total dose of the drug is released in 4 weeks and the remains over the course of the subsequent 2 weeks (Wong and Chan 2004). The second commercially existing DES is the Taxus™ stent (Boston Scientific, Natrick, MA, USA), which has a proprietary platform, the Express™ stent, and is coated with a proprietary polymer (Translute™) loaded with 1 µg of paclitaxel/mm2 of stent surface area. Even though there are three drug-release formulations (slow, moderate, and fast), only reasonable- and slow-release formulations have been confirmed in clinical trials. The moderate-release (MR) form of Taxus stent permits for a preliminary bolus release over the first 48 hours subsequent stenting followed by a low-level release completed at least the subsequent 10 days. In the initial 10 days of drug release, the slow-release (SR) formulation of Taxus stent has a drug release concentration of 8–10 times laser than that of the MR formulation. Only SR formulation is used in Food and Drug Administration Taxus stents (Sanidas, E.A., Golemati, S. and Dangas, G.D., 2015).

13. IMPLANTABLE DRUG DELIVERY

There was a necessity for delivery systems that could maintain a steady release of drug to the specific site of action. Thus, drug delivery systems were established to optimize the therapeutic properties of drug products and render them more safe, effective, and reliable. In comparison with many of the other form of drug delivery systems, such as implantable pumps and implants for tuneable rate delivery are at a crude stage of development. Even though the typical implantable pump consists of various mechanisms to regulate drug delivery. The benefits most frequently provided by the dosage form are predictable to be 1) Implantable devices permit site-specific drug administration where the drug is needed most. Examples include implants used in the treatment of brain prostate cancer or tumours. This may also permit for significantly lower doses of the drug, which can minimize potential side effects. 2) Implantable devices permit for sustained release by the zero-order release rate of a drugs agent. The major advantages of these systems contain targeted local delivery of drugs at a constant rate, less dose needed to treat the disease condition, lowers the probable side effects, and greater efficacy of treatment. Due to the development of such type of sustained release formulations, due to that possible to administer very unstable drugs once a week to once a year that in the past required recurrent daily dosing of the drugs (Govender, T., Choonara, Y.E., Kumar, P., Bijukumar, D., du Toit, L.C., Modi, G., Naidoo, D. and Pillay, V., 2017; Gifford III, H.S. and Reich, C.J., Novartis Ag, 2017).

The Drug development includes designing or discovering, altering molecules to maximize up to desirable therapeutic features while reducing side effects. The orally administered drug must be protected from the denaturation in the gastrointestinal tract and should be accomplished absorption from the across the wall of the stomach or the intestine. After absorption and upon reaching the hepatic portal circulation, it must be resistant to first pass metabolism. The rate of drug elimination and absorption should ensure the drug levels between the therapeutic index. Furthermore, the amount of intact drug that reaches the site of action should be enough to obtain desired pharmacological action but inadequate to cause unpleasant side effects. Implantable drug delivery devices are devoid of above-mentioned restrictions accompanying with oral, IV, topical drug administration by subcutaneously implantable drug delivery devices offer one unique improvement of a retrievable mechanism. (Govender et al, 2017; Gifford et al, 2017).

13.1 Advantages

- **Convenience:** The Effective concentration of drug in the blood can be sustained for the extended period by procedures such as continuous intravenous infusion or Implantation treatment permits patients to get medication outside the hospital setting with negligible medical observation.
- **Compliance:** Compliance enhances by reducing the frequency of drug administration over the total period of treatment improve patient compliance. The patient can fail to recall to take a medicine, but drug delivery from an implant is not dependent on patient input.
- **Stability:** Implants are environmentally inert and stable they should not breakdown under the effect of light, heat, air and moisture. It should be unchanged and harmless and have good mechanical strength.
- **Improved Drug Delivery:** The drug is dispersed locally or in systemic circulation with least interference by biological barriers or metabolic. For example, the drug moiety avoided the GIT and the liver. The by-passing effect is advantageous to drugs, which are either easily deactivated or absorbed poorly in the GIT and the liver earlier systemic distribution.
- **Controlled Release:** The Implants exist which deliver drugs by nearly zero order release kinetics. So that the dosing frequency is reduced, and patient compliance is increased. It leads to enhanced usefulness and reduce side effects.
- **Flexibility:** In the choice of materials, methods of production, capacity of drug loading, rate of drug release, etc. substantial flexibility is possible. From a regulatory viewpoint, it is observed as a new product and can extend the market fortification of the drug.

13.2 Mechanisms

13.2.1 Diffusion Controlled

Reservoir type of system contains of a core of drug enclosed by a polymeric thin layer and diffusion of the drug across the polymer layer is work as the rate limiting step. Zero order release kinetic easily attained. In Matrix type systems the zero order release rate can be achieved by remunerating by the increasing diffusional distance with an increasing area of the drug.

13.2.2 Chemically Controlled

The drug is distributed homogeneously throughout the bio-erodible polymer, which erodes and decreases in geometry with time to permit the drug release. The Zero order kinetics can be attained if the surface area remains unaffected with time

13.2.3 Swelling Controlled

In this type of the release system the rate is equal to the product of surface area and a constant rate equivalent to rate of advance of periphery separating the outer shell from central core.

13.2.4 Osmotically Controlled

This is the matrix type of the system where the core is enclosed by semipermeable membrane that utilizes osmotic pressure as driving force for delivery of drugs.

13.2.5 Magnetically Controlled

This type of system contains of drug and small magnetic beads homogeneously discrete inside a polymer matrix. In the contact with aqueous media, drug is released in diffusion-controlled manner.

13.3 Implantable Drug Delivery Devices

13.3.1 Transdermal Patches

The transdermal patches generally have hollow microneedles made by biocompatible polymer through which the drug is transported across the skin. Transdermal patches have abundant advantages compared with others systems of drug delivery: the drugs are stable in the GIT, these painless, and they releases a persistent dosage without the need for patient's compliance.

13.3.2 Polymer Implants

The Polymer implants are biodegradable polymers loaded with the therapeutics. The polymer degrades when it comes in contact with body fluids and in the process releases therapeutics molecules. The rate of matrix degradation, and hence the drug release, can be adjusted by altering the properties of the polymers. The polymer material which are most extensively used for these application include, but are not restricted to, Polylactic acid (PLA), Polyurethane and Polyglycolic acid (PGA), the combinations of these in different proportions.

13.3.4 Bioadhesives

The bioadhesives are materials which form bonds with biological surfaces. The most common materials which are used in this case are polymer hydrogels. The principle of process is analogous to polymer implants in this that they too are loaded with drugs and release drugs at a precise rate when in contact with body fluids and ECF .

13.3.5 Microencapsulation

The microencapsulation denotes to the method of covering the therapeutic molecule with a material which will extend the time before the drug is resorbed so that it will persist in the active state and that will be released when it reaches the planned destination. There are the variety of ways in which microencapsulation is done. Some of them are use of, liposomes, nanoparticles, polymer microspheres, etc.

13.4 Materials for Drug Delivery

As with all implantable devices, key material considerations for use in drug delivery include biocompatibility, stability and durability (except in the case of biodegradable drug delivery systems), and the ability of the material to control release of the active pharmaceutical ingredient (API). Silicones have long been a material of choice for drug delivery given their extreme chemical inertness, range of stable mechanical properties, and ability to compound various APIs within the matrix. The rate of release is generally proportional to the loading of drug within the silicone, typically 5% to 50% by weight. Ethylene vinyl acetate (EVA) is also finding use in drug delivery application due to the additional ability to control release rate by varying the vinyl acetate content. Like silicone, EVA is processed at relatively low temperatures, typically 150 to 250°F, which helps to minimize risks associated with degradation of the API. Polyurethanes and acrylate hydrogels have also been utilized in select applications (Fend et al, 2017; Bardoli, A.D., Taylor, W.S.J. and Mahmalji, W., 2017).

13.5 Transdermal Spray

A metered-dose transdermal spray (MDTS) device deliberate therapeutics to the open surface of the skin and is absorbed up to the blood circulation on a sustained basis. Its mechanism in a similar way to a transdermal patch, cream or topical gel. The drug is delivered by a suitable device placed softly against the skin and triggered, triggering it to release a light spray holding a proprietary formulation of the therapeutics that rapidly dries on the skin surface and form an invisible drug depot. As it would be from a covering, the drug is then absorbed progressively for a predetermined amount of time (Bardoli et al, 2017).

13.6 Transdermal Implant

The transdermal implants are advanced type of drug delivery in this type of formulation mainly body modification used both in an aesthetic and medical context. In either case, they comprise of an object located partially underneath and partially above the skin layer, thus transdermal. The skin around it normally heals as if it were a penetrating.

When the process is done using a post-like implant, a cut is made a small distance from the site. The skin is then elevated, and the implant is delivered through. Then, a hole is opened at the site for it to pass through, and it is moved so that the top portion fills the hole. The implants used for this are commonly small and not surfaced in any way except rounding.

Table 2.

Product	Company	Material	Active Ingredient	Application	Launch
Vantas	Endopharmaceuticals	N/A	Histerelin	Prostate cancer	2004
NuvaRing	Market&Co	EVA	Etonorgestral Estradiol	Contraception	2002
Eplanon	Market&Co	EVA	Etonorgestral	Contraception	2006
Synchromed	Medtronic	Silicon	Beclofec	Analgesic	1998
Jedelle	Bayer	Silicon	Levonorgestral	Contraception	1996

If an extra graphic implant is anticipated, it is usually done in two fragments. First, the base is introduced the same way a single-part would be, excluding that the base implant is threaded. It may either stick out similar a bolt, or be inward like a nut. When this is done, the top half is screwed on. This type is frequently done for spikes and/or horns. In any case, the portion of the implant which passes under the skin normally is slightly large and has holes. The skin will propagate into them, making it more perpetual (Huizenga, T., Riyaz, F. and Ozog, D.M., 2017).

The micro dermal implants are form of body modification which provides the aesthetic look of a transdermal implant, without the difficulties of the much more complex surgery related with transdermal implants. Mainly micro dermal implants are single point piercings which are a short of surface piercing (Huizenga et al, 2017).

Microdermal implants may place practically everywhere on the surface of the normal skin on the body, but are unalike from conventional piercings in that they are composed of two constituents: an anchor, which is inserted underneath the skin, with a step expanded from (or flush with) the surface of the neighbouring skin, and the transposable jewellery, which is screwed into the threaded hole in the step of the anchor. They should not be implanted in feet, hands, wrists, collarbones or any area where it is not flat or that is near any joint (Huizenga et al, 2017).

14. INTRAUTERINE DEVICE

An intrauterine device (IUD or coil) is a tinny, regularly T-shaped birth control device that is introduced into a woman's uterus to avoid pregnancy. IUDs are one form of long-acting reversible birth control technique. Among all birth control approaches, IUDs, along with contraceptive implants, result in the extreme satisfaction among users. Evidence supports efficiency and safety in youngsters and individuals who have and have not earlier had children. Once removed, even subsequently long-term use, fertility returns to normal rapidly. Failure rates are approximately 0.8% with copper devices and 0.2% with hormonal (levonorgestrel) devices in the first year of use. While Cu IUDs might increase menstrual bleeding and consequence in more painful cramps of uterus, the hormonal IUDs may decrease menstrual bleeding or halt menstruation altogether. Cramping can be cured with NSAIDs. Other potential problems include expulsion (2–5%) and infrequently perforation of the uterus (< 0.7%). IUDs do not affect breastfeeding and may be inserted instantly after delivery. They may also be used immediately afterwards an abortion (Huizenga et al, 2017; Sonalkar, S. and Kapp, N.,2015).

The usage of IUDs as a practise of birth control dates from the 1800s. An earlier model known as the Dalkon shield was accompanied with an increased threat of pelvic inflammatory disease; though, the risk is not affected by current models in those without sexually transmitted infections at the time of time of insertion. The types of intrauterine devices available, and names they go by, differ by the location. In the USA, there are two types available

14.1 Non-Hormonal Cu-IUD

14.1.1 IUD With Progestogen

The WHO ATC tagged both copper and hormonal devices as IUDs. In the United Kingdom, there are over 10 various types of copper IUDs existing. In the UK, the term IUD applies only to these Cu devices.

Hormonal intrauterine contraception is considered to be a different kind of birth control and is tagged with the term as the intrauterine system (IUS) (Sonalkar et al, 2015).

14.1.2 Copper

Cu-IUDs mainly work by disrupting sperm motility and damage to sperm so that they are prohibited from joining with an egg. Cu acts as a spermicide inside the uterus, increasing levels of copper ions, white blood and cells prostaglandins, within the uterus and fallopian tubal fluids. The increased Cu ions in the cervical mucus prevent the sperm's motility and viability, stopping sperm from travelling through cervical mucus, or destroying it as it passes through. Cu can also modify the endometrial lining, but studies show that while this alteration can avoid implantation of the fertilised egg ("blastocyst"), it cannot disrupt one that has already been implanted. Most Cu-IUDs have a plastic T-shaped casing that is wound around with pure electrolytic Cu wire and has Cu collars (sleeves). The arms of the frame hold IUD in place close to the top of the uterus. The Paragard TCu 380a measures, and 35 mm (1.41") vertically (leg of the T) 32 mm (1.25") horizontally (top of the T) (Sonalkar et al, 2015; Cheung, C.S. and Cheung, V.Y., 2016).

14.2 Mechanism of Action

IUDs principally work by blocking fertilization. The progestogen discharged from the hormonal IUDs may avoids ovulation from occurring but only partially. The hormone also increases the thickness of the cervical mucus so that sperm cannot reach the fallopian tubes. Copper IUDs include no hormones, but the copper ions in the cervical mucus cause the toxic effect to sperm. and also toxic for uterus and fallopian tubes due to that its produce a fluid that contains copper ions, white blood cells, prostaglandins, and enzymes. The extremely effectiveness of Cu-releasing IUDs as emergency contraceptives implies they may also act by avoiding implantation of the blastocyst in uterus. In non-emergency use, inhibition of implantation is at most an unusual method of action, not a typical mechanism of action (Cheung et al, 2016).

14.3 Adverse Effects

Further report: IUD with progestogen and IUD with Cu Transvaginal ultrasonography displays a perforated Cu IUD as a hyperechoic (rendered as bright) line at right, 3 cm away from the uterus at left. The IUD is enclosed by a hypoechoic (dark) foreign-body granuloma.

Regardless of comprising copper or progestogen potential side effects of intrauterine devices contain, uterus perforation, expulsion pelvic inflammatory disease (particularly in the first 21 days after insertion), as well as unbalanced menstrual pattern. A small possibility of pregnancy remains after IUD insertion, and when it occurs, there is a greater threat of ectopic pregnancy. Considerable pain with insertion that requires active management occurs in about 17% of nulliparous women and around 11% of parous women (Cheung et al, 2016). In this type of cases, NSAID are the evidenced to be effective. However, no prophylactic analgesic drugs have been found to be effective for routine use for women undergoing IUD insertion (Cheung et al, 2016, Sonalkar et al, 2015).

15. PHONOPHORESIS

In Phonophoresis the ultrasound used for the enhance the topically delivery of applied drugs. Phonophoresis has been used with an aim to enhance the absorption of topically applied drugs such as analgesics and anti-inflammatory molecules through the therapeutic utilization of ultrasound. Phonophoresis has been shown to be ineffective for some treatments, where it did not increase the efficiency of absorption of drugs, or did not change the outcome more than the use of ultrasound alone (Oka

16. OSMOTIC CONTROLLED-RELEASE ORAL

OROS (Osmotic Controlled Release System) is an emerging area in controlled release of oral drug delivery system in the form of a hard tablet with the semi-permeable outer membrane and one or more small laser drilled holes in it. As the tablet passes through the GIT, water is absorbed by the semipermeable membrane via osmosis, and creates osmotic pressure is used to drive forward the active drug through the opening(s) in the tablet. OROS is a trademarked name used by ALZA Corporation, which pioneered the use of osmotic pumps for oral drug delivery (Peppas, N.A., Caldorera-Moore, M.E. and Steichen, S.D.,2015; Mathur, M. and Mishra, R.,2016).

Osmotic release systems have a several of major advantages over others controlled-release system. They are significantly less affected by factors such as food, pH, GI motility, and various intestinal environments. Using an osmotic pump to deliver therapeutics has additional inherent advantages on control over the drug delivery rates. This allows for much very precise drug delivery over a long period, which results in much more anticipated pharmacokinetics. However, osmotic release systems are relatively complex, somewhat difficult to manufacture, and may create irritation or even blockage of the gastro intestinal tract due to extended release of irritating drugs from the non-deformable tablet (Peppas et al, 2015; Mathur et al, 2016).

Figure 6. A diagrammatic representation of OROS system

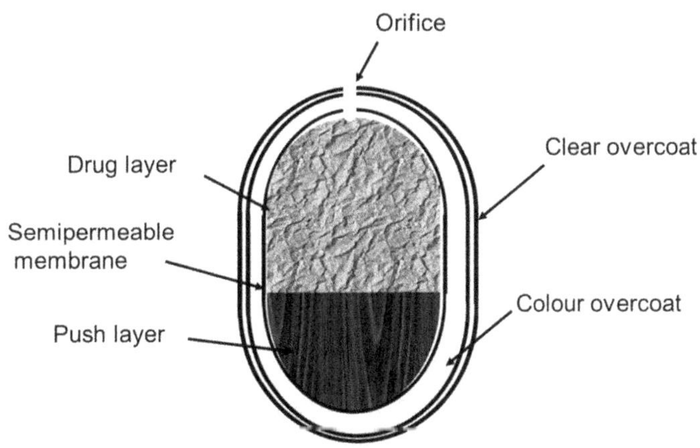

16.1 Single-Layer

The first Elementary Osmotic Pump (EOP) was developed by ALZA Corporation in 1974, and was the first working example of an osmotic pump based drug release system for the oral drug delivery use. It was launched in to the market in the early 1980s in Osmosin withAcutrim (phenylpropanolamine), and (indomethacin) but unexpectedly severe issues with GI irritation and cases of GI perforation led to the withdrawal of Osmosin from the marke (Mathur et al, 2016).

16.2 Multi-Layer

Both the EOP and CPOP were comparatively simple designs and were restricted by their failure to deliver poorly water soluble drugs. This directed to the development of an additional internal layer "push layer" composed of material (a swellable polymer) that would expand as it received water, which then forced the drug layer (which combines a viscous polymer for suspension of poorly soluble drugs) out of the exit hole at a controlled rate. strong Osmotic agents such as NaCl, KCl, or xylitol are added to both the drug and push layers to enhance the osmotic pressure. The initial design formed in 1982 by ALZA corporation was entitled the Procardia XL (nifedipine) and Push-Pull Osmotic Pump (PPOP), was one of the earliest drugs to utilise this PPOP design. (Peppas et al, 2015; Mathur et al, 2016; Liu, X., Wang, S., Chai, L., Zhang, D., Sun, Y., Xu, L. and Sun, J., 2014).

17. MICROBIAL DRUG DELIVERY

Microbial drug delivery is an emerging field of drug delivery and characterized by the help of commensal gut microbes that have been genetically engineered to produce therapeutics for any chronic diseases in humans (Liu, Wang et al, 2014). But only proteinaceous therapeutics can be formed by commensal microbes, as DNA encodes for the particular protein. the Research into microorganism based drug delivery applies to this route of administration as topical since the microbes release the product directly to the surface of affected tissues of the organ, namely the gastrointestinal (GI) epithelium (Liu, Wang et al, 2014; Steidler, L. and Rottiers, P.,, 2006) microorganism based drug delivery is not currently in use as a standard route of drug administration due to its experimental in nature. microorganism based delivery during clinical trials, it has been used to treat forms of inflammatory bowel disease (IBD) (Braat, H., Rottiers, P., Hommes, D.W., Huyghebaert, N., Remaut, E., Remon, J.P., van Deventer, S.J., Neirynck, S., Peppelenbosch, M.P. and Steidler, L., 2003). The most frequent studied vehicles of microbial drug administration are the bacterial species, such as L. *lactis* and B. *ovatus* are used . The usage of the various recombinant microbes (i.e. microorganisms engineered to include DNA from two or more different species) used for treating of chronic diseases (Liu, Wang et al, 2014; Steidler et al, 2006; Braat et al, 2006). In 2006, Braat et al. used microbial drug delivery with L. lacks in clinical trials, and successfully treating the Crohn's disease (CD), a form of IBD that causes the inflammation and ulceration of the large intestines. In this study, the recombinant strain of L. lactic containing complimentary DNA (cDNA) for the human interleukin-10 (IL-10) gene used to treatment for CD with IL-10, an anti-inflammatory cytokines Patients consumed capsules which containing the microbe to populate the in intestines and received therapeutic doses the IL-10 directly from the recombinant bacteria (Braat et al, 2006). As this route of administration is experimental, it is currently not available as a standard treatment option. In a

2013 animal study with B. ovatus as the vehicle for microbial drug delivery, researcher Zaed Hamady suggested that recombinant strains of B. *ovatus* containing transforming growth factor-beta (TGF-β) and keratinocyte growth factor-2 (KGF-2) are ready for clinical trials (Liu, Wang et al, 2014; Steidler et al, 2006; Braat et al, 2006).

18. MICROCHIP BASED DRUG DELIVERY

Abundant research has been ongoing in the journey to find an ideal system for drug delivery within the human body. Drug delivery is a very important feature of medical treatment. The efficiency of many drugs is straightly related to the way in which they are administered. Unfortunately, this may make it very challenging to choice the proper drug delivery system. Some therapies require that the drug be frequently administered to the patient over an extended period, or in precise quantities at a time to maximise drug efficiency. In numerous cases, patients often forget, are unwilling, or are unable to take their medication. Likewise, approximately drugs are too potent for systemic drug delivery and may cause more impairment than good. Consequently, it is of a great advantage to invention a drug delivery device that is accomplished of controlled, pulsatile or continuous release of a wide variety of drugs and other medication that can be securely implanted inside the body. Biocompatibility, material dependability, method of drug release, and processibility, are only a few of the many significant aspects that need to be well thought-out in creating a successful and active drug delivery system of this type. Some drug delivery systems previously exist that endeavour to control the release rate of drugs. One such system contains polymeric devices that have been deliberate to provide drug release for prolong time via diffusion mechanism of the drug out of the polymer and/or degradation of the polymer (Jones, D.A., 1996).

This system, is too simple to have the capacity to precisely control the amount and rate of drug released. But in some cases, the where polymer degrades too fast because of unanticipated environmental conditions inside the body (i.e. in the existence of enzymes that increase the degradation rates of biodegradable polymers matrix). Other devices are ones that are automatic, electromechanically driven and contain features such as inlet and outlet valves and/or micropumps to dispense therapeutic into the body8. These devices comprise tiny power-driven mechanical parts that are mandatory to either, retract, dispense, or pump in order to deliver therapeutics in the body. These devices. Three due to difficulties and size limitations, they are inappropriate to deliver more than a few drugs or drug mixtures at a time. It is necessary to develop a drug delivery device that possess the following features: 1.) one that is easy to use and manufacture, 2.) one that is multi-welled so that drugs and other drug molecules can be delivered for several months, 3.) one that can hold many different drugs or other therapeutics molecules of variable dosages volume and can release these materials in a controlled manner, near to zero order and 4.) One that is biocompatible and very small in size that can be implantable in the human body (i.e. a microchip). The microchip that will be described in this manuscript is based on the invention by Langer et al. at the Massachusetts Institute of Technology.

18.1 Microchip Device Design

The microchip delivery system comprises a substrate containing numerous reservoirs capable of holding therapeutics in the solid, liquid, or gel form. Each reservoir is covered (i.e. with a conductive membrane) and wired with the final circuitry controlled by a microprocessor unit. This central processor should be able to effectively control electrically the exact time of release and the amounts of therapeutics dispersed by controlling the dissolution of the gold membrane. The system should be sensible to manufacture by standard microfabrication techniques and still be cost-effective enough. Device Dimensions: 17mm x 17mm x 315mm Reservoirs 400 total .05 mm spacing (bottom side) 25 nl volume (Espinosa, H., Capito, R.M. and Lucas, L.A., 2000).

18.2 The Designing Approach

18.2.1 Substrate

According to system design, the Substrate and the reservoirs will be located in the substrate. This can be easily be done by standard etching techniques of microfabrication. Any material that can assist as a support is suitable for etching, and is impermeable to the molecules that can be delivered and to the surrounding fluids can be used as a substrate material. For this in vivo application, biocompatibility should be strictly considered. Non-biocompatible materials, however, can also be sealed off within biocompatible materials like poly (ethylene glycol). One example of a strong, non-degradable, easily etched substrate that is impermeable to the delivered therapeutic agent and non-degradable to the surrounding milieu within the body. It should be noted that for some specific applications a material should be degradable over time might be preferred. For example, the brain implants make the removal of a device is very difficult or threatening to the patient and thus this device would not be applicable (Espinsosa et al, 2004; Hovell, C.M., Sei, Y.J. and Kim, Y.,2015).

18.2.2 Release System

The design of a release system mainly depends on the kind of treatment required by the patient whether it is a pulsed or continuous release. Desired drug delivery can be attained by a passive or active release system. In the passive system, the therapeutics diffuse through a membrane or enter to the body by the degradation of the substrate material. The Active systems are activated by a microprocessor and are preferred due to a more precise release profile of the drugs. The exact time release and amounts of therapeutics can then be controlled. The chip can be placed tactically as well for therapeutics that are too potent for a continuous release profile (Hovell et al, 2015; Guidion et al, 2004).

18.2.3 Reservoir Caps

In this devices, the reservoir caps contain thin films of electroconductive material patterned in the shape of anodes enclosed by cathodes. Any electroconductive material that can oxidise and quickly dissolve in solution upon the application of an electric potential may use for the manufacturing of the anodes and cathodes. The oxidation occurs on the anode. The portion of the anode above the reservoir oxidizes and get dissolves into the solution upon the application of a potential between the anode and cathode. This exposes the release system to the covering fluids and results in the release of the molecules or therapeutics. Gold is taken as the typical membrane material because of it is easily deposited and patterned, and having very low reactivity with other substances and resists spontaneous corrosion in many fluids over the entire pH range (Hovell et al, 2015; Guidion et al, 2004).

18.2.4 Control Circuit and Power Source

The control circuit consists of a timer, microprocessor, demultiplexer or an input source. The microprocessor will control the anticipated reservoir to be triggered so that a variety of drugs may be contained in individually specific reservoir. The input source may either be a memory source, remote control device or a biosensor based. A very thin-film microbattery can be used as a power source.

18.2.5 Reservoir Filling

3D printing is capable of constructing complex structures by ink-jet printing liquid binder onto loose, fine powder6. The printing design can be attained from the computer-aided-design model (CAD). Inkjet printing in order with a computer-controlled alignment apparatus is capable of depositing as small as 0.2 nl of a gel or liquid solution of known concentration into individual reservoir2. The volume of the reservoirs can be controlled by specifying the appropriate the print head to deposit a pre-determined amount of binder. The drug is pressed out of the nozzle as the vapour bubble inside the nozzle increases upon heating. The relation between the amounts expanded by the vapour bubble to the heat added follows the ideal gas law relationship (Hovell et al, 2015; Guidion et al, 2004).

18.3 Mimicking Atherosclerosis With Blood Cells on a Microchip

Georgia Institute of Technology investigators has engineered a microchip coated with human blood vessel cells. The objective: learn more about the circumstances under which nanoparticles get accumulate in the plaque-filled arteries of patients with atherosclerosis, the underlying condition of myocardial infarction and stroke. They coated microchips with the fragile layer of endothelial cells, which make up the inner endothelial layer of blood vessels.

In healthy human blood vessels, endothelial cells act as a barrier layer to keep foreign articles out of the bloodstream. But at sites predisposed to atherosclerosis, the endothelial barrier breaks down (Hovell et al, 2015).

Figure 7. A diagrammatic representation of microchip based drug delivery system

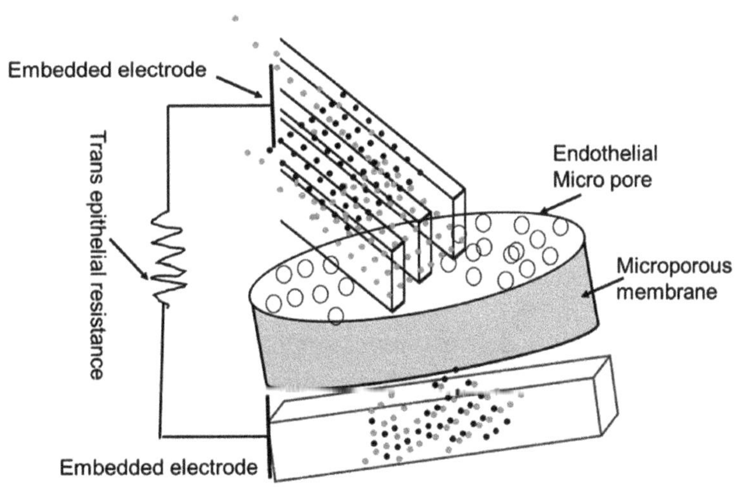

ACKNOWLEDGMENT

Thanks to CSIR for fellowships and thanks to CSIR-CSMCRI to provide me facility for working and learning.

REFERENCES

Bardoli, A. D., Taylor, W. S. J., & Mahmalji, W. (2017). Can the UroLift prostatic implant device treat the symptoms of benign prostatic hypertrophy, avoid sexual dysfunction and reduce hospital TURP waiting times? A single centre, single surgeon experience and review of the literature. *The Aging Male*, 1–6. doi:10.1080/13685538.2017.1336531 PMID:28609136

Barnard, K. D., Lloyd, C. E., & Skinner, T. C. (2007). Systematic literature review: Quality of life associated with insulin pump use in Type 1 diabetes. *Diabetic Medicine*, *24*(6), 607–617. doi:10.1111/j.1464-5491.2007.02120.x PMID:17367304

Barnes, P. J., Rodger, I. W., & Thomson, N. C. (Eds.). (1998). *Asthma: basic mechanisms and clinical management*. Academic Press.

Bønaa, K. H., Mannsverk, J., Wiseth, R., Aaberge, L., Myreng, Y., Nygård, O., ... Bendz, B. (2016). Drug-eluting or bare-metal stents for coronary artery disease. *The New England Journal of Medicine*, *375*(13), 1242–1252. doi:10.1056/NEJMoa1607991 PMID:27572953

Braat, H., Rottiers, P., Hommes, D. W., Huyghebaert, N., Remaut, E., Remon, J. P., ... Steidler, L. (2006). A phase I trial with transgenic bacteria expressing interleukin-10 in Crohn's disease. *Clinical Gastroenterology and Hepatology*, *4*(6), 754–759. doi:10.1016/j.cgh.2006.03.028 PMID:16716759

Brocchini, S., James, K., Tangpasuthadol, V., & Kohn, J. (1998). Structure–property correlations in a combinatorial library of degradable biomaterials. *Journal of Biomedical Materials Research. Part A*, *42*(1), 66–75. doi: PMID:9740008

Cheung, C. S., & Cheung, V. Y. (2016). Response to "Uterine perforation in an adolescent using an intrauterine device with memory function: A case report and review of the published work". *Journal of Obstetrics and Gynaecology Research*, *42*(2), 228–229. doi:10.1111/jog.12836 PMID:26461807

Choi, B., Loh, X. J., Tan, A., Loh, C. K., Ye, E., Joo, M. K., & Jeong, B. (2015). Introduction to in situ forming hydrogels for biomedical applications. In *In-Situ Gelling Polymers* (pp. 5–35). Springer Singapore. doi:10.1007/978-981-287-152-7_2

Di, J., Yao, S., Ye, Y., Cui, Z., Yu, J., Ghosh, T. K., ... Gu, Z. (2015). Stretch-triggered drug delivery from wearable elastomer films containing therapeutic depots. *ACS Nano*, *9*(9), 9407–9415. doi:10.1021/acsnano.5b03975 PMID:26258579

Djupesland, P. G. (2013). Nasal drug delivery devices: Characteristics and performance in a clinical perspective—a review. *Drug Delivery and Translational Research*, 1–21. PMID:23316447

Du, J., & O'Reilly, R. K. (2009). Advances and challenges in smart and functional polymer vesicles. *Soft Matter*, *5*(19), 3544–3561. doi:10.1039/b905635a

Ekroos, H. (2008). *Exhaled nitric oxide: Variability and association with bronchial hyperresponsiveness and atopy*. Academic Press.

Espinosa, H., Capito, R.M., & Lucas, L.A. (2000). *Microchip for Drug Delivery*. Academic Press.

Evans, D. A., & Whitsett, J. A. (1997). Surfactant Replacement Therapies in Children. In The Pediatric Lung (pp. 199-227). Birkhäuser Basel. doi:10.1007/978-3-0348-8960-5_9

Fend, M. (2017). *Fleshing Out Surfaces: Skin in French Art and Medicine, 1650-1850*. Oxford University Press. doi:10.7228/manchester/9780719087967.001.0001

Ferrari, M., & Torchilin, V. (2008). *Fundamental biomedical technologies-Multifunctional pharmaceutical nanocarriers. In Multifunctional polymeric nanosystems for tumor-targeted delivery* (pp. 33–66). New York: Springer Sicences.

Florence, A. T., & Siepmann, J. (Eds.). (2009). *Modern Pharmaceutics: Applications and Advances* (Vol. 2). Informa Healthcare USA.

Gifford, H. S., III, & Reich, C. J. (2017). *Drug delivery treatment device*. U.S. Patent 9,668,917.

Giri, S., Trewyn, B. G., Stellmaker, M. P., & Lin, V. S. Y. (2005). Stimuli-responsive controlled-release delivery system based on mesoporous silica nanorods capped with magnetic nanoparticles. *Angewandte Chemie International Edition*, *44*(32), 5038–5044. doi:10.1002/anie.200501819 PMID:16038000

Govender, T., Choonara, Y. E., Kumar, P., Bijukumar, D., du Toit, L. C., Modi, G., ... Pillay, V. (2017). Implantable and transdermal polymeric drug delivery technologies for the treatment of central nervous system disorders. *Pharmaceutical Development and Technology*, *22*(4), 476–486. doi:10.1080/10837450.2016.1189937 PMID:27268737

Grayson, A. C. R., Choi, I. S., Tyler, B. M., Wang, P. P., Brem, H., Cima, M. J., & Langer, R. (2003). Multi-pulse drug delivery from a resorbable polymeric microchip device. *Nature Materials*, *2*(11), 767–772. doi:10.1038/nmat998 PMID:14619935

Guidoin, M. F., & Guidoin, R. G. (2004). Sélection des matériaux pour la conception et le développement du boîtier d'un cœur artificiel total implantable: Supériorité du titane et de ses alliages. *ITBM-RBM*, *25*(3), 126–138. doi:10.1016/j.rbmret.2004.05.003

Hoffman, A. S. (2008). The origins and evolution of "controlled" drug delivery systems. *Journal of Controlled Release*, *132*(3), 153–163. doi:10.1016/j.jconrel.2008.08.012 PMID:18817820

Hovell, C. M., Sei, Y. J., & Kim, Y. (2015). Microengineered vascular systems for drug development. *Journal of Laboratory Automation*, *20*(3), 251–258. doi:10.1177/2211068214560767 PMID:25424383

Htay, T., & Liu, M. W. (2005). Drug-eluting stent: A review and update. *Vascular Health and Risk Management*, *1*(4), 263–276. doi:10.2147/vhrm.2005.1.4.263 PMID:17315599

Huizenga, T., Riyaz, F., & Ozog, D. M. (2017). Implantable Body Jewelry and Methods for Their Removal. *Dermatologic Surgery*, *43*(5), 761–764. doi:10.1097/DSS.0000000000000979 PMID:27984327

Jewett, W. R., & Williams, R. C., III. (2001). *Metered dose inhaler pump*. U.S. Patent 6,223,746.

Jiang, W., Kim, B. Y., Rutka, J. T., & Chan, W. C. (2007). Advances and challenges of nanotechnology-based drug delivery systems. *Expert Opinion on Drug Delivery*, *4*(6), 621–633. doi:10.1517/17425247.4.6.621 PMID:17970665

Jones, D. A. (1996). Principles and prevention of corrosion. Prentice Hall.

Kost, J., & Langer, R. (2012). Responsive polymeric delivery systems. *Advanced Drug Delivery Reviews*, *64*, 327–341. doi:10.1016/j.addr.2012.09.014 PMID:11259837

Kottayil, S., Crooks, P., Riggs, D., Murty, R., & Kottayil, S. (2001). *Thermal vaporizing device for drug delivery*. U.S. Patent Application 09/984,294.

Kozlovskaya, L., Abou-Kaoud, M., & Stepensky, D. (2014). Quantitative analysis of drug delivery to the brain via nasal route. *Journal of Controlled Release*, *189*, 133–140. doi:10.1016/j.jconrel.2014.06.053 PMID:24997277

Kumaravelrajan, R. (2016). Development and Evaluation of Elementary Osmotic Pump for the Simultaneous Delivery of Nifedipine and Metoprolol Tartrate. *Asian Journal of Pharmaceutics (AJP)*, *10*(4).

Kwatra, S., Taneja, G., & Nasa, N. (2012). Alternatives routes of drug administration-transdermal, pulmonary & parenteral. *Indo Global Journal of Pharmaceutical Sciences*, *2*(4), 409–426.

Kwon, G. S., & Okano, T. (1996). Polymeric micelles as new drug carriers. *Advanced Drug Delivery Reviews*, *21*(2), 107–116. doi:10.1016/S0169-409X(96)00401-2

Labiris, N. R., & Dolovich, M. B. (2003). Pulmonary drug delivery. Part II: The role of inhalant delivery devices and drug formulations in therapeutic effectiveness of aerosolized medications. *British Journal of Clinical Pharmacology*, *56*(6), 600–612. doi:10.1046/j.1365-2125.2003.01893.x PMID:14616419

Li, Y., Shawgo, R. S., Tyler, B., Henderson, P. T., Vogel, J. S., Rosenberg, A., ... Cima, M. J. (2004). In vivo release from a drug delivery MEMS device. *Journal of Controlled Release*, *100*(2), 211–219. doi:10.1016/j.jconrel.2004.08.018 PMID:15544869

Liu, X., Wang, S., Chai, L., Zhang, D., Sun, Y., Xu, L., & Sun, J. (2014). A two-step strategy to design high bioavailable controlled-release nimodipine tablets: The push–pull osmotic pump in combination with the micronization/solid dispersion techniques. *International Journal of Pharmaceutics*, *461*(1), 529–539. doi:10.1016/j.ijpharm.2013.12.023 PMID:24374219

Luo, Z., Cai, K., Hu, Y., Zhao, L., Liu, P., Duan, L., & Yang, W. (2011). Mesoporous Silica Nanoparticles End-Capped with Collagen: Redox-Responsive Nanoreservoirs for Targeted Drug Delivery. *Angewandte Chemie International Edition*, *50*(3), 640–643. doi:10.1002/anie.201005061 PMID:21226142

Luo, Z., Cai, K., Hu, Y., Zhao, L., Liu, P., Duan, L., & Yang, W. (2011). Mesoporous Silica Nanoparticles End-Capped with Collagen: Redox-Responsive Nanoreservoirs for Targeted Drug Delivery. *Angewandte Chemie International Edition*, *50*(3), 640–643. doi:10.1002/anie.201005061 PMID:21226142

Mainardes, R. M., & Silva, L. P. (2004). Drug delivery systems: Past, present, and future. *Current Drug Targets*, *5*(5), 449–455. doi:10.2174/1389450043345407 PMID:15216911

Maisel, W. H., & Laskey, W. K. (2007). Drug-eluting stents. *Circulation*, *115*(17), e426–e427. doi:10.1161/CIRCULATIONAHA.107.688176 PMID:17470700

Mathur, M., & Mishra, R. (2016). A review on osmotic pump drug delivery system. *International Journal of Pharmaceutical Sciences and Research*, *7*(2), 453.

Mura, S., Nicolas, J., & Couvreur, P. (2013). Stimuli-responsive nanocarriers for drug delivery. *Nature Materials*, *12*(11), 991–1003. doi:10.1038/nmat3776 PMID:24150417

Murthy, C. D., Sunkara, G., & Young, D. (Eds.). (2007). *Pharmaceutical product development: in vitro-in vivo correlation*. Taylor & Francis US.

Narasimhan, B., & Langer, R. (1997). Zero-order release of micro-and macromolecules from polymeric devices: The role of the burst effect. *Journal of Controlled Release*, *47*(1), 13–20. doi:10.1016/S0168-3659(96)01611-2

Oktayoğlu, P., Gür, A., Yardımeden, İ., Çağlayan, M., Çevik, F., Bozkurt, M., ... Nas, K. (2014). Comparison of the Efficacy of Phonophoresis and Conventional Ultrasound Therapy in Patients with Primary Knee Osteoarthritis. Erciyes Medical Journal. *Erciyes Tip Dergisi*, *36*(1), 11–18. doi:10.5152/etd.2013.64

Peppas, N. A., Caldorera-Moore, M. E., & Steichen, S. D. (2015). *Historical Survey of Drug Delivery Devices*. Drug-device Combinations for Chronic Diseases.

Pirmoradi, F. N., Jackson, J. K., Burt, H. M., & Chiao, M. (2011). A magnetically controlled MEMS device for drug delivery: Design, fabrication, and testing. *Lab on a Chip*, *11*(18), 3072–3080. doi:10.1039/c1lc20438f PMID:21860883

Pirmoradi, F. N., Jackson, J. K., Burt, H. M., & Chiao, M. (2011). A magnetically controlled MEMS device for drug delivery: Design, fabrication, and testing. *Lab on a Chip*, *11*(18), 3072–3080. doi:10.1039/c1lc20438f PMID:21860883

Preedy, E. C., & Prokopovich, P. (2013). *History of inhaler devices. In Inhaler devices-fundamentals, design and drug delivery* (p. 13). Cambridge, MA: Woodhead Publishing.

Sachan, V. K., Singh, A. K., Jahan, K., Kumbar, S. G., Nagarale, R. K., & Bhattacharya, P. K. (2014). Development of redox-conducting polymer electrodes for non-gassing electro-osmotic pumps: A novel approach. *Journal of the Electrochemical Society*, *161*(13), H3029–H3034. doi:10.1149/2.0071413jes

Sanidas, E. A., Golemati, S., & Dangas, G. D. (2015). Interventional Pharmacology: Stent Based Drug Delivery, Local Drug Delivery Management of Patients Before and After PCI. In PanVascular Medicine (pp. 993-1007). Springer Berlin Heidelberg.

Santini, J. T., Cima, M. J., & Langer, R. (1999). A controlled-release microchip. *Nature*, *397*(6717), 335–338. doi:10.1038/16898 PMID:9988626

Sharma, S., Nijdam, A. J., Sinha, P. M., Walczak, R. J., Liu, X., Cheng, M. M., & Ferrari, M. (2006). Controlled-release microchips. *Expert Opinion on Drug Delivery*, *3*(3), 379–394. doi:10.1517/17425247.3.3.379 PMID:16640498

Sharma, S., Nijdam, A. J., Sinha, P. M., Walczak, R. J., Liu, X., Cheng, M. M., & Ferrari, M. (2006). Controlled-release microchips. *Expert Opinion on Drug Delivery*, *3*(3), 379–394. doi:10.1517/17425247.3.3.379 PMID:16640498

Sonalkar, S., & Kapp, N. (2015). Intrauterine device insertion in the postpartum period: A systematic review. *The European Journal of Contraception & Reproductive Health Care*, *20*(1), 4–18. doi:10.3109/13625187.2014.971454 PMID:25397890

Steidler, L., & Rottiers, P. (2006). Therapeutic drug delivery by genetically modified Lactococcus lactis. *Annals of the New York Academy of Sciences*, *1072*(1), 176–186. doi:10.1196/annals.1326.031 PMID:17057198

Stockmann, C., Roberts, J. K., Yellepeddi, V. K., & Sherwin, C. M. (2015). Clinical pharmacokinetics of inhaled antimicrobials. *Clinical Pharmacokinetics*, *54*(5), 473–492. doi:10.100740262-015-0250-x PMID:25735634

Thomas, D. A., Myers, M. A., Wichert, B., Schreier, H., & Gonzalez-Rothi, R. J. (1991). Acute effects of liposome aerosol inhalation on pulmonary function in healthy human volunteers. *Chest*, *99*(5), 1268–1270. doi:10.1378/chest.99.5.1268 PMID:2019191

Tsals, I., Gross, J., & Lavi, G. (1999). *Cartridge-based drug delivery device*. U.S. Patent 5,858,001.

Vaghefi, F. (1999). *Dry powder inhaler*. U.S. Patent 5,875,776.

Weinstein, L. A., Richards, F. M., Laun, D. A., & Middleton, D. T., Jr. (1999). *Metered dose inhaler spacer*. U.S. Patent D412, 979.

Wolinsky, J. B., Colson, Y. L., & Grinstaff, M. W. (2012). Local drug delivery strategies for cancer treatment: Gels, nanoparticles, polymeric films, rods, and wafers. *Journal of Controlled Release*, *159*(1), 14–26. doi:10.1016/j.jconrel.2011.11.031 PMID:22154931

Wood, K. C., Zacharia, N. S., Schmidt, D. J., Wrightman, S. N., Andaya, B. J., & Hammond, P. T. (2008). Electroactive controlled release thin films. *Proceedings of the National Academy of Sciences of the United States of America*, *105*(7), 2280–2285. doi:10.1073/pnas.0706994105 PMID:18272499

Wu, S. Z., Harish, S., Sanders-Millare, D., & Guruwaiya, J. A. (2001). *Implantable medical device having protruding surface structures for drug delivery and cover attachment*. U.S. Patent 6,254,632.

Zanen, P., Go, L. T., & Lammers, J. W. (1998). The efficacy of a low-dose, monodisperse parasympathicolytic aerosol compared with a standard aerosol from a metered-dose inhaler. *European Journal of Clinical Pharmacology*, *54*(1), 27–30. doi:10.1007002280050415 PMID:9591926

Chapter 6
Low-Cost Body Area Network for Monitoring of Diabetic Patient

Geshwaree Huzooree
Charles Telfair Institute, Mauritius

Kavi Kumar Khedo
University of Mauritius, Mauritius

Noojehan Joonas
Ministry of Health and Quality of Life, Mauritius

ABSTRACT

The confluence of wireless body area network (WBAN) advancement has led to a great shift in the healthcare sector and has enormous potential to reduce long-term costs, social problems, workforce issues, and improve quality of healthcare service. Based on existing literature on WBANs, technologies, and standards, a WBAN is proposed to bridge the gap of information between patients and healthcare professional through sharing of high quality of information (QoI) whereby the latter can have real-time and historical view of patient's condition for effective and timely monitoring. This feature will also address the time and space restriction of healthcare service. Moreover, a best fit glucose prediction model considering various exogenous inputs based on autoregressive (ARX) model is proposed to perform data analytics in a WBAN system. The performance of the model is evaluated through performance metrics. Potential challenges and future research work are pointed out for further development of WBAN.

INTRODUCTION

Diabetes remains a critical plague with the continuous rising of fundamental health challenges associated with it. The International Diabetes Federation (IDF) estimated that Mauritius has the highest adult diabetes prevalence rate of 22.0% in the South-East Asia region (IDF Diabetes Atlas, 2017) and WHO reported that the prevalence might increase by 98% by 2030 (Shaw, Sicree, & Zimmet, 2010). Moreover,

DOI: 10.4018/978-1-5225-4969-7.ch006

diabetes leads to major health complications which ultimately results into national health burden and are associated with very high social and economic costs. There is a high need for real-time monitoring systems that can be provided ubiquitously for better diabetes disease management. Pervasive Healthcare System (PHS) is a promising technology since it enables real-time continuous monitoring and helps to prevent the symptoms of diabetes in patients through timely intervention and provide effective responses during emergency cases. Moreover, with the help of a PHS, patients diagnosed with diabetes can make better informed decisions, self-manage their vital signs, be more patient-centric than doctor-centric and lead a more pleasurable life (Preuveneers & Berbers, 2008; Chiarini, Ray, Masella, & Ganz, 2013). Low-cost is one of the most fundamental factors for the acceptance of real-time diabetic monitoring system using wireless body area network.

This chapter presents an overview of the current state-of-the-art technologies for monitoring patients by classifying the Pervasive Mobile Healthcare Systems (PMHSs) under 4 main classifications namely self-monitoring, assisted-monitoring, supervised-monitoring and continuous-monitoring. It also covers research challenges in the PMHSs such as high dependability, reliability, security and privacy for successful adoption and acceptability. This chapter also outlines the importance for a low-cost Wireless Body Area Network (WBAN) system for real-time diabetes monitoring and proposes the design of a low-cost WBAN system architecture. The data analytics that are used to process the data from the WBAN are described and evaluated through performance metrics.

CURRENT STATE OF TECHNOLOGIES

Recently, many PMHSs have been designed and implemented to manage and monitor different chronic diseases. A recent survey was conducted to evaluate the state-of-the-art PMHSs to identify major technical requirements and design challenges associated with its realization (Huzooree, Khedo, & Joonas, 2017b). The PMHSs were classified into four main categories namely: self-monitoring, assisted-monitoring, supervised-monitoring and continuous-monitoring.

Self-Monitoring

Nowadays, many patients are moving towards a fundamental strategy to promote preventive healthcare by using a vast range of self-monitoring health technologies. This type of disease monitoring is more patient-centric than doctor-centric, thus the patients' commitment and diligence is critical for effective disease management. Very often, patients make use of available off-the-shelf technologies such as invasive and non-invasive sensors and mobile phones to gather, monitor and manage their conditions through mobile applications. Various communication protocols such as Bluetooth, Global System for mobile communication (GSM), Universal Mobile Telecommunication Service (UTMS), Internet and Hypertext Transfer Protocol (HTTP) are used for transferring of information from the sensors to the mobile phones. A recent survey revealed that common diseases that are self-monitored have been chronic obstructive pulmonary diseases (Hofer, Schumacher, & Bromuri, 2015; Joshua, Qian, & Bruce, 2015) and sleep apnea (Thanuja & Balakrishnan, 2013). In this particular type of monitoring, there is usually no interaction with the health care professionals and the patients are in charge.

Assisted-Monitoring

Assisted-monitoring is another common type of disease management whereby the patients do not only self-monitor their conditions but also seek assistance of healthcare professionals in emergency cases. Same communication protocols as self-monitoring are used to transfer information. A recent survey shows that common diseases that are monitored with assistance are asthma (Al-Dowaihi et al., 2013), risks of fall (Horta, Lopes, Rodrigues, & Proenca, 2013), cardiac diseases (Kumar & Ganesan, 2011), and any other chronic diseases (Liu, Wen, Yu, Yang, & Wang, 2011)

Supervised-Monitoring

Patients also seek supervised monitoring periodically from healthcare professionals to manage diseases such as cardiac problems, chronic conditions and hypertension. In such cases, besides handling emergency cases, health professionals also monitor the psychological data of the patients once in a while to ensure that there is no anomaly in their health conditions. In case of any abnormal situation, an urgent message is sent to the healthcare professional's mobile phone to take immediate actions. Some common communication protocols to transfer information among the sensors, mobile phone and servers that are used besides Bluetooth, GSM, UTMS, Internet and Hypertext Transfer Protocol (HTTP) are 2/3G, 3G/4G, Wi-Fi, Universal Asynchronous Receiver-Transmitter (UART), Universal Serial Bus (USB), ZigBee, Extensible Messaging and Presence Protocol (XMPP), Web services, Transport Layer Security (TSL), GPRS and SimpliciTi (Huzooree et al., 2017b).

Continuous-Monitoring

Continuous monitoring goes beyond all the other types of monitoring whereby the patients require real-time active and passive monitoring from healthcare professionals. The patients' health data can be continuously accessed by healthcare professionals to provide timely diagnosis and necessary intervention. This type of monitoring uses intelligent algorithms to facilitate the information transfer among the devices and is mostly used to manage stress, chronic disease of cognitive impairment, dementia or Alzheimer.

SENSORS AND TECHNOLOGIES FOR DIABETES MONITORING

Sensor technologies can maximize the independence for individuals to participate actively in their healthcare. The quality of life and patients' outcome can significantly improve as they are more likely to participate in behavioral changes (Frontino et al., 2013). Health complications can be reduced to a great extent through proper diet, physical exercises, and medications. However, it is also critical to monitor the glucose pattern of diabetic patients in an invasive and noninvasive manner so that timely interventions are performed. Currently, most glucose monitoring devices are invasive, minimally invasive and non-invasive. Despite a wide range of devices have been introduced, it is highly critical to ensure the devices have already sought approval and got clearance from Food and Drug Association (FDA).

Invasive methods to measure blood glucose levels can be done using two traditional invasive methods 1) finger pricking, which uses disposable sample strips, or 2) minimally invasive glucose monitoring systems, which use implanted sensors that need regular replacement.

Despite the prevalent advancements in glucose monitoring biosensors, there are still many challenges related to the achievement of reliable glucose monitoring. Desirable features of a glucose biosensors are accuracy, reliability, ultra-sensitivity, fast response, and low cost per test (Ozana et al., 2014). Although all the revolution, the size, physical compatibility and reliability of body sensors still remain a crucial aspect to their wide acceptance and adoption. With this motivation, there is a high need for novel materials.

Non-Invasive Techniques for Diabetes Monitoring

Various noninvasive technologies are categorized into optical methods, electric methods or other methods shown in Figure 1. One of the major challenges is to perform accurate glucose measurement from the various available technologies since they are highly sensitive to many external factors.

Optical Techniques for Diabetes Monitoring

Blood glucose levels are detected by determining and analyzing the quantity and optical properties of light (wavelength of radiation) which is either absorbed, transmitted or emitted as a function of glucose concentration. The classification of sensors is based on the various optical properties of light which is applied. Moreover, the optical properties of light are used to classify the various sensors available on the market which are employing spectroscopy principle.

Figure 1. Non Invasive technologies

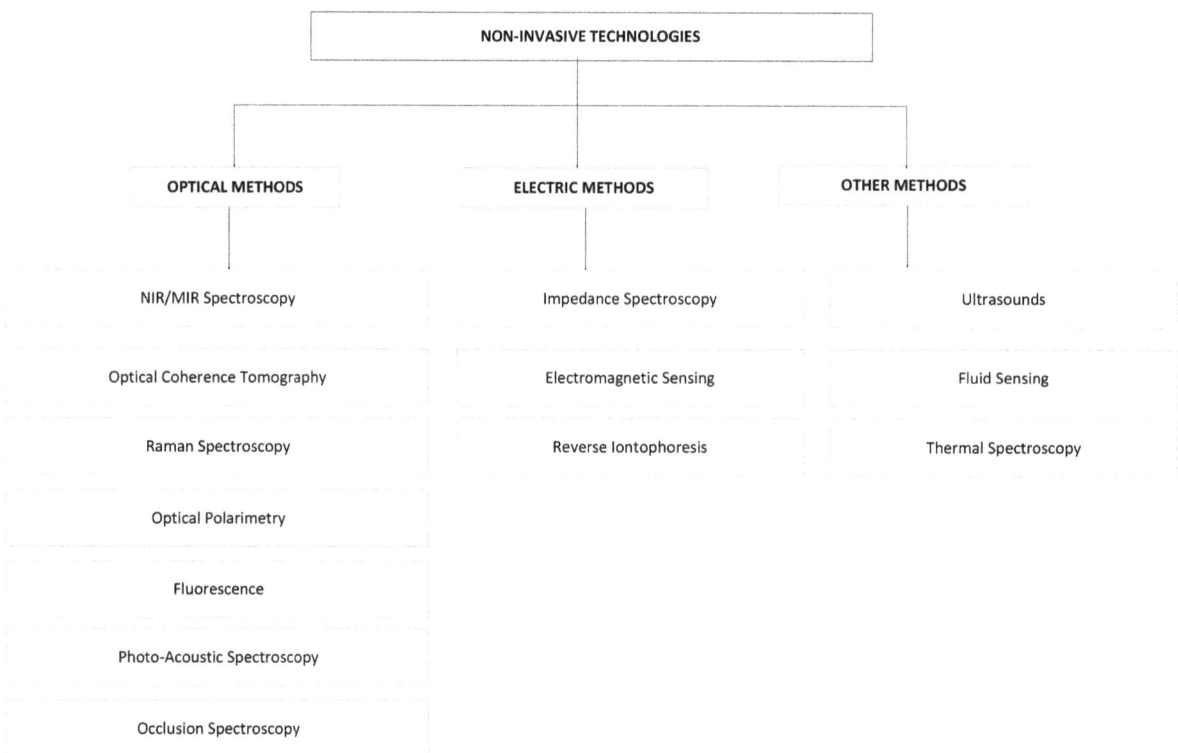

Near Infrared Spectroscopy

Table 1 illustrates some devices using the Near Infrared (NIR) spectroscopy technology. NIR is based on absorption-transmittance photometry and is located in the wavelength region of 730–2500 nm (So, Choi, Wong, & Chung, 2012; Vashist, 2012; Tura, 2008). NIR has been successfully tested with human and was proven to be safe. The technique has some prominent limitations as it is affected by physical and chemical parameters such as body temperature, blood pressure, skin hydration, and concentrations of triglyceride and albumin which interfere strongly with the blood glucose measurements (Tura, Maran, & Pacini, 2007). Moreover, it is sensitive to environmental conditions such as temperature, relative humidity, light, and air quality.

Mid Infrared (MIR) Spectroscopy

MIR uses the same physical principle as NIR, but it is based on light in the spectral range of 2500–10,000 nm. When compared to NIR, however, MIR exhibits reduced scattering phenomena and increased absorption due to the higher wavelengths. Moreover, the penetration through skin is very poor (Oliver, Toumazou, Cass, & Johnston, 2009). On the other hand, MIR has an advantage over NIR since the response peak of biological factors is more precise with MIR than NIR. The technique has been explored for noninvasive glucose measurements, but so far without success (Smith, 2017).

Optical Coherence Tomography

Table 2 represents the device that implemented the Optical Coherence Tomography (OCT) methods. The optical setup consists of a broad bandwidth light source, an interferometer and a photodetector to detect the output images. OCT is regarded as surrogate measure for glucose. However, OCT is very sensitive to motion of individuals and skin temperature which often leads to inaccurate measurement for higher degrees (Tura, 2008 ; Oliver et al., 2009).

Table 1. Optical methods: Near infrared spectroscopy

Device	Company	Technology	Target Tissue	Approval	Status
Diasensor 1000	BioControl Technology Inc.	Uses NIR light of 1640 nm, 1670 nm	Forearm skin	CE approval (2000)	• Device was large in size • Could not detect hypoglycemic events • Discontinued in 2002 due to consistent technological and financial issues
Combo Glucometer	CNoga Medical Ltd	Uses a wavelength range of with the range of 600 nm - 1150 nm	Finger	FDA approval (2011)	• Is used only with patients above 18 years • Lack of clarification on the principles used • Technology did not work as well as planned and might require additional time
SugarTrac™	LifeTrac Systems Inc.	Uses wavelength of 650 - 1300 nm	Earlobe	Not available	• Unsuccessful clinical trials • Difficulties in the mechanical design • Not commercialized
MedOptix™	Medoptix Inc.	Uses ReSense technology (NIR light)	Skin	Not available	• No reliable amount ot glucose was found into sweat, whether the film is thick or thin • Product was discontinued

Table 2. Optical methods

Device	Company	Technology	Target Tissue	Approval	Status
Glucolight Sentris-100TM	GlucoLight Corporation	OCT	Skin dermis	Not available	Project ceased due financial limitations
C8 MediSensors optical glucose monitorTM	C8 MediSensors	Raman Spectroscopy	Finger	CE Approval	Awaiting for clinical studies and trials for further validation
Scout diabetic score	VeraLight Inc.	Fluorescence Technology	Left volar forearm	• CE Approval • Health Canada License for commercial distribution	Issues with regards to portability, wearability and unobtrusiveness as the commercial glucose meter
ApriseTM	Glucon Medical Ltd	Photoacoustic Spectroscopy	Forearm skin	Not available	• Highly sensitive to other physiological substances leading to interferences • Not commercialized
OrSense NBM-200G	OrSense Ltd	Occlusion Spectroscopy	Fingertip	CE mark (2007)	Product is for market awareness purpose only

Raman Spectroscopy

Table 2 illustrates the device implementing Raman spectroscopy, a technique that attempts to circumvent the high absorption of water in the mid-infrared region. Human fluids can be helpful to estimated blood glucose concentration level since the emission of scattered light is sensitive to molecular rotation and vibration (So et al., 2012). Moreover, the light source is proved to be quite harmful to human body. When compared to NIR and MIR spectroscopy, it provides sharper spectra. Nevertheless, it is less sensitive to temperature and water.

Optical Polarimetry

The technique optical polarimetry has been extensively used in pharmaceutical and nutritional industries. It is based on the optical rotary dispersion of polarized light. The rotation is dependent on several factors such as temperature, thickness and concentrations of the samples. With this motivation, there have been many trials to apply this optical technique for non-invasive glucose monitoring. Moreover, the high dispersion coefficients of skin generate complete beam depolarization (Cameron & Cote, 1997). Despite many advancements, no device employing this technology has been developed so far. Nevertheless, researchers have presented a real-time optical polarimetry approach utilizing dual wavelength (Malik & Coté, 2010).

Fluorescence Technology

Table 2 illustrates the device using fluorescence technology, which is based on the principle that human tissue will generate fluorescence when exposed to lights at specific wavelength (Pickup, Hussain, Evans, Rolinski, & Birch, 2005). This technology is highly sensitive and is dependent on other factors such as skin pigmentation, redness, and epidermal thickness besides glucose. However, it could lead to scattering phenomenon and the life span is short (Klonoff, 2012).

Photoacoustic Spectroscopy

Table 2 represents the device using photoacoustic spectroscopy, which uses the principle of ultrasonic waves by the absorption of infrared light to measure the glucose concentration (Tanaka, Tajima, & Seyama, 2017). This method has an advantage over other spectroscopy to determine the glucose level since the acoustic response of blood is better than water. However, it is sensitive to fluctuation of temperature, noise and costly (Salam, bin Mohd Saad, Manap, & Salehuddin, 2016).

Occlusion Spectroscopy

Table 2 represents the device using occlusion spectroscopy, which employs the scattering phenomenon of light. An increase in glucose level results into decreasing the diffusion coefficient of light and enhancing the transmission of light. Moreover, the blood flow at the targeted tissue (the finger) is occluded momentarily to generate an optical signal using light sources and detectors operating at 610 nm and 810 nm (Vashist, 2012).

Electric Methods

Impedance Spectroscopy

Table 3 illustrates the device using impedance spectroscopy, which uses electrical property change of tissue indirectly affected by blood glucose level after applying electric current (Amir et al., 2007). Spectrum in impedance spectroscopy is measured in the frequency range of 0.1 to 100 MHz frequency. The device cost effective and it does not need any statically derived calibration model. However, the calibration process is not trivial and the effect of physical factors such as sweat, movement and temperature is high.

Electromagnetic Sensing

Table 3 illustrates some devices using electromagnetic sensing, which is a technique detects the dielectric properties of blood exploiting the electromagnetic coupling between two inductors turned around the blood sample (Sparacino et al., 2012). The glucose level can be determined since the dielectric properties of the solution are highly sensitive to any changes in glucose. However, the blood glucose is highly sensitive to temperature and consequently the temperature should be measured to ensure that the glucose readings are correctly interpreted. In addition, the blood dielectric parameters are influenced by several components other than glucose which can eventually lead to inaccurate measurements (So et al., 2012).

Reverse Iontophoresis

Table 3 illustrates some devices using reverse iontophoresis, whereby glucose concentration can be extracted through intact skin by electro-osmotic (Potts, Tamada, & Tierney, 2002). While this technology has great potential, the electrodes irritate the skin and need to be in contact with the skin for a minimum of 60 minutes. Consequently, this limitation leads to lack of patience from patients. Moreover, the patient's sweat had a high impact on the glucose readings leading to incorrect diagnoses.

Table 3. Electric methods: Impedance spectroscopy

Device	Company	Technology	Target Tissue	Approval	Status
PENDRA	Pendragon Medical ltd	Impedance Spectroscopy	Wrist	Not available	Withdrawn from the market due to poor reliability
Glucoband®	Calisto Medical, Inc.	Electromagnetic Sensing	Wrist	FDA Approved	• Correlation coefficient of the glucose measurements between Glucoband® and AccuCheck: 0.89 • Device could do data transfer via USB • Durable battery life • Device appeared in 2005 and the commercial pilot was planned for 2011 but was never released
GluControl GC300 ®	ArithMed GmbH	Electromagnetic Sensing	Fingertip skin	Not available	• Portable device, battery-powered with data storage facility • Lack of evidence how the device operates and test of clinical trials were not presented • Company ceased to exist around 2006
TouchTrak Pro 200	Samsung Fine Chemicals Co. Ltd	Electromagnetic Sensing	Fingertip	Not available	• The device was not commercialized due to unknown reasons • Claimed to be a portable device with high cost
GlucoWise™	MediWise Ltd	Electromagnetic Sensing	Finger or ear-lobe	Still waiting for approval	• Measurements can then be wirelessly uploaded via Bluetooth 4.0 using the mobile app • Glucose readings can then be transmitted to the Cloud or to a PC via USB cable. • Still have to demonstrate accuracy and reliability
SugarBEAT®	Nemaura Medical	Electromagnetic Sensing	Arm, leg or abdomen	Not available	• Measurements can be transferred via Bluetooth and also forwarded onto healthcare professionals • Expect market launch in 2017
GlucoWatch® Biographer	Cygnus, Inc.	Reverse Iontophoresis	Wrist	FDA Approval in 2001	• The sale was discontinued in July 2007 following persistent device issues • The device was expensive • Long warm up times (2–3 hour) Disposable pad must be replaced every 12h of monitoring time for accurate result • The readings was highly sensitive to factors such as motion, exercising, sweating or rapid temperature changes and thus leading to faulty readings
GluCall	KMH Co. Ltd	Reverse Iontophoresis		Korean FDA approval	The device was not commercialized due to unknown reasons

Other Methods

Fluid Harvesting

Table 4 illustrates some devices using fluid harvesting, which is a technique is based on the use of a laser light or ultrasounds on the human skin to generate micropores (Tura, 2008). Despite this technique have

Table 4. Other methods: Fluid harvesting

Device	Company	Technology	Target Tissue	Approval	Status
Biophotonics-based NGM	SpectRx Inc.	Fluid Harvesting	Skin	Not available	• Calibration procedure is quite easy • The device supports wireless telemeter • Glucose meter needs calibration • Glucose measurements have a time lag of 2-4 min
Symphony™ CGM	Echo Therapeutics	Fluid Harvesting	Skin	Not available	• Triggers alerts upon rapid changes in glucose concentration • Good correlation coefficient with glucose meters • Aims to launch 2015
CGM device	Infratec Inc.	Thermal Spectroscopy	Ear	Not available	Very limited documentation is available on this device
CCM device	Hitachi Ltd	Thermal Spectroscopy	Not specified	Not available	Not commercialized due to unknown reasons
GlucoTrack™	Integrity Applications Ltd	Ultrasonic, electromagnetic and heat capacity	Ear lobe	CE Mark in 2013	• Demonstrates multi-sensor capabilities, high precision and accuracy • Alerts for hypo and hyperglycemia and shows good correlation with glucose meters • Requires individual monthly re-calibration using invasive basal and post prandial fingertip glucose references (approx. 90-120min) • Claimed to be indiscrete by users to wear on the ear in public

few limitations, it is categorized as minimally invasive and a mismatch between the interstitial fluid and blood can occur and lead to inaccurate readings (Bruen, Delaney, Florea, & Diamond, 2017).

Thermal Spectroscopy

Table 4 illustrates some devices using thermal spectroscopy, which measures absorptive effects of glucose on the infra radiation signals naturally emitted by the human body. However, this technology is also highly sensitive to body temperature and motion (Eadie & Steele, 2017; Salam et al., 2016).

Ultrasonic, Electromagnetic, and Heat Capacity

Table 4 illustrates the device using ultrasonic, electromagnetic and heat capacity, which is a technique that has higher precision and accuracy during glucose sensing as it involves a combination of the 3 non-invasive technologies. Consequently, the noise is significantly reduced during measurements.

Invasive Sensors and Technologies for Diabetes Monitoring

Invasive sensors can be used in the treatment of diabetes. Nowadays, patients' either rely on implantable needle-type enzyme sensor or uses a glucose meter to monitor their glucose levels.

Implantable Needle-Type Enzyme Sensors

Table 5 represents the implantable glucose sensors which act as artificial pancreas and are used to ensure continuous glucose measurements and monitoring. These sensors have several challenges such as ensuring the sensor stability which is difficult especially when a biosensor approach is employed. Moreover, the calibration process for each patients is quite challenging and sometimes there can be issues of sensor compatibility with the patients' body (Frontino et al., 2013; Oliver et al., 2009).

Leading Commercially-Available Glucose Biosensors

Table 6 shows a wide range of leading glucose biosensors that are available off-the-shelf nowadays. For most biosensors, it can be seen that the sample size required to measure the glucose level is around 0.5 microliter. However, the accuracy of the biosensors differs. Most of them have the capacity to store test results.

ISSUES AND CHALLENGES FOR PMHS FOR DIABETIC MONITORING

PMHSs is a promising technology for effectively monitor chronic diseases to provide emergency and preventive healthcare services, however, there are major bottlenecks that need to be addressed at different levels in the system namely the sensor level, network level and human level.

Node-Level Challenges

Sensor Technology

Patients use both minimally invasive sensors and non-invasive ones during their diabetes monitoring and treatment. Therefore, it is critical that these sensors are unobtrusive, physically comfortable and

Table 5. Implantable needle-type enzyme sensors

Device	Company	Target Tissue	Approval	Status
DexCom® SEVEN® PLUS	DexCom, San Diego, CA	Skin		Approved for 7-day wear in 2010
Medtronic MiniMed 670G	Medtronic MiniMed, Northridge, CA	Skin	FDA approved (2012) for Type 1 diabetes (>= 14 years)	• Will launch in 2017 • Cannot be used in children < 7 years • Cannot be used on patients less than eight units of insulin per day
Guardian® REAL- Time	Minneapolis, Minnesota, US	Stomach area	FDA Approved in 2006	• Offer exceptional comfort and continuous support • Alerts the patients' for any unusual measurement • Convenient, smart and comprehensive
Abbott Diabetes Care FreeStyle Navigator	Maidenhead, Berkshire, UK	Implanted sensor with an external monitor	FDA Approved in 2008	Require calibrations at 10, 12, 24, and 72 hours and get the glucose readings

Table 6. Leading commercially-available glucose biosensors

Device	Sample Size (μL)	Target Site	Test Time(s)/ Test Memory	Comm.	Size	Weight	Cost
FORA TN'G (Test N'GO) Blood Glucose Meter	0.5	Fingertip	5 450	Bluetooth	93 x 26.03 x 5.57 mm	26.8g (without battery)	$29.99
FORA TN'G (Test N'GO) Voice Blood Glucose Meter	0.5	Fingertip	5 450	Bluetooth	104.4 x 58 x 23 mm	71.2 g (without battery)	$24.99
Accu-Chek Aviva Connect	0.6	Fingertip	5 750	Bluetooth Micro USB	3.1 x 1.8 x 0.8 inches	6.1 ounces	$49.99
AgaMatrix Wavesense	0.5	Fingertip	6 300	Bluetooth	1.18 x 2.56 x 0.39 inches	18.4 g	$5.00
Contour Next EZ	0.6	Fingertip	5 480	Bluetooth	3.15 x 2.09 x 0.5 inches	1.6 ounces (with battery)	$17.85
FreeStyle Lite	0.3	fingertip, palm and upper arm	4	Bluetooth	1.57 x 2.90 x 0.65 inches	1.4 ounces (with battery)	$19.23
Nova Max	0.3	Fingertips and other sites	5 400	Bluetooth	3.6x2.3x0.9 inches	2.65 oz	$19.94
LifeScan's OneTouch Ultra 2	1	Fingertip, forearm, or palm	5 500	Bluetooth	7.92 x 5.72 x 2.29 cm	1.5 ounce or 42.5gms, with batteries	$16.47
OneTouch Verio IQ	0.4	Fingertip	5 750	USB cable	3.46 x 1.85 x 0.47 inches	1.66 ounces with battery	$15.00
Walgreens True Metrix Air	0.5	Fingertip and other sites	4 500	Bluetooth	1.65x 1.8x 2.7 inches	NA	$21.97

compatible to human tissues. Moreover, the size, form, aesthetic issues and safety concerns of the sensors should be addressed since patients can face discomfort due to the weight, excessive sweating or might also develop rashes since the electronic and magnetic energy are eventually absorbed by human body (Nachman et al., 2010).

Furthermore, novel research must be carried out to have one sensor design that can be used for multiple conditions since patients prefer to wear fewer sensors devices. New developments about miniaturization of sensor design would surely overcome the shortcomings of bulky sensors. Patients are concerned with the visibility and discreteness of the device so that they are comfortable to use it in public. An effective sensor design especially for implanted sensors should also address the issue of battery life time. At the same time, new techniques for sustainability should be explored to make them maintenance free since the cost and patients' inconvenience increases during replacement and re-calibration.

Efficiency/Power Consumption

High amount of energy is consumed during the transfer of information and ensuring minimum power consumption and energy efficiency is one of the main issues about the WBAN. Unfortunately, battery-operated sensor devices have a battery lifetime and need to be recharged or replaced once the battery has depleted. Thus, novel researches on energy efficient advanced sensor designs are important. Further research in energy-harvesting, particle swarm optimization, battery technologies, power scavenging techniques (Abbate, Avvenuti, & Light, 2012, Zhang et al., 2013) will appropriately address these shortcomings.

Proper use of wireless communication during routing and controlling traffic seems a potential way to ensure energy efficiency (Alemdar & Ersoy, 2010). Energy consumption should be considered as a design optimization strategy with very high priority while developing the protocols and algorithms for sensor networks to prolong the network lifetime in BAN systems (Ghamari, Arora, Sherratt, & Harwin, 2015). The mobile computing tier usually have a high processing power, storage capacity and rechargeable battery, thus it can move closer to the sensors which are transmitting information during data collection (Latiff, Latiff, & Ahmad, 2011).

As widely addressed in the literature (Bachir, Dohler, Watteyne, & Leung, 2010), the main reasons leading to energy inefficiency are collisions, overhearing and idle listening. Moreover, low power MAC protocols in sensor network have been widely explored improve energy efficiency by turning the radio on and off periodically to prolong sensor lifetime. However, the protocols proposed such as S-MAC, T-MAC, TRAMA, WiseMAC, B-MAC and SCP-MAC show low network throughput and delay performance at different traffic (Chen, Gonzalez, Vasilakos, Cao, & Leung, 2011). It is still a challenge for low power protocol to synchronize the duty cycles of sensors with different power requirements and traffic characteristics especially in different levels of emergencies.

Network-Level Challenges

Quality of Information (QoI) and Quality of Service (QoS)

There is still a high need to explore effective and optimized way of data collection and data transmission to ensure high QoI and QoS, which are compulsory for an effective disease management for all medical applications (C. Li, Li, & Kohno, 2009). When the QoI is tampered due to delayed, incorrect sensor data, fading and packet loss during data transmission over the network, this ultimately results into wrong diagnosis of patients and untimely decisions. Thus, for a wider acceptance of PMHSs and reliable data transfer, a higher degree of confidence of QoI is fundamental and thus new techniques should be explored. The reliability of information can be considered either end-to-end or on a per link base to ensure in in-order data delivery. Furthermore, messages should be transmitted and delivered within the specified reasonable time and any possible error in this regard may cause fatal results. Therefore, it is highly important to ensure the network reliability as it has a direct impact on the patients' treatment and life.

Despite all the advancement made, there is still the need to adapt the reliability techniques to specific WBAN system to ensure high QoI and QoS.

Security and Privacy

Patients' sensitive health data can be highly vulnerable as these are usually transmitted over different wireless connections and the internet. Ensuring security and privacy of information over the network during data collection and transmission has become an inescapable challenge that cannot be overlooked and has to be guaranteed. Patients' data can be tampered and hijacked with malicious intent (M. Li, Lou, & Ren, 2010). Body sensors can also be faced with security attacks or privacy leak (Srinivasan, Stankovic, & Whitehouse, 2008) by compromising the sensor and WBAN gateway (Uniyal & Raychoudhury, 2014).

Thus, the security and privacy requirements of PMHSs can be categorized as confidentiality, authenticity, integrity, dependability, accountability, required access control, and availability.

Table 7 describes the possible solutions that can be explored for assuring the security and privacy requirements. However, most security and privacy measures usually consume power and should therefore be energy-efficient. Moreover, The Health Insurance Portability and Accountability Act (HIPAA) have established national standards, privacy and security rules to protect the patients' medical records. Commercial applications need to be explicit regarding the extent of their HIPAA compliance (El-gayar, Timsina, Nawar, & Eid, 2013).

Human–Centric Challenges

Technology Acceptance

One of the human-centric challenges that still prevail in promoting a successful PMHSs adoption is technological acceptance. Patients are quite reluctant to embrace new technologies especially if they are technology-naïve, technology-averse or they belong to an elderly population.

Critical qualities of technological acceptance that cannot be compromised are the user-friendliness and usability level of the system. Actions that have been used to increase the usability of the system are user involvement during the modeling of the project and developing natural interfaces with a diverse group of people. It is equally important to seek continuous feedback from the users, assess the level of

Table 7. Possible solutions for security and privacy

Security and Privacy Requirements		Possible Solutions
Data Confidentiality	Data should be private and be stored securely whereby only authorized users have access to it. The confidentiality should remain robust against any node comprise such as hi-jacking.	• Efficient encryption techniques at the network layer. • Access control methods
Data authenticity	Healthcare professional should also ensure that the information belongs only to the appropriate patient for precise diagnosis.	Message authentication codes
Data integrity	Patients data should not be tampered or falsified at any point in time	• Keyed secure hash function • Digital signature
Data dependability	Patients' data should be backup securely so that it is retrievable even under node failure.	
Access control	Patient's medical record should be accessible only to authorized users. The users should have autonomy and control over their data of any type.	• Tamper-proofing • Intrusion detection
Data accountability	A trace should be kept about all patient's transactions.	
Authentication	Proper authentication process should be followed before anyone can access the data. No outside party should be allowed to tamper the data.	• Security protocols • Public key cryptography • Radio frequency identification (RFID) • Random key distribution
Availability	All patients' data should not be compromised and should be available even under denial-of- service attack	• Intrusion detection • Redundancy

user-friendliness of the system and also incorporating the patient's requirements in the system. Moreover, adequate technical support and training is a key requirement to boost the acceptance level.

Other barriers with regards to the adoption of PMHSs include the accuracy of the system whereby the patients are quite concerned to invest in a system if the accuracy of the measurement is not guaranteed. Moreover, unsafe devices or PMHSs lead to reluctance of adoption since patients are apprehensive to encounter other complications such as exposure to lasers or infrared over a prolonged amount of time. Lastly, PMHSs should consider the time taken to generate the result since patients are reluctant to adopt solutions where the processing time is long.

Sensitivity of Sensors

Another major challenge that is open for research is the sensitivity of sensors devices whereby they are easily perturbed by harsh or hostile environmental conditions such as heat or even during exercising. Thus, the rate of device failure or incorrect data might increase. Hence, factoring re-calibration of sensors or development sensitivity algorithms during various environmental changes will bring a major contribution to the advances of PMHSs.

Mobility

Patients' demands are continuously rising as far as PMHSs are concerned. Nowadays, all patients want to access healthcare services anywhere and anytime ubiquitously. Thus, it is mandatory to devise new techniques to provide mobility support for the sensor devices so that they can always be connected to the network systems. There is a high need for new research and synthesis for novel development as far as macro-mobility and micro-mobility are concerned so that patients can be continuously connected to the communication networks without any intervention, irrespective of the movement and change in location (Touati & Tabish, 2013). The change from different networks should be very fluid so as to not to create delays and channel fading during information transfer especially if patients' life are at risk. New advances in multi-hop, multi-modal and ad hoc sensor networks can address these shortcomings.

Standardization

Even though a vast range of on-the-shelf wireless sensors devices are available, the manufacturers and vendors should also address all the process and protocols of standardization to ensure easy integration and enhanced interoperability with any healthcare system. Thus, manufacturers, vendors, network providers, healthcare professionals, researchers and other health organizations should abide by standardizing rules while developing or designing communication interfaces or sensor devices. It is very important that manufacturers abide by the set foundations and specifications while developing their products to reduce the costs for both the vendors and consumers. Moreover, such practices will avoid dependency on a specific vendors and vendor lock in. Besides open standards such as IEEE802.15.4, other standards can also be researched and developed to promote more open architectures.

Interoperability

Interoperability remains a crucial requirement to be met when it comes to integration to existing or new systems since all the patients' information should be readily available for a seamless and continuous monitoring (Hofer et al., 2015). Since there is a vast range of devices available on the market, it is very important that they can be easily and rapidly integrated over a network. As a matter of fact, it is fundamental that different infrastructures, sensor devices, hardware and other medical systems communicate seamlessly via standard format and protocols. Thus, there is a high need for coming up with interoperability protocols so that manufacturers, vendors and health organizations can abide by.

Cost Factors

Self-monitoring of blood glucose (SMBG) is the most common method used by diabetic patients. A recent survey reported that 70% diabetic patients practice SMBG (Kjome, Granas, Nerhus, Roraas, & Sandberg, 2010). With the recent development in glucometers, most of the commercially available ones are quite affordable due to market forces (Bwititi, Angel, & Day, 2008). A glucometer costs around $25 as depicted in Table 14. However, the cost of test strips is highly exorbitant since they need to be disposed after each measurement. The cost of a disposable strip is approximately $1. The operation cost is only feasible if the frequency of measurement is less. However, diabetic patients have to perform their blood glucose measurements around 8-10 times daily. Consequently, the total annual cost of strips comes to $365 assuming that the patients test only once per day. Moreover, patients measuring their glucose level at a higher frequency will undoubtedly incur higher yearly expenses. Zhang et al., reported that the overall market for glucose observing items was assessed 180 billion INR in the year 2000 (as cited in Yadav, Rani, Singh, & Murari, 2015).

Continuous Glucose Monitoring (CGM) solutions are also expensive and patients are reluctant to adopt them. Each CGM includes several direct costs including cost of the receiver, sensors, transmitters and calibration. The recent economic analysis conducted by National Clinical Guideline Centre (2015) on three of the main real time CGMs namely Dexcom G4, Abbott Freestyle, and Medtronic RT Guardian highlighted that the total average cost for the first year is approximately £3,511 and £3,674 for the second year per patient. Consequently, the overall cost of acquisition, operation and maintenance demotivate patients to adopt such strategies.

These cost concerns indeed create a high need for the development of low-cost non-invasive glucose monitoring devices for wider adoption and for accessibility.

SOLUTIONS AND RECOMMENDATIONS

Due all the open challenges mentioned, it is still a major concern to design a cost-effective and reliable WBAN with a higher degree of confidence for QoI for real-time continuous monitoring of patients. A low-cost WBAN for real-time diabetes is further described in this section so that healthcare professionals can continuously monitor patients' physiological parameters remotely, perform diagnosis, suggest appropriate treatments and take timely decisions (Huzooree, Khedo, & Joonas, 2016).

Several key requirements such as the design requirements, architectural design, sensor design, communication architecture, data design and application design are taken into consideration while designing the low-cost WBAN for real-time diabetes monitoring.

Design Requirements

The foremost design requirements for this proposed WBANs is to ensure a higher degree of confidence for QoI/QoS in terms of timeliness, accuracy, reliability, completeness, relevancy, usability and confidentiality. Ensuring high QoI/QoS is one of most important criteria that affect the adoption and acceptability of WBANs since higher QoI/QoS will eventually result into correct interpretation and intervention during the treatment of diseases.

Architectural Design

Figure 2 illustrates a three tier architecture is used design the WBANs since information will be transmitted from the sensor tier to the mobile computing tier and eventually the remote server tier.

The sensor tier consists of both invasive and non-invasive sensors and is mainly responsible to collect the physiological parameters of the patients such as such as the glucose concentration level, temperature and blood pressure to be transmitted over the network using short-range transmission communication protocols such as ZigBee or Bluetooth to the mobile computing tier. The sensors can form a body area network (BAN) using a star topology to transmit the sensed information. The sensor tier consists of two main modules. The *data sensing module* is mainly responsible to capture patients' physiological data and vital signs from each sensor, while the *data acquisition module* supplies efficient mechanisms to serialize and de-serialize the data.

The mobile computing tier acts as the gateway and consists of a smart phone, PDA or a pocket PC which provides a user friendly interface for the patients to log in his personal details and daily eating habits. He can also use the interface to track his past glucose levels or check future possible trends. Besides aggregating and storing all the sensed data, the mobile computing tier also process energy consumption and optimize the energy usage during information transmission to the remote server at a specified time interval. Several technologies can be used such as wireless local area network (WLAN), global system for mobile communication (GSM), general packet radio service (GPRS), universal mobile telecommunications system (UMTS), worldwide interoperability for microwave access (WiMAX) and 4G to offer wide coverage and ubiquitous network access (Pantelopoulos & Bourbakis, 2010).

The mobile computing tier consists of a software that has seven main modules which includes the *Communication module* that provides effective short-range communication and traffic control from the sensor nodes to the mobile phones. It also provides long-range communication with the remote server and ensure data synchronization The *Local Signal Storage module* to store all the information received from the sensor nodes, the *Data Representation module* is responsible for the compression and filtering of the information, the *Data Pre-Processing module* is responsible to filter noise from data, get useful information to enhance data integrity and reliability. Moreover, this module is responsible for filtering noise from the data and preparing it for further processing, feature selection, classification and decision support algorithms in case of emergencies. The *Data Aggregation module* is responsible for applying the appropriate data fusion techniques to reduce data redundancy, reduce the communication overhead and

Figure 2. Modular representation of WBAN architecture

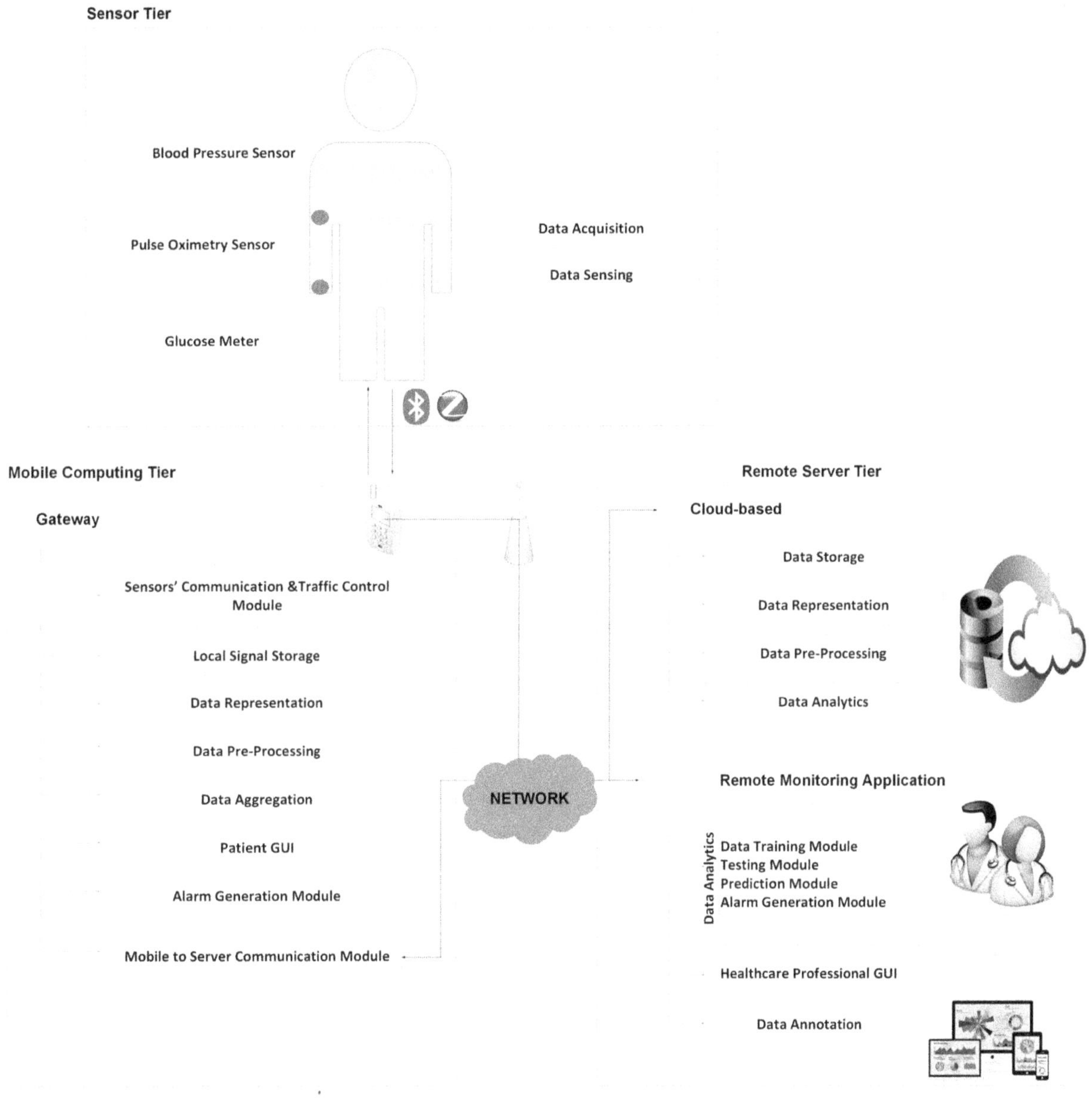

energy consumption, and consequently extending the network lifetime, the *Patient GUI module* offers a user-friendly visualization interface for user to log on his personal details and view his health trends and statistics and, finally, the *Alarm Generation module* aims at detecting any anomaly measurement and sending immediate messages to the healthcare providers in emergency cases.

The remote server tier consists of the remote servers and healthcare professionals' phones.

The cloud-based system stores all the patients' information and health parameters and is responsible to synchronize the real-time measurements. This cloud-based set up offers a secure distribution system and offers a tremendous benefit, especially during times of medical emergencies. Moreover, it consists of four main modules and includes the *Data Storage module* helps which store patients' medical background, medical imaging reports, and lab tests, the *Data Representation module* is responsible to further filter the information. The *Data Pre-Processing module* is used further extract reliable features from the patient details, transmit them over networks, and aggregate them before delivering them to the healthcare professionals for further diagnosis and decision making.

The patient's remote monitoring server application has a three main modules.

Firstly, the *Data Analytics module* includes other sub modules such as the *Data Training module*, which trains the patient's dataset, the *Testing Model module*, which assess the model's reliability by checking if the model is able to predict glucose measurements within the 95% interval of confidence, the *Prediction module*, responsible for the glucose prediction based on past glucose measurements, the *Alarm generation module,* sends immediate feedback to the patients.

Secondly, the *Healthcare Professional GUI module* consists of a web interface that the healthcare professional and administrators can access through an authentication mechanism to ensure the security of the system. The healthcare professional can view/manipulate patients' records that are assigned only to them so as to maintain the privacy of other patients. They can see some graphical representation of the patient physiological signs that can be used to diagnose and monitor patients' condition, suggest possible treatments or validate patients' medication and confirm diagnosis. The administrators can view/manipulate patients' details and doctors' details, manage the healthcare professionals' right, and database for medical information.

Thirdly, the *Data Annotation module* is used by healthcare professional to include all their observations such as clinical analysis and data, disease, medication, patients' status, and patients' risk level.

Sensor Design

The use of invasive, minimally invasive and non-invasive sensor devices can significantly aid diabetic patients to self-manage and record their daily blood glucose levels. A vast range of off the shelf sensor devices are now available on the market which are wearable, implantable and portable (Chan, Estève, Fourniols, Escriba, & Campo, 2012). Many glucometers can be used by patients depending on their cost and accuracy of measurement as depicted in Table 14. LifeScan's OneTouch Ultra 2 glucose meter manufactured by LifeScan, Inc. has widely been used to measure the blood glucose level with a reasonable degree of accuracy (Mohan, Marin, Sultan, & Deen, 2008; Mamykina & Mynatt, 2008; Pai, Sanki, & Banerjee, 2015). Patients can also use minimally invasive glucose measuring techniques (real-time CGMs) which are FDA approved such as Dexcom G4, Abbott Freestyle, and Medtronic RT Guardian (Frontino et al., 2013; Matuleviciene et al., 2014).

Non-invasive glucometers such as Combo Gluco meter or GlucoTrack can be used to sense the glucose levels by placing them directly on the finger. Moreover, the non-invasive sensors are gaining more prevalence since they highly sensitivity and promote better patient compliance compared to invasive ones (Frontino et al., 2013).

Moreover, although blood remains the most accurate method for glucose measurement, new developments using other biological fluids such as interstitial fluid, urine, sweat, breath, saliva and ocular fluid are currently being investigated (Eadie & Steele, 2017). Clinical trials and approval for clearance are yet to come. Companies such as Google, Novartis and Microsoft believe that new approaches of glucose monitoring will really create significant market potential (Bruen et al., 2017).

Communication Architecture

A reliable PMHSs requires a highly robust and reliable network that can be accessible anywhere and anytime anytime to perform real-time patients monitoring. The network reliability is highly influenced by network failures, database failures, coverage limitations and uninterruptable access.

Short-Range Communication Protocols

Table 8 shows the short-range communication protocols for the proposed WBAN design, the most common protocols that are used in PMHSs which are IEEE 802.15.1 (Bluetooth) and IEEE 802.15.4 (ZigBee).

IEEE 802.15.4- ZigBee

ZigBee standard is a low-power wireless specification based on the Institute of Electrical and Electronics Engineers (IEEE) Standard 802.15.4. Nowadays, it is also considered as a de-facto standard for the implementation of WSNs. It specifies the two bottom layers of ISO/OSI protocol stack, namely PHY and the MAC layers for short-range wireless communications and support a maximum transmission distance of 100 m. The key features are low cost, low bit rate transmissions, simple protocol complexity, low power consumption, with multi month-to-multiyear battery life, relaxed latency, enhanced throughput and is well suited with cheap fixed and moving sensor devices. It operates in a total of 27 half-duplex channels across three frequency bands. The first frequency consists of one channel in the 868 MHz band (20 kb/s, BPSK modulations), the second frequency consist of 10 channels in the 915 MHz band (40 kbps, BPSK modulation) and the third one has 16 physical channels in the 2.4 GHz industrial, scientific, and medical ISM band (250 kb/s, Orthogonal QPSK modulation).

The network topologies supported include star, tree cluster and mesh. It utilizes two different channel access schemes at the MAC layer namely the beacon-enabled (collision detection (CSMA-CA) channel access) and non-beacon-enabled (synchronized channel access). The CSMA-CA protocol allows multiple use of the same channel at different intervals without collisions. Moreover, ZigBee uses a direct sequence spread spectrum (DSSS) coding which is resistant to noise and interference. Moreover, it provides coding gain to enhance network reliability. ZigBee ensures message privacy, integrity and security by making use of advanced encryption standard (AES) algorithm having 128-bit keys.

Finally, with the concerns of battery life, cost, high reliability and scalability, ZigBee was claimed to be the most suitable standard for WBSN systems.

IEEE 802.15.1- Bluetooth

Bluetooth is one of the popular choices with a max data rate mode of 3 Mb/s and a range of less than 10 m. IEEE 802.15.1 wireless technology also exhibits some key features such as energy efficiency and cost effectiveness during operation. It uses an adaptive fast frequency hopping and operates in a total of 79 channels in the ISM band in 2.4 GHz spectrum. Bluetooth ensures message privacy, integrity and security by making use of advanced encryption standard (AES) algorithm having 128-bit keys.

Table 8. Short-range communication protocols

Technology	ZigBee	Bluetooth
Standard	IEEE 802.15.4	IEEE 802.15.1
Operating frequency	2.4 GHz 868 MHz 915 MHz	2.4 GHz
Distance	10–200 m	10 to 100 m
Cost per chip	$2	$3
Battery Life (days)	100-1000+	1-7
Protocol Complexity	Simple	High
RF Data Rate Distance	868 MHz: 20 Kb/s 915 MHz: 40 Kb/s 2.4 GHz: 250 Kb/s	1–3 Mbps
Number of Physical Channels	A total of 27 channels: 2.4 GHz:16 channels 915 MHz:10 channels 868 MHz: 1 channel	23 79
Modulation Type	868/915 MHz: BPSK(Binary Phase Shift Keying) 2.4 GHz: OQPSK(Orthogonal QPSK) Uses DSSS to convert bits/symbols to chips	Gaussian FSK / FHSS (Gaussian Frequency Shift Keying)
Network size (Nodes / Active Slaves)	> 65000	>7
Power Consumption	< 15 mA	< 30 mA
Robustness	DSSS, Uses 16 Channels ISM (2.4 GHz) band only	Adaptive Fast Frequency Hopping, FEC, fast ACK
Security	128b AES and application layer user defined	64b/128b AES and application layer user defined
Channel Bandwidth	Each channel is 2 MHz wide with a wasteful 5 MHz spacing	Each channel is up to 1 MHz
Multiple Access Scheme	CSMA-CA, slotted CSMA-CA	FH-TDD-TDMA
Network Topology	P2P, Star, Cluster Tree, Mesh	Scatter net
Spread Spectrum Techniques	Direct Spread Spectrum technique (the original signal is mixed and extracted from a pseudo random code at transmitter and receiver, respectively)	Frequency Hopping Spread Spectrum technique (carrier signal vary in terms of frequencies)
Single-hop / Multi-hop	Multi-hop	
Media	Data	Voice Data
Reliability	High Reliability and used for M2M	Reliability is low when devices is more than 10
Latency	30ms-1s	10 s
Extendibility	Yes	No
Success Factors	Battery Life, Cost, Reliability, Scalability	Cost, Convenience

Long-Range Communication Protocols

Long-range communication medium such as IEEE 802.11 / Wi-Fi/ GPRS are used to transmit information from the mobile computing tier to the remote server tier and vice-versa since they are widely used protocols which exhibits a good operating frequency and a reasonable data rate distance.

Data Design

The challenges present at the node-level, network-level and human-centric level such as node failures, inaccurate and low-powered sensors have a direct impact on the level of the QoI. Thus, to monitor the patient's health status in real-time, it a fundamental to guarantee a high QoI by properly modeling the sensor network data from the time of raw data collection at the sensor tier till the operations at remote server are conducted. QoI has been defined as a collection of attributes (Rodríguez, Riveill, & Antipolis, 2010) including timeliness, reliability, completeness, relevancy, usability and confidentiality.

At the sensor tier, the sensor devices are responsible to collect the raw data based on the specified user requirements such as different time intervals so that effective monitoring can be done. A high sensor quality and adequate sampling rate alleviates contamination of the data set with temporal effects and allows the user to set their requirements for data collection. Thus, the appropriate sampling rate that results in a higher QoI should be tested so that the data-driven model is not overburden and there is no overuse of power consumption.

As the sensed data are being processed at the mobile computing tier from raw data into useful and actionable information, the different QoI attributes for sensed data are affected. Assuring the quality of these sensed data is a prime concern and it is critical to ensure that attributes such as 1) how fast the information was processed and 2) the probability of correct detection and false alarm. The accuracy of the information can be determined through metrics such as probability of error detection and signal noise ratio. Moreover, several network-processing techniques can be used such as aggregation, filtering, compression, and suppression (Hunkeler & Scotton, 2008)

At the remote server tier, reliability of message delivery can also be ensured through several techniques such as (a) multicast or broadcast to enable multipath routing, (b) amplified power transmission, (c) optimized network or middleware protocols' design for reliability.

Application Design

The main aim while designing the application for both the patients and the healthcare professionals is to ensure they are user friendly and easy to use for better adoption. The sequence diagram in Figure 3 shows the flow of information from the sensor to the mobile phone and eventually to the cloud-based system and finally to the healthcare professionals.

Patient's GUI

The mobile application is developed mainly to communicate the sensor devices remotely over ZigBee and Bluetooth technology and to provide an interface to the patients. The application is developed in

Figure 3. Sequence diagram of communication flow

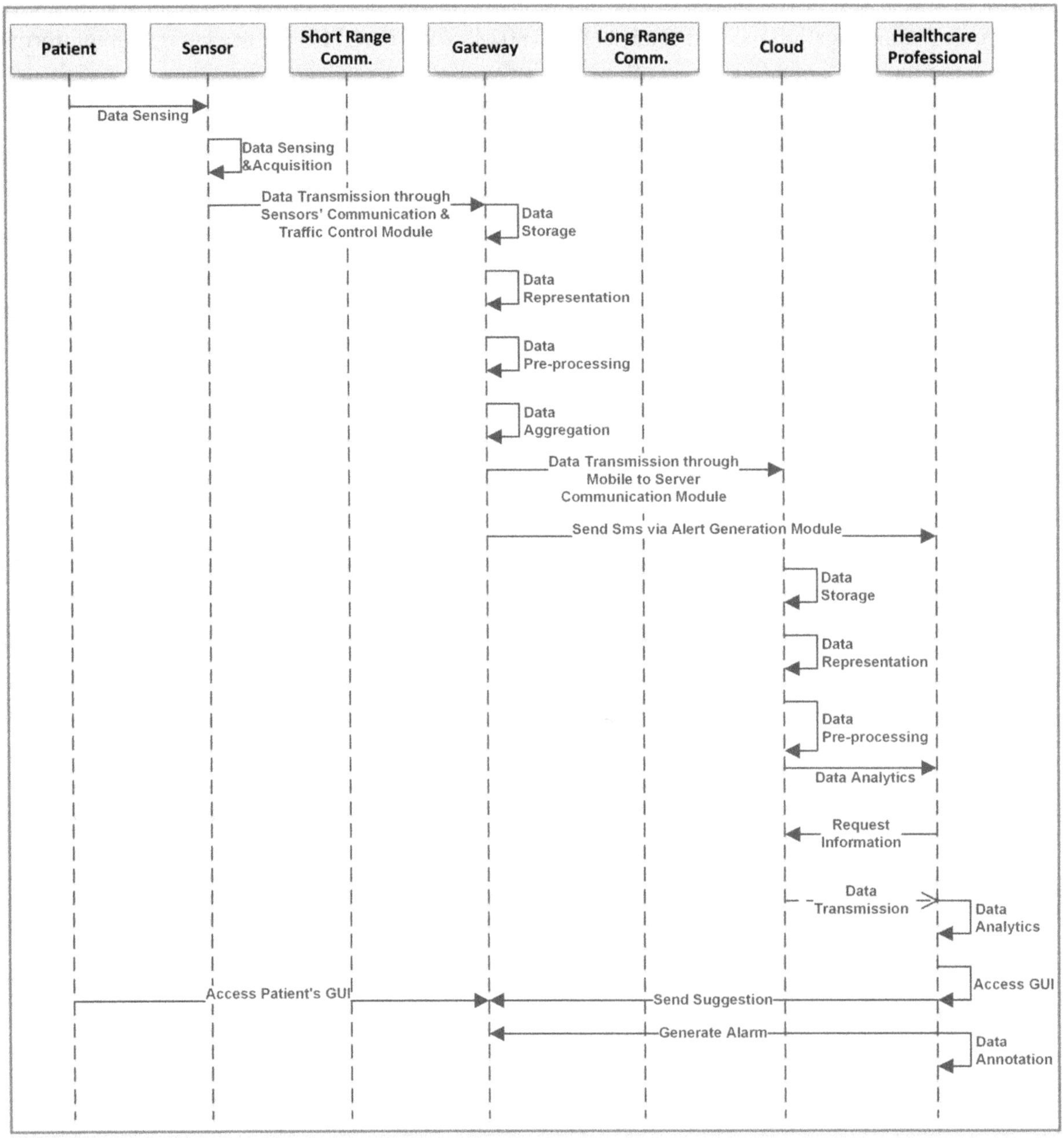

Android SDK using Java since it is can exhibit high security and confidentiality. It receives the sensed data, processes and displays it using a user friendly GUI to the patients despite the limited screen space of smart phones. The GUI is also responsible to display generated alerts to patients if any anomalous data is encountered by the sensors. The usability of system is increased through the use of a color coding scheme whereby patients can easily track their health status and perform better self-monitoring. The navigation flow of the patients' GUI is represented in Figure 4.

Figure 4. Patient's GUI

Login : Send the health data to server
View Health Data : View Blood Glucose Graphs and Past Measurements
Contact Doctor : Send glucose measurements to healthcare professional
Alert Generation : Receive alert when healthcare professional is received
Alarm Generation : Trigger alarm and send message to the healthcare In emergency cases
View Doctor Appointment : Receive appointment date with doctor

Healthcare Professional GUI

The healthcare professional can access the remote monitoring application. The remote application is a web based application that is developed using Microsoft Visual Studio 2013. The database is based on SQL Server 2014 and contains relational tables. The navigation flow of the healthcare professional's GUI in Figure 5.

Data Analytics for Prediction of Glucose Level

Table 9 is a representation of the data used to evaluate and test the model is from the diabetes dataset used by Efron et al.,. This dataset includes 442 sets of data recorded on diabetes patients (Huzooree, Khedo, & Joonas, 2017a).

Present glucose values can be estimated as linear combinations of past glucose measurements using the ARX model expression. The glucose prediction model to perform data analytics for is described as equation 1.

$$G(t) = b_0 + b_1 X_{1t} + b_2 X_{2t} + \ldots + b_k X_{kt} + \gamma + e(t) \quad (1)$$

A clear correlation was demonstrated between the actual and predicted glucose levels. Moreover, the computed Residual Q-Q Plot also demonstrated that the model is fit for glucose prediction. Finally, three performance metrics were evaluated namely 1) MAE: mean absolute error between the predicted BG level and the actual BG level, 2) RMSE: root-mean-square error that measures the standard deviation

Figure 5. Healthcare professional's GUI

View Records : View patient's diabetes reports
Update Records : Assign appropriate risk level
Prescription : Sends e-prescription/feedback to patient

Table 9. Dataset characteristics

Input Parameters	Values	Input Parameters	Values
Patient Baseline Characteristics		Descriptive Statistics of the Glucose Dataset	
Gender	235F / 207M	Total Cholesterol (TC)	189±34.6
Age	48.5±13a	Low-density lipoprotein Cholesterol (LDL)	115±30.4
BMI	26.4±4.4	High Density Lipoproteins (HDL)	49.8±12.9
Blood Pressure	94.6±13.8	Ratio (TC/HDL)	4.0±1.29
		Glucose	91.2±11.5

of the differences in the predicted BG level and the actual BG level and 3) R^2: measures the proportion of the variance of the BG level. All the three metrics confirmed that the model can be used for glucose prediction. Moreover, Figure 6 shows that all the forecasted values falls within the 95% interval of confidence therefore demonstrating that the model is reliable.

FUTURE RESEARCH DIRECTIONS

PMHSs have immense opportunities in monitoring chronic diseases, but at the same time, such systems give rise to several challenges. These systems are very critical and complex since they demand high dependability, reliability, security and privacy for successful adoption and acceptability. Due to these complexities, many research challenges are still open. The challenges are discussed in this section below and are categorized under the node-level, network-level and human-centric level. Node-level challenges are related with the sensors design and energy consumption without violating their unobtrusiveness. More optimized data quality algorithm can be developed to increase the QoI attributes for a higher degree of confidence. Moreover, privacy-preserving mechanisms, authentication protocol, advanced algorithms

Figure 6. Glucose prediction graph

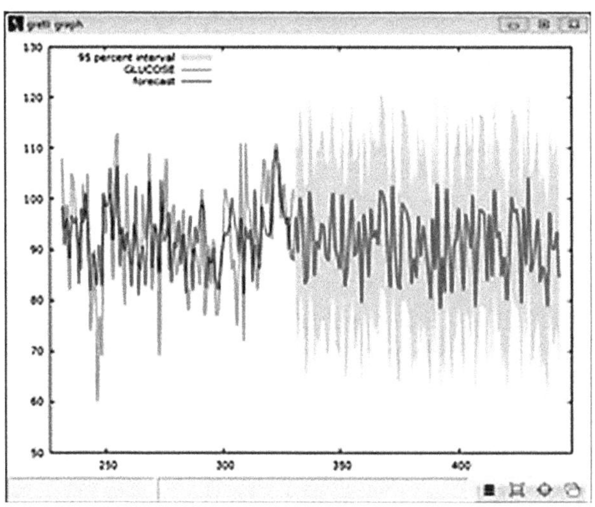

encrypted and cryptography techniques can be further explored to address the issues at the network-level. Lastly, new technology acceptance models can be developed and used to get constructive feedback on their acceptance levels by patients. These models can be used to address the issues at human-centric level. Moreover, energy aware protocols can be developed to ensure that nodes can negotiate their transmission power to extend their battery life.

Furthermore, the glucose prediction model can be further enhanced and tested through the Error Grid Analysis so as to achieve a perfect compromise in terms of performance and accuracy. Advanced prediction algorithms can be developed to maintain the prediction performance as the prediction horizon increases. The prediction model can be further enhanced by accommodating other exogenous inputs apart from CGM data for more accurate data analysis and reliable decision making. Advanced powerful data analytics and modeling techniques are required to detect correlation from the diverse range of raw data to extract clinically meaningful knowledge and to be widely accepted for clinical practice. Moreover, there is limited research conducted on glucose prediction models applicable to patient suffering from both Type 1 and Type 2 diabetes.

CONCLUSION

Despite all the challenges, advancement in PMHSs development can lead to numerous advantages in the healthcare sector such as a shift in healthcare delivery model. Based on the different design considerations outlined in this chapter and the comparison of sensor devices conducted, a low cost WBAN system architecture for real-time diabetes monitoring was proposed to ensure a higher degree of confidence in Quality of Information (QoI) and to enhance the communication channel between healthcare professionals and patients. The proposed WBAN allows physicians to easily access and continuously monitor the health records of diabetic patients from any remote location. Moreover, patients will have an effective platform to record and monitor their health status as compared to the traditional way of frequent hospital visits. Furthermore, accessibility to the real-time and historical information of patients allows healthcare professionals to perform more accurate diagnosis, timely intervention and effective decision making in emergency situations.

Future work is required for the software on the mobile computing tier by including advanced signal processing algorithms for noise filtering and data compression to promote efficient power consumption. Another future work includes the analysis and further optimization of the performance of the glucose prediction algorithm by using bigger prediction horizon.

REFERENCES

Abbate, S., Avvenuti, M., & Light, J. (2012). MIMS: A Minimally Invasive Monitoring Sensor Platform. *IEEE Sensors Journal*, *12*(3), 677–684. doi:10.1109/JSEN.2011.2149515

Al-Dowaihi, D., Al-Ajlan, M., Al-Zahrani, N., Al-Quwayfili, N., Al-Jwiser, N., & Kanjo, E. (2013). mBreath: Asthma monitoring system on the go. In *Proceedings of the International Conference on Computer Medical Applications (ICCMA)* (pp. 5–8). Sousse, Tunisia: Academic Press. 10.1109/ICCMA.2013.6506169

Alemdar, H., & Ersoy, C. (2010). Wireless sensor networks for healthcare: A survey. *Computer Networks*, *54*(15), 2688–2710. doi:10.1016/j.comnet.2010.05.003

Amir, O., Weinstein, D., Zilberman, S., Less, M., Perl-Treves, D., Primack, H., ... Karasik, A. (2007). Continuous Noninvasive Glucose Monitoring Technology Based on "Occlusion Spectroscopy.". *Journal of Diabetes Science and Technology*, *1*(4), 463–469. doi:10.1177/193229680700100403

Bachir, A., Dohler, M., Watteyne, T., & Leung, K. K. (2010). Article. *MAC Essentials for Wireless Sensor Networks*, *12*(2), 222–248.

Bruen, D., Delaney, C., Florea, L., & Diamond, D. (2017). Glucose sensing for diabetes monitoring: Recent developments. *Sensors (Basel)*, *17*(8), 1866. doi:10.339017081866

Bwititi, P., Angel, L., & Day, S. (2008). Self-monitoring of Blood Glucose Levels Using Glucometers in Riverina NSW: Patients' Perspectives. *Australian Journal of Medical Science*, *29*(1), 3.

Cameron, B. D., & Cote, G. L. (1997). Noninvasive glucose sensing utilizing a digital closed-loop polarimetric approach. *IEEE Transactions on Biomedical Engineering*, *44*(12), 1221–1227. doi:10.1109/10.649993

Chan, M., Estève, D., Fourniols, J., Escriba, C., & Campo, E. (2012). Artificial Intelligence in Medicine Smart wearable systems : Current status and future challenges. *Artificial Intelligence in Medicine*, *56*(3), 137–156. doi:10.1016/j.artmed.2012.09.003

Chen, M., Gonzalez, S., Vasilakos, A., Cao, H., & Leung, V. C. M. (2011). Body Area Networks: A Survey. *Mobile Networks and Applications*, *16*(2), 171–193. doi:10.100711036-010-0260-8

Chiarini, G., Ray, P., Akter, S., Masella, C., & Ganz, A. (2013). mHealth technologies for chronic diseases and elders : A systematic review. *IEEE Journal on Selected Areas in Communications*, *31*(9), 6–18. doi:10.1109/JSAC.2013.SUP.0513001

IDF Diabetes Atlas. (2017). *IDF Diabetes Atlas*. 10.1017/CBO9781107415324.004

Eadie, M., & Steele, R. J. (2017). Non-invasive Blood Glucose Monitoring and Data Analytics. In *Proceedings of the International Conference on Compute and Data Analysis* (pp. 138–142). Lakeland, FL: ACM. 10.1145/3093241.3093283

El-gayar, O., Timsina, P., Nawar, N., & Eid, W. (2013). Mobile Applications for Diabetes Self-Management. *Status and Potential*, *7*(1), 247–262.

Frontino, G., Meschi, F., Bonfanti, R., Rigamonti, A., Battaglino, R., Favalli, V., ... Chiumello, G. (2013). Future Perspectives in Glucose Monitoring Sensors. *European Endocrinology*, *9*(1), 21–26. doi:10.17925/EE.2013.09.01.21

Ghamari, M., Arora, H., Sherratt, R. S., & Harwin, W. (2015). Comparison of low-power wireless communication technologies for wearable health-monitoring applications. In *2015 International Conference on Computer, Communications, and Control Technology (I4CT)* (pp. 1–6). Kuching, Malaysia: Academic Press. 10.1109/I4CT.2015.7219525

Hofer, T., Schumacher, M., & Bromuri, S. (2015). COMPASS : an Interoperable Personal Health System to Monitor and Compress Signals in Chronic Obstructive Pulmonary Disease. In *Proceedings of the 9th International Conference on Pervasive Computing Technologies for Healthcare* (pp. 304 – 311). Istanbul, Turkey: Academic Press. 10.4108/icst.pervasivehealth.2015.259186

Horta, E. T., Lopes, I. C., Rodrigues, J. J. P. C., & Proenca, M. L. (2013). A mobile health application for falls detection and biofeedback monitoring. In *2013 IEEE 15th International Conference on e-Health Networking, Applications and Services (Healthcom 2013)* (pp. 36–40). Lisbon, Portugal: IEEE. 10.1109/HealthCom.2013.6720634

Hunkeler, U., & Scotton, P. (2008). A Quality-of-Information-Aware Framework for Data Models in Wireless Sensor Networks. In *2008 5th IEEE International Conference on Mobile Ad Hoc and Sensor Systems* (pp. 742–747). Atlanta, GA: IEEE. 10.1109/MAHSS.2008.4660118

Huzooree, G., Khedo, K. K., & Joonas, N. (2016). Wireless Body Area Network System Architecture for Real-Time Diabetes Monitoring. In *Emerging Trends in Electrical* (pp. 262–271). Electronic and Communications Engineering. ELECOM.

Huzooree, G., Khedo, K. K., & Joonas, N. (2017a). Glucose Prediction Data Analytics for Diabetic Patients Monitoring. In *2017 1st International Conference on Next Generation Computing Applications (NextComp)* (pp. 188–195). Academic Press. 10.1109/NEXTCOMP.2017.8016197

Huzooree, G., Khedo, K. K., & Joonas, N. (2017b). Pervasive mobile healthcare systems for chronic disease monitoring. *Health Informatics Journal*, 1 –25. 10.1177/1460458217704250

Joshua, J., Qian, C., & Bruce, S. (2015). A Natural Walking Monitor for Pulmonary Patients Using Mobile Phones. *IEEE Journal of Biomedical and Health Informatics*, *19*(4), 1399–1405. doi:10.1109/JBHI.2015.2427511

Kjome, R. L. S., Granas, A. G., Nerhus, K., Roraas, T. H., & Sandberg, S. (2010). The Prevalence of Self-Monitoring of Blood Glucose and Costs of Glucometer Strips in a Nationwide Cohort. *Diabetes Technology & Therapeutics*, *12*(9), 701–705. doi:10.1089/dia.2010.0056

Klonoff, D. C. (2012). Overview of Fluorescence Glucose Sensing: A Technology with a Bright Future. *Journal of Diabetes Science and Technology*, *6*(6), 1242–1250. doi:10.1177/193229681200600602

Kumar, T. S., & Ganesan, R. (2011). Sharon: Tension free mobile incorporated with health care system using Christina heart card. *3rd International Conference on Advanced Computing, ICoAC 2011*, 46–51. 10.1109/ICoAC.2011.6165217

Latiff, N. A. A., Latiff, N. M. A., & Ahmad, R. B. (2011). Prolonging lifetime of wireless sensor networks with mobile base station using particle swarm optimization. In *2011 Fourth International Conference on Modeling, Simulation and Applied Optimization* (pp. 1–6). Kuala Lumpur, Malaysia: Academic Press. 10.1109/ICMSAO.2011.5775487

Li, C., Li, H.-B., & Kohno, R. (2009). Performance Evaluation of IEEE 802.15.4 for Wireless Body Area Network (WBAN). In *IEEE International Conference on Communications (ICC) Workshops, 2009.* (pp. 1–5). Dresden, Germany: IEEE. 10.1109/ICCW.2009.5208087

Li, M., Lou, W., & Ren, K. (2010). Data Security and Privacy in Wireless Body Area Networks. *IEEE Wireless Communications*, *17*(1), 51–58. doi:10.1109/MWC.2010.5416350

Liu, C. H., Wen, J., Yu, Q., Yang, B., & Wang, W. (2011). HealthKiosk: A family-based connected healthcare system for long-term monitoring. In *2011 IEEE Conference on Computer Communications Workshops (INFOCOM WKSHPS)* (pp. 241–246). Shanghai, China: IEEE. 10.1109/INFCOMW.2011.5928816

Malik, B. H., & Coté, G. L. (2010). Real-time, closed-loop dual-wavelength optical polarimetry for glucose monitoring. *Journal of Biomedical Optics*, *15*(1), 1–6. doi:10.1117/1.3290819

Mamykina, L., & Mynatt, E. (2008). MAHI: investigation of social scaffolding for reflective thinking in diabetes management. In *Proceedings of the SIGCHI Conference on Human Factors in Computing Systems* (pp. 477–486). Florence, Italy: ACM. 10.1145/1357054.1357131

Matuleviciene, V., Joseph, J. I., Andelin, M., Hirsch, I. B., Attvall, S., Pivodic, A., ... Lind, M. (2014). A clinical trial of the accuracy and treatment experience of the Dexcom G4 sensor (Dexcom G4 system) and Enlite sensor (guardian REAL-time system) tested simultaneously in ambulatory patients with type 1 diabetes. *Diabetes Technology & Therapeutics*, *16*(11), 759–767. doi:10.1089/dia.2014.0238

Mohan, P., Marin, D., Sultan, S., & Deen, A. (2008). MediNet: Personalizing the Self-Care Process for Patients with Diabetes and Cardiovascular Disease Using Mobile Telephony. In *2008 30th Annual International Conference of the IEEE Engineering in Medicine and Biology Society* (pp. 755–758). Vancouver, Canada: IEEE.

Nachman, L., Baxi, A., Bhattacharya, S., Darera, V., Deshpande, P., & Kodalapura, N., … Acharya, R. (2010). Jog Falls : A Pervasive Healthcare Platform for Diabetes Management. In *8th International Conference, Pervasive Computing* (pp. 94–111). Helsinki, Finland: Academic Press. 10.1007/978-3-642-12654-3_6

National Clinical Guideline Centre. (2015). *Type 1 diabetes in adults: diagnosis and management*. National Institute for Health and Care Excellence.

Oliver, N. S., Toumazou, C., Cass, E. G., & Johnston, D. G. (2009). Glucose sensors: A review of current and emerging technology. *Diabetic Medicine*, *26*(3), 197–210. doi:10.1111/j.1464-5491.2008.02642.x

Ozana, N., Arbel, N., Beiderman, Y., Mico, V., Sanz, M., Garcia, J., ... Zalevsky, Z. (2014). Improved noncontact optical sensor for detection of glucose concentration and indication of dehydration level. *Biomedical Optics Express*, *5*(6), 1926–1940. doi:10.1364/BOE.5.001926

Pai, P. P., Sanki, P. K., & Banerjee, S. (2015). A Photoacoustics based Continuous Non-Invasive Blood Glucose Monitoring System. In *IEEE International Symposium on Medical Measurements and Applications* (pp. 106–111). Turin, Italy: IEEE. 10.1109/MeMeA.2015.7145181

Pantelopoulos, A., & Bourbakis, N. G. (2010). A Survey on Wearable Sensor-Based Systems for Health Monitoring and Prognosis. *IEEE Transactions on Systems, Man and Cybernetics. Part C, Applications and Reviews*, *40*(1), 1–12. doi:10.1109/TSMCC.2009.2032660

Pickup, J. C., Hussain, F., Evans, N. D., Rolinski, O. J., & Birch, D. J. S. (2005). Fluorescence-based glucose sensors. *Biosensors & Bioelectronics*, *20*(12), 2555–2565. doi:10.1016/j.bios.2004.10.002

Potts, R. O., Tamada, J., & Tierney, M. J. (2002). Glucose monitoring by reverse iontophoresis. *Diabetes/Metabolism Research and Reviews*, *18*(S1), 49–53. doi:10.1002/dmrr.210

Preuveneers, D., & Berbers, Y. (2008). Internet of things: A context-awareness perspective. In L. Yan, Y. Zhang, L. T. Yang, & H. Ning (Eds.), *The Internet of Things: From RFID to the Next-Generation Pervasive Networked Systems* (pp. 287–308). Auerbach. doi:10.1201/9781420052824.ch13

Salam, N. A. B. A., bin Mohd Saad, W. H., Manap, Z. B., & Salehuddin, F. (2016). The Evolution of Non-invasive Blood Glucose Monitoring System for Personal Application. *Journal of Telecommunication Electronic and Computer Engineering*, *8*(1), 59–65.

Shaw, J. E., Sicree, R., & Zimmet, P. Z. (2010). Global estimates of the prevalence of diabetes for 2010 and 2030. *Diabetes Research and Clinical Practice*, *87*(1), 4–14. doi:10.1016/j.diabres.2009.10.007

Smith, J. L. (2017). *The Pursuit of Noninvasive Glucos : Hunting the Deceitful Turkey*. Retrieved December 8, 2017, from https://www.researchgate.net/publication/317267760_The_Pursuit_of_Noninvasive_Glucose_5th_Edition

So, C. F., Choi, K. S., Wong, T. K. S., & Chung, J. W. Y. (2012). Recent advances in noninvasive glucose monitoring. *Medical Devices: Evidence and Research*, *5*(1), 45–52. doi:10.2147/MDER.S28134

Sparacino, G., Zanon, M., Facchinetti, A., Zecchin, C., Maran, A., & Cobelli, C. (2012). Italian contributions to the development of continuous glucose monitoring sensors for diabetes management. *Sensors (Basel)*, *12*(10), 13753–13780. doi:10.3390121013753

Srinivasan, V., Stankovic, J., & Whitehouse, K. (2008). Protecting your Daily In-Home Activity Information from a Wireless Snooping Attack. In *Proceedings of the 10th International Conference on Ubiquitous Computing* (pp. 202–211). Seoul, South Korea: Academic Press. 10.1145/1409635.1409663

Tanaka, Y., Tajima, T., & Seyama, M. (2017). Acoustic Modal Analysis of Resonant Photoacoustic Spectroscopy with Dual-Wavelength Differential Detection for Noninvasive Glucose Monitoring. *IEEE Sensors Letters*, *1*(3), 1–4. doi:10.1109/LSENS.2017.2698062

Thanuja, R., & Balakrishnan, R. (2013). Real Time Sleep Apnea Monitor Using ECG. In *2013 IEEE Conference on Information Communication Technologies* (pp. 973–976). IEEE. 10.1109/CICT.2013.6558237

Touati, F., & Tabish, R. (2013). U-healthcare system: State-of-the-art review and challenges. *Journal of Medical Systems*, *37*(3), 9949. doi:10.100710916-013-9949-0

Tura, A. (2008). Noninvasive glycaemia monitoring: Background, traditional findings, and novelties in the recent clinical trials. *Current Opinion in Clinical Nutrition and Metabolic Care*, *11*(5), 607–612. doi:10.1097/MCO.0b013e328309ec3a

Tura, A., Maran, A., & Pacini, G. (2007). Non-invasive glucose monitoring: Assessment of technologies and devices according to quantitative criteria. *Diabetes Research and Clinical Practice*, *77*(1), 16–40. doi:10.1016/j.diabres.2006.10.027

Uniyal, D., & Raychoudhury, V. (2014). *Pervasive Healthcare-A Comprehensive Survey of Tools and Techniques, 48*. Retrieved from http://arxiv.org/abs/1411.1821

Vashist, S. K. (2012). Non-invasive glucose monitoring technology in diabetes management: A review. *Analytica Chimica Acta*, *750*, 16–27. doi:10.1016/j.aca.2012.03.043

Yadav, J., Rani, A., Singh, V., & Murari, B. M. (2015). Comparative Study of Different Measurement Sites Using NIR Based Non-invasive Glucose Measurement System. In *Proceedings of the 4th International Conference on Eco-friendly Computing and Communication Systems (ICECCS)* (*Vol. 70*, pp. 469–475). Academic Press. 10.1016/j.procs.2015.10.082

Zhang, Y., Zhang, F., Shakhsheer, Y., Silver, J. D., Klinefelter, A., Nagaraju, M., ... Otis, B. P. (2013). A Batteryless 19μW MICS/ISM-Band Energy Harvesting Body Sensor Node SoC for ExG Applications. *IEEE Journal of Solid-State Circuits*, *48*(1), 199–213. doi:10.1109/JSSC.2012.2221217

Chapter 7
Advances in MEMS and Micro-Scale Technologies for Application in Controlled Drug-Dosing Systems:
MEMS-Based Drug Delivery Systems

Ranjit Barua
Indian Institute of Engineering Science and Technology Shibpur, India

Sudipto Datta
Indian Institute of Engineering Science and Technology Shibpur, India

Amit Roy Chowdhury
Indian Institute of Engineering Science and Technology Shibpur, India

Pallab Datta
Indian Institute of Engineering Science and Technology Shibpur, India

ABSTRACT

Implantable drug delivery devices have shown promise for drug administration for management of several diseases spanning chronic diseases to emergency medicine as they overcome the limitations of continuous monitoring by medical physician or paramedical professional. Micro-electro mechanical systems (MEMS) technologies are they key enabling technology platform that allow fabrication of miniature devices with precise control over drug dosing rates. Recently, many of these technologies are also finding applications in microfluidic chips applications. MEMS are composed of microvalves, microchannels, microsensors, and micropumps within a miniaturized control device. Among these, micropumps play a dynamic role in determining the extent of control over drug dispensation. In this chapter, principles and developments of MEMS-based drug delivery systems with micropumps are presented, which may allow future development of affordable technologies based on this principle.

DOI: 10.4018/978-1-5225-4969-7.ch007

INTRODUCTION

Controlled drug delivery systems help to release the drug in a pre-determined rate in the body. The Micro-Electro Mechanical Systems (MEMS) technology employment has been increasing promptly in the field of biomedical applications and in drug delivery processes because it construct microfluidic devices (Maillefer, Lintel, Mermet, Hirschi, 1999; Bhom, Timmer, Olthuis, Bergveld, 2000; Gao, Mantell, Polla, 2000; Tao, Lubeley, Desai, 2003) and the most important and remarkable elements of MEMS are microactuators, micro sensors and microfluidic systems (Reynaerts, Peirs, Brussel, 1997). In microfluidic systems the fluid flows in tiny amounts, usually in microlitres (μL). The main functions of microfluidics systems are basically drug transport, purification, sample preparation, separation, reaction, detection labeling, and biosensing. In MEMS technology, micropumps are considered as the miniature of pumping devices which are fabricated by micromachining technologies (Grayson, Shawgo, Johnson, Flylnn, Yawen, Cima, Langer, 2004; Karman, Ibrahim, Soin, 2007) and widely used in chemical processing, microelectronics and biomedical industries. In biomedical field, the demand of micropump is extensive. The most important features of micropump is to dispense small as well as fixed amount of fluid which will able to meet the medical and biomedical requirements of the target pathologies with enormous technical along with marketable possibilities. Apart from micropump, there are several other components of the whole delivery system. This includes micro-sensor to monitor certain physiological parameters and may be optionally for feedback control of drug dispensation through analysis by microcontroller and closed loop algorithms, a drug reservoir attached to the micropump and a single or array of microchannels to transport the drug to the site of delivery. It is indeed appreciable that development in MEMS (1 mm to 100 mm size scale) has enabled realization of such sophisticated biomedical systems.

Micropump

Micropumps are used for different kinds of applications such as flow fluids, carrying fluids from one point to another, mixing tiny amount of fluids or dosages and also safe handling of precarious fluid. In drug delivery systems, these pumps are mostly responsible for transferring drug from reservoir to the target place. Micropumps are classified in to two main individual categories: Displacement or mechanical micropumps and dynamic or non-mechanical micropumps (Tsai, Sue, 2007). A comparison of different properties of representative micropumps of different categories is given in Table 1.

Mechanical Micropumps

A mechanical micropump basically requires a corporal actuation for performing the medications purpose. Mechanical displacement micropumps are also known as diaphragm pumps where various actuation mechanisms are involved. A physical internal controller (actuator) is required for driving and transferring drugs. Mechanical micro dosing systems are further categorized into displacement micro-dosing system and dynamic micro-dosing system (Woias, 2001). In displacement micro-dosing system, pressure is generated in to the drug reservoir at scheduled time periods. Applied pressure helps to overcome the mechanical opposition of the outlet valve, discharging the drug to the outer space. In contrast, dynamic mechanical micro-dosing system is designed to exert continuous pressure inside drug reservoir and the drug is continuously delivered to the outer location (Staples, Daniel, Cima, Langer, 2006). The most popular examples of mechanical micropumps used in drug delivery devises are thermo-pneumatic,

Table 1. A comparison of representative MEMS based micropumps

Micropump Technology	Pumping Medium Reported	Size	Voltage (V)	Flow Rate	Frequency	Application	Ref.
Thermo-pneumatic	Compressed air	NA	NA	96 μL/min	10 Hz	Microfluidic devices	(16)
Piezoelectric	Insulin	15 × 8 mm	36	6.23×10^{-5} mL/min	200 Hz	Insulin therapy System	(21)
Electrostatic	Gas	NA	NA	0.29–0.07 SCCM	2.2–2.8 KHz	Drug delivery	(23)
ICPF	Water	25 × 25 × 10 mm	4	1260 μL/min	0.5 Hz	Biomedical devices	(27)
SMA	DI water	8 × 8 × 1.8 mm	NA	235 μL/min	80 Hz	NA	(43)
Bimetallic	Gas/Water	13 × 7 × 2 mm	15	5.6 μL/s	NA	NA	(32)
Electro-wetting	Mercury	Not reported	2.3	70 μL/min	25 Hz	Biomedical Devices	(35)
Electrochemical	Water	5.6 × 16 × 26 mm	±1.5	52 μL/min	NA	Microfluidic	(39)

piezoelectric, electrostatic, Ionic conductive polymeric film (ICPF), bimetallic and shape memory alloy (SMA) micropumps.

Thermo-Pneumatic Micropump

In thermo-pneumatic micropump, basically a compartment full of air is intermittently compressed and expanded by a cyclic use of twosome of heater and cooler (Zimmerman, Frank, Liepmann, Pissano, 2004). Intermittent variation in the volume of the compartment delivers the film a recurrent impetus for fluid flows. Figure 1 shows a schematic diagram of thermo-pneumatic micropump. This type of micropump creates a comparatively large induced pressure (Chen, Kwon, Tan, 2008), and also consequently displacement of membrane. The increasing pressure in the liquid is expressed in equation 1.

$$\Delta P = E\left(\beta \Delta T - \frac{\Delta V}{V}\right) \quad (1)$$

where,

ΔP= Pressure variation,
E=Young's modulus,
β= Coefficient of thermal expansion,
ΔT= Variation of temperature,
$\frac{\Delta V}{V}$= Variation in volume percentage.

Figure 1. A diagrammatic representation of thermo-pneumatic micropump

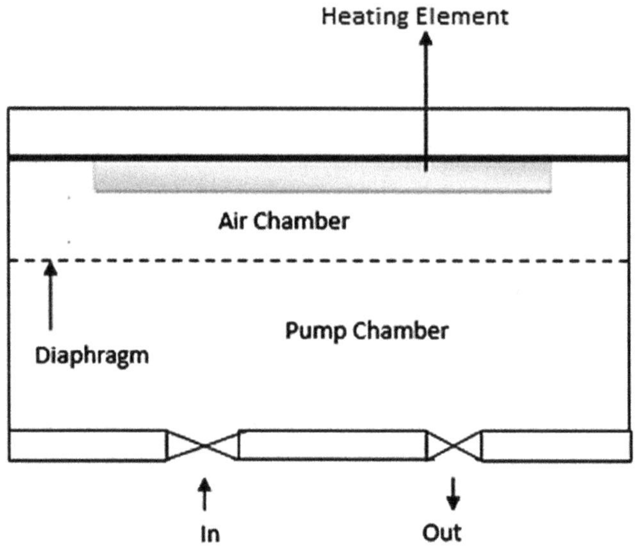

Van De Pol et al. (1990) described the first thermo-pneumatic micropump based on micro fabrication where fluid flow was 34μL/min be detected around 6 V in addition to nearly 30°Celsius. A thermo-pneumatic micropump (Jeong, Yang, 2000) was developed with the flow rate around 14 μL/min with working voltage at 8 V and frequency of 4 Hz. Cooney et al. (Cooney, Towe, 2004) proposed a thermo-pneumatic micropump containing one thin film heater; flow stricter along with two tanks were achieved at highest flow rate around 1.4 μL/min till 4.5 h and the mean power was 200 mW. A peristaltic micropump was fabricated (Johari, Yunas, Yeopamjlis, 2009) with the attachment of microchannels to the PDMS poly(dimethyl siloxane)/PMMA poly(methyl methacrylate) division, PDMS functioned like pneumatic actuator. The highest flow rate of 96 μL/min was reached. Thermo-pneumatic micropump creates quite larger induced pressures along with film displacement. The key for the driving power to sustain at a continuous and exact plane and the lengthy reaction are the drawbacks of this micropump.

Piezoelectric Micropump

Piezoelectric effect is known as the conversion of electronic energy (voltage) to mechanical energy or vice versa. A stress is applied on materials which cause the break up among the positive and the negative charges, effecting exterior surface net polarization. Equation (2) represents the effects of piezoelectric.

$$\varepsilon = S^{E}\sigma + dE \quad (2)$$

where,

S^{E} = Compliance tensor,
$\sigma = Stress$,
d = piezoelectric-charge constant tensor,

E= electric field.

As soon as an electric voltage is applied in through the piezoelectric material, the length of the material changes consistently and the amount of the displacement is function of the value of the given voltage (Johari, Yunas, Yeopamjlis, 2009). When the voltage is made zero i.e open circuit, the material comes back towards its initial shape. When the piezoelectric material coating is placed on a film, the induced voltage generates a certain amount of distortion which behaves like a thrust plate by releasing the liquid out of the compartment of a micropump. Figure 2 represents a schematic diagram of micropump based on piezoelectric effect.

V. Lintel et al. (1988) constructed a piezoelectric micropump using micromachining technology and the micropump contained a pumping compartment, passive silicon verification valve, and thin glass film controlled via piezo disk. Utmost flow rate of approx 8 μL/min along with reverse pressure at 9.8 kPa were noted near 125 V with frequency of 1 Hz. On silicon membrane, screen printing of Lead Zirconate Titanate based piezoelectric micropump (Koch, Harris, Evans, White, 1998) was described, where the flow rate was about 120 μL/min plus reverse pressure of 2 kPa were observed near given 600 V in addition to frequency of 200 Hz. A piezostack actuated peristaltic micropump was reported by Trenkle et al. (2009). The flow rate of water was around 40 μL/min along with frequency of 28.6 Hz. The rate of flow was examined for freeing of reverse pressure of almost 7 kPa, in addition to a highest reverse pressure of 45 kPa near 140 V. A non reusable high functioning piezoelectric micropump in addition to four compartments in serial bonding for blocked loop insulin therapy system has been subsequently demonstrated by Liu et al. (2010) and they observed the release resolution of 6.23×10^{-5} μL/ pulse. The highest reverse pressure of 22 kPa was noted near given voltage of 36 V in addition to 200 Hz frequency. The advantages of piezoelectric actuators are, they provide large actuation forces, quick response and simple structures. The major disadvantage of piezoelectric micropump is their complex fabrication.

Figure 2. A diagrammatic representation of micro-pump based on piezoelectric effect

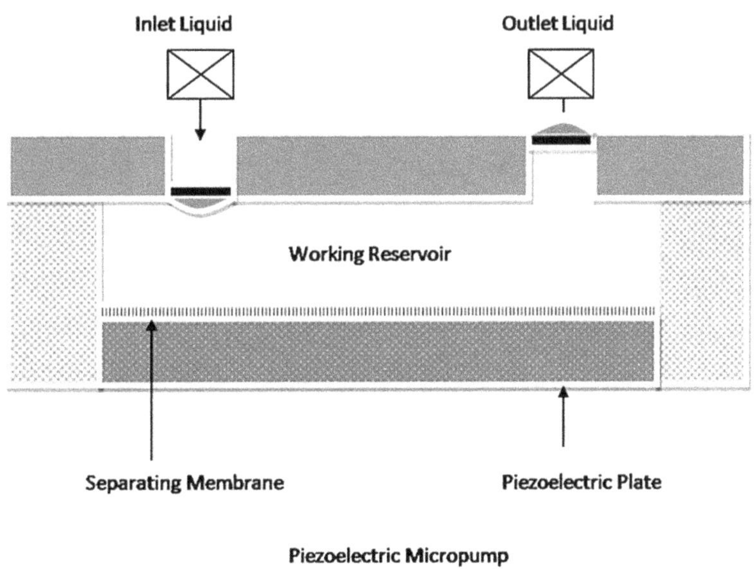

Electrostatic Micropump

The main actuation mechanism of electrostatic micropump is electrostatic forces (Koch et al, 1998). Figure 3 represents a diagrammatic representation of electrostatic micropump. When the membrane is bent, alteration pressures are created inside the pump compartment which causes pumping of liquid from the compartment. Equation (3) represents the electrostatic force applied on the electrostatic plates and the relationship with dispensing rate of applied voltage.

$$F = \frac{dw}{dx} = \frac{1}{2}\left(\varepsilon A \frac{V^2}{X^2}\right) \tag{3}$$

where,

F= Electrostatic force,
A= Surface area of the electrode,
ε= Dielectric constant,
X= Electrode spacing,
V= Applied voltage

Several authors have tried to fabricate such pumps for drug delivery application. For example, Cabuz et al. (2001) reported a double diaphragm electrostatic micropump through injection molding method where a flow rate of 30 µL/min was noted at a given voltage of 160 V in addition to 30 Hz frequency and power of 8 mW. Fluidic resonance for high rate of flow plus multi stage peristaltic arrangement was used in an electrostatic gas micropump (Lee, Yee, Besharatian, Kim, Bernal, Najafi, 2009). The pressure varied in the range 7.3 to 3.3 kPa along with rate of flow from 0.29 to 0.07cubic cm/min with

Figure 3. A diagrammatic representation of electrostatic micropump

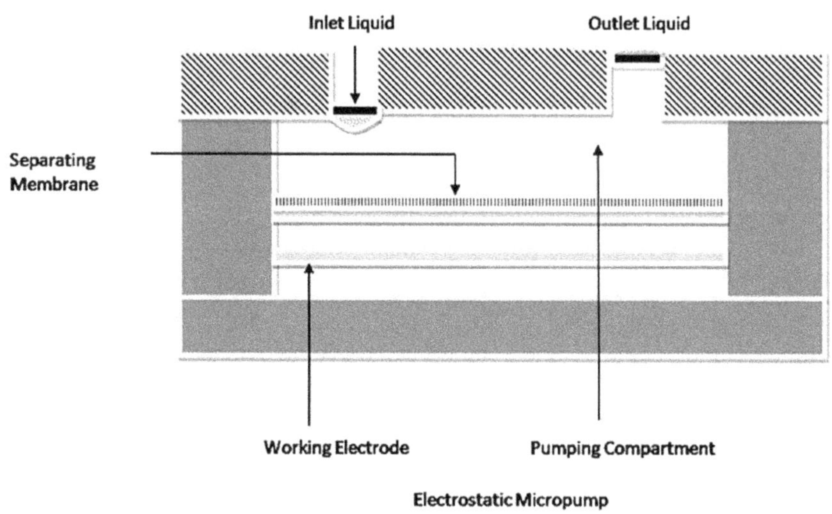

time interval ranging between 0.05 and 0.35 cycles for valves gaping. Electrostatic micropump widely use in microfluidic applications as their main advantages is they require low power consumption for (Byun, Park, Hahn, 2002) micropump applications.

ICPF (Ionic Conductive Polymeric Films) Micropump

This type of micro-pump usually contains a polyelectrolyte film, each faces of which are chemically plated by platinum. These films have good electrical conductivity and are attached to one end immobile diaphragm. The diaphragm is controlled by turning it upward otherwise downward in definite applied voltages to the electrodes for a definite period. To step to the cathode the electric field generates the ions in each faces of the polymer molecule chain. Concurrently, positive charged ions will join few molecules of water and directs on the way to cathode. This transfer of ions creates cathode swelling and anode contraction (Liu, 2010) and the signal of voltage will turn the films alternately. An ICPF micro-pump (Chen, Kwon, Tan, 2008) was used for manufacturing of a flap valve ionic polymer-metal composite micropump along with the diaphragm maintained by a bendy material where the highest flow rate of 760 μL/min and negative pressure of 1.5 kPa were achived at applied voltage of 3 V and 3 Hz frequency. Fang et al. (2008) fabricated an organized adjusted model for visualizing the bending of the diaphragm along with the rate of flow. The polypyrole (PPy) actuated micropump displayed highest flow rate of 1260 μL/min for near 4 V. ICPF actuators provide certain advantages like driving voltage is low, high biocompatibility and rapid reaction; plus it can be operated out in the aqueous environments. The drawback is low levels of reproducibility during batch manufacturing (Lil, Zhu, Zhou, Ren, 2010). Figure 4 represents a schematic diagram of ICPF micro-pump.

Shape Memory Alloy Micro-Pump

Shape-memory effect can be described as the phenomenon of a material recovering its original shape from its distorted shape when heated or cooled (Benard, Kahn, Heuer, Huff, 1998). This effect includes a phase alteration process inside two solid phases: (i) austenite high temperature phase and (ii) martensite low temperature phase. Figure 5 represents a schematic diagram of shape memory alloy micro-pump.

Figure 4. A diagrammatic representation of ICPF micro-pump

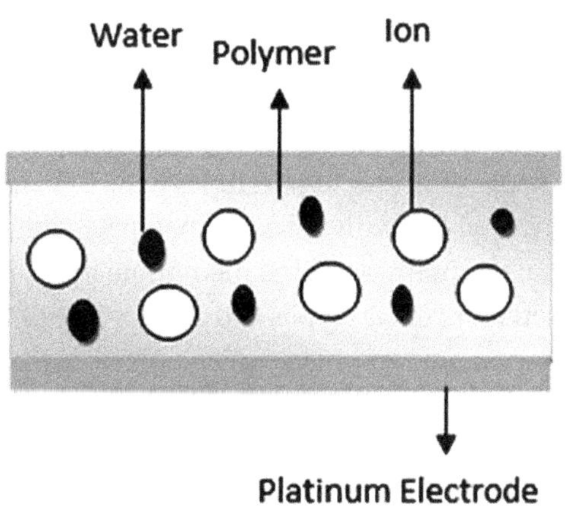

Figure 5. A diagrammatic representation of shape memory alloy micro-pump

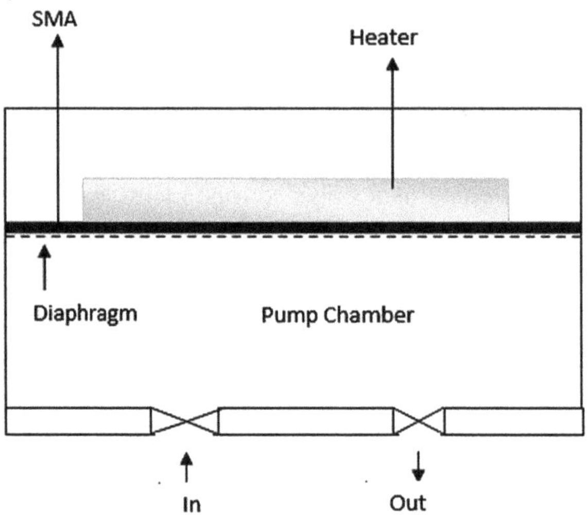

SMA micro-pump diaphragm (Machado, Savi, 2003) is commonly made by Titanium-Nickel alloy (TiNi), a extremely appropriate material for micro-pump actuators since its actuation force is capable of producing high pumping rates and great recoverable strain as well as high working pressures (Cabuz, Herb, Cabuz, Lu, 2001).A SMA micro-pump (Makino, Mitsuya, Shibata, 2000) has been reported, with the total size of almost 10mm×20mm×1.4 mm plus the volumetric flow rate along with the reverse pressure of the pump are almost 34 μL/min and 100 kPa, correspondingly. The advantages shape of memory alloy micro-pump are large force-to-volume ratio, capability to recover high stress, strain transformation in processes of heating and cooling, extremely chemical inertness along with being biocompatible. The main disadvantages of shape memory alloy materials based micro-pump are that they need comparatively greater power utilization and of irresistible distortion of the effect due to temperature sensitivity.

Bimetallic Micropump

The bimetallic diaphragm micro-pump is of basically composed of two dissimilar metals with different coefficients of thermal expansion (CTE). Their bonding mechanism and enslavement of the temperature variations generates thermal stresses as the metals coefficients fluctuate, in case of actuation. A bimetallic micro-pump (Zou, Ye, Zhou, Yang, 1997) has been reported of both bimetallic thermal actuation as well as thermal pneumatic actuation procedures, wherein the bimetallic actuator was made of Al/Si membrane. When heat was given on the membrane, the membrane is distorted downward and the gas in the air compartment is inflated because of the high temperature to bear bimetallic actuation. The flow rate about 336 μL per minute was attained with 0.5 kPa open pressure. Yang et al. (1996) reported that the main constituents of bimetallic thermally actuated membrane micro-pump are the two types of chips, pump compartment, bimetallic actuators of two types and check valve of two types. A maximum flow rate around 43 μL/ min has been reported next to given voltage of 16 V plus frequency of 0.9 Hz. Benefits of the bi-metallic micro-pump are of relatively low voltage required than the other type of micropumps and the disadvantage is their unsuitability for large frequency operation (Tadokoro, Yamagami, Ozawa, 1999). Figure 6 shows bimetallic micro-pump schematic representation.

Figure 6. A schematic representation of bi-metallic micro-pump

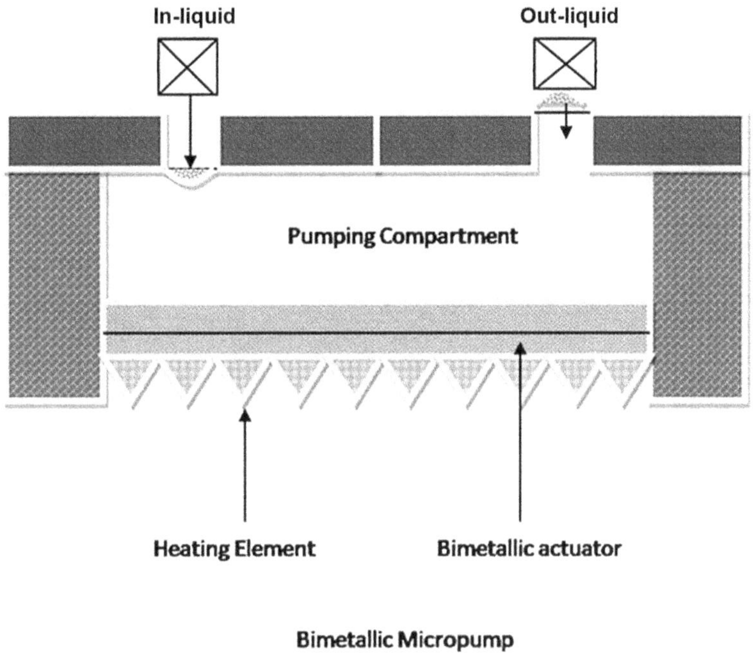

Non Mechanical Micro-Pumps

Non mechanical micro-pumps convert the mechanical energy into the kinetic momentum, which can assist to drive the fluid into the micro channel. Examples of non-mechanical micropumps are electro wetting micro-pump, electro chemical micro-pump, electro-hydrodynamic (EHD) micro-pump, bubble type micro-pump etc.

Electro-Wetting (EW)Micro-Pump

In EW, the wettability is altered in response to a given electric potential. Liquid is fused by surface tension, which is energies governing at the micro scale. Applied voltage at dielectric layer reduces the energy of liquid and solid surfaces interfacial triggering in starting fluid flow. A continuous EW micropump was reported by Yun et al. (2002), with the volumetric flow rate of 70 µl/min along with driving voltage of 2.3 V plus power utilization of around 170 µW. The highest pressure was nearly 800 Pa by applying a voltage of 2.3 V at 25 Hz frequency. For the examination of EW, a full model (Yun et al, 2002) of instrument was represented by applying liquid flow via a small canal. EW provides pumping of fluid directly without use of any movable mechanical components which may be advantageous for several fields of application in micro-electronic instruments. The results illustrate that EW may be utilized for obtaining the pressures of around 0.01 MPa in a channel of radius of 10 µm. The advantages of this micropump are quick response times and less power consumption. Figure 7 signifies electro wetting micropumps schematic diagram.

Figure 7. A schematic representation of electrowetting micropump

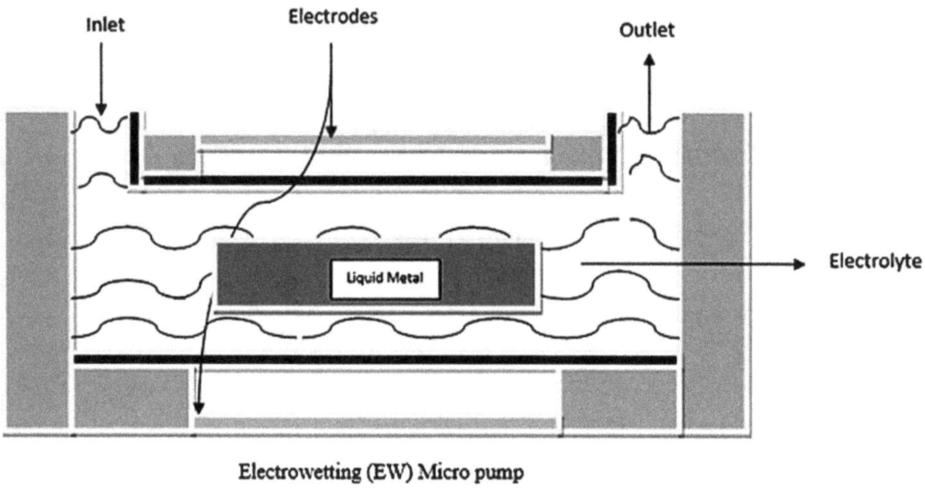

Electro-Chemical Micropump

Electrochemical micropump produces bubbles by electrolysis process of water, which results in generation of in hydrogen (H_2) as well as oxygen gas (O_2). The reservoir is filled by a redox electrolyte solution which generates the bubble force during electrolysis process. This micropump has electricity supplying electrodes, electrolysis chamber, liquid channels, and inlet and outlet reservoirs (Olsson, Stemme, Stemme, 1995). The electrolysis reaction is explained by:

Reaction on Anode $2H_2O \rightarrow 4H^+ + 4e^- + O_2$

Reaction on Cathode $2H_2O + 2e^- \rightarrow 2OH^- + H_2$

An electro chemical micro-pump made-up of electrochemical syringe through micromachining with minimal voltage of operation or power utilization has been reported (Yoshimi, Shinoda, Mishima, Nakao, Munekane, 2004). This microfludic structure is made by a valve checking which is controlled by electrochemically produced hydrogen bubble. Thin film electrodes were employed by means of a platinum black operating electrode. To produce flow canals and storage place for electrolyte mixtures, PDMS substrate was utilized. A polypyrrole membrane based microfludic pump (Kim, Laua, Shepherd, Wu, Wallace, Diamond, 2008). comprising of two dyes was also reported, and the pumping function was conducted by an electrochemical actuated Polypyrrole-PDMS film. Flow rate was controlled via check valves. A maximum flow rate of 52 μL/min was attained at ± 1.5 V through entrance power around 55 mW. The representation of such a micropump is shown in Figure 8.

Electro-Hydrodynamic (EHD) Micropump

In EHD micropump, depicted in Figure 9, the fluid flow can be generated by applying the electrostatic forces on dielectric liquids. In the dielectric solution the flow is operated by the charges which are induced by the electric field interface. When the DC charge was applied on the EHD micro-pump, on the

Figure 8. A schematic representation of electro chemical pump

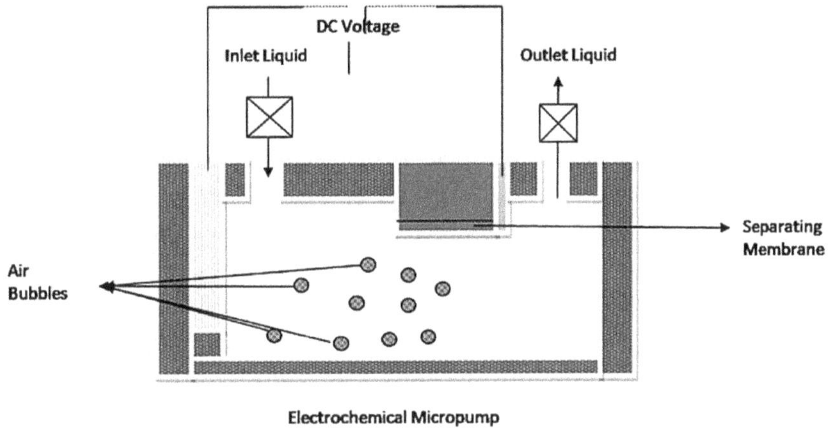

Figure 9. A schematic representation of electro-hydrodynamic (EHD) micropump

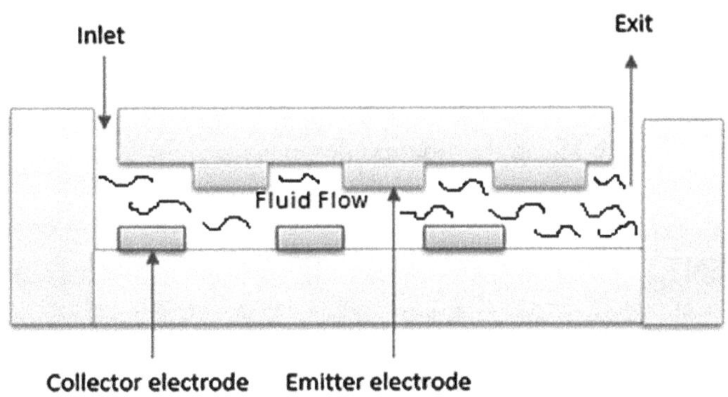

permeable electrodes the columbic force was applied in straight connection with the liquid to be impelled. With the help of electrochemical reactions the infusion of the ion occurs on one or both of the electrodes.

EHD micro-pump was first developed by Fuhr et al. (1992) which was based upon the travelling wave-induced electro convection and achieved a flow rate 0.05 to 5 µL/min. The EHD micropump of ejection type are also reported where indium-tin-oxide (ITO) was used as a planar electrode to solve aging problems (Darabi, Ohadi, DeVoe, 2001) and shown to drive ethyl alcohol with a flow rate of 356 µL/min at applied DC voltage of 61 V. Analysis of numerical micro cooling for EHD micropump was reported (Singhal, Garimella, 2007) where the micropump presented the pumping power by means of the dipole moment force produced as of molecules of the fluid which are polarized where the pressure head was noted 13 kPa, and at 500 V the wall heat flux was generated 10 W/cm^2.

CONCLUSION

MEMS-based systems are a powerful micro-scale platform to meet the technical challenges of meeting greater functionality and patient usability in drug delivery. Indeed these technologies enable efficient miniaturization, allowing for higher degree of precision and automation of the process, while including the scope for personalization) and reducing discomforts associated with invasive administration. However, applied voltage required in range of 5 to 12 V is a constraint factor, especially for electrostatic and piezoelectric micro pumps. On the other hand, MHD and EHD essentially require certain electric conductivity of the fluid solution. The non-mechanical micropumps display a longer delay and slower response times, though they do not require physical actuation for operations. Biocompatibility and relatively lower flow rates have been the main concerns for shape memory based micropumps. Since many of these devices are required for implantation applications, biocompatibility also becomes a principal factor for clinical applications. In this regards, ICPF technology shows better biocompatibility and they can also be operated at low driving voltage with fabrication flexibility. The issues of manufacturing flexibility and biological acceptance are a bottleneck for the bimetallic micropumps, which however, show superior flow rates. Increasingly, these technologies will be integrated with Internet-of-Things (IoT), digital and wireless data transmission technologies to achieve greater and remote functionalities.

MEMS based drug delivery is finding applications in the treatment of hemorrhagic shock, ophthalmic disorders, diabetes, osteoporosis and cancer. There is a greater demand to for developing affordable and low-cost systems requiring minimal surgical invasion due to economic considerations and insurance reimbursements and integration of MEMS with micro-needle technologies may become a key enabler in that direction. If the present limitations of the existing systems can be further improved, these technologies are expected to find newer applications to improve the treatment outcomes with greater patient compliance and customized closed loop therapeutic devices.

ACKNOWLEDGMENT

Sudipto Datta thanks IIEST, Shibpur for Institute Scholarship. Pallab Datta acknowledged SERB DST, Govt. of India for FAST Track research funding.

REFERENCES

Benard, Kahm, Heuer, & Huff. (1998). Thin-Film Shape-Memory Alloy Actuated Micropumps. *Journal of Microelectromechanical Systems, 7*(2), 245-251.

Bohm, S., Timmer, B., Olthuis, W., & Bergveld, P. (2000). A closed-loop controlled electrochemically actuated micro-dosing system. *Journal of Micromechanics and Microengineering*, *10*(4), 498–504. doi:10.1088/0960-1317/10/4/303

Cabuz, C., Herb, W. R., Cabuz, E. I., & Lu, S. T. (2001)The dual diaphragm pump. In *Proceedings of the 14th IEEE International Conference on Micro Electro Mechanical Systems* (pp. 519–522). Interlaken, Switzerland: IEEE.

Chen, Z., Kwon, K., & Tan, X. (2008). Integrated IMPC/PVDF sensory actuator and its validation in feedback control. *Sensors and Actuators. A, Physical*, *144*(2), 231–241. doi:10.1016/j.sna.2008.01.023

Cooney, C. G., & Towe, B. C. (2004). A thermopneumatic dispensing micropump. Sens. Actuators A, 116, 519–524.

Darabi, J., Ohadi, M. M., & DeVoe, D. (2001). An Electrohydrodynamic polarization micropump for electronic cooling. *Journal of Microelectromechanical Systems*, *10*(1), 98–106. doi:10.1109/84.911097

Fang, T., & Tan, X. (2010). A novel diaphragm micropump actuated by conjugated polymer petals: Fabrication, modeling, and experimental results. *Sensors and Actuators. A, Physical*, *158*(1), 121–131. doi:10.1016/j.sna.2009.12.012

Fuhr, G., Hagedorn, R., Muller, T., Benecke, W., & Wagner, B. (1992). Pumping of Water Solutions in Microfabricated Electrohydrodynamic Systems. *Proceedings of IEEE Micro Electro Mechanical Systems. An Investigation of Micro Structures, Sensors, Actuators, Machines and Robots MEMS,Travemunde*, 25–30. 10.1109/MEMSYS.1992.187685

Gao, L., Mantell, S., & Polla, D. (2000). Implantable medical drug delivery systems using micro-electro-mechanical systems technology. *First IEEE-EMBS Special Topic Conference on Microtechnologies in Medicine and Biology*, 487–490.

Grayson, A. R., Shawgo, R. S., Johnson, A. M., Flynn, N. T., Yawen, L., Cima, M. J., & Langer, R. (2004). A BioMEMS review: MEMS technology for physiologically integrated devices. *Proceedings of the IEEE*, *92*(1), 6–21. doi:10.1109/JPROC.2003.820534

Jeong, O. C., & Yang, S. S. (2000). Fabrication and test of a thermopneumatic micropump with a corrugated p+ diaphragm. *Sensors and Actuators. A, Physical*, *83*(1-3), 249–255. doi:10.1016/S0924-4247(99)00392-1

Jin-kyu, B., Il-han, P., & Song-yop, H. (2002). Topology optimization of electrostatic actuator using design sensitivity. *Magnetics. IEEE Transactions*, *38*, 1053–1056.

Johari, J., Yunas, J., & Yeopmajlis, B. (2009). Piezoeletric Micropump for Drug Delivery System Fabricated Using Two Optical Masks. *Advanced Materials Research*, *74*, 279–282. doi:10.4028/www.scientific.net/AMR.74.279

Karman, S., Ibrahim, F., & Soin, N. (2007). A review of MEMS drug delivery in medical application, Biomed 06. *Proc. IFMBE* 15, 312–315. 10.1007/978-3-540-68017-8_80

Kim, J. H., Laua, K. T., Shepherd, R., Wu, Y., Wallace, G., & Diamond, D. (2008). Performance characteristics of a polypyrrole modified polydimethylsiloxane (PDMS) membrane based microfluidic pump. *Sensors and Actuators. A, Physical*, *148*(1), 239–244. doi:10.1016/j.sna.2008.07.029

Koch, M., Harris, N., Evans, A. G. R., White, N. M., & Brunnschweiler, A. (1998). Brunnschweiler, A. A novel micromachined pump based on thick film piezoelectric actuation. *Sensors and Actuators. A, Physical*, *70*(1-2), 98–103. doi:10.1016/S0924-4247(98)00120-4

Lee, S., Yee, S. Y., Besharatian, A., Kim, H., Bernal, L. P., & Najafi, K. (2009). Adaptive gas pumping by ontrolled timing of active microvalves in peristaltic micropumps. In Proceedings of Transducers (pp. 21–25). Academic Press.

Lil, L., Zhu, R., Zhou, Z., & Ren, J. (2010). Modeling of a Micropump Membrane with Electrostatic Actuator. *Proceedings of 2nd International Conference on Advanced Computer Control (ICACC)*, 27–29.

Liu, G., Shen, C., Yang, Z., Cai, X., & Zhang, H. (2010). A disposable piezoelectric micropump with high performance for closed-loop insulin therapy system. *Sensors and Actuators. A, Physical, 163*(1), 291–296. doi:10.1016/j.sna.2010.06.030

Liu, W. (2010). Research on Electrostatic Micropump Pull-in Phenomena Based On Reduced Order Model. *Proceedings of International Conference on Intelligent Computation Technology and Automation*, 11–12. 10.1109/ICICTA.2010.99

Machado, L., & Savi, M. (2003). Medical applications of shape memory alloys. *Brazilian Journal of Medical and Biological Research, 36*(6), 683–691. doi:10.1590/S0100-879X2003000600001 PMID:12792695

Maillefer, D., Lintel, H. V., Mermet, G. R., & Hirschi, R. (1999). A high-performance silicon micropump for an implantable drug delivery system. *Proceedings of IEEE MEMS*, 212–215. 10.1109/MEMSYS.1999.746886

Makino, E., Mitsuya, T., & Shibata, T. (2000). Micromachining of NiTi shape memory thin-film for fabrication of micropump. *Sensors and Actuators. A, Physical, 79*(3), 251–259. doi:10.1016/S0924-4247(99)00290-3

Olsson, A., Stemme, G., & Stemme, E. (1995). A valve-less planar fluid pump with two pump chambers. *Sensors and Actuators. A, Physical, 47*(1-3), 549–556. doi:10.1016/0924-4247(94)00960-P

Reynaerts, D., Peirs, J., & Brussel, H. V. (1997). An implantable drug-delivery system based on shape memory alloy micro-actuation. *Sensors and Actuators. A, Physical*, 488–562.

Richter, A., & Sandmaier, H. (1990). An Electrohydrodynamic Micropump. *Proceedings of IEEE Microelectromechanical Systems,* 99–104.

Singhal, V., & Garimella, S. V. (2007). Induction electrohydrodynamics micropump for high heat flux cooling. *Sensors and Actuators. A, Physical, 134*(2), 650–659. doi:10.1016/j.sna.2006.05.007

Staples, M., Daniel, K., Cima, M. J., & Langer, R. (2006). Application of micro and nano electromechanical devices to drug delivery. *Pharmaceutical Research, 23*(5), 847–863. doi:10.100711095-006-9906-4 PMID:16715375

Tadokoro, S., Yamagami, S., & Ozawa, M. (1999). Soft Micromanipulation Device with Multiple Degrees of Freedom Consisting of High Polymer Gel Actuators. In *Proceedings of IEEE International Conference on Microelectromechanical Systems* (pp. 37–42). Orlando, FL: IEEE. 10.1109/MEMSYS.1999.746748

Tan, H. Y., Loke, W. K., & Nguyen, N. (2010). A reliable method for bonding polydimethylsiloxane (PDMS) to polymethylmethacrylate (PMMA) and its application in micropumps. *Sensors and Actuators. B, Chemical, 151*(1), 133–139. doi:10.1016/j.snb.2010.09.035

Tao, Lubeley, & Desai. (2003). Bioadhesive poly(methyl methacrylate) microdevices for controlled drug delivery. *J. Control. Rel.,* 215–228.

Trenkle, F., Haeberle, S., & Zengerle, R. (2009). Normally-closed peristaltic micropump with re-usable actuator and disposable fluidic chip. *Procedia Chemistry, 1*(1), 1515–1518. doi:10.1016/j.proche.2009.07.378

Tsai, N. C., & Sue, C. Y. (2007). Review of MEMS based drug delivery and dosing systems. *Sensors and Actuators*, *134*(2), 555–564. doi:10.1016/j.sna.2006.06.014

Van de Pol, F. C. M., & van Lintel, H. T. G. (1990). A thermopneumatic micropump based on microengineering techniques. *Sensors and Actuators. A, Physical*, *21*, pp198–pp202. doi:10.1016/0924-4247(90)85038-6

van den Berg, A., & Lammerink, T. (1998). Micro total analysis systems: microfluidic aspects, integration concept and applications. In Microsystem technology in chemistry and life science (pp. 21-49). Springer.

Van Lintel, H. T. G., Van de Pol, F. C. M., & Bouwstra, S. (1988). A piezoelectric micropump based on micromachining of silicon. *Sensors and Actuators. A, Physical*, *15*(2), 153–168. doi:10.1016/0250-6874(88)87005-7

Woias, P. (2001). *Micropumps: summarizing the first two decades*. Micromachining and Microfabrication.

Yang, Y., Zhaoying, Z., Xiongying, Y., & Xiaoning, J. (1996). Bimetallic Thermally Actuated Micropump. Proceedings of International Mechnical Engineering Congross and Exposition (ASME 1996), 17–22.

Yoshimi, Y., Shinoda, K., Mishima, M., Nakao, K., & Munekane, K. (2004). Development of an artificial synapse using an electrochemical micropump. *Journal of Artificial Organs*, *7*(4), 210–215. doi:10.100710047-004-0269-5 PMID:15739055

Yun, K. S., Cho, I. J., Bu, J. U., Kim, C. J., & Yoon, E. (2002). A surface tension driven micropump for low voltage and low power operations. *Journal of MEMS.*, *11*(5), 454–461. doi:10.1109/JMEMS.2002.803286

Zhang, H. J., & Qiu, C. J. A. (2006). TiNiCu thin film micropump made by magnetron Co-sputtered method. *Materials Transactions*, *47*(3), 532–535. doi:10.2320/matertrans.47.532

Zimmermann, S., Frank, J. A., Liepmann, D., & Pisano, A. P. (2004). A planar micropump utilizing thermopneumatic actuation and in-plane flap valves. In *17th IEEE International Conference on Micro Electro Mechanical Systems (MEMS): Maastricht MEMS 2004 Technical Digest* (pp. 462–465). IEEE. 10.1109/MEMS.2004.1290622

Zou, J. X., Ye, Y. Z., Zhou, Y., & Yang, Y. (1997). A Novel Thermally Actuated Silicon Micropump. *Proceedings of International Symposium on Micromechatronics and Human Science*.

Chapter 8
Optimization Techniques Applications in Biochemical Engineering and Controlled Drug Delivery:
Current Practices and Forthcoming Challenges

Satya Eswari Jujjavarapu
National Institute of Technology Raipur, India

Bikesh Kumar Singh
National Institute of Technology Raipur, India

ABSTRACT

Before starting semi-pilot/pilot production plants for biochemical metabolites production, it is essential to optimize the fermentation media. This chapter discusses the classical and advanced techniques of media optimization. The statistical approaches save experimental time for developing processing and improving quality. Recent years have seen the growth of integrated approaches of microbial cultures. Optimization techniques such as response surface methodology, artificial neural network, genetic algorithms, differential evolution, ant colony optimization, etc. have received attention recently because of their major applications in various fields. Controlled release formulations have so many versatile applications in the field of pharmaceutical drugs that they have become important tools to apply the modern concept of therapeutic treatment. Process optimization of such formulations, mathematical modelling can play an important role. This chapter discusses various methodologies for optimization of formulation conditions for drug delivery.

DOI: 10.4018/978-1-5225-4969-7.ch008

INTRODUCTION

Application of Optimization Techniques in Controlled Drug Delivery

There have been a lot of advancements, over the past few years, in the field of drug delivery. These advances can be mainly attributed to the improvement of meticulous drug discharge dosage. Most of these advances have been done in the controlled drug discharge of oral quantity, by controlling the conditions that influence drug discharge. The drug release patterns can be fined into 2 groups; i) formulations that release drug at a slow, (0 or 1st order) rate and ii) sustained release formulations that afford a first amount of dose, followed by slow (zero or first order) release of active drug (Dash et al., 2010). Sustained release formulations allow us to maintain desired drug absorption in the plasma or in any target tissue for a lengthy period of time (Langer and Wise, 1984). The specific sustained release formulations allow controlling the rate of drug release and its duration (Li and Lee, 1987). These formulations generally release only a part of the active drug initially, to achieve the active tonic concentration of the drug in a short time. After that, the drug release kinetics follows a well-defined behaviour so as to attain and maintain the desired drug concentration. Designing and developing the controlled discharge formulations needs engineers and pharmacists to work composed to produce more effective products. The procedure of modelling may allow us to predict the release kinetics without or with minimum experimental data, which is an important step to develop formulations. Also mathematical modelling might improve the quantity of certain imperative parameters such as the drug diffusion coefficient and resorting to model fitting on experimental release data. Thus, for the process optimization of such formulations, mathematical modelling is having a significant role. The development of mathematical models needs the understanding of all the factors affecting drug release kinetics (Cartensen, 1996). The mathematical models involved in drug release kinetics can be viewed as mathematical metaphors of some aspects of reality which controls the phenomena ruling the discharge kinetics (Dressman and Fleisher, 1986). Because of these general aspects, mathematical modelling is widely employed in varied fields of science and technology ranging from genetics to medicine, psychology to economy, biology, and obviously engineering. In this article we explained about the RSM, design of experiments, ANN, RBFN, GRNN methodologies for the application of drug delivery process.

Advancements of Optimization Techniques for Biochemical Production

Advancements in biochemical production require better understanding of the bioprocesses involved in biochemical production from different raw materials, agro-industrial by-products and waste streams, as well as possibility to predict the outcomes of these processes in terms of biochemical yield and substrate utilization (Olsson, 2007). Optimization of biochemical production processes is also important from the aspect of yield increase and bioprocess cost reduction. Optimization techniques such as Design of experiments (DOE), fuzzy logic (FL), Particle swarm optimization (PSO), genetic algorithms (GA), differential evolution (DE) neural networks (NN) and Multi objective optimization (MOO), could be used as a tool for biochemical production modelling and optimization. The basic characteristics and applications of ANN in modelling and optimization of biochemical production processes have been experimentally proven (Ivana et al., 2017). Figure 1 shows about the flow chart of various optimization methods.

Figure 1. Advancement of optimization techniques in bioprocesses

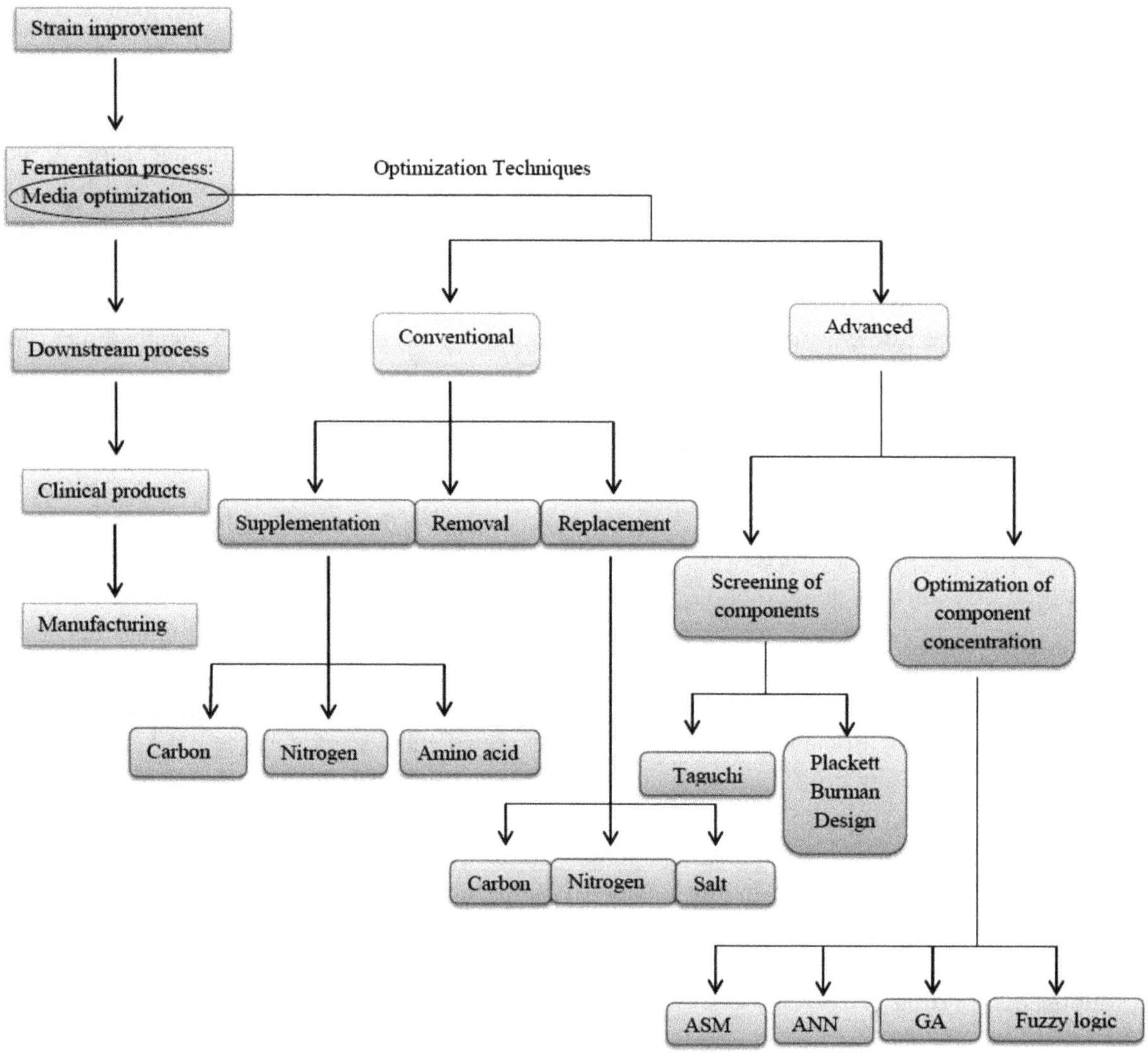

CONTROLLED DRUG DELIVERY, OPTIMIZATION

In a condition of surgery or in case of patients in intensive care unit, certain drugs are administered to the patients generally to maintain vital physiological parameters, such as body temperature, blood pressure etc. The concentration of such drugs has to be maintained by experienced personnel on the basis of physiological conditions. It is a tedious and laborious process and thus prone to human errors. Therefore, there is a need to make the process at least partially automated by the use of computational tools. This might improve the intensive care of patients. At present computational tools such as optimization methods are used to restrict the increasing cost of health care. The drug delivery system has not been automated till date because the mathematical models describing the effects of drugs on the physiological parameters are not accurate. This has been a difficult step because of the non-linear response, the difference in response by different patients, the effects of outer conditions, and the interaction amongst different drugs. Various models such as Response surface models; artificial neural network models can be developed and can be used as models in controlled drug delivery also further can be evaluated experimentally.

Response Surface Methodology (RSM) Application in Controlled Drug Delivery

RSM can be used to optimise the drug delivery systems, since drug delivery depends on various factors, including physical, chemical, and physiological factors. RSM has been successfully used by research groups for optimisation of drug delivery. Kumari et al. (2009) optimised the delivery of chlorpheniramine maleate (CPM) by using RSM. The CPM drug was loaded in chitosan-alanine beads for controlled release; and was cross linked using glutaraldehyde as cross-linker. Four components were used as formulating agents and regression models were developed. The response variable (i.e. drug release) was optimised on the basis of formulation variables, which were, chitosan concentration, % of cross-linker, concentration of drug, and release time (RT). Factorial design (FD) analysis was castoff to find the effect of each parameter. The authority of the model was appraised by analysis of variance (ANOVA). All the 4 factors were said to have important effect on CPM release. The optimum values for the variables were found to be 0.42 g, 10-18%, and 100 mg respectively for X_1, X_2, and X_3. Release time (X_4) has a linear effect on drug release. Here they used linear regression models for controlled drug delivery process.

Placket Burman (PB) Methodology in Controlled Drug Delivery (CDD)

Placket Burman (PB) can be used for designing controlled drug delivery (CDD) systems. Porous type tablets were intended as an osmotic drug delivery system, to invent out the better formulation (Patel et al., 2016). Three categories of polymers were screened for designing of the porous osmotic pump tablets. Six independent variables, namely osmotic agent sodium chloride (OASC) and microcrystalline cellulose (MCC), sodium lauryl sulphate (SLL) and sucrose, and ethyl cellulose (EC) and cellulose acetate (CA) were selected for screening. The drug release was mainly affected by osmotic agent and pore former. The porous osmotic pump tablets contained dicloxacillin sodium and amoxicillin trihydrate as the active antibiotic drugs. The optimised drug delivery system was designed by using sodium chloride (150 mg) as osmotic agent, sodium lauryl sulphate (15 mg) as pore former, and cellulose acetate (2%) as coating agent. Thus Placket Burman design was successfully used for optimisation of drug delivery system.

Neural Network (NN) Methodology in Controlled Drug Delivery

The release profile of a new formulation of drug is a time consuming process because the many drug compositions and other linked variables are also to be considered account. The common procedure includes repeated stages of random experiments based on the experience of the drug formulators. An investigational study in trans-skin treatment was performed to assess the applicability of an NN-model in modelling and predicting drug release profiles (Lim et al. 2003). Gaussian mixture model (GMM) is an intelligent learning system based on neural-networks, which was used to model and predicts the drug release profiles using experimental data. The simultaneous effect of three process variables (pH and ionic strength of the buffer, and the magnitude of electrical current) on iontophoresis process was examined. The bootstrap method was used to prove the reliability of GMM for prediction. Brier et al.

(1995) reported the prediction of peaks and troughs of gentamicin serum concentrations based on a set of empirical data using an ANN system and the results were comparable with those using nonlinear mixed effect modelling. They predicted serum drug concentration for more than 100 patients of various physical parameters. The aptitude of NN in predicting the output of patients paining from a disorder to a particular drug was demonstrated (Valafar and Valafar 1999). Also they validated and response of the drug hydroxyurea was predicted by the neural network on 23 sickle cell anaemic patients. They reported 86 to 100% accuracy in predicting the response of patients. Some pharmacokinetic models based on ANNs have been developed to predict plasma drug concentration and to estimate heparin concentrations in patients undergoing haemodialysis treatment (Valafar and Valafar 1999). Some research groups reported the release of corticosteroid drug that can be controlled by an implant. The drug delivery system was based on the use of a biodegradable polymer. NN is used for modelling of the drug release data was examined by Rutkowski 2004. ANN classes are multilayer perceptron (MLP), radial basis function network (RBFN), and generalized regression neural network (GRNN) were used. The overhead stated NNs have potential of modelling and determining the relation among nonlinear data, approximating any arbitrary function between input and output vectors from training samples (Rutkowski 2004). They also mentioned the effectiveness of NNs in optimizing release drug profiles for designing controlled release formulations. Many recent articles (Barmpalexis et al., 2011a; Barmpalexis et al., 2011b; Petrović et al., 2012; Chansanroj et al., 2011; Tan et al., 2012) indicate that, in future NNs can be integrated with additional soft computing, such as fuzzy logic (FL), genetic programming (GP), decision trees (DT), self-organizing maps (SOM)a, etc.

OPTIMIZATION OF BIOPROCESSES

Design of Experiments and Response Surface Method Methodology Application for Bioprocess

The experimental analysis of any bioprocess generally requires expensive materials to extract the product or to analyse the concentration of any particular metabolite or even a drug molecule or its degradation product. Hence optimization tools can play vital role to reduce experimental efforts. Various advanced optimization techniques can be dealt in the following sections.

Fuzzy Logic Methodology Application for Bioprocess

Fuzzy logic is a qualitative approach to modelling for bioprocess control. Biochemical processes can be controlled by specially designed fuzzy controllers (FLC). Fuzzy logic control based on the Takagi-Sugeno inference (TKI) is useful for control of the baker's yeast fermentation. Strongly non-linear processes and processes that are difficult to model because of complicated reaction kinetics can be successfully controlled by fuzzy control; this gives an advantage to fuzzy logic to other control methods. But tuning of controllers working on fuzzy control designs is very time consuming process (Vasičkaninová et al., 2017). The use of fuzzy logic – a machine-learning algorithm - to assess cancer risk in screening oral potentially malignant disorders have also been proposed by Scrobota et al.(2017).

Genetic Algorithms (GA) Methodology Application for Medical Signals

Genetic algorithms can be efficiently used in biomedical applications such as extraction and classification of data. Cardiac diseases can be diagnosed automatically only after successful extraction of features and for classifying signals of electrocardiogram (ECG) which can be achieved using wavelet packet decomposition (WPD) by the method neural network (GA-NN). This approach was projected by Li et al. (2017). The extraction of the effective features of ECG signals can be performed by WPD combined with the statistical method. The applications of GA include reduction in the dimensions of the feature sets; optimization of weights as digits and biases which is generally one NN. NN classifier with GA optimization is able to classify six types of ECG signals. The GA-NN system has been used with the database of arrhythmia, which was able to reduce dimensions by 50% and the classification results were accurate up to 97.78%. Some studies have shown the use of GA-BPNN method to achieve a much accuracy of up to 99.33%. Thus, it can be capably useful in the instinctive identification of arrhythmias.

Particle Swarm Optimisation (PSO) Methodology Application for Medical Signals

PSO is yet another algorithm which can be used for biomedical data extraction and optimisation. It is a quite interesting heuristic method that has produced promising results for solving complex optimization problems. An ANN and PSO are used to ECG heartbeats are classified of a patient into 5 signals by Shadmand and Mashoufi (2016). A block established from 2-D array of interconnected blocks, was used as the classifier. PSO was used for the optimisation of the structure of network along with the weights. The input of the NN is a vector with its decision values as the features extracted from the ECG signals. The optimisation of NN parameters by PSO algorithm has an advantage to overwhelm the likely variations of signals of ECG variations. The trained NN has a distinctive structure for each person. A more accuracy of classification is 97% was reported by using the arrhythmia database.

Differential Evolution (DE) Methodology Application for Bioprocess

There have been numerous developments area of bioprocess for better model development and validation, with current modern algorithms is insignificant. In case of fermentation, there are transformations detected amid model predictions and real conditions which may follow unreliable effects. An evolutionary algorithm of evolutionary optimization multiobjective (MOO) problems includes differential evolution (DE) and genetic algorithm (GA) yield optimal elucidations. Rocha et al. (2007) recited the 2 algorithms fit in Evolutionary Algorithms (EA) based on their optimal control. The advantages of DE include identical effects after associated models of mathematically represented process. Another advantage is that it treaties in terms of state variable noise which is the property of flowing decrease. On the other hand, when noisier settings are considered other optimisation methods prove superior to the differential evolution (DE). DE has been used for culture conditions optimization for the production of CHO cells which are Chinese hamster ovaries. According to the authors, involvement of trepidations in the components of the medium for growth and component composition optimization is the most flavour for any type of cell productivity. They have taken experimental model for the CHO cells growth metabolic flux analysis (MFA)-DE. They concluded that this method is an excellent for connecting input spaces and output variables (Satya Eswari and Venkateswarlu, 2012). Evolutionary algorithms (GA and DE) linked RSM models are constructed. For this purpose, numerous sets of goals analogous to the populace the variable space are generated after calculating with RSM. Since does not take part of nonlinearities hence the ANN based RSM used. MOO strategies derived by either RSM model or an ANN-RSM-DE used for high formation of rhamnolipid by *Pseudomonas aeruginosa* AT10. Carbon (*X*1, gdm^{-3}), nitrogen ($NaNO_3$) (*X*2, gdm^{-3}), the phosphate content (K_2HPO_4/KH_2PO_4) (*X*3, gdm^{-3}) and the iron ($FeSO_4.7H_2O$) (*X*4, g dm^{-3}) were considered critical components. The responses are the biomass (*Y*1, gdm^{-3}) rhamnolipid (*Y*2, g dm^{-3}). Pilot production of rhamnolipids the factors of the components-medium need to be optimized (Satya Eswari et al., 2013).

Ant Colony Optimisation (ACO) Methodology Application for Bioprocess

Ant colony optimisation (ACO) algorithm can be applied as an optimisation method for bioprocesses. The kinetic and film thickness factors for treatment of wastewater in an anaerobic fixed bed biofilm reactor (AFBR) assessed by an inverse modelling (IM) ant colony optimization (ACO). Experimental data of treatment of industrial pharmaceutical waste water (PWW) can be determined the factors of model. Different modelling patterns resulting from the combination of mathematical prototypes, time wise data of expressions different optimization flow charts were assessed and 2D models with kinetic haldane was shown to be best treatment of the PWW. The mathematical and kinetic prototypes are worthwhile PWW (Satya Eswari and Venkateswarlu, 2013). Obtaining reliable models from experimental data is important are influenced by number of decision factors and best decision factors are identified. The Ant Colony Optimization (ACO) algorithm can be used efficiently for variable selection. Pessoa et al. (2015) used *Saccharomyces cerevisiae* fermentation data to select various variables for trail update and model comparison. ACO has also been used with flux balance analysis to optimize gene knockout identification by Salleh *et al.* (2015). Growing claim of biochemical supply for various industries which has led to designing of microbial cell factories. Natural producers mostly have very low product yields. Gene knockout strategy can improve the metabolite production. Some optimal microbial strains, to be used as cell factories, have been designed by the use of computational algorithms, developed specifically for the purpose. However, the large genome size of microorganisms, poses difficulties in finding the optimal combination of genes to be knocked out. A hybrid of Genetic Ant Colony Optimization (G-ACO) and Flux Balance Analysis (FBA) namely G-ACO-FBA was established to invention the optimal gene knockout to intensify biochemical production. Best optimal genes ate used to raise the production of four tested metabolites while taking care of the optimal growth rate in *E. coli* and *S. cerevisiae* genome scale model. It was shown to be more actual present methods.

Neural Network (NN)

The selection of cell disruption technique depends on many factors such as type of cell, its growth status, molecules to be detected, etc. The most common lysis inducing chemical agents used are EDTA, lysozyme, Triton X, and polymyxin B. The degree of cell lysis is generally detected by the soluble protein concentration in the lysate. An experiments-with the strategy for efficient cell disruption protocols was designed by Glauche et al. (2016). Monitoring of a bioprocess can be done by using a feed-forward neural network in combination with 2-D fluorescence spectroscopy. In traditional approach, for the training the neural network, an offline measurement was needed. But in this method there is no need of any offline measurement; instead a theoretical model of the process can be used to simulate the process state at a given time.

Multi Objective Optimization (MOO) Methodology Application for Bioprocess

Naïve slow Genetic algorithms (NSGA) and Naïve slow Differential evolution (NSDE) The industrial bioprocesses mainly produce more than one product in a batch. Such processes need to be optimized for better utilization of substrate and obtaining more favourable products. MOO concerns with simultaneously optimizing two or more objectives. In case of conflicting objectives, optimizing one objective results in compromising with other objectives. The non-dominated objectives in this case are called as Pareto optimal or non-inferior solutions. These Pareto optimal solutions refer to different optimal operating conditions and called as Pareto set. Different methods are employed for solving the problems on conflicting multi-objective optimization. Classical methods of multiobjective optimization, namely weighting and e-constraints, convert the multi-objective problem into a single objective one and solve further to obtain Pareto optimal solutions (Chankong and Haimes, 1983; Ray, 1989). The problem with this approach is that they iteratively change the solution to get a single point optimized solution by using a point by point approach. MOO approach, on the other hand, uses EA, namely DE and GA to yield many Pareto solutions. Deb (2001), Rajesh et al. (2001) and Ohh et al. (2002) provide detailed information on the use of evolutionary algorithms (EA) for MOO. MOO strategies have been developed by integrating an EA algorithm with soft computing tools for formulation of pharmacological products. J. Satya Eswari et al., 2017 developed RBFN-NSDE (radial basis function network - non-conquered sorting differential evolution) and applied for optimal formulation of a trapidil product concerning conflicting output (OP) features. RBFN models are established by means of orthogonal designs (OD) of trapidil formulation variables on behalf of the amounts of MCC (microcrystalline cellulose), HMC (hydroxypropyl methylcellulose) and CP (compression pressure), and the analogous OP (output) distinctive data of RO (release order) and RC (rate constant).

CONCLUSION

Experimental efforts of a biological concern are always laborious and cumbersome. Hence it is always easy to avoid experiments by using design of experiment and modelling of a bioprocess. Optimization concepts in controlled drug delivery and bioprocess optimization can reduce many experimental efforts and cost also. Before going for large production of biochemical and animal trials for controlled drug delivery, it is essential to optimize the fermentation media and formulation conditions. This chapter discusses about the classical and advanced techniques of optimization methodologies which are applied on biological concepts. The statistical approaches save experimental time for developing processing and improving quality. Optimizing a process leads to reduction in overall cost of production. The methods for optimization depend on simplicity, efficiency and time consumption. This chapter elaborately explains about the flavour of various optimization techniques in bioprocess engineering and controlled drug delivery formulations.

REFERENCES

Barmpalexis, P., Kachrimanis, K., & Georgarakis, E. (2011a). Solid dispersions in the development of animodipine floating tablet formulation and optimization by artificial neural networks and genetic programming. *European Journal of Pharmaceutics and Biopharmaceutics*, *77*(1), 122–131. doi:10.1016/j.ejpb.2010.09.017 PMID:20934511

Barmpalexis, P., Kachrimanis, K., Tsakonas, A., & Georgarakis, E. (2011b). Symbolic regression via genetic programming in the optimization of a controlled release pharmaceutical formulation. *Chemometrics and Intelligent Laboratory Systems*, *107*(1), 75–82. doi:10.1016/j.chemolab.2011.01.012

Brier, E., Zurada, J. M., & Aronoff, G. R. (1995). Neural network predicted peak and trough of gentamicin concentrations. *Pharmaceutical Research*, *12*(3), 406–412. doi:10.1023/A:1016260720218 PMID:7617529

Cartensen, J. T. (1996). *Modeling and data treatment in the pharmaceutical sciences*. New York: Technomic Publishing Co. Inc.

Chankong, V., & Haimes, Y. Y. (1983). *Multiobjective Decision making theory & methodology*. New York: Elsevier.

Chansanroj, K., Petrović, J., Ibrić, S., & Betz, G. (2011). Drug release control and system understanding of sucrose esters matrix tablets by artificial neural networks. *European Journal of Pharmaceutical Sciences*, *44*(3), 321–331. doi:10.1016/j.ejps.2011.08.012 PMID:21878388

Cheng, K. K., Wu, J., Lin, Z. N., & Zhang, J. A. (2014). Aerobic and sequential anaerobic fermentation to produce xylitol and ethanol using non-detoxified acid pretreated corncob. *Biotechnology for Biofuels*, *7*(1), 166. doi:10.118613068-014-0166-y PMID:25431622

Dash, S., Murthy, P. N., Nath, L., & Chowdhury, P. (2010). Kinetic modelling on drug release from controlled drug delivery systems. *Acta Poloniae Pharmaceutica-Drug Research*, *67*(3), 217–223. PMID:20524422

Deb, K. (2001). *Multi-objective optimization using evolutionary algorithms*. New York: John Wiley & Sons Limited.

Dressman, J. B., & Fleisher, D. (1986). Mixing-tank model for predicting dissolution rate control or oral absorption. *Journal of Pharmaceutical Sciences*, *75*(2), 109–116. doi:10.1002/jps.2600750202 PMID:3958917

Glauche, F., Pilarek, M., Bournazou, M. N. C., Grunzel, P., & Neubauer, O. (2016). Design of experiments based high-throughput strategy for development and optimization of efficient cell disruption protocols. *Engineering in Life Sciences*, 1–7.

Huang, L., Shi, Y., Wang, N., & Dong, Y. (2014). Anaerobic/aerobic conditions and biostimulation for enhanced chlorophenols degradation in biocathode microbial fuel cells. *Biodegradation*, *25*(4), 615–632. doi:10.100710532-014-9686-1 PMID:24902896

Ivana, P., Jovana, G., Jelena, D., & Aleksandar, J. (2017). Applicaton of artificial neural networks in modelling and optimization of biofuels production. *Journal on Processing and Energy in Agriculture*, *21*(2), 66–70. doi:10.5937/JPEA1702066P

Kumari, K., Prasad, K., & Kundu, P. P. (2009). Optimization of chlorpheniramine maleate (CPM) delivery by response surface methodology – four component modeling using various response times and concentrations of chitosan-alanine, glutaraldehyde and CPM. *Express Polymer Letters*, *3*(4), 207–218. doi:10.3144/expresspolymlett.2009.27

Langer, R. S., & Wise, D. L. (Eds.). (1984). *Medical Applications of Controlled Release, Applications and Evaluation* (Vols. 1-2). Boca Raton, FL: CRC Press.

Li, H., Yuan, D., Ma, X., Cui, D., & Cao, L. (2017). Genetic algorithm for the optimization of features and neural networks in ECG signals classification. *Scientific Reports*, 7. PMID:28139677

Li, V. H. K., & Lee, V. H. L. (1987). Controlled drug delivery: Fundamentals and applications (2nd ed.). Marcel Dekker Inc.

Lim, C. P., Quek, S. S., & Peh, K. K. (2003). Prediction of drug release profiles using an intelligent learning system: An experimental study in transdermal iontophoresis. *Journal of Pharmaceutical and Biomedical Analysis*, *31*(1), 159–168. doi:10.1016/S0731-7085(02)00573-3 PMID:12560060

Nair, G., Jungreuthmayer, C., & Zanghellini, J. (2017). Optimal knockout strategies in genome-scale metabolic networks using particle swarm optimization. *BMC Bioinformatics*, *18*(1), 78. doi:10.118612859-017-1483-5 PMID:28143607

Oh, P. P., Rangaiah, G. P., & Ray, A. K. (2002). Simulation and multi-objective optimization of an industrial hydrogen plant based on refinery off-gas. *Industrial & Engineering Chemistry Research*, *41*(9), 248–2261. doi:10.1021/ie010277n

Olsson, L. (2007). *Biofuels*. Berlin, Germany: Springer-Verlag. doi:10.1007/978-3-540-73651-6

Patel, A., Dodiya, H., Shelate, P., Shastri, D., & Dave, D. (2016). Design, Characterization, and Optimization of Controlled Drug Delivery System Containing Antibiotic Drug/s. *Journal of Drug Delivery*, *2016*, 9024173. doi:10.1155/2016/9024173 PMID:27610247

Pessoa, C. M., Ranzan, C., Trierweiler, L. F., & Trierweile, J. O. (2015). Development of Ant Colony Optimization (ACO) Algorithms Based on Statistical Analysis and Hypothesis Testing for Variable Selection. *IFAC-PapersOnLine*, *48*(8), 900–905. doi:10.1016/j.ifacol.2015.09.084

Petrović, J., Ibrić, S., Betz, G., & Djurić, Z. (2012). Optimization of matrix tablets controlled drug release using Elman dynamic neural networks and decision trees. *International Journal of Pharmaceutics*, *428*(1-2), 57–67. doi:10.1016/j.ijpharm.2012.02.031 PMID:22402474

Rafieniaa, M., Amirib, M., Janmalekic, M., & Sadeghiand, A. (2010). Application of artificial neural networks in controlled drug delivery systems. *Applied Artificial Intelligence*, *24*(8), 807–820. doi:10.1080/08839514.2010.508606

Rajesh, J. K., Gupta, S. K., Rangaiah, G. P., & Ray, A. K. (2001). Multi-objective optimization of industrial hydrogen plants. *Chemical Engineering Science*, *56*(3), 999–1010. doi:10.1016/S0009-2509(00)00316-X

Ray, W. H. (1989). *Advanced Process Control*. New York: Butterworths.

Rocha, M., Pinto, J. P., Rocha, I., & Ferreira, E. C. (2007). Evaluating Evolutionary Algorithms and Differential Evolution for the Online Optimization of Fermentation Processes. In E. Marchiori, J. H. Moore, & J. C. Rajapakse (Eds.), Lecture Notes in Computer Science: Vol. 4447. *Evolutionary Computation, Machine Learning and Data Mining in Bioinformatics. EvoBIO 2007*. Berlin: Springer. doi:10.1007/978-3-540-71783-6_23

Rutkowski, L. (2004). Generalized regression neural networks in time-varying environment. *IEEE Transactions on Neural Networks*, *15*(3), 576–596. doi:10.1109/TNN.2004.826127 PMID:15384547

Satya, E. J., & Ch, V. (2012). Optimization of Culture Conditions for Chinese Hamster Ovary (CHO) Cells Production Using Differential Evolution. *International Journal of Pharmacy and Pharmaceutical Sciences*, *4*(1), 465–470.

Satya, E. J., & Ch, V. (2013). Evaluation of Kinetic Parameters of an Anaerobic Biofilm Reactor Treating Pharmaceutical Industry Wastewater by Ant Colony Optimization. [PubMed]. *Environmental Engineering Science*, *30*(9), 527–535. doi:10.1089/ees.2012.0158

Satya Eswari, J., & Mohan, A. (2013). Optimum Culture Medium Composition for Rhamnolipid Production by Pseudomonas Aeruginosa AT10 Using a Novel Multiobjective Optimization Method. *Journal of Chemical Technology and Biotechnology (Oxford, Oxfordshire)*, *88*(2), 271–279. doi:10.1002/jctb.3825

Scrobotă, I., Băciuț, G., Filip, A. G., Todor, B., Blaga, F., & Băciuț, M. F. (2017). Application of Fuzzy Logic in Oral Cancer Risk Assessment. *Iranian Journal of Public Health*, *46*(5), 612–619. PMID:28560191

Sendrescu, D. (2013). Parameter Identification of Anaerobic Wastewater Treatment Bioprocesses Using Particle Swarm Optimization. *Mathematical Problems in Engineering*, *2013*, 103748. doi:10.1155/2013/103748

Shadmand, S., & Mashoufi, B. (2016). Personalized ECG signal classification using block-based neural-network and particle swarm optimization. *Biomedical Signal Processing and Control*, *25*, 203–208. doi:10.1016/j.bspc.2015.10.008

Tan, C., & Degim, I. T. (2012). Development of sustained release formulation of an antithrombotic drug and application of fuzzy logic. *Pharmaceutical Development and Technology*, *17*(2), 242–250. doi:10.3109/10837450.2010.531739 PMID:21062232

Valafar, H., & Valafar, F. (1999). Prediction of a patient's response to a specific drug treatment using artificial neural networks. IEEE, 3694–3697.

Vasičkaninová, A., Bakošová, M., & Mészáros, A. (2017). Control of a biochemical process using fuzzy approach. *2017 21st International Conference on Process Control (PC)*, 173-178.

Chapter 9
Segmentation of Liver From 3D Medical Imaging Dataset for Diagnosis and Treatment Planning of Liver Disorders

Gajendra Kumar Mourya
North Eastern Hill University, India

Dinesh Bhatia
North Eastern Hill University, India

Akash Handique
North Eastern Indira Gandhi Regional Institute of Health and Medical Sciences, India

ABSTRACT

CT- and MRI-based imaging modalities are non-invasive, fast, and accurate in the diagnosis of different anatomical and pathological disorders. As such, there is a pertinent requirement for segmentation of the large organs such as liver and lungs to give proper visual information on the extent of involvement of morphological and pathological changes. The aim of this chapter is to discuss and implement different liver segmentation techniques on the 3D medical data set to determine best feasible technique for the purpose. The localization and detection of liver tumor will be easier for a radiologist with the extraction of the liver margins from other adjoining organs and its localization within the anatomical segments. It is found that active contour technique provides satisfactory results and also the validation results are well outlined in the case of active contour techniques.

INTRODUCTION

The liver is the largest and heaviest internal organ and a gland in the human body and is usually located in the right side of upper abdominal cavity, related to the right hemi-diaphragm above, surrounded by lower right thoracic cage to protect from external trauma. One pint (13%) of the body's blood supply at any given moment is hold by the Liver. Inferior surface comes in contact with the right kidney, gall

DOI: 10.4018/978-1-5225-4969-7.ch009

bladder, stomach and adjacent small and large intestines. It is a wedge shaped dark reddish-brown organ that weighs about 1.44-1.66 kilograms in a healthy adult (See Figure 1). The hepatic portal system is responsible for directing blood from parts of the gastrointestinal tract carrying nutrients from food to the liver. In the hepatic portal system, the liver receives a dual blood supply from the portal vein and hepatic arteries. Also, hepatic portal vein used to it supplies 75% of the liver's blood and carries venous blood drained from the gastrointestinal tract, spleen and to the associated organs, The hepatic arteries supply arterial blood to the liver and account for the remainder 25% of its blood flow.

Lobes of Liver

The liver consists of two main lobes the right lobe (largest) and the left lobe along with two smaller quadrate (Part of left lobe) and the caudate lobe. Entire liver consist of eight (8) segments based on Couinaud's classification that consist of 1,000 lobules (small lobes) as shown in Figure 2. Each lobule and subsequently a segment is an independent functional unit with its own portal vein, bile duct, hepatic artery in the center and a draining hepatic vein in the periphery. These lobules are connected to small bile ducts (tubes) that connects with larger ducts to ultimately form the common hepatic duct. The common hepatic duct transports the bile produced by the liver cells to be stored temporarily in the gallbladder finally draining to the duodenum (the first part of the small intestine) via the common bile duct along with pancreatic duct which joins at its distal end and drains via a common duct called ampulla of Vater which is routinely identified as a projection from inside the duodenum called Papilla during endoscopic retrograde cholangiopancreatography or ERCP.

Figure 1. Location of liver
Retrieved 2017 from https://commons.wikimedia.org/wiki/File:Liver_and_nearby_organs.jpg

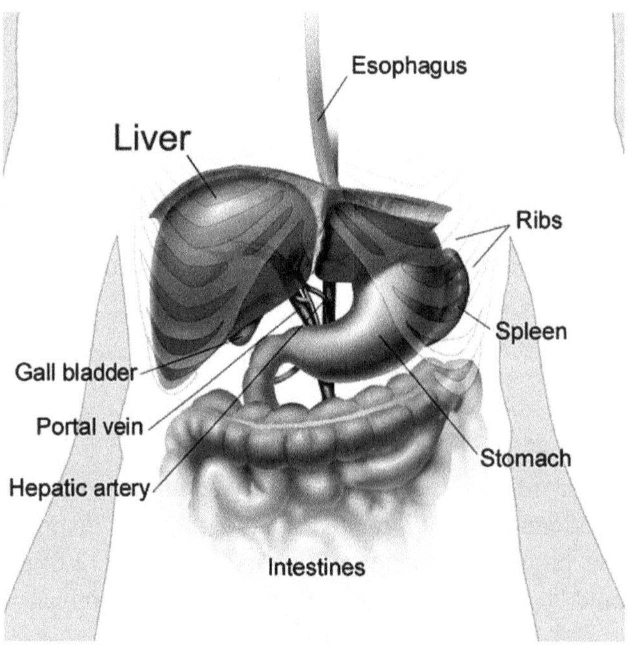

Figure 2. Segmental anatomy of the liver
Retrieved 2017 from https://commons.wikimedia.org/wiki/File:Liver_04_Couinaud_classification_animation.gif

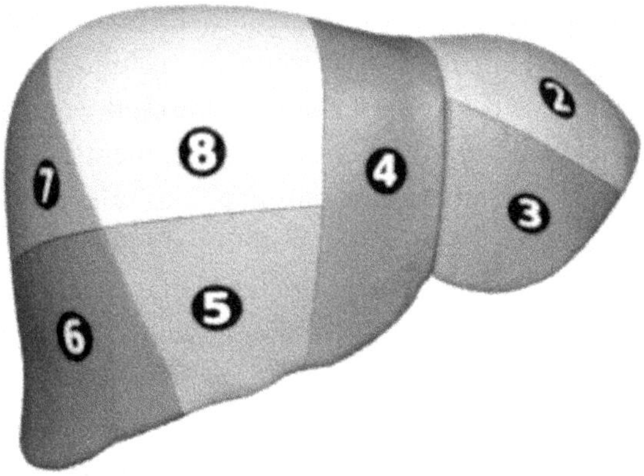

Anatomical Liver Lobe Classification

Grossly the liver is divided into two distinct lobes first one is right lobe and second is left lobe as shown in Figure 3. The right and left lobes are separated by falciform ligament. The right lobe is larger than the left lobe. This classification is not preferred for radiological reporting and surgical planning of liver tumors.

This classification is system was first described by the French Surgeon Claude Couinaud in 1957. The fissure for the round ligament of the liver (ligamentum teres) separates the medial and lateral segments. The medial segment, also called the quadrate lobe is considered a part of left lobe. Caudate lobe is a

Figure 3. Anterior and posterior view of liver
Retrieved 2017 from https://wiki2.org/en/Liver

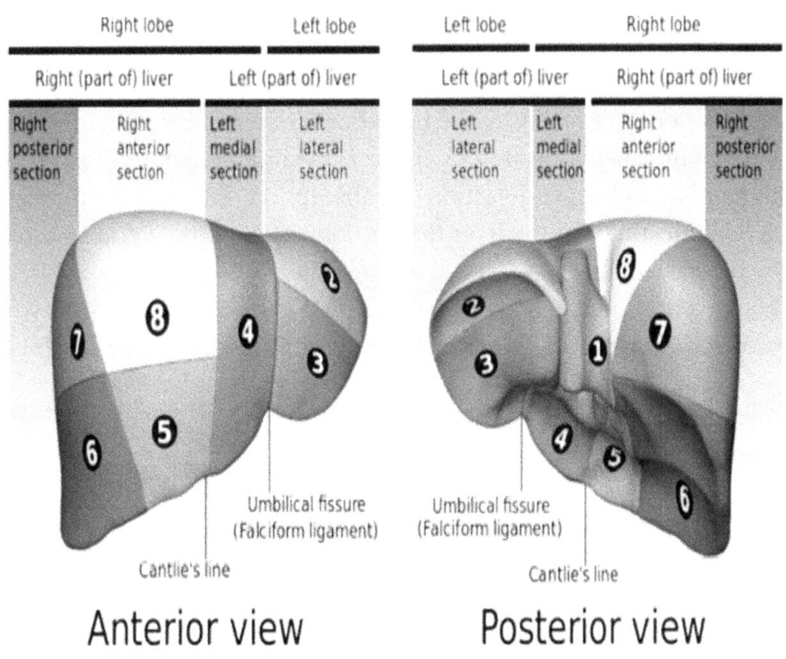

separate unit that receives blood from both right- and left-sided of the vascular branches. Classification of couinaud of the liver anatomy divides into eight functionally independent segments. Each segment has its own vascular inflow, outflow, and biliary drainage. In the centre of each segment there is a branch of the portal vein, hepatic artery, and bile duct. Also, there is vascular outflow through the hepatic veins inthe periphery of each segment. The division of the liver into independent units means that segments can be surgically resected without damaging the remaining segments.

The Couinaud classification is the preferred anatomical classification system as it divides the liver into eight functional units rather than relying on the traditional morphological description based on the external appearance of the liver. The segments are numbered in roman numerals as discuss below. Right and left lobe is divided by a plane along the middle hepatic vein superiorly (cranially) and gall bladder inferiorly (caudally).

1. Segment I is the caudate lobe and is situated posteriorly (dorsally) and it may receive its supply from both the right and the left branches of portal vein
2. Segments II and III lie lateral to the falciform ligament on left side with II superior (cranial) to the portal venous supply and III inferior (caudal) to it.
3. Segments IV lies medial to the falciform ligament and is subdivided into IV-a (superior) and IV-b (inferior) and is anatomically part of left lobe of liver.
4. Segments V to VIII make up the right part of the liver.
5. Segment V is the most medial and inferior and closely related to the gall bladder.
6. Segment VI is located more posteriorly and laterally below the right portal vein branch
7. Segment VII is located above Segment VI and right portal vein branch. It is also located lateral and posterior.
8. Segment VIII lies superior to the Segment V and right portal vein branch in the superior-medial position anterior to segment VII.

Functions of Liver

The liver is responsible for the regulation of levels of several chemicals in the blood and excretes bile. Bile along with pancreatic enzymes helps in the breakdown of water insoluble fat. Fats such as Triglycerides are emulsified by bile and hydrolyzed by the enzyme lipase, resulting in a mixture of fatty acids and monoglycerides helping for further digestion and absorption. Through the liver all of the blood used to pass the stomach and intestines. In the liver the nutrients (fat, carbohydrates, proteins, vitamins and minerals) carried by blood from intestines reach through the portal system are stored, metabolized and broken down into components that the body can use. It metabolizes drugs into active form for obtaining desired therapeutic effect. Some of the more well-known functions include the following (Ballard. & Oliver., 1965).

Carbohydrate Metabolism

The liver performs the following functions, in carbohydrate metabolism:

1. Storage of excess carbohydrate as glycogen
2. Breakdown of galactose and fructose into glucose

3. Gluconeogenesis
4. Formation of various chemical compounds from intermediate products of carbohydrate metabolism.

The liver helps mainly in maintaining a normal blood glucose concentration. In the liver, the storage of glycogen allows to remove excess glucose from the blood, store it, and then return it to the blood when the blood glucose concentration begins to fall too low. This is called the glucose buffer function of the liver. In a person with poor liver function, blood glucose concentration after a meal rich in carbohydrates may rise two to three times as much as in a person with normal liver function (Ballard. & Oliver., 1965).

Fat Metabolism

Though most cells of the body metabolize fats, certain aspects of fat metabolism occur mainly in the liver. The main function of the liver in fat metabolism is mentioned below:

1. Oxidation of fatty acids for the supply of energy form several body functions
2. Synthesis of large quantities of cholesterol, phospholipids, and most lipoproteins
3. Synthesis of fat from proteins and carbohydrates

Protein Metabolism

Protein metabolism is important functions of the liver and the function are as follows:

1. Formation of urea for removal of ammonia from the body fluids
2. The removal of an amino group from an amino acid
3. Formation of plasma proteins
4. Inter-conversions of the various amino acids
5. Synthesis of other compounds from amino acids

Before they can be used for energy or converted into carbohydrates or fats, removal of amino acids is required. A small amount of deamination can occur in the other tissues of the body, especially in the kidneys, but this is much less important than the deamination of amino acids by the liver.

Other Functions

- It helps in the production of certain proteins for blood plasma. Also, it helps in making bile that helps to carry away waste and break down fats in the small intestine during digestion.
- Production of cholesterol and special proteins to help carry fats through the body
- It stores and releases glucose when required
- Processes haemoglobin for use of its iron content (the liver stores iron)
- Clearing the blood of drugs and other harmful substances
- Helps in regulating blood clotting
- Clearance of bilirubin (if there is a build-up of bilirubin, the skin and eyes turn yellow)

Problems Associated With Liver

It is a potentially fatal condition that demands urgent medical care. When wide range of the liver become damaged beyond repair and is no longer able to function properly then the Liver failure occurs. Most often, the liver failure occurs gradually and over many years called chronic liver disease or cirrhosis. However rarely fulminant liver failure can occurs rapidly in as little as 48 hours and can be cause rapid deterioration of liver function needing urgent liver transplant as only option.

Hepatitis

Hepatitis is not a disease but an inflammation of the liver. Inflammation is body's natural reaction to injury and can often result in swelling and tenderness due to edema or accumulation of excess water within the liver. Hepatitis can be mild and self limiting or it may result in severe damage, causing permanent and life-threatening damage to the liver. Hepatitis can chronic and can causing cirrhosis leading to chronic liver failure and resultant portal hypertension leading to bleeding ascites and even death. Hepatitis, or liver inflammation, can be caused by several factors including viral infections, alcohol abuse and other toxic agents, autoimmune diseases (rare). Hepatitis can be caused by Infection caused by hepatitis A, B, C, D and E viruses; Epstein-Barr virus (Hall., 2007), cytomegalovirus; adenovirus; and rarely, herpes simplex virus can result in acute mild self resolving disease to chronic hepatitis which can lead to cirrhosis and chronic liver failure. Toxic agents such as alcohol, recreational drugs, prescription medicines or other chemicals can result mild self resolving hepatitis to life threatening fulminant liver failure.

Figure 4. Helical CT scan of hepatitis B e antigen-positive chronic hepatitis B
Retrieved 2017 from https://commons.wikimedia.org/wiki/File:Fundusvarizen.jpg

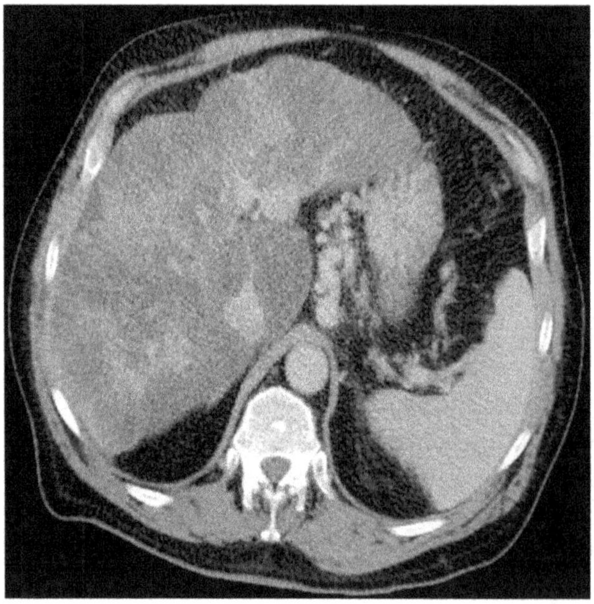

Fibrosis

Fibrosis is the build-up of scar tissue within the liver after on-going inflammation from viral infection, alcohol abuse, fat, toxins, damaged to the bile ducts or autoimmune diseases. As liver inflammation continues, normal liver cells are replaced by scar tissue which becomes dense enough to interfere with the structure of the liver. This in turn interferes with the metabolic functions and blood flow to the liver.

Liver fibrosis occurs more rapidly in men than in women and in people over 50 years of age. Excessive alcohol abuse and fatty liver are also associated with worse fibrosis. *Figure 5* shows an image of liver suffering from Liver fibrosis.

Cirrhosis

In chronic hepatitis, serious fibrosis usually leads to cirrhosis, a condition in which the liver is severely scarred, its blood flow is restricted, and its ability to function is damaged. The process can take up to 20 to 30 years of accumulated damage and scarring to the liver. Cirrhosis can also be the result of autoimmune hepatitis, some inherited diseases that cause high levels of certain minerals to accumulate in the liver such as copper (Wilson's disease) or iron (Hemochromatosis), blocked or inflamed bile ducts, long exposure to environmental toxins and some drug reactions (including prescription drugs Figure 6 shows CT image of a Patient with cirrhosis showing tortuous hepatic arteries in addition to enlarged left lobe and caudate.

Liver Cancer

Most common cancer found in the liver is metastatic cancer, which means it has spread (metastasized) from other parts of the body, mostly from the gut (Stomach and intestines). Malignant cells detach from the primary cancer and travel to the liver in the bloodstream. Cancers that most commonly spread to the liver include colon, lung and breast cancers. Second most common cancer is primary cancer of liver or hepatocellular carcinoma or HCC. HCC is common in preexisting cirrhosis of liver from any cause

Figure 5. Liver fibrosis
Retrieved 2017 from https://en.wikipedia.org/wiki/Fibrosis

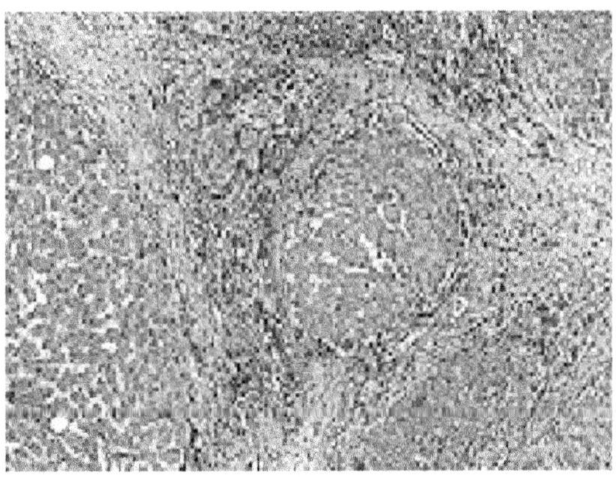

Figure 6. CT image of liver with cirrhosis
Retrieved 2017 from https://hi.wikipedia.org/wiki/%E0%A4%9A%E0%A4%BF%E0%A4%A4%E0%A5%8D%E0%A4%B0:CT_abdomen_-_liver_cirrhosis_-_01.JPG

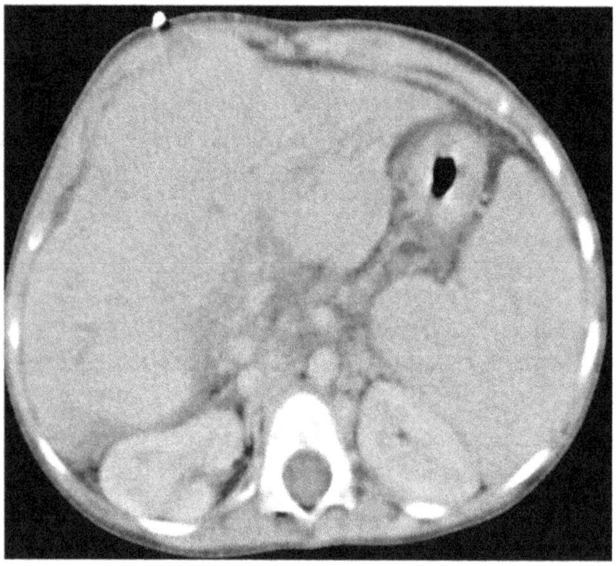

however it can occur in normal liver too. Diagnosis of both primary HCC and Metastatic disease is at an advanced stage where most patients cannot be offered curative surgery. Moreover even if curative surgery is possible in tumors presenting at an early stage, pre-existing cirrhosis prevents safe resection as residual liver might not have enough hepatic function compatible with life. (Göran., 1981)

Figure 7. CT scan image through the liver that shows a liver cancer (arrow)
Retrieved 2017 from https://commons.wikimedia.org/wiki/File:Neuroblastoma_liver.jpg

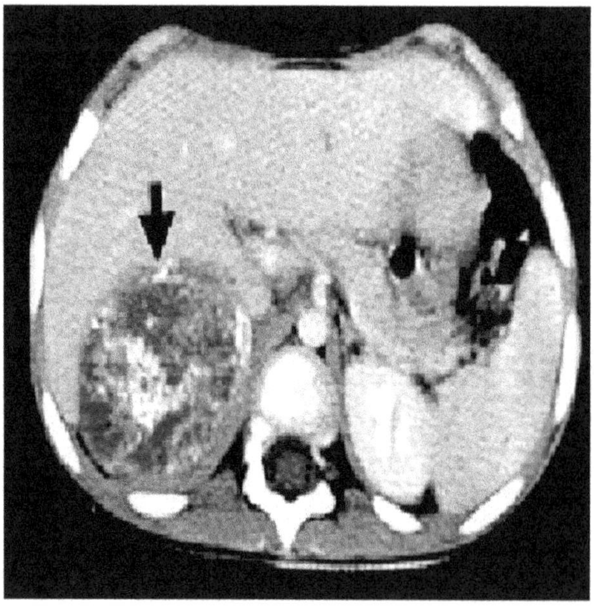

Mortality Rate Cause of Liver Disorder

Global liver cirrhosis deaths have increased from around 676,000 in 1980 to over 1 million (1,029,042; 670,216 to 1,554,530) in 2010 (about 2% of the global total). Over the same period, the age-standardized cirrhosis mortality rates have decreased by 22%. By decreasing cirrhosis mortality rates this was largely driven in China, the US and countries in Western Europe. In the year 2010, the highest age-standardized cirrhosis mortality rates in some of the country are Egypt, followed by Moldova, the rate are: 72.7 and 71.2 deaths per 100,000, respectively, while Iceland had the lowest. In Egypt, almost one-fifth (18.1%) of all deaths in males 45 to 54-years old were due to liver cirrhosis. Also in Mexico the Liver cirrhosis mortality is the highest in Latin America. Whereas, in France & Italy the liver cirrhosis mortality drop by 50% to 60%. Conversely, in the United Kingdom, mortality increased by about one-third. Also, Mortality of the liver cirrhosis was compare high in several parts of Central Asia countries (like: Uzbekistan, Kyrgyzstan and Mongolia) and in sub-Saharan Africa, notably Gabon. According to the World Health Organization in India disease in the liver is the tenth most common cause of death. Around 10 lakh new patients of liver cirrhosis are diagnosed every year in India.

IMAGING MODALITIES

Ultrasound

Ultrasound waves are sound waves having frequencies greater than normal human audible range i.e. 20-20KHz. In case of medical field, these sound waves play a major role in the radiology field. Diagnostic imaging techniques based on application of these ultrasounds are widely used and is termed as medical ultrasonography. Ultrasonic images known as sonograms are made by sending pulses of ultrasound to the body tissues through the transducer probe. This technique is similar to echolocation used by bats Principle of ultrasound. To generate images of internal body structures the medical ultrasound imaging consists of using high pitched sound bouncing off tissues. The sound echoes off the tissue with different tissues reflecting varying degrees of attenuation of sound which are recorded and displayed as a 2D image to the operator.

To calculate the depth of the tissue interface causing the echo, the time taken for the echo to travel back to the probe is used. Higher the echo is, higher the difference between acoustic impedances. If the pulse hits gases or bones, it is not possible to see deeper because of the larger density difference and most of the sound energy is reflected back. For the generation of the 2-D image the ultrasonic beam is swept. Most of the modern equipments use electronic steering however; transducer may be swept mechanically by rotating or swinging. To construct the image, the received data is processed and used. Then the 2D representation of the slice into the body. Ultrasound travels at a slightly different speed through different tissues. A rough average of 1540m/s is used, but the velocity through fat (~1460m/s) and water (~1480m/s) is somewhat slower. Structures deep to a large fluid collection can therefore appear a little further away than their actual position.

Ultrasound applications in Obstetric and Gynecologic Imaging, measuring the size of the foetus to determine the due date, checking the foetus's growth rate by making many measurements over time, detecting ectopic pregnancy, safely guiding specialized procedures such as visualizing and avoiding the needle injury to the fetus during amniocentesis or taking sample of amniotic fluid for analysis or for therapy and seeing tumors of the ovaries, uterus and breast. Ultrasound is utilized routinely to see abdominal organs, blood vessels and its flow within, heart morphology and function (echocardiography), neck, musculoskeletal system and other superficial organ imaging. Ultrasound can be used for guiding biopsies, draining pus, obstructed bile and urine etc.

Disadvantages of ultrasound imaging include, artifacts which are certain conditions causing abnormalities which affect the final image. These include abnormal low signal in tendons and ligaments if beam is not perpendicular due to anisotropy arising from linear orientation of the collagen fibers reflecting ultrasound waves, Specular of mirror reflection at highly reflecting surfaces such as air containing lungs and bones, abnormal brightness of objects behind fluid containing structures such as urinary bladder and eye due to low attenuation of ultrasound waves. Other disadvantages include, being operator dependant, inability to look structures deep to the reflecting surfaces such as bones gas filled intestines and lungs (poor acoustic window), However additional advanced functions such as liver and breast elastography have been developed to quickly assess nature of lesions within them based on ability of tissues to deform on application of external pressure. Ultrasound elastography is invaluable to calculate liver hardness in early cirrhosis for early diagnosis and treatment.Image of Ultrasound Machine and the output of Ultrasound Machine can be seen in Figure 8 (a),(b).

CT Scan

CT scan or computed tomography is used to determine normal or abnormal structures in the body based on differences in X-ray attenuation of various tissues. A highly collimated beam of X-rays are passed through a ssection of the body to an array of detectors at multiple angles along the circumference at a

Figure 8. (a) Ultrasound machine (b) Liver image of ultrasound
Retrieved 2017 from https://commons.wikimedia.org/wiki/File:Liver_ultrasound_0530115943921.jpg

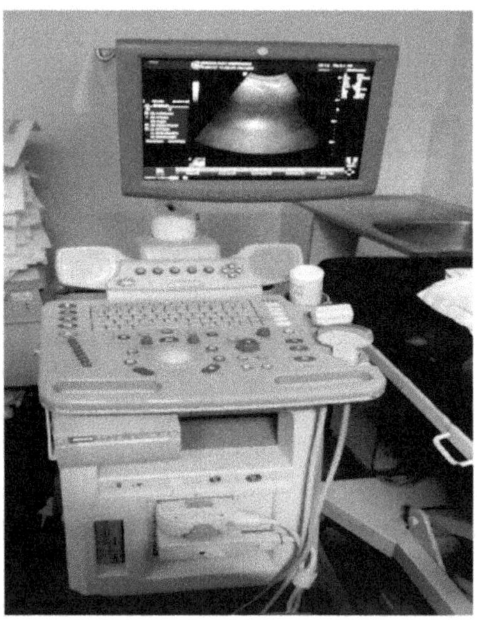

(a)

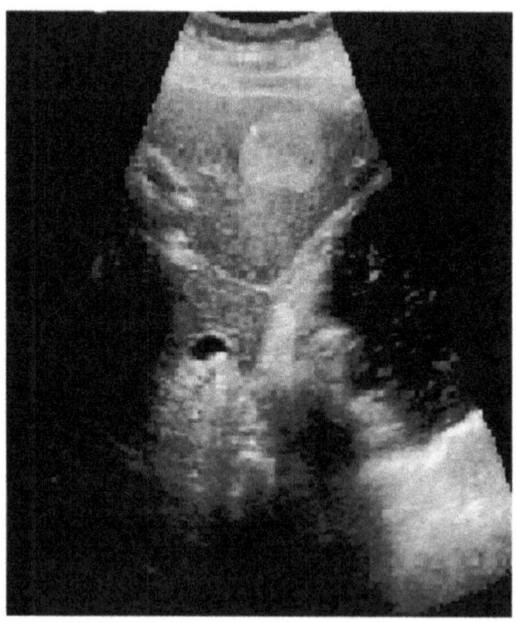

(b)

very high speed to determine the degree of attenuation of X-rays as they pass through various tissues depending on the angle. The attenuation data set undergoes complex mathematical iterations to construct a single image or a series of images or slices in the onboard computer and displayed in appropriate window and level setting in varying shades of grey, higher attenuation denoting lighter shades and lower attenuation darker. Most modern CT scanners have multi slice capability (2 to up to 640 slices) enabling rapid spiral acquisition of 3D volume data set which can be used to construct images in any orthogonal plane. Most CT scans are performed as outpatient procedure. The Advantages of CT scan are that it enables direct imaging and differentiation of soft tissue structure for (e.g. liver, lung tissue) based on attenuation. Attenuation difference can be enhanced with the use of iodinated contrast medium which is administered intravenously immediately before CT acquisition. Iodine is a highly radiopaque and hence contrast medium increases the attenuation of tissue wherever it is distributed. CT acquisition can be repeated at different phases to see the contrast transit along the blood vessels and its uptake in various organs and within the lesions. Usually highly vascular lesions such as tumors or inflammation having significant blood flow and therefore take up contrast more avidly and appear brighter.

CT is especially useful for detecting space occupying lesions such as tumors, abscess etc. and measuring its size, location, presence of fat and or calcification and extent of invasion of the tumour. It is also used for detecting orbital, neck., thoracic, blood vessels and lung abnormalities. CT imaging is used extensively in orthopedics for imaging subtle and complex bone fracures, bony protrusion of vertebra (osteophytes) and joint imaging. The 3-D CT is an invaluable tool for surgical reconstruction following facial trauma. CT angiography is can visualize renal arteries, carotid vessels, thoracic and abdominal aorta. Cardiac CT of the heart, its function and heart vessels is possible in modern mutislice (64 and above) CT Scanners. CT imaging techniques are also used in forensic sciences. Disadvantages of CT scan is higher radiation dose as compared to plain X-rays

With the advancement in generation of CT machine the radiation dose per procedure has not significantly diminished. CT scans are contraindicated for pregnancy, due to the risk radiation exposure and its adverse event on the fetus. In addition contrast agents are also contraindicated in pregnant mothers.

Figure 9. (a)CT machine (b) Abdominal region image of CT
Retrieved 2017 from https://commons.wikimedia.org/wiki/File:CT_scan_autosomal_dominant_polycystic_kidney_disease.jpg

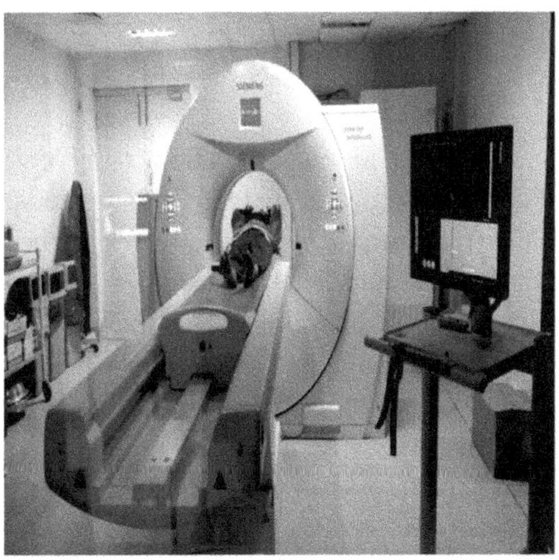

(a)

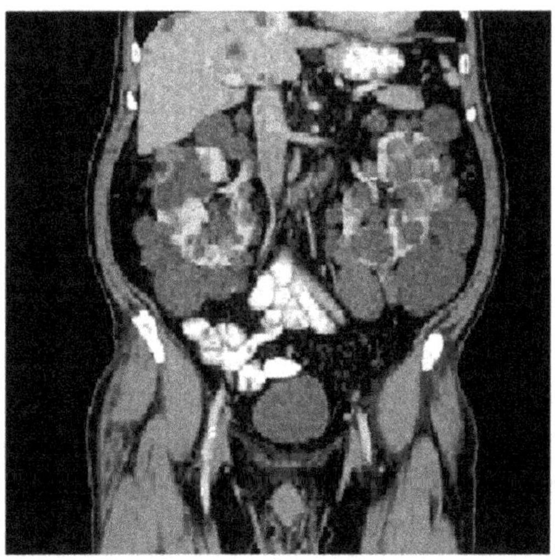

(b)

CT examination requires voluntary immobilization and breath hold by the patient which is usually well tolerated. CT imaging of the Brainstem and posterior fossa is relatively inferior due to presence of surrounding dense bones of the skull base. Similarly metallic implants can degrade CT images significantly.

MRI

Magnetic resonance imaging (MRI) is a machine which utilizes strong magnetic fields and radio waves to produce detailed images of the inside of the body. An MRI scanner is a large tube that contains powerful, often superconducting magnet and where the patient lies inside the tube during the scan. Magnetic resonance imaging (MRI) obtains high quality images of the soft tissues of the human body. It is based on the principles of nuclear magnetic resonance (NMR) of hydrogen nucleus which is abundant in our body, a spectroscopic technique used earlier to obtain microscopic chemical and physical information about molecules.

The person is positioned inside an MRI scanner which creates a strong magnetic field around the area to be imaged. Hydrogen atoms in tissues containing water molecules are used to create a signal that is processed to form an image of the body and this is used in medical application. The radio signal can be made to encode spatial or position information by varying the main magnetic field using gradient coils. The repetitive noise of an MRI scan is also produce when these coils are rapidly switched on and off they create the characteristic. The contrast between different tissues is determined by the rate at which excited hydrogen nuclei return to the equilibrium state. A magnetic field is required in MRI that is both strong and uniform. The field strength of the magnet is measured in tesla and while the majority of systems operate at 1.5T, commercial systems are available between 0.2T–7T. Most clinical magnets are superconducting which requires liquid helium to keep them cool. Lower field strengths can be achieved with permanent magnets, which are often used in MRI scanners to suffering from claustrophobia patients. MRI for imaging anatomical structures or blood flow can be done without contrast agents as the varying properties of the tissues or blood provide natural contrasts. For more specific types of imaging the most commonly used intravenous contrast agents are based on chelates of gadolinium and used similar to iodinated contrast use in CT.

When a human body is placed in a large magnetic field, free hydrogen nuclei align themselves with direction of the magnetic field and start to process similar to a spinning top around the magnetic field at certain frequency specific to the strength of the magnetic field. The frequency of the precession is known as Larmor frequency, which is given by $\Omega 0 = \gamma B0$ Where, $\Omega 0$ = precession frequency (Hz) γ= gyroscopic constant, B0= magnetic field strength (T).

The advantages of MRI are its ability to image without the use of ionizing radiation (x-ray) unlike CT scanning. Images may be acquired in multiple planes (Axial, Sagittal, Coronal, or Oblique) and even as 3D volume dataset without repositioning the patient. CT images have only relatively recently been able to be reconstructed in multiple planes with the same spatial resolution. MRI images demonstrate superior soft tissue contrast over CT and plain X-rays making it the ideal examination of the brain, spine, joints and other soft tissue body parts. Some angiographic images can be obtained without the use of contrast material, unlike CT or conventional angiography. Functional MRI allows visualization of active parts of the brain during certain activities and understanding of the underlying networks. Disadvantages and challenges to implementing MRI scanning are being more expensive than CT scans and longer time to acquire images so patient comfort is sometimes an issue and uncooperative patients may need sedation.

Additionally images are subject to unique artefacts that must be recognized and abated such as presence of ferromagnetic materials in implants and jewelry. MRI scanning is not safe for patients with certain metal implants and foreign bodies. Careful attention to safety measures is necessary avoid serious injury to patients and staff and this requires special MRI compatible equipment and stringent adherence to safety protocols. Image of MRI Machine and the output of MRI Machine can be seen in Figure 10.

BACKGROUND

Medical image segmentation approaches can be grouped in two classes, the first one being fully automatic techniques, and other one being semi-automatic techniques. Automatic image segmentation techniques are not employed regularly for medical images for the following reasons. First, the acquired CT images usually have blurred edges and low contrast due to the partial volume effects resulting from spatial averaging, patient movement, beam hardening, and reconstruction artifacts. Secondly, the fact that different organs/tissues may have similar grey levels creates an additional difficulty for segmentation between adjacent organs/tissues (Campadelli et al., 2009).As a result, it is anticipated that the general grey- level dependent image segmentation techniques for edge detection and image classification may not clearly separate overlapped organ regions and correctly extract the desired organs. Thirdly, due to the administration of contrast media and/or different machine setup conditions, the same organ may exhibit different grey-level values in different cases or in different image slices of the same case. Such grey-level variations are sometimes significant, making it impossible to apply a simple thresholding technique. Fourthly, the anatomical structures of an organ in different image slices are different. Even for the same slice position, its shape may vary significantly from patient to patient. Thus, proper identification of organs cannot be easily accomplished by using the traditional shape-based pattern recognition technique.

Figure 10. (a)MRI machine (b) Abdominal region image of CT
Retrieved 2017 from https://commons.wikimedia.org/wiki/File:MRI_of_abdomen_showing_GamnaGandy_bodies_in_schistosomiasis.gif

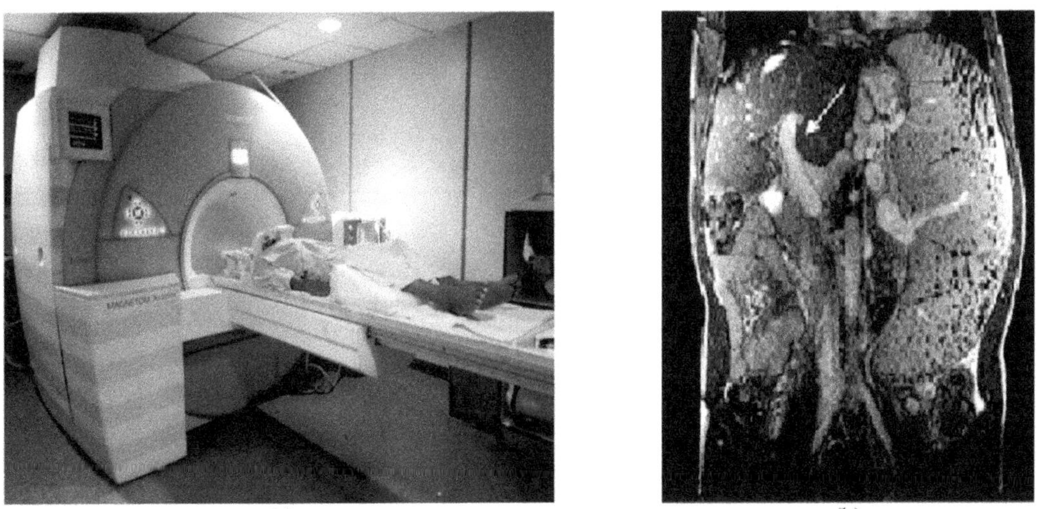

(a) (b)

In the Table 1, a brief literature review is given showing the Pre-processing and the segmentation technique used and their evaluation results are also indicated. It can be seen that paper with the title 'Liver segmentation with new supervised method to create initial curve for active contour has the highest percentage of sensitivity and accuracy.

METHODOLOGY

To achieve objective such as proper segmentation of liver for detecting different diseases such as liver cirrhosis and liver cancer, there are many methods and techniques that can be used. Following various steps are involved in the segmentation of liver from abdominal images as shown in Figure 11 and Figure 12.

Table 1. Literature review for liver segmentation

Paper Title	Preprocessing Technique	Segmentation Method	Evaluation	Sensitivity and Accuracy	References
Segmentation of cancerous regions in liver using an edge- based and phase congruent region enhancement method.	Edge-based, Region enhancement, thresholding	Active counter, based level set	Quantitative evaluation, Volume overlap error, Average surface distance.	89% of sensitivity & 96% of Accuracy	Campadelli et al., (2009)
Liver segmentation with new supervised method to create initial curve for active contour.	Watershed, thresholding, Gradient vector flow (GVF)	Level Set Methods, Active Contour	Quantitative evaluation, Average contour distance (ACD), Area overlapping error (AOE), Volume overlapping error (VOE), Relative volume difference (RVD).	99.5% of sensitivity& 98% of Accuracy	Saito et al.,(2016)
A new unified level set method for semi-automatic liver tumor segmentation on contrast-enhanced CT images.	Edge based, region-based, Edge enhancement, fuzzy Clustering.	Quasi-Monte Carlo, active appearance model, live wire, bottleneck based Method	Volumetric overlap error (VOE), Relative absolute volume difference, Average symmetric surface distance (ASD), Root-mean-square of symmetric surface distance, Maximum symmetric surface distance.	75% of sensitivity	Li et al.,(2013)
Liver Segmentation Using Location and Intensity Probabilistic Atlases	Thresholding, Region Growing	Probabilistic atlas	Dice and Jaccard volume	58% of Accuracy	Zhou and Bai, (2007)
The study and implementation of liver volume measuring method based on 3-dimensional reconstruction technology.	Thresholding, Region Growing.	Quasi-Monte Carlo, Closed surface mesh, Active Counter.	Standard-volume integral Direct volume measurement.	67% of Sensitivity	Wolz et al., (2013)
Adaptive local window for level set segmentation of CT liver lesions.	Threshold Based, Graph cut, Region	Level set, Adaptive	Maximum symmetric surface distance, average volume difference standard deviation.	94% of sensitivity	Selver (2015)

Figure 11. Block diagram of proposed methodology

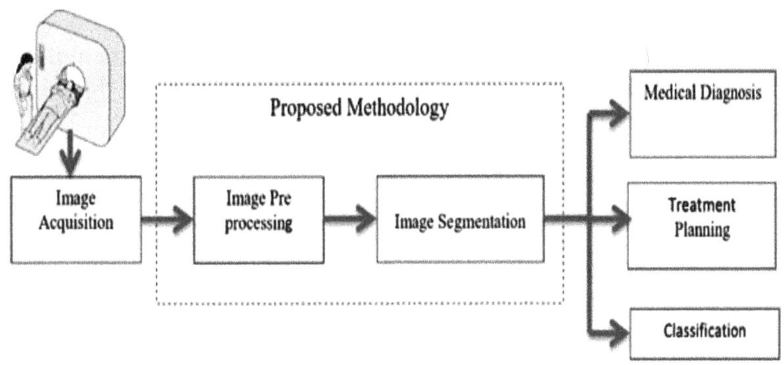

Figure 12. Plan of work

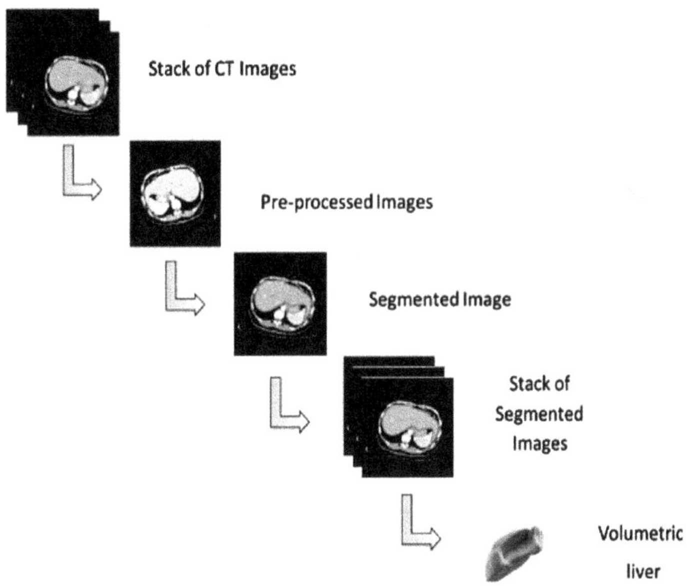

Image Acquisition

We collected CT image data sets from Radiology and Imaging Department, North Eastern Indira Gandhi Regional Institute of Health &Medical Sciences (NEIGRIHMS), Shillong, INDIA. CT data sets are mainly classified into two types, first is non-contrast enhanced and another is contrast enhanced CT data sets. CT images acquired without injecting contrast agent to the subject is known as non-contrast CT imaging data sets and if intravenous contrast agent is injected into the subject before acquiring the CT image data sets it is known as contrast CT data sets. In case of contrast enhanced image data sets, contrast agent administered to the subject after that images acquired with the time interval. Contrast enhanced CT data sets further classified into time dependant categories viz. Arterial Phase, Portal Phase, Venous Phase and sometimes delayed phases.

Image Pre-Processing

The image pre-processing is the primary procedure of medical image segmentation. Image-processing is based on a combination of several techniques such as threshold-based segmentation, morphological operators, border detection, border thinning, border reconstruction, and region filling. Apart from these operations, we should first make the resolution of the image in different directions as the same, or make the image isotropic. To reduce the noise and in homogeneity in the image, we can use the anisotropic diffusion filter. This filter will reduce the noise as well as enhance the edges of the image.

Image Segmentation

Segmentation is one of the most important techniques for image processing. The purpose of segmentation is to partition an image into distinct, semantically meaningful entities by defining boundaries between features and objects in an image based on some constraint, or homogeneity predicate. Segmentation can also be defined as partitioning an image sufficiently into non-overlapping regions.

Image segmentation facilitates higher-level image analysis, description, recognition, quantitative measurement, and visualization of objects of interest. Realizing the importance of image segmentation in image analysis, a great number of breakthroughs have been made in the past several decades. However, image segmentation remains acutely problem-centric. Achieving a generic segmentation method that is universally applicable for a broad range of problem domains is difficult.

Segmentation can be done by two approaches semi-automatic and fully automatic segmentation. Automatic segmentation refers to the process whereby segment boundaries are assigned automatically by an algorithm. Semi-automatic segmentation refers to the process whereby this automatic segmentation is complimented or assisted by manual marking of the segment boundaries. In this research study, we plan to use the deformable model (active contour) based energy minimization techniques for automatic segmentation of abdominal organs.

An active contour is an energy minimizing spline guided by external constrains forces and influence by image forces that pull it toward features such as lines and edges. Active contour models also commonly known as snakes lock onto nearby edges thus, localizing them accurately. Scale space based enhancement techniques can be used to enlarge the capture region surrounding a feature. For this research work, we will combine active contour model with machine intelligence techniques for achieving accurate results.

LIVER SEGMENTATION TECHNIQUES

Adaptive Thresholding

Adaptive thresholding is a technique used when a several threshold is employed in different regions of the image. This are often referred to as local or dynamic thresholding. This technique, usually subdivide original image into small areas and utilize a different threshold to segment each sub images. As the threshold employed for each pixel depends on the precise location of the pixel with regards to the sub images, this type of thresholding is adaptive. An approach to handling situations in which single value thresholding will not work is always to divide a picture into sub images and threshold these individually because the threshold for every pixel is dependent upon its location in an image as this technique is believed to adaptive. The adaptive thresholding can be utilized for segmentation of liver tumour in CT images. The thresholding process convert CT image directly into binary image. The process of adaptive thresholding is the following:

- Adaptive Thresholding divide original CT image into sub images
- Utilize a different threshold to segment each sub images
- Difficulties occur in subdivision and subsequent threshold estimation (Singh, 2015).

Region Growing

Region Growing is an image segmentation method, it can be classified as a pixel-based as it involves the choice of initial seed points. This technique starts with initial "seed points" and then examines neighboring pixels to find out perhaps the pixel neighbors ought to be added with the region. The method is iterated on, in the exact same manner as general data clustering algorithms. The different process used in region growing algorithm can be described as: (i) Select several seed points: These point selection is decided by user like: pixels in a particular gray-level range, pixels evenly spaced on a grid, etc. The first region begins as the complete precise location of the seeds. (ii) Then growing of the regions are from these seed points to adjacent points according to a location membership criterion.

The criterion could be pixel intensity, gray level texture, or colour. Due to the fact the regions are grown on the building blocks of the criterion, the image information itself is important. For instance, if the criterion were pixel intensity, examine the adjacent pixels of seed points. If they've the same intensity value with the seed points, classify them to the seed points. It is surely an iterated process until there's no change in two successive iterative stages. (Rajagopal and Subbaiah, 2015)

Region Splitting and Merging

The split-and-merge algorithm is composed by two steps. In the step one the entire image is subdivides into smaller regions following a dissimilarity criterion. Different strategies can be adopted such as a quad tree partition and a binary space partition (BSP) for divide the image. In step two, the merging is done of the neighbor regions obtained from the splitting step if they verify a similarity criterion.

These matching and mismatching criteria can be based on gradient, intensity range, region statistics, contrast or texture. The merging of splitting and combination steps lead for the segmentation of arbitrary shapes. The subdivide an image initially into a set of arbitrary when region splitting and merging is done, disjoint regions and then merge and/or split the regions in an attempt to satisfy the necessary conditions. (Singh, 2015)

Watershed Segmentation

The main objective of image segmentation is to partition an image into important regions with respect to a particular application. Watershed segmentation produces good results for gray level images with different minima and catchment basins. Here, the gray level of a pixel is interpreted as its altitude in the relief and the length of the gradient is interpreted as elevation information. For binary images, there are only two gray levels 0 and 1 standing for black and white. One minimum and catchment basin are formed in the topographic surface, if two black blobs connected together in a binary image. To segment the connected blobs, distance transforms is used to pre-process the image to make it suitable for watershed segmentation. The Euclidean distance transform is used to take the distance from every pixel of the object component, black pixel to the nearest white pixel. (Sudhamani, M. V. and Raju, G. T.,2014)

K-Means Clustering

K-means is an unsupervised learning algorithms, it is used for classifying the given data set into certain quantity of clusters (assume k clusters) fixed a priori. The main aim is always to define k centroids, one for each single cluster. These centroids must certainly be put right into a cunning way, because different location causes different result. So, the greater choice is to position them as much as possible far from each other. After this each point belonging to a given data set and associate it to the nearest centroid is taken. When no point is pending, the first step is completed and an early on grouping is done. Again re-calculate k new centroids of the clusters (resulting from the final step). After having these k new centroids, a fresh binding needs to be performed between the same data set points and the nearest new centroid. Repeat the strategy until centroids don't move any more. The k centroids change their location feature by feature, in the successive loops. The K-mean algorithm uses the following distance formula to compute the distance of the n data points from their respective jth cluster centre. (Singh, 2015)

Advantages of Liver Segmentation

- Reduce clinician time
- Help in surgery planning. Clinician can plan before making actual incision and cut.

Results won't depends of individual subject or technician, parallax error can be remove Helpful in the measurement of the liver volume, which is an important index in cases of living donor liver transplantation, and the 3D liver volume rendering, which has been shown to be helpful for surgical planning prior to hepatic resection.

Limitation of Liver Segmentation

CT images have low contrast and blurred edges, due to the partial volume effects resulting from spatial averaging, patient movement, beam hardening, and reconstruction artifacts. The gray tones in CT images are related to the tissue density that might be similar in different organs, like: liver, spleen and stomach. Besides, the same organ may exhibit different gray level values both in the same patient, due to the administration of contrast media, and in different ones, for different machine setup conditions. (Shi et al., 2016)

SOLUTIONS AND RECOMMENDATIONS

Computer Assisted Surgery

Computer assisted surgery (CAS) technology guides a surgeon on the patient's anatomy during a procedure. CAS is usually referred to as surgical navigation. The use of this technology is to employs the latest software to aid in intra-operative planning and pre-operative guidance of surgical instrumentation. CAS technology creates a virtual 3D model of the patient's anatomy, generating a digital, interactive map for the surgeon to follow throughout the surgical procedure. In real time, the surgeon is able to track the exact position of instruments and implants in relation to the patient's anatomy, enhancing the overall precision of the procedure.

Computer assisted surgery (CAS) is taking visualization and surgical accuracy to new heights in the operating room. The utmost importance in neurosurgical procedures, CAS technologies are now being utilized in trauma, Neuro, ENT, spine, and orthopedic surgeries. Some advantages of using CAS are ability to plan surgery with a 3D computer model of the patient's anatomy, potentially saving valuable time in the operating room, allows better visualization of anatomy which is particularly important when minimally invasive techniques are used. Provides the surgeon with real-time feedback on the exact location of instruments and implants and offers the ability to correct potential errors during surgery CAS does not replace the surgeon's skills. CAS in the operating room may aid in the surgeon's confidence, especially when operating in and around delicate anatomy.

CAS technology may also offer potential benefits to the patient: Allows for minimally invasive techniques which may lead to smaller incisions, shorter post-operative rehabilitation and less blood loss

A 3D computer model of the patient's anatomy is created, guiding the surgeon to more accurately place implants based on the patient's unique anatomy In procedures where multiple X-rays might be used (such as spine and trauma surgeries), CAS may limit the number of X-rays taken and lessen the amount of radiation exposure Computer assisted surgery is cutting-edge medical technology that offers many benefits to both the surgeon and the patient. (Campadelli et al., 2009)

As shown the Figure 13 represent Computer-assisted surgery (CAS), for surgical planning that uses computer technology, and for performing or guiding surgical interventions. Navigation in surgery relates to stereotactic principles, based on ability to locate a given point using geometric references (Adams et al., 1990. Development of an accurate model of the patient is the most important component for CAS. This can be conducted through a number of medical imaging technologies including CT, MRI, x-rays, ultrasound plus many more. Region to be operated has to be scanned and uploaded into the computer system for the generation of CAS model. 3D models of liver segmented images can be uploaded which resembles the exact geometrical situation of the normal and pathological tissues and structures of that region.

Graphical User Interface

A graphical user interface (GUI) is an interface through which a user interacts with electronic devices such as computers, hand-held devices and other appliances. This interface uses icons, menus and other visual indicator (graphics) representations to display information and related user controls, unlike text-based interfaces, where data and commands are in text. GUI representations are manipulated by a pointing device such as a mouse, trackball, stylus, or a finger on a touch screen.

The need for GUI became apparent because the first human/computer text interface was through keyboard text creation by what is called a prompt (or DOS prompt). Commands were typed on a keyboard at the DOS prompt to initiate responses from a computer. The use of these commands and the need for exact spelling created a cumbersome and inefficient interface.

In this GUI we have used three buttons for loading of image, liver segmentation and exit. In Figure 15 if we press the load image button the original image will be displayed.

Figure 13. Computer assisted surgery (2017)
Retrieved 2017 from https://media.defense.gov/2017/Feb/07/2001695993/-1/-1/0/170131-F-JC454-105.JPG

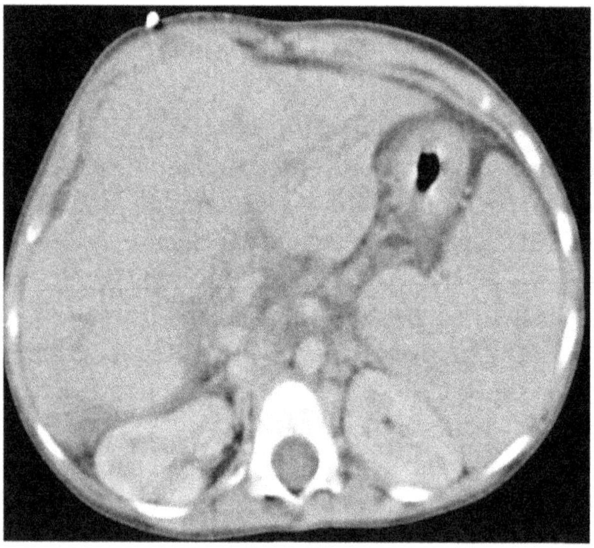

Figure 14. Loading of original image

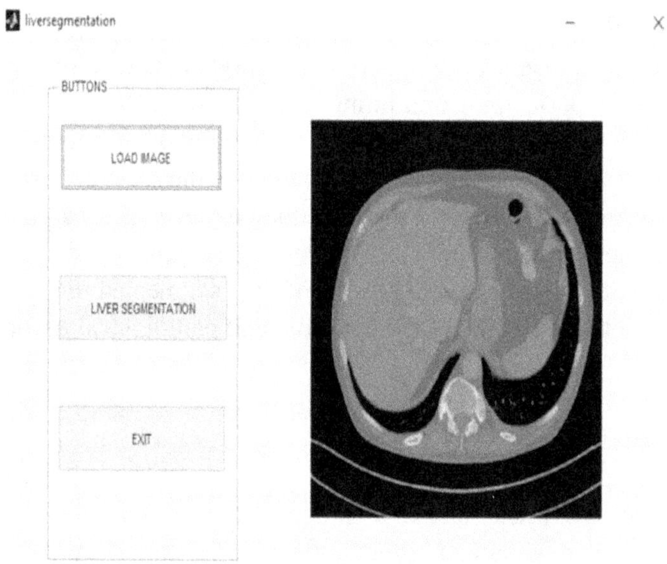

RESULTS AND DISCUSSION

Evaluation Measurements

The evaluation of liver segmentation methods is done by comparing the liver segmentation method results to ground truth data sets created by radiologists and similar other segmentation technique. Following common measures can be used for the validation of segmentation algorithms:

Figure 15. Liver segmented image

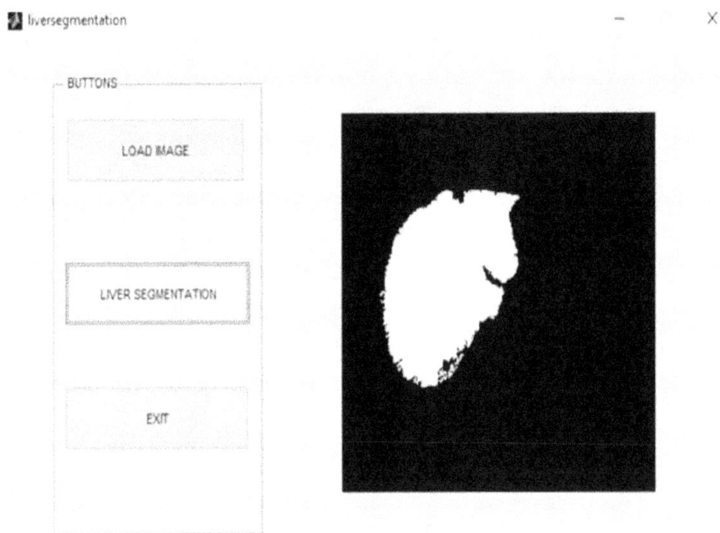

- Jaccard Similarity Coefficient (Casciaro et al., 2012)
- Dice similarity coefficient (Shimizu et al., 2010)
- Mean Squared Error(Chai1 and Draxler, 2014)

Jaccard Similarity Coefficient

The Jaccard Similarity Coefficient Also known as the Jaccard index, the Jaccard similarity coefficient is a statistical measure of similarity between sample sets of image. For two sets of image, it is defined as the cardinality of their intersection divided by the cardinality of their union. Mathematically,

$$J(X,Y) = \frac{|X \cap Y|}{|X \cup Y|} = \frac{|X \cap Y|}{|X| + |Y| - |X \cap Y|} \tag{1}$$

(For 1 perfect segmentation and 0 for a completely failed one.)

$0 \leq J(X,Y) \leq 1$

Dice Similarity Coefficient

The Dice similarity coefficient (DSC) is a statistical validation metric to access the performance of the reproducibility of manual segmentations and the spatial overlap precision of automated probabilistic fractional segmentation of CT images. One assigns to a perfect segmentation and 0 to a completely failed one. Mathematically,

$$DSC = \frac{2\left|X \cap Y\right|}{\left|X\right| + \left|Y\right|} \tag{2}$$

Mean Squared Error

The mean squared error tells how close a regression line is to a set of points. This is done by taking the distances between the points and the regression line (these distances are the "errors") and squaring them. The squaring is necessary to remove any negative signs. It also gives more weight to larger differences. It's called the mean squared error as finding the average of a set of errors. If X is a vector of n predictions, and Y is the vector of observed values correlating with the inputs to the function which generated the predictions, then the MSE of the predictor can be calculated as shown below.

$$MSE = \frac{1}{n}\sum_{i=1}^{n}\left(X - Y\right)^2 \tag{3}$$

Experimental Results

The abdominal CT data used in this study was acquired from one CT scanner and abdominal contrast and non-contrast images were acquired from 20 patients. Table one is showing result for the various evaluation measures.

For better results, values of DSC and JI should be close to 1 and for MSE, the value should be close to 0.

In the Table 2, we can see the evaluation and Mean$\pm$ Standard Deviation results of six patients. It can be seen that in all the cases Dice Similarity Coefficient (DSC) results are giving more accurate results as compared to Mean Square Error (MSE) and Jaccard Index (JI) validation techniques. However, it can be inferred from the following table that overall output of our segmentation technique gives near accurate results in all the cases. However, it can be inferred from the Table 2 that overall output of our segmentation technique gives near accurate results in all the cases.

There are many approaches which are used for segmentation where we found that graph cut can also prove to be good in the segmentation of the images. In future, we would like to use the multiple atlas based technique as a hierarchical model and evaluate graph cut as it can show more accurate results in abdominal organ segmentation. The use of other techniques such as Random Forest and Fuzzy Clustering based technique will be incorporated.

Future work will be to focus on a more accurate validation of the segmented liver dataset. To incorporate other techniques to segment the liver from CT images in 2D and 3D with an aim to compare the results with other existing techniques.

CONCLUSION

In this chapter, we presented the automatic segmentation of liver. After thorough reviewing the research done earlier, our first focus of segmentation is on the liver organ due to its important functionality, large

Table 2. Validation results

Patient ID	Evaluation	Mean ± Standard Deviation
Subject 1	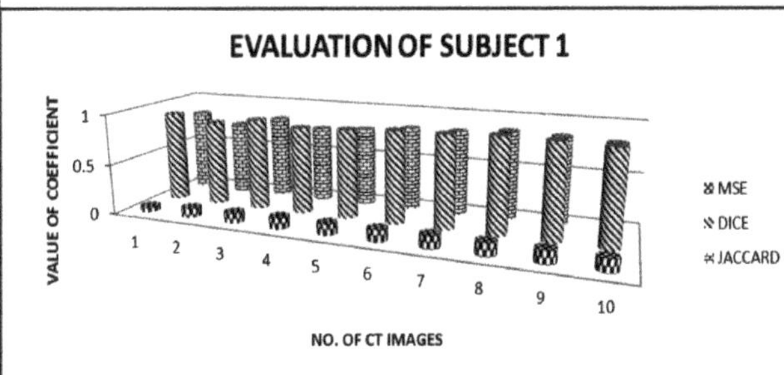	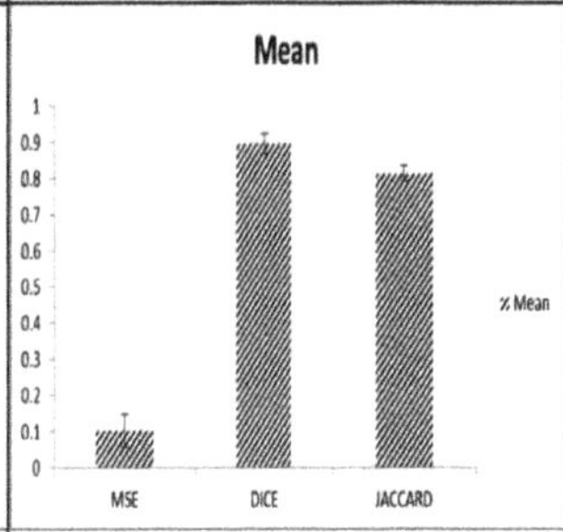
Subject 2	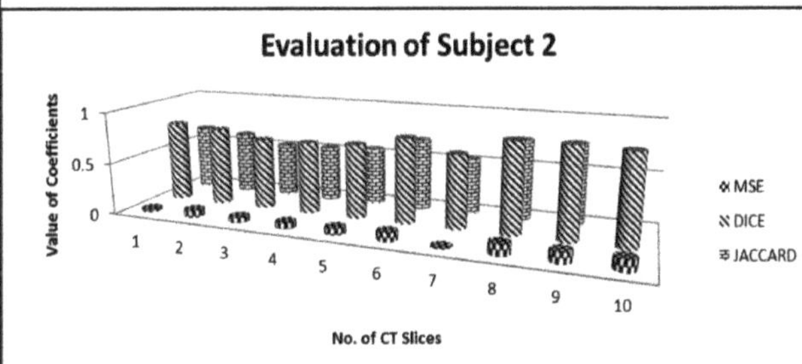	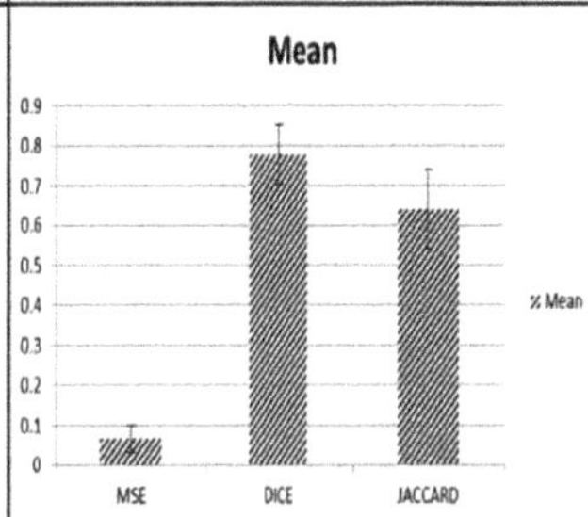
Subject 3	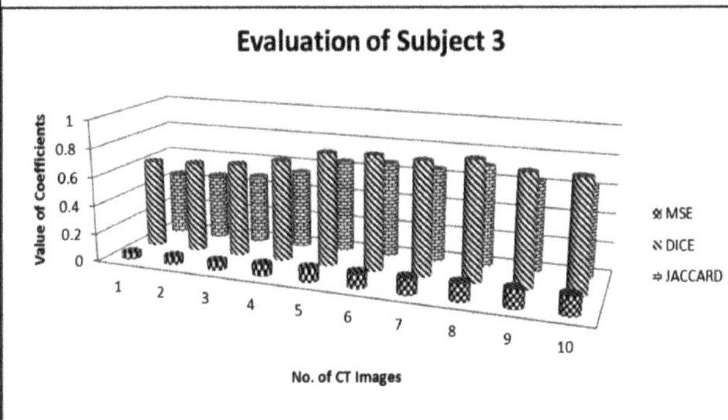	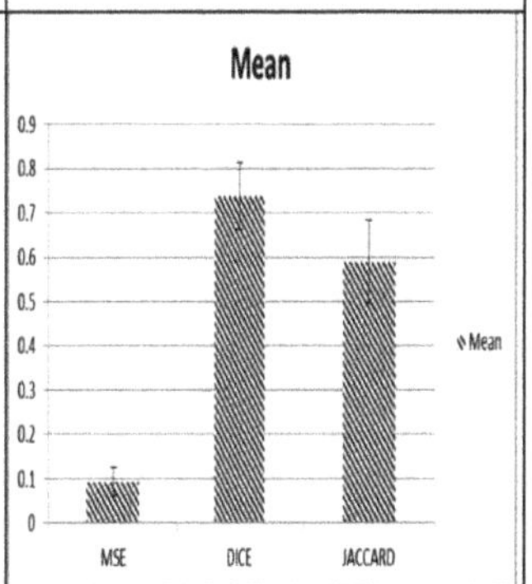
Subject 4	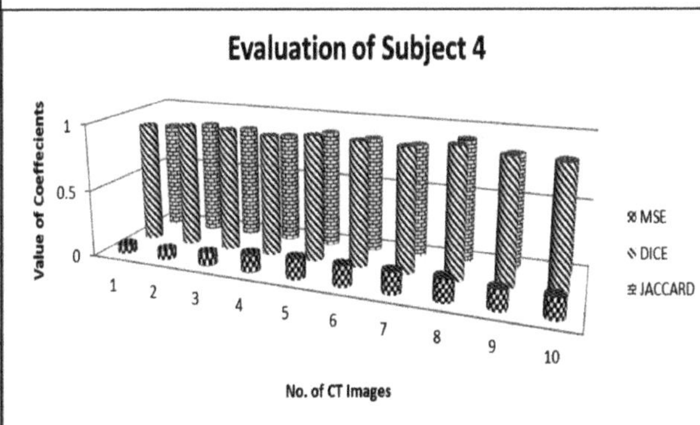	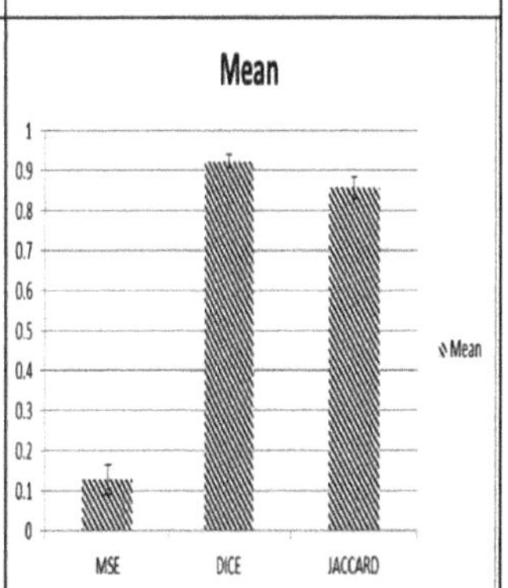

continued on following page

Table 2. Continued

Subject 5	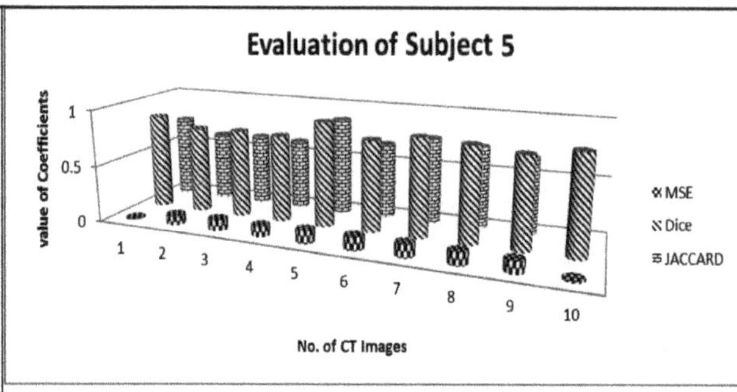	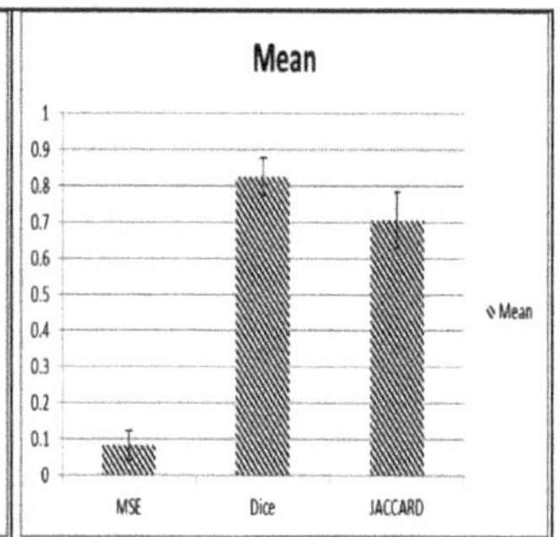
Subject 6	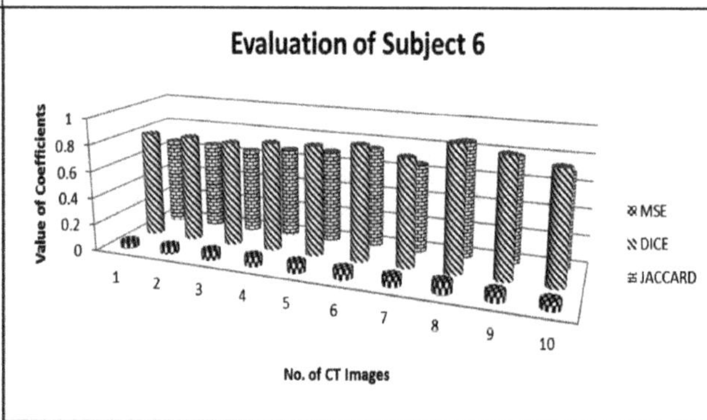	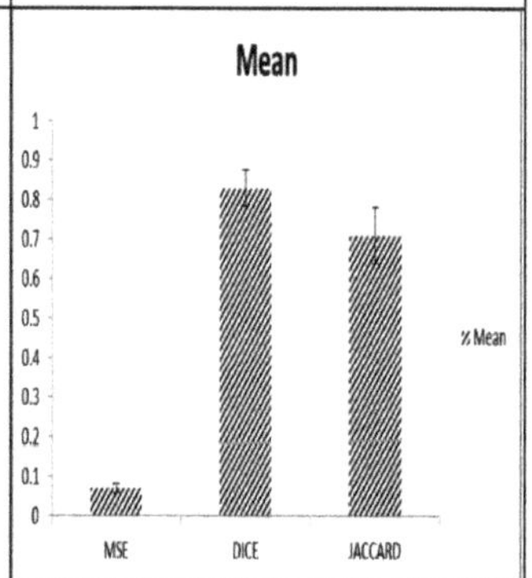

structure, and sharp edges. We have used the active contour segmentation technique for segmentation of liver from CT images which can prove to be useful for radiologist for further diagnosis and treatment planning.

ACKNOWLEDGMENT

Authors are thankful to Department of Radiology, North Eastern Indira Gandhi Regional Institute of Health and Medical Sciences (NEIGRIHMS), Shillong for providing 3D medical data sets and also for helping in validation of the output CT images for this study. Also, we are thankful to the SERB, Department of Science and Technology (DST), Government of India, New Delhi for financial assistance (Grant: SERB/EMEQ-433/2014).

REFERENCES

Adams, L., Krybus, W., Ebrecht, D. M., & Rueger, R. (1990). Computer-assisted surgery. *IEEE Computer Graphics and Applications*, *10*(3), 43–52. doi:10.1109/38.55152

Anatomy and Function of the Liver. (n.d.). Retrieved 2017 from http://www.stanfordchildrens.org/en/topic/default?id=anatomy-and-function-of-the-liver-90-P03069.(2017).

Ballard, F. J., & Oliver, I. T. (1965). Carbohydrate metabolism in liver from foetal and neonatal sheep. *The Biochemical Journal*, *95*(1), 191–200. doi:10.1042/bj0950191 PMID:14333556

Bojwani, D. (2017). *Cervical Di 3 level cer* [Online image]. Retrieved 2017 from. http://www.dheerajbojwani.com/computer-assisted-surgery-India-low-cost-benefits.html

Campadelli, P., Casiraghi, E., Campadelli, P., & Casiraghi, E. (2009). Liver Segmentation from CT Scans : A Survey Liver Segmentation from CT Scans : A Survey. *Artificial Intelligence in Medicine*, *45*, 185–196. doi:10.1016/j.artmed.2008.07.020 PMID:19059767

Casciaro, S. (2012). Fully Automatic Segmentations of Liver and Hepatic Tumors From 3-DComputed Tomography Abdominal Images. *Comparative Evaluation of Two Automatic Methods.*, *12*, 464–473.

Chai, T., & Draxler, R. R. (2014). *Root mean square error (RMSE) or mean absolute error (MAE)? –Arguments against avoiding RMSE in the literature*. Copernicus Publications.

Cirrhosis (Liver). (n.d.). Retrieved 2017 from http://www.medicinenet.com/cirrhosis/article.htm

CT Scan or CAT Scan: How Does It Work? What is a CT scan? When is a CT scan used? (2017). [Online image]. Retrieved 2017 from http://www.lumen.luc.edu/lumen/MedEd/Radio/curriculum/Surgery/Hepatic_mass.htm

Foregut, D. (2017). *For other uses, see Liver (disambiguation)* [Online image]. Retrieved 2017 from https://wiki2.org/en/Liver

Freudenrich, C. C. (n.d.). *How Ultrasound Works*. Retrieved 2017 from https://www.physics.utoronto.ca/~jharlow/teaching /phy138_0708/lec04/ultrasoundx.htm

Göran, B. M. D. (1981). Natural history of patients with untreated liver metastases from colorectal cancer. *American Journal of Surgery*, *141*(5), 586–589. doi:10.1016/0002-9610(81)90057-X PMID:7223955

Hall, G. F. (2007). Hepatitis A, B, C, D, E, G: an update. *Ethn Dis. Spring, 17*(2 Suppl 2), S2-40-5. Retrieved 2017 from http://www.hopkinsmedicine.org/healthlibrary/conditions/liver_biliary_and_pancreatic_disorders/liver_anatomy_and_functions_85,P00676/

InnerBody- Liver Anatomy Explorer. (n.d.). Retrieved 2017 from http://www.innerbody.com/image_digeov/card10-new2.html

Li, C., Wang, X., Li, J., Eberl, S., Fulham, M., Yin, Y., & Feng, D. D. (2013). Joint probabilistic model of shape and intensity for multiple abdominal organ segmentation from volumetric CT images. *IEEE Journal of Biomedical and Health Informatics*, *17*(1), 92–102. doi:10.1109/TITB.2012.2227273 PMID:23193317

Liver Anatomy and Functions Anatomy of the liver. (2017). [Online image]. Retrieved 2017 from http://www.hopkinsmedicine.org/healthlibrary/conditions/liver_biliary_and_pancreatic_disorders/liver_anatomy_and_functions_85,P00676/

Liver Cancer (Hepatocellular Carcinoma). (n.d.). Retrieved 2017 from http://www.medicinenet.com/liver_cancer_hepatocellular_carcinoma/article.htm

Liver fibrosis. (n.d.). [Online image]. Retrieved 2017 from http://www.meddean.luc.edu/lumen/meded/orfpath/fibrosis.htm

MRI. A Guided Tour. (2003). [Online image]. Retrieved 2017 from http://www.medscape.org/viewarticle/488088

Untitled. (n.d.). [Online image]. Retrieved 2017 from https://en.wikipedia.org/ wiki/Liver#/media/File:Liver_04_Couinaud_classification.svg.

Rajagopal, R., & Subbaiah, P. (2015). a Survey on Liver Tumor Detection and Segmentation. *Journal of Engineering and Applied Sciences (Asian Research Publishing Network)*, *10*(6), 2681–2685.

Saito, A., Nawano, S., & Shimizu, A. (2016). Joint optimization of segmentation and shape prior from level-set-based statistical shape model, and its application to the automated segmentation of abdominal organs. *Medical Image Analysis*, *28*, 46–65. doi:10.1016/j.media.2015.11.003 PMID:26716720

Science Education Computed Tomography (CT). (n.d.). Retrieved 2017 from https://www.nibib.nih.gov/science-education/science-topics/computed-tomography-ct

Selver, M. A. (2015). Exploring brushlet based 3d textures in transfer function specification for direct volume rendering of abdominal organs. *IEEE Transactions on Visualization and Computer Graphics*, *21*(2), 174–187. doi:10.1109/TVCG.2014.2359462 PMID:26357028

Sentul Medical Centre Kuala Lumpur. (2017). [Online image]. Retrieved 2017 from https://www.absolutemed.com/ultrasound-machines/

Shi, C., Cheng, Y., Liu, F., Wang, Y., Bai, J., & Tamura, S. (2016). A hierarchical local region-based sparse shape composition for liver segmentation in CT scans. *Pattern Recognition*, *50*, 88–106. doi:10.1016/j.patcog.2015.09.001

Shimizu, A., Nakagomi, K., Narihira, T., & Kobatake, H. (2010). Automated Segmentation of 3D CT Images Based on Statistical Atlas and Graph Cuts. In *International MICCAI Workshop on Medical Computer Vision*. Springer Berlin Heidelberg.

Singh, I. (2015). A Study of Effective Segmentation Techniques for Liver Segmentation. *International Journal of Advanced Research in Computer Engineering & Technology*, *4*(4), 1661–1666.

Smithuis, R., & Lange, E. E. (2015). *Anatomy of the Liver*. Retrieved 2017 from http://www.radiologyassistant.nl/en/p4375bb8dc241d/anatomy-of-the-liver-segments.html

Sudhamani, M. V., & Raju, G. T. (2014). Segmentation and Classification of Tumour in Computed Tomography Liver Images for Detection, Analysis and Preoperative Planning. *International Journal of Advanced Computer Research*, *4*(1), 166–171.

Ultrasound Machines. (2017). [Online image]. Retrieved 2017 from http://site.sentulmedical.com.my/main/3138/index.asp?pageid=138470&t=ultrasound

Web, M. D. (n.d.). *Picture of the Liver*. Retrieved 2017 from http://www.webmd.com/digestive-disorders/picture-of-the-liver#2.(2005-2017)

Wolz, R., Chu, C., Misawa, K., Fujiwara, M., Mori, K., & Rueckert, D. (2013). Automated abdominal multi-organ segmentation with subject-specific atlas generation. *IEEE Transactions on Medical Imaging*, *32*(9), 1723–1730. doi:10.1109/TMI.2013.2265805 PMID:23744670

Zhou, Y., & Bai, J. (2007). Multiple abdominal organ segmentation: An atlas-based fuzzy connectedness approach. *IEEE Transactions on Information Technology in Biomedicine*, *11*(3), 348–352. doi:10.1109/TITB.2007.892695 PMID:17521085

Chapter 10
Development of a Text-to-Speech Scanner for Visually Impaired People

Minerva Sarma
A. D. Y. Patil University, India

Anuskha Kumar
A. D. Y. Patil University, India

Aditi Joshi
A. D. Y. Patil University, India

Suraj Kumar Nayak
National Institute of Technology Rourkela, India

Biswajeet Champaty
A. D. Y. Patil University, India

ABSTRACT

In this chapter, a low-cost, efficient, and real-time wearable text-to-speech scanner has been proposed that can enable blind persons to hear the contents of a text material. The device captures the images of the text and converts them to speech. The hardware of the device has been realized using Raspberry Pi 3, Pi camera, and an earphone. Optical character recognition (OCR) and text-to-speech synthesis (TTS) have been implemented using Raspberry Pi 3 to accomplish the working of the device. OCR technology converted the captured text images to editable text, whereas the TTS technology scanned the alphanumeric characters in the processed image and converted them to speech. The proposed technology imitates the ability of the human sensory organs and the nervous system, where the camera mimics human eye and the image processing in Raspberry Pi 3 substitutes the human brain. This proposed device can also help people suffering from diseases like dyslexia and nyctalopia, and inability to see in dim light or at night.

DOI: 10.4018/978-1-5225-4969-7.ch010

INTRODUCTION

As per the survey report published by Pascolini *et al.* (2011), the total number of visually-impaired individuals across the globe in the year 2010 is nearly 285 million (Pascolini & Mariotti, 2011). Cataract, glaucoma, corneal scarring from various causes, diabetic retinopathy, macular degradation due to age, birth defects and uncorrected refractive have been reported to be the main reasons of blindness (Foster & Resnikoff, 2005). It is a common belief that the blind persons can partially indemnify the loss of vision through the development of augmented capability with the residual senses (Stronks, Nau, Ibbotson, & Barnes, 2015). In comparison to auditory perception and touch, vision divulges better spatial information regarding the distant environment (Capodanno et al., 2015). A study done with blind persons reveals that numerous difficulties are faced by them like alignment, focus, accuracy, mobility, and efficiency while reading using braille. Nearly 74% of the blind and 72% of the partially sighted people cannot read the normal information provided by their care givers or physicians (Lightstone, 2007). And, more than half (52%) of them would feel awkward to make someone else reading out the results of their medical test. However, numerous recent studies have proposed that the use of contemporaneous speech can be a valid alternative while scanning for the required material (Guerreiro & Gonçalves, 2015). Speech technologies are currently considered to be the most crucial for providing accessibility to the visually-impaired people (Massof, 2003). Most auditory assistive devices for the blind persons employ synthetic speech. These include talking devices, human-computer interfaces, reading-machines, and a wide range of talking appliances (Massof, 2003). Current technologies allow softwares to be effectively dispersed and realized on hand-held devices, even when using of computers are important. Therefore, electronic travel aids, navigational assistance equipments, text-to-speech mobile applications as well as virtual audio displays, which combine audio with haptic channels, are being integrated to make ideal portable devices (Csapó, Wersényi, Nagy, & Stockman, 2015). Text to speech scanner is such a device that can be easier for the visually impaired people to use. This device may not only help the blind people but also the people with low vision to recognise letters and numbers without having to struggle or strain their remaining vision. These advancements will allow the people with visual impairments to compete successfully with sighted people and to have equal access to printed information (Russotti, Shaw, & Spungin, 2004). Therefore, the current study discusses the development of an inexpensive and portable text to speech scanner device to assist the visually impaired persons to read the required text material.

BACKGROUND

The work done by Akhlagi *et al.* (2003) on reader pen scanner is a major technological advancement for learning alphabets and is highly useful for people suffering from hindrance in reading such as dyslexia patients. The device is portable and pocket sized. It has an in-built dictionary and converts the text from Spanish to English and vice-versa. The user needs to pass the nib across a line and the pen will read the words aloud. The main drawback of this device is that it is not suitable for a visually impaired person (Akhlagi, Lonn, & Wittrup, 2003). Sung Wook Park (2008) developed the Voice Stick, which is a text scanning device and converts text to voice. The voice stick is shaped like a wand, which when filtered in the printed text material, the OCR perceives the content and changes the data into voice. The limitation of the device is that it is not user-friendly, especially for blind people. This may be attributed to the fact that the device has to be in contact with the text material and placing the device horizontally on every line properly is not an easy task (Park, 2008).

Shilkrot *et al.* (2014) proposed a Finger Reader that assists the visually-challenged people in reading text materials. It is basically a finger ring with an attached tiny camera that the user wears on the index finger. When the user wants to read some text, he/she has to point the index finger at the surface of the text material and the gadget reads the text loudly. The device has an installed feedback mechanism which gives feedback on the progression of the scan. The feedback mechanism also helps in placement of the device with proper angle and keeping it in line with the text. The finger-wearable assistive device is useful not only for the blind but also for the children and others. The only frailty is that though the device has a real-time feedback for the proper alignment, the blind user will find it difficult to place his/her finger on the correct line for the device to scan the text (Shilkrot, Huber, Liu, Maes, & Nanayakkara, 2014).

Siqueira *et al.*(2016) proposed the need of Braille symbols on mobile screens, as the use of smart phones are increasing day by day. However, those devices are difficult to be accessed by the blind people as they cannot feel the letters on the normal mobile screen (Siqueira et al., 2016). Taking a note of the above-mentioned facts, we have proposed the development of a text to speech scanner device that can overcome the limitations of the previously invented devices. Our device need not be in contact with the text material. It can scan the text material placed in front of the user from a distance (about 40-50 cm). Hence, it will be more user-friendly.

MAIN FOCUS OF THE CHAPTER

It is difficult for visually-challenged people to access text documents in various situations (e.g. low lighting, different layout, non-perpendicular page orientations). The inability to access the day-to-day text materials greatly hampers the freedom and the mobility of visually challenged people outside their home.

Nowadays many devices and softwares are available for conversion from text to speech (TTS). But most of the softwares require a computer and sometimes even a scanner to read text aloud. But it's not possible to carry such a giant set up everywhere. Also, conversion from text to an image requires a lot of steps. It requires lots of buttons to be pressed to complete the whole conversion from text to speech, which is not possible for a visually impaired person. So, most of the devices wouldn't be practical for blind people or people with low vision. There are also many TTS mobile applications that come for free on Google play store. But, the blind people cannot use them because it will require them to operate the application and focus on the textual material, which they wish to read. Hence, though these applications are for free of cost, it is not useful for them.

This paper introduces a TTS scanner device, which converts the contents of a text image into voice. This allows people to hear the textual material instead of reading through it. The system is based on Raspberry Pi 3 (model B), which is a small sized, affordable computer. The proposed system mainly requires two softwares, namely, Tesseract OCR software and Espeak-TTS software, which are installed in Raspberry Pi 3. This device basically captures the image of the textual material, converts it into text format, which is done by using Tesseract OCR software. This text is then sent to the TTS software, which converts this text to voice. The proposed device consists mainly of two modules, namely, image processing module and voice processing module. It provides an innovative and inexpensive method to convert the contents of the textual material into voice. Individuals who have vision disabilities will be benefited from the proposed device. This can help them in reading books, legal contracts, cheques, newspapers, etc. The proposed device may further help the visually-impaired people to interact with computers effectively through voice interface.

This device is not only helpful for the people visual impairment, but also for the normal people. This device gives the proper pronunciation for each word, and hence can help people to learn proper pronunciation for different words. Also, the device will help in reducing the strain on the eyes as the user does not need to keep the eyes open and concentrate on the text. The text material just needs to be in the proper range of the device so that it can be converted into voice and the user will comfortably hear the speech of the text without stressing the eyes. Apart from protecting the eyes, it allows people to sit back and read text materials without straining their body. This device will also make the editing of documents easy.

A few devices have been proposed to facilitate the visually challenged users to read printed text as discussed in the background section. However, most of the devices require the person to focus on the printed material properly. It is difficult for the blind person to exactly point at the appropriate place to read the textual material. This device can overcome this limitation as it does not require focusing on an exact position to read the text and reads text over a range of area. Exhaustive training is not required to operate this device.

REQUIREMENTS

Hardware

Raspberry Pi 3.0 (Model B, Raspberry Pi Foundation, United Kingdom), SD card (SanDisk, US), Ethernet cable (Quantum), HDMI cable (BlueRigger, India), battery (9.0 V-2.0 A) or a DC power adapter (9V, 2Amp), Pi camera (Raspberry Pi Foundation, UK), earpiece/speakers, push-button switch, laptop (DELL, India), and jumper wires. The authors have mentioned the make and model of these hardware components which were used in this study. This is not necessarily meant that only these products were required to develop this product.

Software

Raspbian operating system (OS), Tesseract OCR, Espeak-Text to Speech synthesizer, PuTTY, Win32 Disk Imager, Advanced IP Scanner, Xming X server, OpenCV were used

METHODOLOGY

Configuration of Raspbian OS

To connect the Raspberry Pi 3 to a laptop display, an Ethernet cable was used. This was done because the Raspberry Pi's desktop GUI (Graphical User Interface) can be viewed through the laptop display using an Ethernet connection between the two (Figure 1). Also, the internet was shared from the laptop

Figure 1. Laptop connected to Raspberry Pi 3 with Ethernet cable and HDMI cable

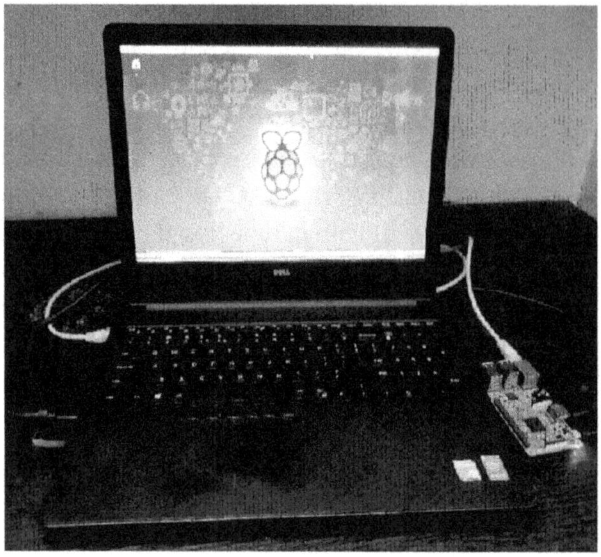

through the Ethernet cable to install some of the libraries and softwares. This also allowed to access internet on the Raspberry Pi apart from connecting it to the laptop display. In the "network and sharing centre", IP address 192.168.137.1 and the subnet mask 255.255.255.0 of the Ethernet cable were allotted. The HDMI port is required to run the Raspberry Pi for the first time when using a monitor.

Raspbian is the Foundation's official supported operating system, which has thousands of pre-built libraries to perform various tasks and optimize the OS. Before connecting Raspberry Pi to laptop display, initially, Raspbian Jessie was downloaded from the official Raspberry Pi website then the Raspbian Jessie was extracted directly to the formatted Micro SD card with the win32 Disk Imager (Figure 2).

Figure 2. Extracted file with win32Disk Imager

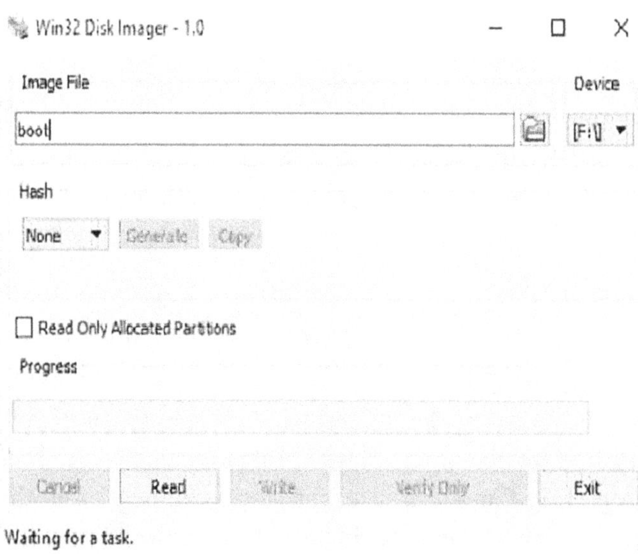

The IP address of the Raspberry Pi 3 was found with the help of the “Advanced IP Scanner” by setting the range to 192.168.137.1-192.168.137.255 (Figure 3). Since, Raspberry Pi 3 does not have a static IP address the IP address keeps changing after a certain interval of time.

The PuTTY software was downloaded from GitHub. *via* Secure Shell (SSH), which is a secure network protocol for data communication.. It can quickly copy text or files across the Raspberry Pi’s command line instead of typing it *via* SSH. The laptop acts as the server and the Raspberry Pi 3 serves as the client.

With the help of the LX Terminal, Raspbian OS was opened in the laptop. As, Raspberry Pi 3 has its own Operating System (Raspbian OS), a different server was to be opened if laptop has been used. However, it was not required if a monitor was used without any other OS already running. In this study, “Xming X” server was used to open Raspbian OS. Since, we have connected from a windows machine, X11 forwarding was enabled by navigating the configuration tree through “Connection/SSH/X11”. The LX Terminal window was opened to get logged in as a ‘pi’ (which is the default user name through the software) into the Raspberry Pi’s IP Address (Figure 4). Then, the command “sudo raspi-config” was given in the LX Terminal to open “Software configuration tool” (Figure 5(a)). The command aims

Figure 3. Found IP address of Raspberry Pi

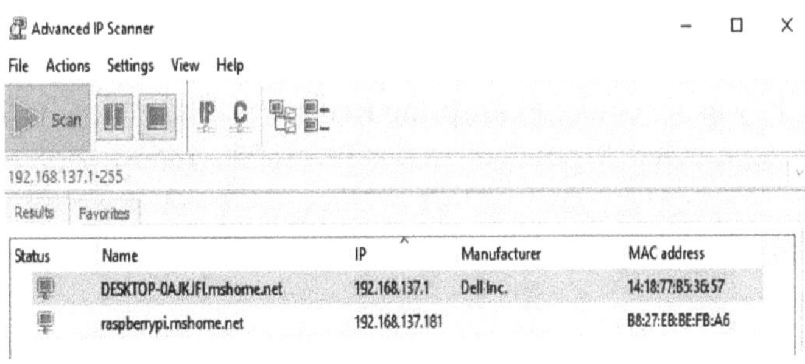

Figure 4. (a) PuTTY software; (b) LX Terminal opened

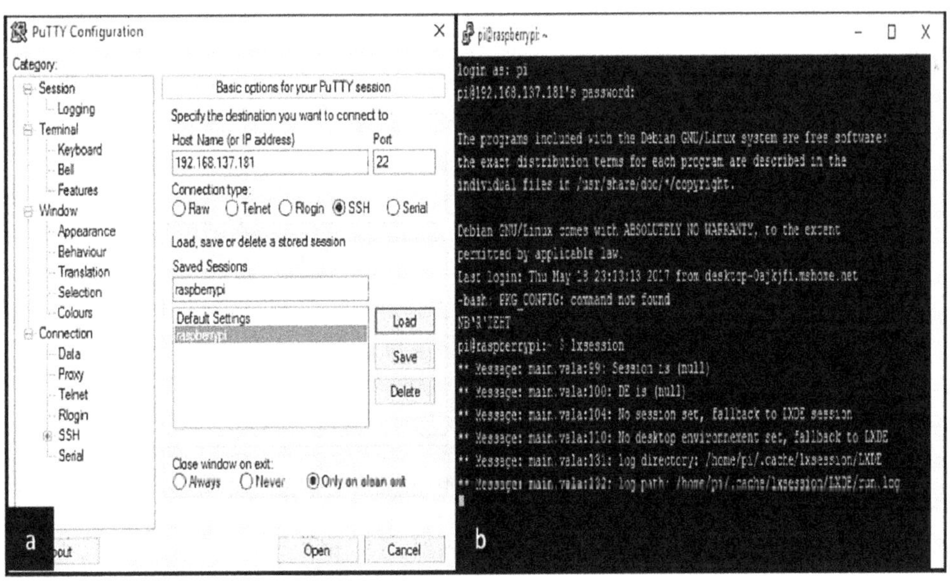

Figure 5. (a) Configuration tool box; (b) Raspbian OS opened

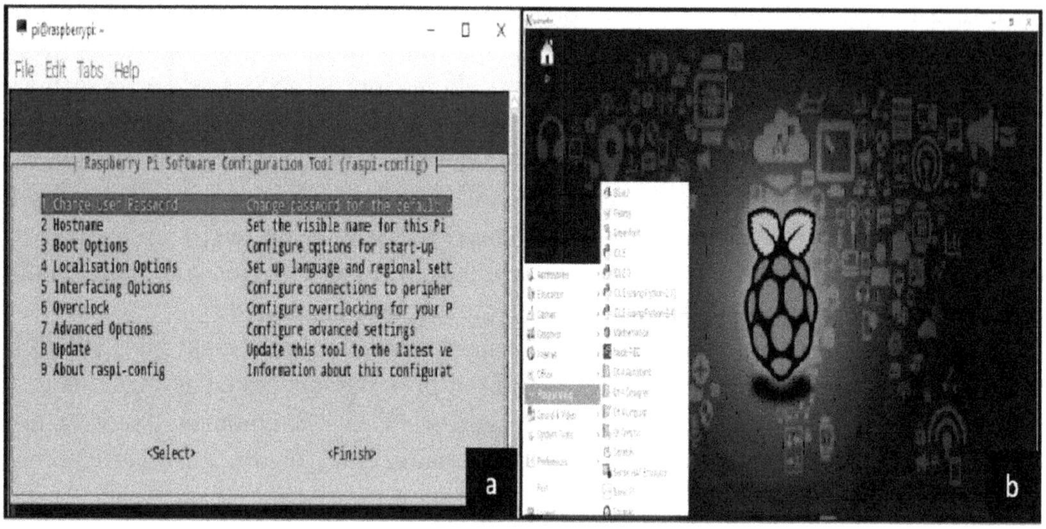

to provide the functionality to make the common changes as a Raspberry Pi user. This resulted in the automated edits to '/boot/config.txt' and various standard Linux configuration files. After making the changes, the Raspberry Pi was rebooted. Finally, the Raspberry Pi desktop itself appears as an Xming X Server after giving the command "lxsession" in the Terminal window (Figure 5(b)).

Configuration of the Pi Camera

Pi camera was attached to the Raspberry Pi via a flat cable. The cable was slotted into the connector situated between the Ethernet and HDMI ports of the Raspberry Pi, with the silver connectors facing towards the HDMI port. After booting the Raspberry Pi 3, "sudo raspi-config" command was given through LX Terminal. Navigating to the "Camera" option and enabling it, the camera was activated successfully (Figure 6). The Raspberry Pi 3 was then rebooted.

Figure 6. Enabled camera through configuration tool box

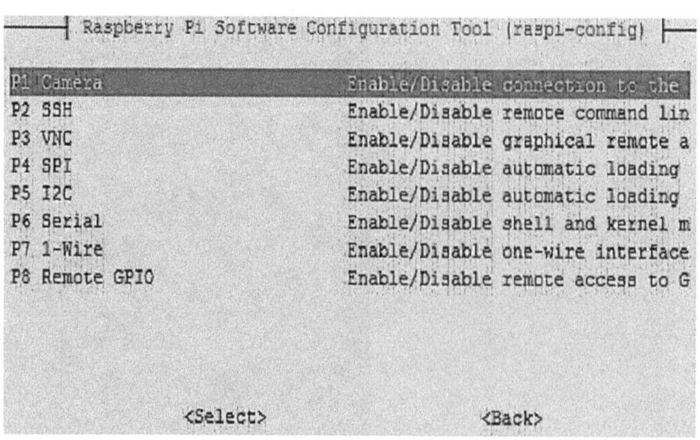

After the rebooting of the Raspberry Pi, the Raspbian OS was reopened in Xming X server. The proper capturing of an image was tested by giving the commands in the LX Terminal and the Python shell.

Designing of the Image Processing Module

An image processing module was designed to convert the required image into text format. Initially, it captured the image of the text material placed in front of the user using a Pi camera (5 megapixels). The Pi camera was kept at a certain predefined distance to capture the image properly. The text material can be any printed documents such as books, legal contracts, cheques and newspaper. After the image was taken in the .jpg/.png file format, it was converted into .txt file format using OCR technology. The OCR was an important element in this module. The OCR technology recognises the character automatically through the optical mechanism. Pytesseract-OCR engine was used in this study. The selection of Pytesseract OCR was done because of its flexibility and extensibility (Lakshmi & Rao, 2016). It is quite simple and easy to use and can detect most languages with 97.8% accuracy. Pytesseract OCR takes less time for character recognition from any image as compared to other OCR engines (Patel, Patel, & Patel, 2012). Pytesseract OCR can support over 248 different languages. In this study, the software was used to identify English alphanumeric characters. Before sending the image to the OCR, the image was converted to grey scale image. The grey scale image was then converted into binary form to increase the recognition accuracy. This process was regarded as digitalization of the image (binarization) (Figure 7). Practically, any captured or scanned image may not be perfect. It may have some noise or blur. By applying suitable techniques and designing algorithms, the noise or the blurring present in the image were removed and a denoised image was produced. The denoised image, thus obtained, was saved as a .txt file in the memory card of the Raspberry Pi 3 for further processing.

The OpenCV software, which is designed to solve computer vision problem by converting the image into text format, has the ability to recognise text as well as face and different symbols. It lets the Pytesseract software to recognize the text from any captured image. In this study, a line finding algorithm was prepared for this purpose. The line recognising algorithm was designed in such a way that a skewed page can be recognised without the need to de-skew, therefore, avoiding the loss of image quality. After detecting the lines, each single character in the image was recognised by the software. After all the characters were recognised, the text was stored as a .txt file (Smith, 2007).

Designing the Voice Processing Module

A voice processing module was designed to convert the text into voice using TTS technique. TTS (Text-to-Speech) is a form of speech synthesis that converts text into a voice output. For this purpose, Espeak TTS software was used. This software was chosen because it allows the user to be more flexible during its usage. Espeak uses a "Format synthesis" method. This type of synthesizers synthesises the artificial voice by using a specific acoustic model for speech generation (Hamiti & Kastrati, 2014).

After converting the image from .jpg/.png format to .txt format, it was sent to the voice processing module, which then created a spoken sound version of the text and saved it as an audio file (.mp3). For doing so the software will first access the text file passed to it. And then convert this text to voice.

The TTS software contains recordings of many types of speech units like political news, poetry sports etc. in an acoustic database, which comprise of almost every possible form of diaphones, morphemes, syllables, phrases, words, and sentences in a particular language (Swetha & Anuradha). When the text

Figure 7. Programme designed for removing noise and thresholding the image

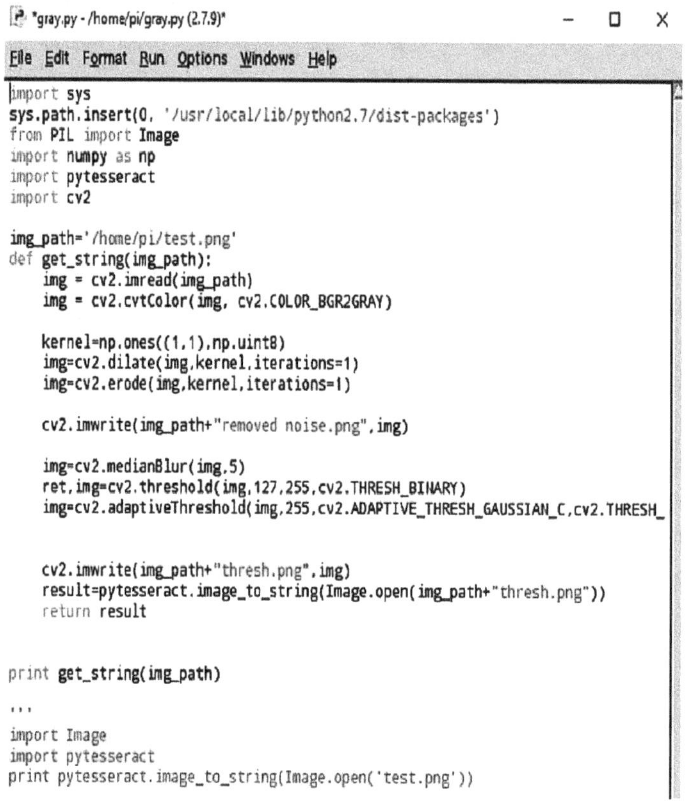

```
*gray.py - /home/pi/gray.py (2.7.9)*
File Edit Format Run Options Windows Help
import sys
sys.path.insert(0, '/usr/local/lib/python2.7/dist-packages')
from PIL import Image
import numpy as np
import pytesseract
import cv2

img_path='/home/pi/test.png'
def get_string(img_path):
    img = cv2.imread(img_path)
    img = cv2.cvtColor(img, cv2.COLOR_BGR2GRAY)

    kernel=np.ones((1,1),np.uint8)
    img=cv2.dilate(img,kernel,iterations=1)
    img=cv2.erode(img,kernel,iterations=1)

    cv2.imwrite(img_path+"removed noise.png",img)

    img=cv2.medianBlur(img,5)
    ret,img=cv2.threshold(img,127,255,cv2.THRESH_BINARY)
    img=cv2.adaptiveThreshold(img,255,cv2.ADAPTIVE_THRESH_GAUSSIAN_C,cv2.THRESH_


    cv2.imwrite(img_path+"thresh.png",img)
    result=pytesseract.image_to_string(Image.open(img_path+"thresh.png"))
    return result


print get_string(img_path)

'''
import Image
import pytesseract
print pytesseract.image_to_string(Image.open('test.png'))
```

was given as input into the TTS engine to reproduce words from the recognised text, the TTS system began by carrying out a sophisticated linguistics analysis that transformed the printed text into phonetic text. The phonetic text meant the visual representation of the speech sounds.

A grammatical and syntax analysis then enabled the system to elucidate how to pronounce each word in order to renovate the sense of the speech. This process was defined as prosody. It provided the intonation and rhythm in a sentence. Finally, the system gave information associating the phonetic text with the tone and the required length of the pronunciation. The overall analysis ended here and the sound was generated by selecting the best units present in the acoustic database (Figure 8). ("How does text-to-speech work?,"). In this way, the text was converted into sound, which was then heard through earphones or speakers by connecting to the audio jack of the Raspberry Pi 3 (Figure 9).

The volume in this device has been set in such a range that it will be appropriate for the users. The volume can be increased or decreased by making changes in the program of the voice processing module.

Designing of the Prototype

The prototype of the proposed device was a wearable one and can be easily used without any internet connection and a display screen. The device contained a rechargeable battery, a switch, a Raspberry Pi 3, an earpiece, and electrical wires (Figure 10).

Figure 8. Flowchart showing the overall functioning of the device

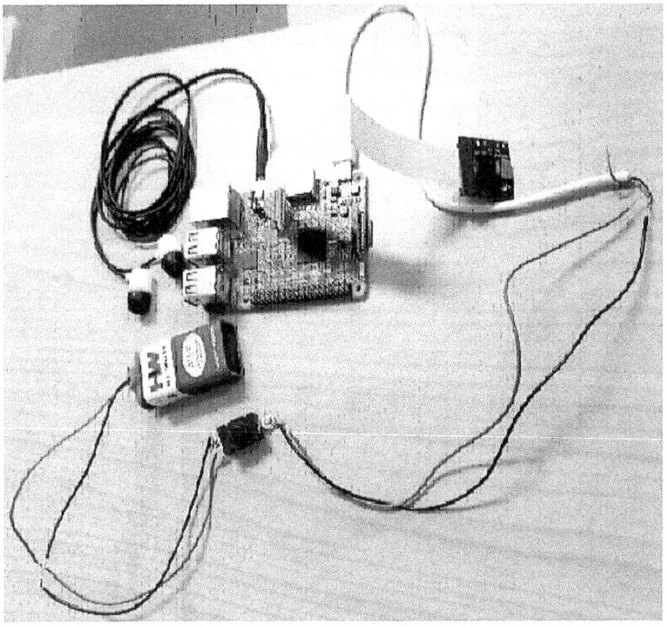

Figure 9. Raspberry Pi 3 connected with Pi camera, Earpiece and power supplied by 9 V battery

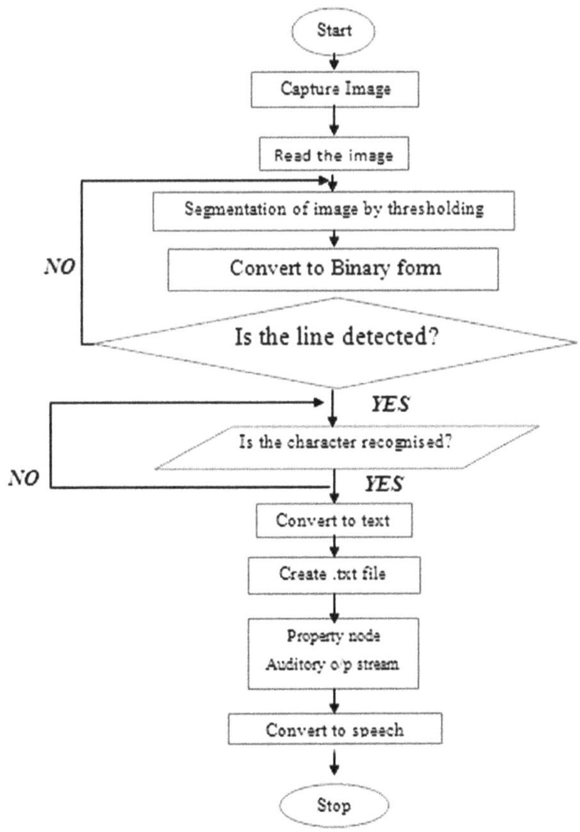

Figure 10. Overall prototype of the device

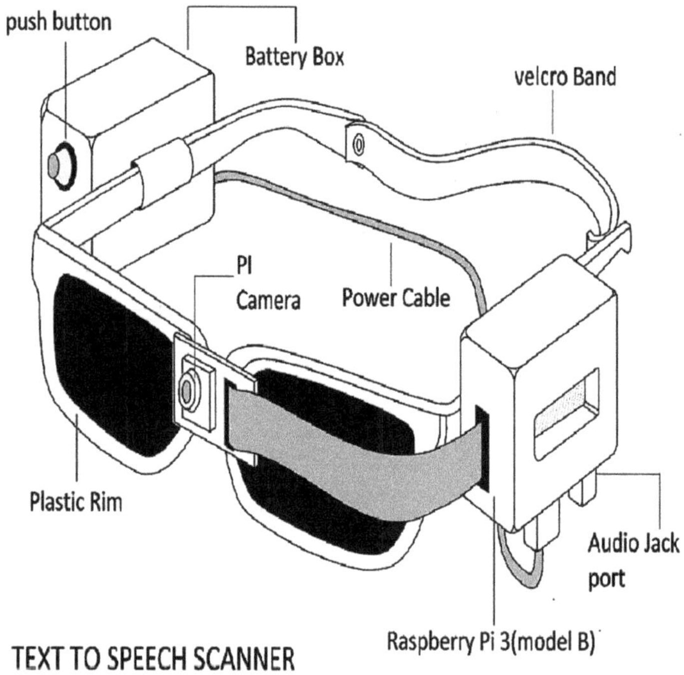

The prototype of the device looked like a goggle. The intuitive and functional design of the prototype device made it easy for the users to operate the device using only the right hand. The goggle was supported by a velcro band attached to the rims of the goggle. The Raspberry Pi 3 was attached on the left side of the goggle. A switch and a battery was connected on the right side of the goggle for power supply to the Raspberry Pi 3. The battery, the switch and the Raspberry Pi were connected in series.

When the device was switched on, the Pi camera captured the image of the text material kept in front of the user. The image was sent to the Pytesseract-OCR software, and then to Espeak-TTS synthesizer. Within 4-5 seconds, the image got scanned and the text was converted into voice. The voice was then heard with the help of an earpiece or speakers, attached to the audio jack of the Raspberry Pi 3.

RESULT AND DISCUSSION

Mainly, the device consists of two modules: Image processing module and Voice processing module.

Working of the Image Processing Module

As soon as the switch beside the Raspberry Pi 3 was pressed, the camera got the command to capture the text document placed in front of the user. The text document can be anything like a newspaper, a novel, a legal document, a simple A4 size sheet, etc. This image was saved in .jpg/ .png format. After that, the image was converted into grey scale during which the image was sharpened by designing a proper algorithm for better recognition of the letters/words. After the image was converted to grey scale, the image was converted to binary form and segmented by thresholding (through designing a proper algorithm in python) (Figure 11). With the help of OpenCV, the text was recognised in the image. Then, the result was fed to Pytesseract-OCR, which was used as the OCR engine. It converted the image into text format which was then stored as a .txt file in the Raspberry Pi 3 memory for further processing (Figure 12). The image processing module was designed for recognizing both English alphabets as well as numbers.

Working of the Voice Processing Module

The output of the image processing module was text, which was stored in Raspberry Pi as a .txt file. The text was then given as input to the voice processing module to convert it into speech. In this module, the Espeak-TTS software was allowed to access the text file and provide pronunciation phonemes to each character after segmenting the words. Espeak is an open source TTS software, which is available in various languages and voice can be generated in both male and female tone from it. In this study, English TTS software was used for reading English alphabets and numbers. It analysed the text using

Figure 11. (a) The original image; (b) Image converted into grey scale; (c) Image after thresholding

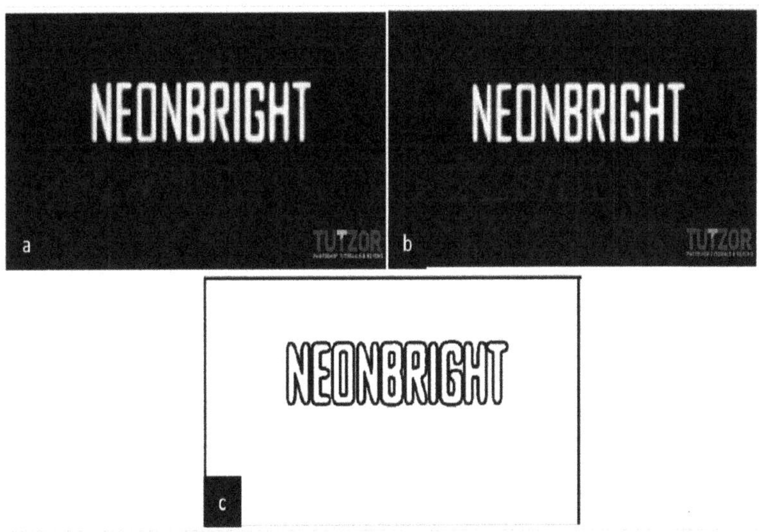

Figure 12. Result shown after the image (after the thresholding) was sent to Pytesseract-OCR

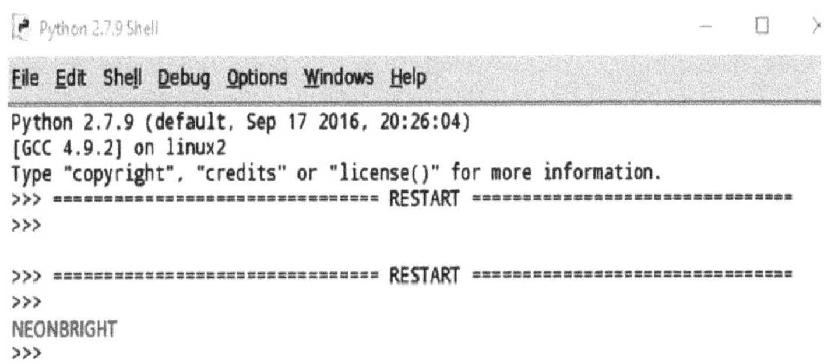

a system of phonics and other word identification rules, and then the text was read aloud through the speech synthesis process. Finally, the voice was sent to the audio jack and was heard through earpiece or speakers by the user.

Overall Working of the Proposed Device

The proposed device was developed using a Raspberry Pi in conjunction with a Pi camera and a pushbutton. The developed prototype was mounted on a goggle and was supported by an adjustable velcro strap for comfortable wearing. The Pi camera and the pushbutton were placed on the bridge and the temple of the goggle, respectively. The reading material was kept at the front side of the pi camera at a distance of 40-50 cm. The perfect alignment of the material was followed by switching the device on to start capturing the image. The captured image was processed and converted to voice statements which were audible by the user through the earphone. The process of capturing the image was completed in 3 seconds. The approximate time required by the device to read a normal A4 sheet with 30 numbers of lines was 85 seconds. The device can be made off by pressing the same pushbutton. The device weights 156g and costs Rs.5500. The device is cost-effective, portable and user-friendly.

CASE STUDY

A group of five volunteers (4 male and 1 female) participated in this study to validate the functionality of the device. All the volunteers were visually impaired due to various acute medical or accidental conditions. Prior to the experiment, a consent form was signed from all the volunteers. Figure 13 shows the practical use of the device by the volunteer. The volunteer details with the reasons of their blindness are given in Table 1.

All the volunteers were explained about the operation of the device through several demos. During the demonstration, personal assistant was given to clear individual doubts. An A4-sized paper with 30 number of lines (spacing 1.5) printed on it was given to all the volunteers as a reading material. During the experiment, no instructions were given to the volunteers. Each volunteer was tested with the device three times, once in a day. The time taken to wear the device, align the paper, and initiating the device were noted and summed up to find out the total time taken in setting up the device.

The study revealed that the volunteers were familiarized in using the device due to repetitive use. The average time taken for device setup to read the text of the hand-out was 15.6 sec. The time can be minimized further with frequent usage of the device. During the first trail, each volunteer faced some difficulty in aligning the hand-out. But with repeated use, this problem was minimized. The volunteers found the device convenient, user-friendly with reasonable-weight for long-term wearing and robust. Many volunteers suggested adding cushion effects for soothing the glabella and preferably a female voice for better interpretation.

FUTURE RESEARCH DIRECTION

There are many future possibilities with this device. Currently, the proposed device converts the text into voice in real time. But, many modifications can be incorporated into this device to further improve

Figure 13. Volunteer wearing the developed device

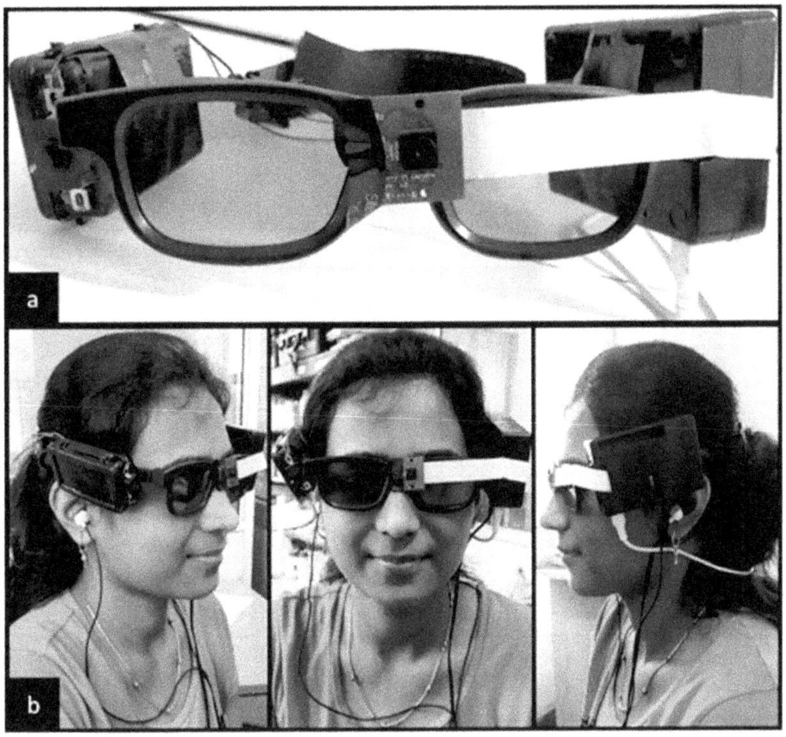

Table 1. Volunteer details

Volunteer	Sex	Age	Reasons of Blindness
1	Male	18	Glaucoma
2	Male	23	Severe head injury
3	Male	27	Stroke
4	Male	30	Subarachnoid haemorrhage
5	Female	35	Diabetic retinopathy

its functionality. The device has a range of about 40-50 cm to capture the image of the text material. A wedge can be made with a stand horizontally attached to it, which will be about 40 cm apart from the user so that when the user will pull the stand and as soon as the stand touches the user, the user will get to know that the camera is in the range to capture the proper image of the required text material on the table (Figure 14).

Another modification can be the conversion of the text into voice and saving it instead of hearing the converted voice at the same instant. This can facilitate the users to hear the particular textual material whenever they want. A play and pause button can be incorporated so that the users can pause the voice whenever they want and resume it from where they left. Two volume buttons can also be added so that the users can increase or decrease the volume as per their needs. Provisions can be included into the proposed device so that it can read the text in many different languages and convert the text from one

Table 2. Performance evaluation of the proposed device

Volunteer	Day	Time Taken (sec)			Total Time Taken (Sec)	Average Time Taken (Sec)	Remark
		Wear the Device	Align the Paper	Initiate the Device			
Volunteer 1	1	7	4	4	15	11.67	1. Difficult in aligning the hand-out. 2. The pronunciation was bothering the user. 3. The user preferred a female voice
	2	5	3	3	13		
	3	4	1	2	7		
Volunteer 2	1	11	7	5	23	16.67	1. The user preferred the weight of the Raspberry Pi to be on the right side of the device to make it wearable for a longer duration. 2. No pain in wearing the device. 3. The voice could be a little less robotic.
	2	8	5	3	16		
	3	6	3	2	11		
Volunteer 3	1	15	10	4	29	19	1. The pronunciation of the voice was proper. 2. The speed was bothering the user. 3. Needed a voice adjustment button
	2	9	6	3	18		
	3	6	3	1	10		
Volunteer 4	1	12	7	5	24	16.67	1. Preferred to be a bit less robotic for better understandable. 2. Cushiony nose-pad needed
	2	8	5	4	17		
	3	5	2	2	9		
Volunteer 5	1	12	6	4	22	14	1. Preferred a different accent. 2. Weight balance is proper. 3. Handy and useful
	2	7	4	2	13		
	3	4	2	1	7		
Average time taken						15.6	

Figure 14. A future modification

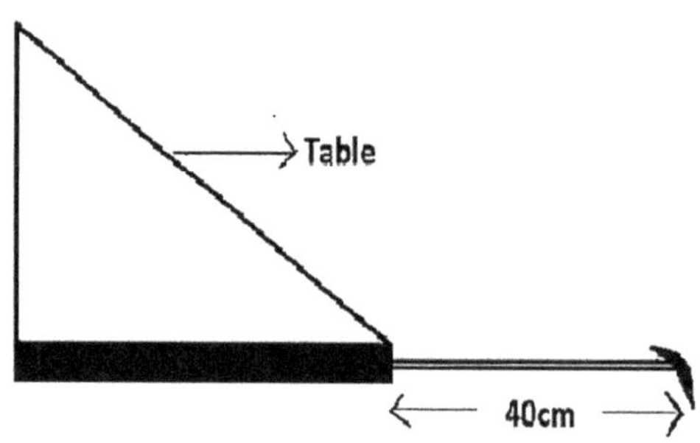

language to another. So, the proposed device will also work as a translator along with TTS scanner. The device can be further modified to detect faces and objects. This will be helpful for the blind people to recognize people objects. The lens of the Pi camera can also be modified. This may help to improve the image quality as well as the range of the device. An obstacle detection sensor may be embedded within the device. This can inform the blind person about the obstacles in the way while walking. This device may also be used for currency note detection. This can be achieved by incorporating modifications in the image processing module so that the acquired image of a currency note will be compared with a standard currency template. It will also help in identifying the currency in real time.

CONCLUSION

There are braille books available for the blind people so that even they can read books. But a lot of times blind people do not even know how to read braille and it can be cumbersome for them to learn braille. Many times the textual material they want to read is not even available in the braille format and printing of braille books is a laborious process. Also, they can be quite expensive. Multimodal devices have also been proposed by researchers in the last few decades to enable the visually-impaired people to read textual information (Akhlagi et al., 2003) (Park, 2008) (Shilkrot et al., 2014). However, most of these devices are costly and/or require extensive training. Many people cannot even afford this kind of gadgets. Also, many voice-based mobile and computer applications are available that can be used to read the textual material. But it is impractical for the visually impaired person to operate the application and focus it on the textual material. These applications are only befitting for people with normal vision. The aim of this study was to develop a text to speech device that is portable, inexpensive, and user-friendly and can overcome all these problems and provide an economical and handy alternative. The prototype of the proposed device has been implemented using Raspberry Pi, which is a small computer. In the prototype model, a Pi camera has been used for capturing the required image. The device reads the textual material in front of the user. It captures the image of the textual material, removes noise and marking the area of interest converts it into text, which is then converted into voice. The device is quite facile and does not require any special training, which makes it easy for any person to use it. All they need to do is keep the text in an appropriate range so proper image can be captured by the camera. And this device can also be used by people with normal vision so as to avoid straining their eyes.

ACKNOWLEDGMENT

The authors would like to thank the Department of Biomedical and Mechatronics Engineering, Ajeenkya DY Patil University, Pune for providing the facility for the development of the device. Special thanks to Harsh Atmaramani, undergraduate student at Ajeenkya DY Patil University, Pune, for helping in the designing of the prototype model.

REFERENCES

Akhlagi, N. N., Lonn, F., & Wittrup, P. (2003). *Reading pen*. Google Patents.

Capodanno, D., Gori, T., Nef, H., Latib, A., Mehilli, J., Lesiak, M., ... Colombo, A. (2015). Percutaneous coronary intervention with everolimus-eluting bioresorbable vascular scaffolds in routine clinical practice: Early and midterm outcomes from the European multicentre GHOST-EU registry. *EuroIntervention*, *10*(10), 1144–1153. doi:10.4244/EIJY14M07_11 PMID:25042421

Csapó, Á., Wersényi, G., Nagy, H., & Stockman, T. (2015). A survey of assistive technologies and applications for blind users on mobile platforms: A review and foundation for research. *Journal on Multimodal User Interfaces*, *9*(4), 275–286. doi:10.100712193-015-0182 7

Foster, A., & Resnikoff, S. (2005). The impact of Vision 2020 on global blindness. *Eye (London, England), 19*(10), 1133–1135. doi:10.1038j.eye.6701973 PMID:16304595

Guerreiro, J., & Gonçalves, D. (2015). Faster Text-to-Speeches: Enhancing Blind People's Information Scanning with Faster Concurrent Speech. *Proceedings of the 17th International ACM SIGACCESS Conference on Computers & Accessibility*. 10.1145/2700648.2809840

Hamiti, M., & Kastrati, R. (2014). Adapting eSpeak for converting text into speech in Albanian. *International Journal of Computer Science Issues, 11*(4), 21.

How does text-to-speech work? (n.d.). Retrieved 08/07/2017, from http://www.acapela-group.com/voices/how-does-it-work/

Lakshmi, K., & Rao, M. T. C. S. (2016). Design and implementation of text to speech conversion using Raspberry Pi. *IJITR, 4*(6), 4564–4567.

Lightstone, A. (2007). Eye health and sight loss: The UK Vision Strategy. *The Journal of Family Health Care, 18*(5), 162–164. PMID:18973088

Massof, R. W. (2003). *Auditory assistive devices for the blind*. Academic Press.

Park, S. (2008). *The Voice Stick*. Retrieved from http://www.yankodesign.com/2008/08/21/voice-stick/

Pascolini, D., & Mariotti, S. P. (2011). Global estimates of visual impairment: 2010. *British Journal of Ophthalmology*.

Patel, C., Patel, A., & Patel, D. (2012). Optical character recognition by open source OCR tool tesseract: A case study. *International Journal of Computers and Applications, 55*(10).

Russotti, J., Shaw, R., & Spungin, S. J. (2004). *When you have a visually impaired student in your classroom: a guide for paraeducators*. American Foundation for the Blind.

Shilkrot, R., Huber, J., Liu, C., Maes, P., & Nanayakkara, S. C. (2014). *FingerReader: a wearable device to support text reading on the go*. Paper presented at the CHI'14 Extended Abstracts on Human Factors in Computing Systems. 10.1145/2559206.2581220

Siqueira, J., de Melo Nunes, F. A. A., Silva, C. R. G., de Oliveira Berretta, L., Ferreira, C. B. R., Félix, I. M., & Luna, M. M. (2016). *BrailleÉcran: A Braille Approach to Text Entry on Smartphones*. Paper presented at the Computer Software and Applications Conference (COMPSAC), 2016 IEEE 40th Annual. 10.1109/COMPSAC.2016.5

Smith, R. (2007). *An overview of the Tesseract OCR engine*. Paper presented at the Document Analysis and Recognition, 2007. ICDAR 2007. Ninth International Conference on. 10.1109/ICDAR.2007.4376991

Stronks, H. C., Nau, A. C., Ibbotson, M. R., & Barnes, N. (2015). The role of visual deprivation and experience on the performance of sensory substitution devices. *Brain Research, 1624*, 140–152. doi:10.1016/j.brainres.2015.06.033 PMID:26183014

ADDITIONAL READING

Ajuwon, P. M., Meeks, M. K., Griffin-Shirley, N., & Okungu, P. A. (2016). Reflections of Teachers of Visually Impaired Students on Their Assistive Technology Competencies. *Journal of Visual Impairment & Blindness*, *110*(2), 128–134.

Alshbatat, N., & Ilah, A. (2013). Automated Mobility and Orientation System for Blind or Partially Sighted People. *International Journal on Smart Sensing and Intelligent Systems*, *6*(2).

Bhargava, A., Nath, K. V., Sachdeva, P., & Samel, M. (2015). Reading Assistant for the Visually Impaired. *Dimensions, 85*, x56mm.

Bhatlawande, S. S., Mukhopadhyay, J., & Mahadevappa, M. (2012). *Ultrasonic spectacles and waist-belt for visually impaired and blind person.* Paper presented at the Communications (NCC), 2012 National Conference on. 10.1109/NCC.2012.6176765

Bigham, J. P., Jayant, C., Ji, H., Little, G., Miller, A., Miller, R. C., . . . White, S. (2010). *VizWiz: nearly real-time answers to visual questions.* Paper presented at the Proceedings of the 23nd annual ACM symposium on User interface software and technology. 10.1145/1866029.1866080

Bourbakis, N. (2008). Sensing surrounding 3-D space for navigation of the blind. *IEEE Engineering in Medicine and Biology Magazine*, *27*(1), 49–55. doi:10.1109/MEMB.2007.901780 PMID:18270050

Brady, E., Morris, M. R., Zhong, Y., White, S., & Bigham, J. P. (2013). *Visual challenges in the everyday lives of blind people.* Paper presented at the Proceedings of the SIGCHI Conference on Human Factors in Computing Systems. 10.1145/2470654.2481291

Ch, S., Mahna, S., & Kashyap, N. (2015). Optical Character Recognition on Handheld Devices. *International Journal of Computers and Applications*, *115*(22).

Choi, Y., & Hong, K.-H. (2012). User requirements for camera-based mobile applications on touch screen devices for blind people. *Computers Helping People with Special Needs*, 48-51.

Cook, A. M., & Polgar, J. M. (2014). *Assistive Technologies-E-Book: Principles and Practice*. Elsevier Health Sciences.

Croxford, S., & Rundle, C. (2013). *Blind people and apps on mobile phones and tablets-Challenges and possibilities.* Paper presented at the Contemporary Ergonomics and Human Factors 2013: Proceedings of the international conference on Ergonomics & Human Factors 2013, Cambridge, UK, 15-18 April 2013. 10.1201/b13826-74

Dell, A. G., Newton, D. A., & Petroff, J. G. (2016). *Assistive technology in the classroom: Enhancing the school experiences of students with disabilities*. Pearson.

Domingo, M. C. (2012). An overview of the Internet of Things for people with disabilities. *Journal of Network and Computer Applications*, *35*(2), 584–596. doi:10.1016/j.jnca.2011.10.015

Dusane, S., Ahuja, M., Ghodke, R., & Kothawade, P. (2016). Text To Speech Synthesizer. *Imperial Journal of Interdisciplinary Research, 2*(5).

Fong, S. L., & Elfaki, A. O. bin Md Johar, M. G., & Aik, K. L. T. (2011). *Mobile language translator.* Paper presented at the Software Engineering (MySEC), 2011 5th Malaysian Conference in.

Hahn, J., & Ryckman, N. (2012). *Optical character recognition software in library mobile apps.* Paper presented at the IFLA World Library and Information Congress, 78th IFLA General Conference and Assembly, Conference Session 103: Usability and Accessibility-the mobile challenge, Information Technology with Library and Research Services for Parliaments.

Hakobyan, L., Lumsden, J., O'Sullivan, D., & Bartlett, H. (2013). Mobile assistive technologies for the visually impaired. *Survey of Ophthalmology, 58*(6), 513–528. doi:10.1016/j.survophthal.2012.10.004 PMID:24054999

Kang, J.-H., Kim, C.-G., Lee, S.-H., & Song, B.-S. (2007). Development of walking assistance robot for the blind. *Journal of Sensor Science and Technology, 16*(4), 286–293. doi:10.5369/JSST.2007.16.4.286

Kang, J.-H., Kim, C.-G., & Song, B.-S. (2007). *Design of a Walking Guide Robot for the Blind People.* Paper presented at the ITC-CSCC: International Technical Conference on Circuits Systems, Computers and Communications.

Khairnar, S., Khairnar, P., Gulave, S., Baviskar, V., & Deshmukh, S. (2016). Smart Phone Based Personal Assistant System with Voice Narration. *International Journal (Toronto, Ont.), 1*(7).

Kim, C.-G., & Song, B.-S. (2007). *Design of a wearable walking-guide system for the blind.* Paper presented at the Proceedings of the 1st international convention on Rehabilitation engineering & assistive technology: in conjunction with 1st Tan Tock Seng Hospital Neurorehabilitation Meeting. 10.1145/1328491.1328523

Kim, C.-G., & Song, B.-S. (2007). *A Guide System for the Blind People Using Bone Conduction Hearing Interface.* Paper presented at the ITC-CSCC: International Technical Conference on Circuits Systems, Computers and Communications.

Kim, C.-G., & Song, B.-S. (2008). Object search using synchronous ultrasonic wave emission for the blind guide system. *Journal of Biomedical Engineering Research, 29*(5), 384–391.

Kim, C.-G., & Song, B.-S. (2009). *Evaluation of a Wearable Walking Guide System.* Paper presented at the ITC-CSCC: International Technical Conference on Circuits Systems, Computers and Communications.

Maidenbaum, S., Hanassy, S., Abboud, S., Buchs, G., Chebat, D.-R., Levy-Tzedek, S., & Amedi, A. (2014). The "EyeCane", a new electronic travel aid for the blind: Technology, behavior & swift learning. *Restorative Neurology and Neuroscience, 32*(6), 813–824. PMID:25201814

Martins, M. M., Santos, C. P., Frizera-Neto, A., & Ceres, R. (2012). Assistive mobility devices focusing on smart walkers: Classification and review. *Robotics and Autonomous Systems, 60*(4), 548–562. doi:10.1016/j.robot.2011.11.015

Maruyama, M., & Yamaguchi, T. (2009). *Extraction of characters on signboards in natural scene images by stump classifiers.* Paper presented at the Document Analysis and Recognition, 2009. ICDAR'09. 10th International Conference on. 10.1109/ICDAR.2009.147

Mulloy, A. M., Gevarter, C., Hopkins, M., Sutherland, K. S., & Ramdoss, S. T. (2014). *Assistive technology for students with visual impairments and blindness Assistive technologies for people with diverse abilities* (pp. 113–156). Springer. doi:10.1007/978-1-4899-8029-8_5

Nicolau, H., Nunes, R., & Jorge, J. (2010). *Personal mobile controller for blind people.* Paper presented at the Proceedings of the 12th international conference on Human computer interaction with mobile devices and services.

Nilesh, J., Alai, P., Swapnil, C., & MR, B. (2014). Voice Based System in Desktop and Mobile Devices for Blind People. *International Journal of Emerging Technology and Advanced Engineering (IJETAE)*, 404-407. Pi, R. model B. *Available onlin e:* https://www. raspberrypi. org/products/raspberry-pi-2-model-b/(accessed on 24 October 2016)

Sharma, F. R., & Wasson, S. G. (2012). Speech recognition and synthesis tool: Assistive technology for physically disabled persons. *International Journal of Computer Science and Telecommunications*, *3*(4), 86–91.

Song, B.-S., & Kim, C.-G. (2013). *Obstacle Searching Method Using a Simultaneous Ultrasound Emission for Autonomous Wheelchairs Multimedia and Ubiquitous Engineering* (pp. 561–566). Springer.

Terven, J. R., Salas, J., & Raducanu, B. (2014). New opportunities for computer vision-based assistive technology systems for the visually impaired. *Computer*, *47*(4), 52–58. doi:10.1109/MC.2013.265

Torabi, K., Durgan, J., & Tarpley, B. (2013). *Early modern OCR project (eMOP) at Texas A&M University: using Aletheia to train Tesseract.* Paper presented at the Proceedings of the 2013 ACM symposium on Document engineering. 10.1145/2494266.2494304

Venkateswarlu, S., Kamesh, D., Sastry, J., & Rani, R. (2016). Text to Speech Conversion. *Indian Journal of Science and Technology*, *9*(38).

Virgili, G., Acosta, R., Grover, L. L., Bentley, S. A., & Giacomelli, G. (2013). Reading aids for adults with low vision. *The Cochrane Library*. PMID:24154864

White, G. R., Fitzpatrick, G., & McAllister, G. (2008). *Toward accessible 3D virtual environments for the blind and visually impaired.* Paper presented at the Proceedings of the 3rd international conference on Digital Interactive Media in Entertainment and Arts. 10.1145/1413634.1413663

Ye, H., Malu, M., Oh, U., & Findlater, L. (2014). *Current and future mobile and wearable device use by people with visual impairments.* Paper presented at the Proceedings of the SIGCHI Conference on Human Factors in Computing Systems. 10.1145/2556288.2557085

Yi, C., Flores, R. W., Chincha, R., & Tian, Y. (2013). Finding objects for assisting blind people. *Network Modeling and Analysis in Health Informatics and Bioinformatics*, *2*(2), 71–79. doi:10.100713721-013-0026-x PMID:23894729

KEY TERMS AND DEFINITIONS

OpenCV: OpenCV stands for open source computer vision. It is a computer vision library with APIs that let us to setup a pipeline for a computer vision project.

Optical Character Recognition: Optical character recognition (OCR) is a technology that allows us to convert different types of documents, such as PDF and images captured by a digital camera into text.

Pi Camera: The Pi camera is a camera module that utilizes the OV5647 chip. It is able to capture five MP resolution images, or 1080 p HD video recording at 30fps.

PuTTY: PuTTY is the name of a software that allows for a secure connection to the UNIX (and Linux) terminals for Windows users. A program called PSFTP.exe is used to copy files to and from the terminal. This program makes it possible to copy files from host computer to the local machine and vice versa. PuTTY is a very versatile tool for remote access to another computer, though that is only one of its many uses.

Raspberry Pi 3.0: Raspberry Pi 3.0 is the third generation of the single board computer developed by Raspberry Pi foundation. It works on the Debian-based GNU/Linux operating system named Raspbian.

Raspbian: Raspbian is a Debian, which is a Linux (UBUNTU-MATE) distribution-based computer OS for Raspberry Pi. It is officially provided by the Raspberry Pi Foundation, as the primary OS for the family of Raspberry Pi SBC (single board computer). Rasbian comes with over 35,000 packages.

Text-to-Speech Synthesizer: Text-to-speech synthesizer is the artificial creation of human speech from text.

Xming X Server: Xming is the leading X Window System Server for Microsoft Windows®. It is fully featured, reliable, fast, and easy to install.

Chapter 11
Analysis of ECG Signals to Investigate the Effect of a Humorous Audio-Visual Stimulus on Autonomic Nervous System and Heart of Females

Karan Pande
National Institute of Technology Rourkela, India

Seemadri Subhadarshini
National Institute of Technology Rourkela, India

Deepanjali Gaur
National Institute of Technology Rourkela, India

Suraj Kumar Nayak
National Institute of Technology Rourkela, India

Kunal Pal
National Institute of Technology Rourkela, India

ABSTRACT

This chapter is an attempt to understand the effect of audio-visual stimulus with a humorous content on the cardiac electrophysiology. Electrocardiogram (ECG) signals were acquired from 11 female volunteers under the pre- and the post-stimulus conditions. Artificial neural network (ANN)-based classification of the ARMA model coefficients computed from the RR interval signals suggested significant variation in the autonomic nervous system activity. Analysis of the Gabor denoised ECG signals indicated a change in the electrical activity of the heart in the post-stimulus condition, which was confirmed by the ANN-based classification. Recurrence analysis of the RR interval suggested plausible differences of the cardiac activity amongst both the conditions. The audio-visual stimulus has resulted in significant alterations in the ANS and the cardiac physiology.

DOI: 10.4018/978-1-5225-4969-7.ch011

INTRODUCTION

The sinoatrial (SA) node, located in the upper region of the right atrium, is a collection of self-excitatory cells. These cells are responsible for the rhythmic contraction of the heart. Because of this unique property, SA node is also known as the natural pacemaker of the heart. This regulation is achieved by the nerve innervations of the Autonomic Nervous System (ANS) into the SA node. Based on the various external stimuli sensed by the sense organs and the internal conditions, ANS issues either excitatory or inhibitory signals to the SA node through sympathetic or parasympathetic nerves. This helps in achieving the required alteration in the heart rate and the duration of the consecutive cardiac cycles. The variation in the cardiac cycles can be measured by monitoring the variations in the time duration of the consecutive 'R' peaks. Such a recording with respect to time is regarded as RRI (RR interval) time series. The ECG signals divulge information about the electrical activity of the heart (Zaidi, Ahmed, & Bakibillah, 2017) and the RRI time series has been reported to describe the ANS activity noninvasively (Salvioli, et al., 2015).

Exposing an individual to stimuli like audio-visual clips has been reported to alter the physiological activities of the individual, including the ANS and the cardiac activities (S. Nayak, Champaty, Ray, & Pal, 2014; S. K. Nayak, et al., 2016; Proverbio, et al., 2015). Studies have been preformed to assess the human emotions like sadness, happiness, fear, disgust and neutral in volunteers due to their exposure to audio-visual clips by analyzing their ECG signals (Murugappan, Murugappan, & Zheng, 2013). Some researchers have employed stressful audio-visual stimulus to understand and estimate the measurable physiological changes that occurs in body as part of the "fight-or-flight" response (Bloomer, Hitt, Olson, & Wruck). It has been shown that stress activates sympathetic nervous system by releasing stress hormones (Hayashi, et al., 2008; Kemeny, 2003) that causes the physiological changes in the conduction pathway of the heart. The audio-visual stimuli have also been exploited to evaluate the effect of weeping and laughing on the ANS activity and the mood states (Sakuragi, Sugiyama, & Takeuchi, 2002). Many researchers around the world have hypothesized that the audio-visual stimulus elicits a greater change in the heart rate, galvanic skin response and respiration as compared to the auditory stimulus, due to a larger baseline deviation but only a few studies have been conducted in the support of this hypothesis (Tkaczyszyn, et al., 2013).

In this study, we report the effect of a humorous audio-visual clip on the ANS and the heart physiology of females. In normal healthy females, the gonadotropic hormone levels undergo continuous change during the menstrual cycle. A change in the level of these hormones not only affects the reproductive organ, but also influences the ANS. In order to maintain the effect of this hormonal changes constant, all the females involved in the study were exposed to the audio-visual stimulus when they were on the day 1 of phase-1 (i.e. follicular phase) of their menstrual cycle.

BACKGROUND

Sakuragi *et al.* (2002) conducted an experiment with 10 female volunteers in order to estimate the effect of comic and tragic videos on the mood states and the autonomic nervous system of the volunteers (Sakuragi, et al., 2002). The above stimuli caused the participants to laugh and weep. Both the respiration curve and ECG of the participants were recorded before and after watching the videos. In order to evaluate the mood states, they were asked to fill out profiles of mood states (POMS). Spectral analysis of HRV was performed and an increase in the vigor score and a decrease in the anger hostility score of PMOS were observed following the comic audio-visual stimuli. In contrast, the depression dejection score increased significantly after watching the tragic videos. Llera *et al.* (2010) examined 38 volunteers having generalized anxiety disorder (GAD) along with a control group of 35 non-anxious participants on exposure to emotions like fear, happiness, calm and relaxation, elicited *via* audio-visual clips (Llera & Newman, 2010). The ECG recordings of the participants were acquired, and their vagal activity was measured throughout the experiment. The study tried to understand the effect of worry *vs.* relaxation in both the groups. The results suggested a more reduction in the vagal activity of the persons suffering from GAD as compared to the control group on exposure to fear emotion. Herring *et al.* (2011) studied the difference in the behavioural, cardiovascular and respiratory properties of two positive emotions, namely, amusement and joy. A more positive facial expression, greater increase in respiratory amplitude and a smaller deceleration of heart rate was observed in case of amusement clip as compared to the joy clip (Herring, Burleson, Roberts, & Devine, 2011). Bong *et al.* (2012) worked on the classification of the emotional stress using the analysis of the ECG signals. The authors extracted mean R peak amplitude (MRAmp), heart rate (HR) and mean R-R intervals (MRRI) from ECG recording of 5 healthy subjects who were induced with emotional stress by audio-visual stimuli. These statistical features were then mapped into emotional state classification using Support Vector Machine (SVM) and k-nearest neighbor (KNN) (Bong, Murugappan, & Yaacob, 2012). Murugappan *et al.* (2013) analyzed the heart rate variability (HRV) (i.e., the RRI time series variability) of twenty healthy university students (with an average age of 23 years) in order to estimate human emotions like happiness, disgust, fear, sadness, and neutral (Murugappan, et al., 2013). The study was accomplished by showing the volunteers the audio-visual clips to induce the above-mentioned five emotions. The statistical features were extracted from the HRV signals using Discrete Wavelet Transform (DWT). These statistical features were then mapped successfully into the corresponding emotions using k-nearest neighbor (KNN) and linear discriminant analysis (LDA). The authors suggested that HRV can act as a suitable tool to detect the changes in the emotional states of the persons and can find applications in the development of real-time, intelligent emotion assessment systems. Jantaro *et al.* (2014) investigated the effect of comic video clip as a stimulus to understand the autonomic nervous system response and subjective happiness in 40 healthy Thai adults, aged between 18- 26 years (Jantaro, et al., 2014). The study was performed by measuring the heart rate (HR), the skin temperature, the respiration rate and the SpO2 level before and after the stimulus. The control condition included a neutral video clip. A significant increase in the SpO2 level along with a decrease of the skin temperature was detected after watching comedy clips. Nayak *et al.* (2014) conducted a similar study on Indian volunteers using HRV and ECG signal analyses. Their results indicated a sympathetic dominance after watching the comic film and a corresponding alteration in the conduction pathwayof the heart (S. Nayak, et al., 2014). Tsai *et al.* (2015) measured heart rate while the volunteers were involved in two activities, i.e., adventure riding and watching movies. This was done by the use of wearable ECG devices. The fluctuations in the emotions resulted in physiological changes in the ANS which was detected by an algorithm. They found that the heart rate and the excitation level are positively related (Tsai & Yi, 2015). Mokashi *et al.* (2016) investigated the effect of sound or audio of a horror movie clip on the autonomic regulation of the cardiac activity. They confirmed these changes in the cardiac conduction pathway using time domain and joint time- frequency analysis of ECG recordings of volunteers (Mokashi, et al., 2016). Roonizi (2017) designed a generalized framework that comprises of some innovative approaches for model-based ECG decomposition, waveform characterization and feature extraction. As a case study, the framework was used to design a model for the characterization of atrial fibrillation. For better estimation of ventricular activity, sum of Gaussian kernels was used and sinusoidal model was used for modeling the atrial activity. The proposed model provided better tracking of the atrial activity, ventricular activity and fibrillatory frequency simultaneously compared to other reported methods (Kheirati Roonizi, 2017). Pham and Wang (2017) used an another method to understand the emotional responses to audio-visual mobile video advertisements. They used physiological signal sensing by recording photoplethysmography (PPG) signals and also by analyzing the facial expression. The attention, sentiment and engagement of the participants were taken into account for the above purpose while watching the audio-visual clip (Pham & Wang, 2017).

In this study, the RRI time series and the ECG signals obtained in the pre and the post-stimulus conditions were analyzed to understand the effect of a humorous audio-visual stimulus on the ANS and the cardiac physiology of the reproductively active female volunteers, respectively. The RRI time series were examined using recurrence analysis and ARMA modeling and the Gabor-based de-noising of the ECG signals was performed prior to its time domain analysis that distinguished this work from all the related studies discussed above.

MAIN FOCUS OF THE CHAPTER

Various methods and techniques have been proposed to analyze the effect of different stimuli on the emotional as well as physiological parameters of the human body. However, very few studies have been performed on the reproductively active females. The main focus of this study is to analyze and estimate the effect of a humorous audio-visual stimulus on the physiology of the ANS and the heart of the reproductively active female volunteers. This study uses two popular techniques, i.e., recurrence analysis and ARMA modelling for the extraction of the parameters from the RRI time series. Further, Gabor denoising technique is implemented to remove the high-frequency noise contained in the ECG prior to its time domain analysis. Artificial neural network based classification has been performed to confirm the alterations in the physiology of the ANS and the heart due to the humorous audio-visual stimulus.

MATERIALS

Acquisition of the ECG signals was performed using EKG sensor (Vernier Software and Technology, USA). Disposable ECG electrodes (BPL Medical Technologies Pvt. Ltd, India) were used to acquire the ECG signals in the lead-I configuration. The ECG signals were digitized and stored in a laptop using DAQ USB-4704 multifunction USB module (Advantech Corporation, Taiwan), and a LabVIEW (V13, National Instruments, USA) program. Analysis of the RR interval was initially carried out using Bios Analyzer (Holan, Lund, & Davis, 2010), and ARMA modelling was done using system identification toolbox of MATLAB R2014a (MathWorks Inc., USA). Statistical analysis and ANN based classification were carried out using Statistica (trial version, V13.2, Dell Inc., USA). Gabor transformation based denoising of the ECG signals and subsequent feature extraction was performed in LabVIEW.

METHODS

Volunteers

Eleven female students of NIT Rourkela volunteered for the study. All the volunteers belonged to the age group of 20-24 years. Detailed information about the nature and the purpose of the study was provided to all the participants. Once, they were satisfied with all the information provided and had agreed to take part in the study, a written consent regarding the same was obtained from all the participants as per the WHO guidelines. Institutional Ethical Clearance Committee (IEC) of NIT Rourkela provided the ethical clearance for the acquisition of the ECG signals in our lab vide its letter no NITRKL/IEC/FORM/2/25/4/11/001, dated 13-12-2013. The volunteers visited our lab between 7 pm to 8 pm on the first day of phase 1 of their menstrual cycle. They were allowed to settle down comfortably in a chair and the ECG signal was acquired for 6 min before exposing them to the humorous audio-visual stimulus. Then, they were exposed to the audio-visual stimulus and the ECG signal was acquired for 6 min, immediately after viewing the audio-visual stimulus. RR interval time series data was extracted using Biomedical Workbench (LabVIEW, V13.0, National Instruments, USA).

Recurrence Analysis of RRI Time Series

Recurrence analysis has been reported as a tool to analyse certain biomedical processes like cardiac activity (Li & McLeod, 1981; McLeod & Li, 1983). The main advantage offered by the recurrence analysis over other non-linear methods is its capability to successfully analyse the data available for short-time duration and those which are non-stationary in nature (Brockway & Brockway, 2013). Bios Analyser software was used to perform recurrence analyses of the pre- and the post-stimulus RRI series (da Costa, Ortigueira, Batista, & Paiva, 2013). Bios is a non-stationary and aperiodic process exhibiting properties of short-time patterns, novelty and diversification. Various natural, physical and biological processes like changes in the weather conditions, movement of animal population in their habitat, distribution of quasars and galaxies in space and cardiac activity are Biotic in nature. Recurrence analysis of a time series data involves quantifying isometry, consecutive isometry, and novelty. Recurrence and embedding plots were used to qualitatively ascertain time-specific variations in the time series data. Recurrence stands for repetition of an event. Repetition of an event in a time scale indicates a pattern and consecutive recurrence suggests order in the time series data.

ARMA Modelling of RRI Time Series

Resampling of 5 sec RRIs was performed at 4 Hz (Graupe & Cline, 1975). As ARMA modelling can be done only on stationary time series data, hence stationarity of the RRI time series data was ascertained by Dicky-Fuller test. Non-stationary time series data were made stationary by a single differencing procedure (MathWorks). This stationary time series was then loaded into the System Identification Toolbox of MATLAB and the 4th order ARMA polynomial models of the RRI time series were obtained. Statistically important coefficients of the A and the C polynomials of the ARMA model were used as inputs for ANN classification to distinguish the pre-stimulus time series data from the post-stimulus time series data.

Analysis of Gabor Denoised ECG

Clinically relevant ECG signals, in general have a frequency range between 0.05 Hz to 100 Hz (Lee, Nam, McManus, & Chon, 2013). Hence, Gabor transform based thresholding technique was used to remove the frequency components above 100 Hz. 12 features were obtained from the Gabor denoised 5 sec ECG signals. Among the 12 features, statistically important ones were obtained using t-test, Classification and Regression Tree (CART), Boosted Tree (BT), and Random Forest (RF). These statistically important features were used as inputs for ANN classification to classify the pre-stimulus ECG signals from the post-stimulus ECG signals.

RESULTS AND DISCUSSION

Recurrence Analysis of RRI Time Series

Recurrence is one of the basic properties exhibited by the dynamic processes enabling their representation in the phase space (Pardey, Roberts, & Tarassenko, 1996). The space consisting of all the possible values that a dynamic process can achieve is known as its phase space. Recurrence can be defined in various ways. Isometry and similarity are two such examples. In this study, we used isometry (recurrence isometry) to quantify recurrence in RRI time series (Weisstein, 2002). Sequences of adjacent elements of a time series generated by a dynamic process are known as vectors. Square root of the sum of squares of the elements of a vector gives its length. The number of elements of the time series included in a vector is known as embedding. Two vectors are isometric when the absolute difference of their lengths is less than a cut-off radius, which is predefined in terms of percentage of the range of the time series. Total number of isometric recurrences in percentage of the total number of vector pairs compared in the time series sample gives %isometry. An embedding plot is a plot of %isometry or any other parameter derived from %isometry with respect to number of embedding. Figure 1(a) shows embedding plot of %isometry of pre-stimulus and post-stimulus RRI time series data. The %isometry was more in pre-stimulus condition than the post-stimulus condition. This suggested a more patterned behaviour during the pre-stimulus condition.

Numbers of adjacent recurrences are measured as consecutive isometry. Consecutive isometry is an indicator of causality. Figure 1(b) shows embedding plot of %consecutive isometry of pre-stimulus and post-stimulus RRI time series. It can be observed that the pre-stimulus %consecutive isometry is greater than the post-stimulus %consecutive isometry over the range of embedding, indicating that the pre-stimulus RRI time series to be more causal in comparison to the post-stimulus time series.

Variations in the isometry due to the change of the cut-off radius are known as radial isometry. Similarly, variations in the consecutive isometry due to change of the cut-off radius is known as consecutive radial isometry. Figure 1(c) and 1(d) show bar graphs of %radial isometry and %consecutive radial isometry with respect to the cut-off radius (%). It can be observed that both %radial isometry and %consecutive radial isometry in the pre-stimulus condition are more than that in the post-stimulus condition (for cut-off radius $\geq$1%).

Novelty is fundamental property of a creative process. If the ratio of the isometry of the shuffled time series to isometry of the original time series is greater than one, then the time series is said to be novel. RRI time series demonstrates the property of novelty. Figure 1(e) shows the embedding plot of novelty

Figure 1. (a) Bar graph of % isometry vs embedding, (b) Bar graph of % consecutive isometry vs embedding, (c) Bar graph of % radial isometry vs cutoff radius, (d) Bar graph of % consecutive radial isometry vs cutoff radius, (e) Bar graph of Novelty vs embedding.

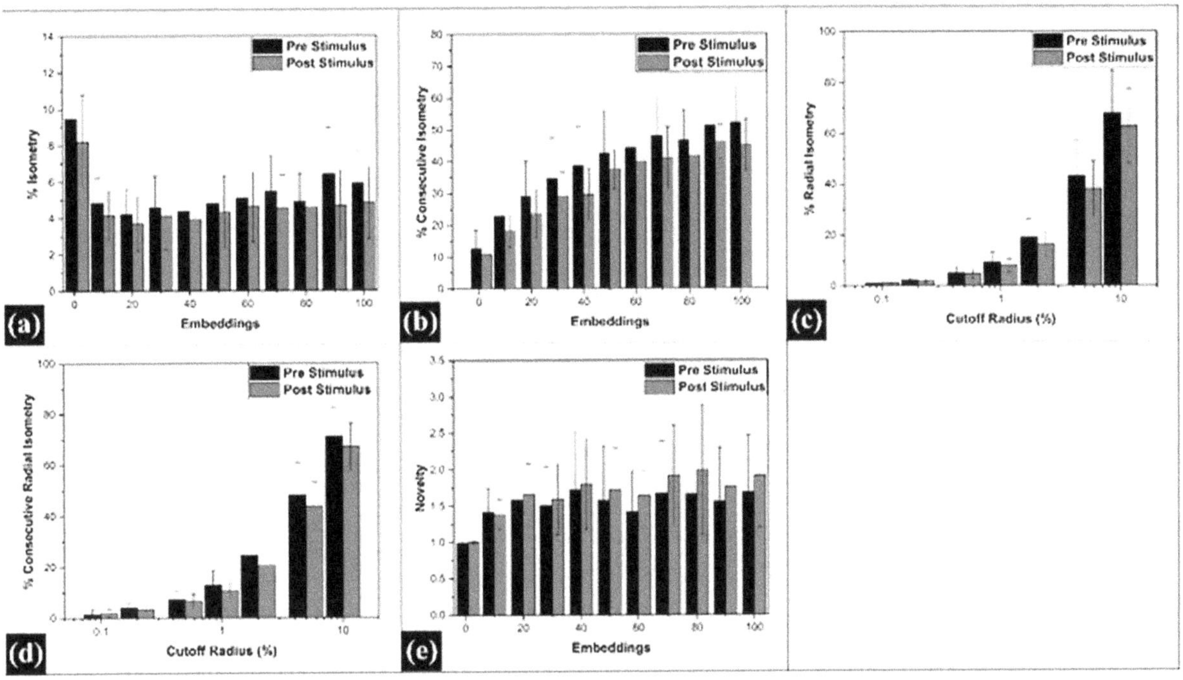

of the pre- and the post-stimulus RRI time series. It can be observed that both the time series exhibited the property of novelty. However, the novelty in the post-stimulus condition is greater than that in the pre-stimulus condition (except for the embedding ≤10).

The recurrence plots give insight into the behavioural dynamics of a system. Figure 2 shows recurrence plots of the pre- and the post-stimulus RRI time series. These recurrence plots were plotted with

Figure 2. (a) Recurrence plot of pre-stimulus RRI, (b) Recurrence plot of post-stimulus RRI

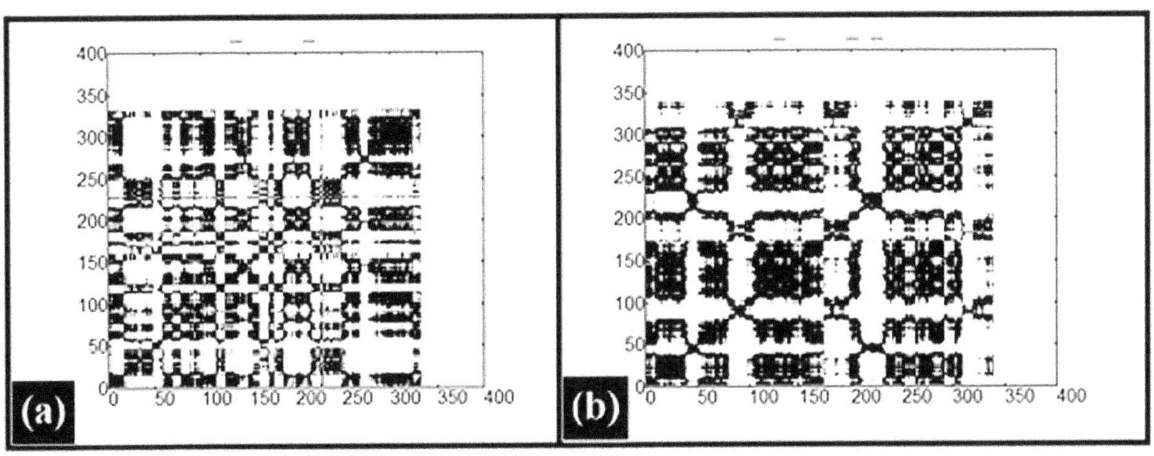

10 embedding and 10% cut-off radius. Specific patterns in the recurrence plots indicate recurrence. Recurrence free or white regions in the recurrence plot indicate either increment or decrement of heart rate while the recurrence rich regions, i.e., the regions rich in definite patterns indicate steady heart rate. From Figure 2, we can observe that the post-stimulus recurrence plot has more recurrence rich regions than the pre-stimulus recurrence plot suggesting a more stable heart rate during the post-stimulus condition. In gist, a variation in the recurrence behavior of the RRI time series was observed in the pre- and the post-stimulus conditions.

ARMA Modelling of RRI Time Series

ARMA models have been reported to parsimoniously (i.e. using least number of parameters possible) represent stationary time series data sets with adequate accuracy (Baselli, Bolis, Cerutti, & Freschi, 1985; Ge, Srinivasan, & Krishnan, 2002). Many researchers have used ARMA modelling technique to model RRI time series and used them to detect specific abnormalities in the autonomic regulation of the cardiac activity (Orini, Bailón, Mainardi, & Laguna, 2012). ARMA models have also been used to model EEG and EMG signals for various clinical and biomedical applications (Graupe & Cline, 1975). In this study, we intended to classify the pre-stimulus and the post-stimulus RRI time series data using ARMA model coefficients. As ARMA modelling can be implemented only on the stationary time series data, hence, stationarity of the RRI time series data was checked using Dicky-Fuller test (Ge, et al., 2002). If any time series was found to be non-stationary, it was made stationary by performing one differencing operation (Christini, et al., 1995). As reported in the literature, we also found that an increase in the model order did not result in appreciable improvement in model accuracy or Fit percent. Also, FPE (Akaike's Final Prediction Error) performs similar to AIC (Akaike's Information Criterion) as an ARMA model quality metric. Hence, any one of them can be used interchangeably. MATLAB uses FPE, LossFcn, MSE and Fit Percent to ascertain the quality of the ARMA model generated (Weisstein, 2002). In our study, 4th order ARMA models (i.e. $ARMA_{(4,4)}$) of the pre-stimulus RRI time series data had average Fit Percent of 79.87%, average FPE of 0.0022, average LossFcn of 0.0011 and average MSE of 0.001. On the other hand, the respective values for $ARMA_{(4,4)}$ models of the post-stimulus RRI time series data were 61.80%, 0.0044, 0.0022 and 0.0034. The coefficients of the polynomials A and C of the ARMA models of the pre- and the post-stimulus RRI time series were tested for statistical significance by t-test, CART, BT and RF. The C4 coefficient was found to be statistically important by t-test (Table 1). CART suggested C1, A2 and A3 to be important parameters while BT suggested C4 as the only important parameter. MLP and RBF ANN networks were implemented using C1, C4, A2 and A3 coefficients as classifying

Table 1. Statistically significant features of ARMA model of the RRI time series

Classifiers	ARMA Model Coefficients	Mean ± SD		Predictor Importance	p-Value
		Pre-Stimulus	Post-Stimulus		
t-test	C4	0.25±0.60	-0.35±0.52	----------	0.04
CART	A2	2.00±1.29	2.21±1.23	1.00	----------
	A3	-1.13±0.88	-1.35±1.36	1.00	----------
	C1	0.36±1.65	0.61±0.89	0.91	----------
BT	C4	0.25±0.60	-0.35±0.52	1.00	----------

parameters. MLP (5-6-2) ANN network provided a 100% classification efficiency using these parameters (Table 2) and RBF 8-6-2 provided 82% efficiency (Table 3). The architecture details of the implemented ANN networks along with their training and testing performances have been tabulated in Table 4. The occurrence of the statistically important ARMA model parameters, computed from the RRI time series of the pre- and the post-stimulus conditions, suggested the alteration in the ANS physiology due to the audio-visual stimulus, which was further confirmed by the results of the ANN classification (Mokashi, et al., 2016).

Time Domain Analysis of Gabor Denoised ECG

Hungarian Nobel laureate, D. Gabor introduced the Gabor transform. Gabor transform modifies (Equation 1) the well-established Fourier transform by introducing a local time-window function, also known as the time-frequency window. Gabor transform brings about localization of Fourier transform at t = b. Gabor transform finds its application in various engineering fields.

Table 2. Classification summary of MLP 5-6-2 network

	Pre-Stimulus	Post-Stimulus	Overall
Total	8.00	9.00	17.00
Correct	8.00	9.00	17.00
Incorrect	0.00	0.00	0.00
Correct (%)	100.00	100.00	100
Incorrect (%)	0.00	0.00	0.00

Table 3. Classification summary of RBF 5-6-2 network

	Pre-Stimulus	Post-Stimulus	Overall
Total	8.00	9.00	17.00
Correct	6.00	8.00	14.00
Incorrect	2.00	1.00	3.00
Correct (%)	75.00	88.89	81.94
Incorrect (%)	25.00	11.11	18.06

Table 4. Details of MLP and RBF networks

Networks	ARMA Coefficients Used	Classification Efficiency (%)	Training Performance (%)	Test Performance (%)	Algorithm	Error Function	Hidden Activation Function	Output Activation Function
MLP 8-6-2	A2. A3,C1 and C4	100.00	100.00	100.00	BFGS 41	Entropy	Logistic	Softmax
RBF 8-6-2	A2. A3,C1 and C4	81.94	75.00	88.00	RBFT	Entropy	Gaussian	Softmax

Mathematically, the Gabor transform is defined as:

$$G_b^{\alpha} f(\omega) = \int_{-\infty}^{\infty} \left[e^{-i\omega t} f(t)\right] g_{\alpha}\left(t - b\right) dt \quad (1)$$

where,

$$f(\omega) = \int_{-\infty}^{\infty} e^{-i\omega t} f(t) dt$$

represents the Fourier transform of the signal and

$$g_{\alpha}(t) = \frac{1}{2\sqrt{\pi\alpha}} e^{-t^2/4\alpha}, \alpha \geq 0$$

indicates the Gaussian function.

Advanced Signal Processing Toolkit of LabVIEW allows application of Discrete Gabor Transform and Discrete Gabor Expansion for signal de-noising applications (LabVIEW). Advanced Signal Processing Toolkit of LabVIEW was used to remove frequency components above 100 Hz from the ECG signals using Gabor transform-based thresholding (Figure 3). The denoised ECG signals were used to obtain 12 features (namely, Energy Density (ED), Shanon Energy (SE), Log Energy (LE), Arithmetic Mean (AM), Root Mean Square (RMS), Standard Deviation (SD), Variance, Kurtosis, Median, Mode, Skewness, Summation). Statistical methods were used to obtain features having statistical significance. AM, Kurtosis and Summation were indicated as statistically significant by CART (Table 5). BT indicated AM and summation to be the important parameters. Skewness was indicated to be important by RF. These statistically significant features were used as inputs for MLP and RBF ANN networks to differentiate pre-stimulus ECG signals from post-stimulus ECG signals. MLP (4-13-2) network achieved a classification accuracy of 95.45% (Table 6). The network architecture details have been summarized and tabulated below in Table 7.

FUTURE RESEARCH DIRECTION

Although the results obtained by the above techniques are quite significant, the study can be further extrapolated by including more female volunteers and the ECG recording can be acquired in all the three stages of menstrual cycle, i.e., follicular phase, ovulatory phase and luteal phase to detect the changes in the physiological parameters due to the hormonal changes during the menstrual cycle. Moreover, other established techniques such as Support Vector Machine (SVM) and K-nearest neighbor (K-NN) can be used for the classification of the acquired ECG signals. By doing so, the study can be made more extensive and the results can be more conclusive.

Figure 3. ECG Signal Spectral Analysis at various thresholding values. (a) threshold at 0 (b) threshold at 0.28, (c) threshold at 0.5, (d) threshold at 0.8, and (e) threshold at 1

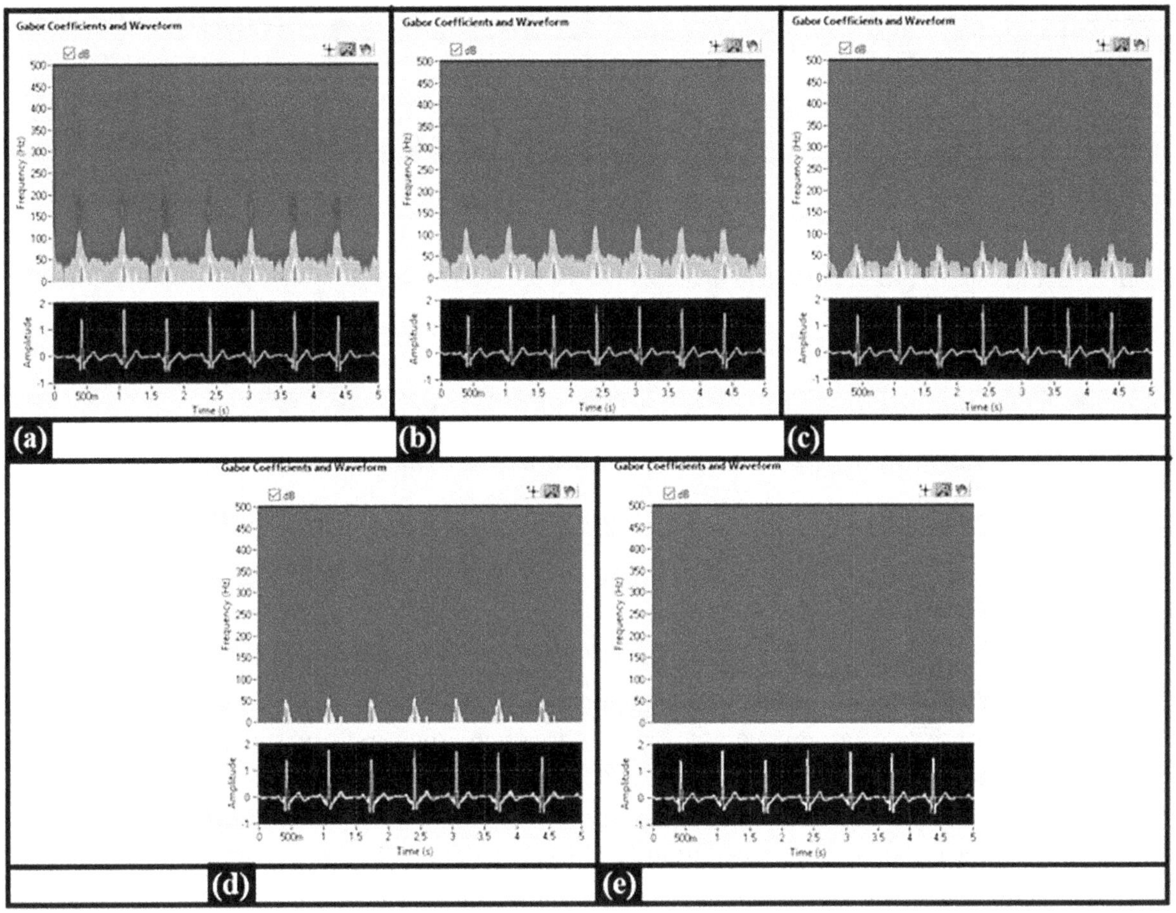

Table 5. Statistically significant features of Gabor-denoised ECG

Classifiers	Time Domain Features	Mean ± SD		Predictor Importance
		Pre-Stimulus	Post-Stimulus	
CART	Arithmetic Mean	-0.00±0.00	0.00±0.00	1.00
	Kurtosis	11.89±4.53	12.45±4.28	0.96
	Summation	-1.64±2.46	0.09±4.49	1.00
BT	Arithmetic Mean	-0.00±0.00	0.00±0.00	1.00
	Summation	-1.64±2.46	0.09±4.49	1.00
RF	Skewness	2.34±0.80	2.37±0.73	1.00

Table 6. Classification summary of MLP 4-13-2 network

	Pre-Stimulus	Post-Stimulus	Overall
Total	11.00	11.00	22.00
Correct	10.00	10.00	20.00
Incorrect	1.00	1.00	2.00
Correct (%)	90.90	90.90	90.90
Incorrect (%)	9.09	9.09	9.09

Table 7. Details of MLP and RBF networks

Networks	Features Used	Classification Efficiency (%)	Training Perf. (%)	Test Perf. (%)	Algorithm	Error Function	Hidden Act	Output Act
MLP 4-13-2	Arithmetic Mean, Summation, Kurtosis, Skewness	95.45	100.00	100.00	BFGS 63	SOS	Exponential	Logistic

CONCLUSION

In the present study, we have studied the changes occurring in the ANS activity and the electrophysiology of the heart of females after they were exposed to a humorous audio-visual stimulus. Recurrence analysis suggested a difference in the dynamic nature of the pre- and the post-stimulus RRI time series. Also, the pre- and the post-stimulus RRI signals were classified with 100% classification accuracy using statistically significant features, obtained from the ARMA model coefficients. Further, the ECG signals were de-noised using Gabor transform. The classification of the statistically significant features of the de-noised ECG signals showed classification efficiency of >95%. This study suggested a probability of definitive change in the ANS and the cardiac electrophysiology during the post-stimulus condition. However, a detailed analysis is required to understand the actual changes occurring in the cardiac electrophysiology.

REFERENCES

Baselli, G., Bolis, D., Cerutti, S., & Freschi, C. (1985). Autoregressive modeling and power spectral estimate of RR interval time series in arrhythmic patients. *Computers and Biomedical Research, an International Journal, 18*(6), 510–530. doi:10.1016/0010-4809(85)90027-8 PMID:4075786

Bong, S. Z., Murugappan, M., & Yaacob, S. (2012). *Analysis of electrocardiogram (ecg) signals for human emotional stress classification.* Paper presented at the First International Conference on Trends in Intelligent Robotics, Automation, and Manufacturing, Kuala Lumpur, Malaysia. 10.1007/978-3-642-35197-6_22

Christini, D. J., Bennett, F., Lutchen, K., Ahmed, H., Hausdorff, J., & Oriol, N. (1995). Application of linear and nonlinear time series modeling to heart rate dynamics analysis. *IEEE Transactions on Biomedical Engineering*, *42*(4), 411–415. doi:10.1109/10.376135 PMID:7729840

da Costa, J. C., Ortigueira, M. D., Batista, A., & Paiva, T. (2013). *ARMA modelling for sleep disorders diagnose.* Paper presented at the Doctoral Conference on Computing, Electrical and Industrial Systems.

Ge, D., Srinivasan, N., & Krishnan, S. M. (2002). Cardiac arrhythmia classification using autoregressive modeling. *Biomedical Engineering Online*, *1*(1), 5. doi:10.1186/1475-925X-1-5 PMID:12473180

Graupe, D., & Cline, W. K. (1975). Functional separation of EMG signals via ARMA identification methods for prosthesis control purposes. *IEEE Transactions on Systems, Man, and Cybernetics*, *SMC-5*(2), 252–259. doi:10.1109/TSMC.1975.5408479

Hayashi, T., Mizuno-Matsumoto, Y., Okamoto, E., Ishii, R., Ukai, S., & Shinosaki, K. (2008). *Anterior brain activities related to emotional stress.* Paper presented at the Automation Congress, 2008. WAC 2008. World.

Herring, D. R., Burleson, M. H., Roberts, N. A., & Devine, M. J. (2011). Coherent with laughter: Subjective experience, behavior, and physiological responses during amusement and joy. *International Journal of Psychophysiology*, *79*(2), 211–218. doi:10.1016/j.ijpsycho.2010.10.007 PMID:21034782

Holan, S. H., Lund, R., & Davis, G. (2010). The ARMA alphabet soup: A tour of ARMA model variants. *Statistics Surveys*, *4*(0), 232–274. doi:10.1214/09-SS060

Jantaro, S., Sayowan, W., Kotchabhakdi, N., Iamsupasit, S., Wankum, N., Hongsranagon, P., & … . (2014). Effect of Comedy Video Clip on Autonomic Response and Subjective Happiness of Thai Early Adults. *J Health Res-vol*, *28*(4).

Kemeny, M. E. (2003). The psychobiology of stress. *Current Directions in Psychological Science*, *12*(4), 124–129. doi:10.1111/1467-8721.01246

Kheirati Roonizi, E. (2017). *Adaptive models-based cardiac signal analysis and feature extraction.* Università degli Studi di Milano.

LabVIEW. (2014). *Discrete Gabor Transform and Expansion (Advanced Signal Processing Toolkit) - LabVIEW 2014 Advanced Signal Processing Toolkit Help - National Instruments.* Retrieved 25 May, 2017, from http://zone.ni.com/reference/en-XX/help/372656C-01/lvasptconcepts/tfa_discrete_gabor_trans_exp/

Lee, J., Nam, Y., McManus, D. D., & Chon, K. H. (2013). Time-varying coherence function for atrial fibrillation detection. *IEEE Transactions on Biomedical Engineering*, *60*(10), 2783–2793. doi:10.1109/TBME.2013.2264721 PMID:23708769

Li, W., & McLeod, A. (1981). Distribution of the residual autocorrelations in multivariate ARMA time series models. *Journal of the Royal Statistical Society. Series B. Methodological*, 231–239.

Llera, S. J., & Newman, M. G. (2010). Effects of worry on physiological and subjective reactivity to emotional stimuli in generalized anxiety disorder and nonanxious control participants. *Emotion (Washington, D.C.)*, *10*(5), 640–650. doi:10.1037/a0019351 PMID:21038947

MathWorks. (n.d.). *Differences and Approximate Derivatives*. Retrieved 23 May, 2017, from https://in.mathworks.com/help/matlab/ref/diff.html?searchHighlight=diff&s_tid=doc_srchtitle

McLeod, A. I., & Li, W. K. (1983). Diagnostic checking ARMA time series models using squared-residual autocorrelations. *Journal of Time Series Analysis*, *4*(4), 269–273. doi:10.1111/j.1467-9892.1983.tb00373.x

Mokashi, C., Nayak, S. K., Pradhan, A., Rout, S. K., Pal, K., & Champaty, B. (2016). *Effect of sound in a horror movie clip on the physiology of the ANS and the conduction pathway of the heart.* Paper presented at the India Conference (INDICON), 2016 IEEE Annual. 10.1109/INDICON.2016.7839020

Murugappan, M., Murugappan, S., & Zheng, B. S. (2013). Frequency band analysis of electrocardiogram (ECG) signals for human emotional state classification using discrete wavelet transform (DWT). *Journal of Physical Therapy Science*, *25*(7), 753–759. doi:10.1589/jpts.25.753 PMID:24259846

Nayak, S., Champaty, B., Ray, S. S., & Pal, K. (2014). *A study on the changes in the autonomic nervous system and cardio-electric physiology after viewing comedy movie clip: A case study.* Paper presented at the Control, Instrumentation, Communication and Computational Technologies (ICCICCT), 2014 International Conference on. 10.1109/ICCICCT.2014.6993113

Nayak, S. K., Shukla, R. D., Panda, I., Champaty, B., Thakur, G., & Mohapatra, B. (2016). Effect of Slow and Fast Music on the Autonomic Nervous System and Cardiac Health: A Preliminary Investigation. *Classification and Clustering in Biomedical Signal Processing*, 198.

Orini, M., Bailón, R., Mainardi, L., & Laguna, P. (2012). Synthesis of HRV signals characterized by predetermined time-frequency structure by means of time-varying ARMA models. *Biomedical Signal Processing and Control*, *7*(2), 141–150. doi:10.1016/j.bspc.2011.05.003

Pardey, J., Roberts, S., & Tarassenko, L. (1996). A review of parametric modelling techniques for EEG analysis. *Medical Engineering & Physics*, *18*(1), 2–11. doi:10.1016/1350-4533(95)00024-0 PMID:8771033

Pham, P., & Wang, J. (2017). *Understanding Emotional Responses to Mobile Video Advertisements via Physiological Signal Sensing and Facial Expression Analysis.* Paper presented at the Proceedings of the 22nd International Conference on Intelligent User Interfaces. 10.1145/3025171.3025186

Proverbio, A. M., Manfrin, L., Arcari, L. A., De Benedetto, F., Gazzola, M., Guardamagna, M., & … . (2015). Non-expert listeners show decreased heart rate and increased blood pressure (fear bradycardia) in response to atonal music. *Frontiers in Psychology*, 6. PMID:26579029

Sakuragi, S., Sugiyama, Y., & Takeuchi, K. (2002). Effects of laughing and weeping on mood and heart rate variability. *Journal of Physiological Anthropology and Applied Human Science*, *21*(3), 159–165. doi:10.2114/jpa.21.159 PMID:12148458

Salvioli, B., Pellegatta, G., Malacarne, M., Pace, F., Malesci, A., Pagani, M., & Lucini, D. (2015). Autonomic nervous system dysregulation in irritable bowel syndrome. *Neurogastroenterology and Motility*, *27*(3), 423–430. doi:10.1111/nmo.12512 PMID:25581440

Tkaczyszyn, M., Olbrycht, T., Makowska, A., Soboń, K., Paleczny, B., Rydlewska, A., & Jankowska, E. A. (2013). The influence of the sounds of crying baby and the sounds of violence on haemodynamic parameters and autonomic status in young, healthy adults. *International Journal of Psychophysiology, 87*(1), 52–59. doi:10.1016/j.ijpsycho.2012.10.017 PMID:23142485

Tsai, H.-H., & Yi, C.-W. (2015). *Wearable ECG for Tension Assessment in Movie Watching and Adventure Riding.* Paper presented at the Moile Ad-hoc and Sensor Networks (MSN), 2015 11th International Conference on. 10.1109/MSN.2015.45

Weisstein, E. W. (2002). *CRC concise encyclopedia of mathematics*. CRC Press. doi:10.1201/9781420035223

Zaidi, A. M. A., Ahmed, M. J., & Bakibillah, A. (2017). *Feature extraction and characterization of cardiovascular arrhythmia and normal sinus rhythm from ECG signals using LabVIEW.* Paper presented at the Imaging, Vision & Pattern Recognition (icIVPR), 2017 IEEE International Conference on. 10.1109/ICIVPR.2017.7890871

ADDITIONAL READING

Aguila, J., Arias, E., Artigao, M., & Miralles, J. (2011). A prediction of electrocardiography signals by combining arma model with nonlinear analysis methods. *Recent Researches in Applied Computer and Applied Computational Science, World Scientific and Engineering Academy and Society (WSEAS)*, 31-37.

Akselrod, S., Gordon, D., Madwed, J. B., Snidman, N., Shannon, D., & Cohen, R. (1985). Hemodynamic regulation: Investigation by spectral analysis. *American Journal of Physiology. Heart and Circulatory Physiology, 249*(4), H867–H875. doi:10.1152/ajpheart.1985.249.4.H867 PMID:4051021

Argenti, F., Facheris, L., & Giarré, L. (2016). *Adaptive quadratic regularization for baseline wandering removal in wearable ECG devices.* Paper presented at the Signal Processing Conference (EUSIPCO), 2016 24th European. 10.1109/EUSIPCO.2016.7760542

Avina-Cervantes, J., Torres-Cisneros, M., Martínez, J. S., & Pinales, J. (2006). *Frequency, time-frequency and wavelet analysis of ECG signal.* Paper presented at the Electronics and Photonics, 2006. MEP 2006. Multiconference on. 10.1109/MEP.2006.335676

Bartoli, F., Baselli, G., & Cerutti, S. (1985). AR identification and spectral estimate applied to the RR interval measurements. *International Journal of Bio-Medical Computing, 16*(3-4), 201–215. doi:10.1016/0020-7101(85)90055-8 PMID:3891637

Begg, R. (2006). *Neural Networks in Healthcare: Potential and Challenges: Potential and Challenges.* Igi Global. doi:10.4018/978-1-59140-848-2

Benitez, D., Gaydecki, P., Zaidi, A., & Fitzpatrick, A. (2001). The use of the Hilbert transform in ECG signal analysis. *Computers in Biology and Medicine, 31*(5), 399–406. doi:10.1016/S0010-4825(01)00009-9 PMID:11535204

Berger, R. D., Saul, J. P., & Cohen, R. J. (1989). Transfer function analysis of autonomic regulation. I. Canine atrial rate response. *American Journal of Physiology. Heart and Circulatory Physiology*, *256*(1), H142–H152. doi:10.1152/ajpheart.1989.256.1.H142 PMID:2912176

Boudraa, A.-O., & Cexus, J.-C. (2006). Denoising via empirical mode decomposition. *Proc. IEEE ISCCSP*, *4*, 2006.

Brockway, B., & Brockway, M. (2013). ECG sensing with noise filtering: Google Patents.

Chon, K. H., & Cohen, R. J. (1997). Linear and nonlinear ARMA model parameter estimation using an artificial neural network. *IEEE Transactions on Biomedical Engineering*, *44*(3), 168–174. doi:10.1109/10.554763 PMID:9216130

Giuliani, N. R., McRae, K., & Gross, J. J. (2008). The up-and down-regulation of amusement: Experiential, behavioral, and autonomic consequences. *Emotion (Washington, D.C.)*, *8*(5), 714–719. doi:10.1037/a0013236 PMID:18837622

Goel, V., & Dolan, R. J. (2007). Social regulation of affective experience of humor. *Journal of Cognitive Neuroscience*, *19*(9), 1574–1580. doi:10.1162/jocn.2007.19.9.1574 PMID:17714017

Herring, D. R., Burleson, M. H., Roberts, N. A., & Devine, M. J. (2011). Coherent with laughter: Subjective experience, behavior, and physiological responses during amusement and joy. *International Journal of Psychophysiology*, *79*(2), 211–218. doi:10.1016/j.ijpsycho.2010.10.007 PMID:21034782

Hubert, W., & de Jong-Meyer, R. (1991). Autonomic, neuroendocrine, and subjective responses to emotion-inducing film stimuli. *International Journal of Psychophysiology*, *11*(2), 131–140. doi:10.1016/0167-8760(91)90005-I PMID:1748588

Kam, A., & Cohen, A. (1999). *Detection of fetal ECG with IIR adaptive filtering and genetic algorithms.* Paper presented at the Acoustics, Speech, and Signal Processing, 1999. Proceedings., 1999 IEEE International Conference on. 10.1109/ICASSP.1999.758406

Kathirvel, P., Manikandan, M. S., Prasanna, S., & Soman, K. (2011). An efficient R-peak detection based on new nonlinear transformation and first-order Gaussian differentiator. *Cardiovascular Engineering and Technology*, *2*(4), 408–425. doi:10.100713239-011-0065-3

Korürek, M., & Doğan, B. (2010). ECG beat classification using particle swarm optimization and radial basis function neural network. *Expert Systems with Applications*, *37*(12), 7563–7569. doi:10.1016/j.eswa.2010.04.087

Lin, C.-C. (2008). Enhancement of accuracy and reproducibility of parametric modeling for estimating abnormal intra-QRS potentials in signal-averaged electrocardiograms. *Medical Engineering & Physics*, *30*(7), 834–842. doi:10.1016/j.medengphy.2007.10.001 PMID:17997342

Lu, G., Brittain, J.-S., Holland, P., Yianni, J., Green, A. L., Stein, J. F., ... Wang, S. (2009). Removing ECG noise from surface EMG signals using adaptive filtering. *Neuroscience Letters*, *462*(1), 14–19. doi:10.1016/j.neulet.2009.06.063 PMID:19559751

Martín-Martínez, D., Casaseca-de-la-Higuera, P., Martín-Fernández, M., & Alberola-López, C. (2014). *ECG Signal Reconstruction Based on Stochastic Joint-Modeling of the ECG and the PPG Signals.* Paper presented at the XIII Mediterranean Conference on Medical and Biological Engineering and Computing 2013. 10.1007/978-3-319-00846-2_245

Martis, R. J., Acharya, U. R., Lim, C. M., & Suri, J. S. (2013). Characterization of ECG beats from cardiac arrhythmia using discrete cosine transform in PCA framework. *Knowledge-Based Systems, 45*, 76–82. doi:10.1016/j.knosys.2013.02.007

Min, H., Yuan, L. G., Chang-wei, M., & Jing, C. (2009). *An application of electrocardiography to emotion recognition.* Paper presented at the Natural Computation, 2009. ICNC'09. Fifth International Conference on. 10.1109/ICNC.2009.338

Moavenian, M., & Khorrami, H. (2010). A qualitative comparison of artificial neural networks and support vector machines in ECG arrhythmias classification. *Expert Systems with Applications*, *37*(4), 3088–3093. doi:10.1016/j.eswa.2009.09.021

Pande, K., Nayak, S. K., Gaur, D., Ray, S. S., Pal, K., Patel, S. J., ... (2017). *Effect of a humorous audio-visual stimulus on autonomic nervous system and heart of females.* Paper presented at the Signal Processing Conference (EUSIPCO), 2017 25th European. 10.23919/EUSIPCO.2017.8081243

Prasad, G. K., & Sahambi, J. (2003). *Classification of ECG arrhythmias using multi-resolution analysis and neural networks.* Paper presented at the TENCON 2003. Conference on Convergent Technologies for the Asia-Pacific Region. 10.1109/TENCON.2003.1273320

Sohn, J.-H., Sokhadze, E., & Watanuki, S. (2001). Electrodermal and cardiovascular manifestations of emotions in children. *Journal of Physiological Anthropology and Applied Human Science*, *20*(2), 55–64. doi:10.2114/jpa.20.55 PMID:11385939

Thakor, N. V., & Zhu, Y.-S. (1991). Applications of adaptive filtering to ECG analysis: Noise cancellation and arrhythmia detection. *IEEE Transactions on Biomedical Engineering*, *38*(8), 785–794. doi:10.1109/10.83591 PMID:1937512

Übeyli, E. D. (2007). ECG beats classification using multiclass support vector machines with error correcting output codes. *Digital Signal Processing*, *17*(3), 675–684. doi:10.1016/j.dsp.2006.11.009

Übeyli, E. D. (2008). Recurrent neural networks with composite features for detection of electrocardiographic changes in partial epileptic patients. *Computers in Biology and Medicine*, *38*(3), 401–410. doi:10.1016/j.compbiomed.2008.01.002 PMID:18275945

Übeyli, E. D. (2009). Combining recurrent neural networks with eigenvector methods for classification of ECG beats. *Digital Signal Processing*, *19*(2), 320–329. doi:10.1016/j.dsp.2008.09.002

Übeyli, E. D. (2010). Recurrent neural networks employing Lyapunov exponents for analysis of ECG signals. *Expert Systems with Applications*, *37*(2), 1192–1199. doi:10.1016/j.eswa.2009.06.022

Xiong, Y., & Yeung, D.-Y. (2004). Time series clustering with ARMA mixtures. *Pattern Recognition*, *37*(8), 1675–1689. doi:10.1016/j.patcog.2003.12.018

Zheng, B. S., Murugappan, M., & Yaacob, S. (2012). *Human emotional stress assessment through Heart Rate Detection in a customized protocol experiment.* Paper presented at the Industrial Electronics and Applications (ISIEA), 2012 IEEE Symposium on.

KEY TERMS AND DEFINITIONS

ARMA: ARMA or autoregressive moving average model is a method to describe a weakly stationary time series using two different polynomials where one represents auto regression and the other indicates the moving average.

Artificial Neural Network: Artificial neural network or ANN is a machine learning technique, inspired from the working of human brain, that uses neurons and dendrites. It consists of nodes interlinked to each other just like the neurons. It is in fact a computer simulation that can be used for classification, clustering, pattern recognition, etc.

Autonomic Nervous System: A branch of the peripheral nervous system, regulated by the hypothalamus, that itself branches into sympathetic and parasympathetic nervous systems and controls involuntary activities like heart rate, respiration rate, digestion, papillary response, etc.

Electrocardiography: A simple technique to measure the electrical activity of the heart which is painlessly done using ECG or EKG sensors.

Gabor Denoising: A high frequency noise interference reduction technique that uses discrete Gabor transform (DGT). It can be implemented by selecting the time varying filter palette in LabVIEW with suitable thresholding.

Heart Rate Variability: The beat-to-beat variability in the time duration measured between subsequent R peaks is regarded as heart rate variability. It is an important parameter to understand the physiological changes taking place in the ANS.

SA Node: The element in the conduction pathway of the heart that generates the electrical stimulation.

Chapter 12
Wavelet Packet Analysis of ECG Signals to Understand the Effect of Cannabis Abuse on Cardiac Electrophysiology of Indian Women Working in Paddy Fields

Suraj Kumar Nayak
National Institute of Technology Rourkela, India

Soumanti Das
National Institute of Technology Rourkela, India

Ashirbad Pradhan
National Institute of Technology Rourkela, India

Gitika Yadu
National Institute of Technology Rourkela, India

Salman Siddique Khan
National Institute of Technology Rourkela, India

Shankar Jaykishan Patel
Jagnyaseni Hospital, India

Shikshya Nayak
Veer Surendra Sai University of Technology, India

Champak Bhattacharyya
National Institute of Technology Rourkela, India

Kunal Pal
National Institute of Technology Rourkela, India

ABSTRACT

This chapter is aimed at identifying the variation in the cardiac electrophysiology due to the abuse of the cannabis products (bhang) in a non-invasive manner. ECG signals were acquired from 25 Indian women working in the paddy fields. Amongst them, 10 women regularly abused bhang and the rest 15 women never abused bhang. The ECG signals were preprocessed and subjected to wavelet packet decomposition (WPD) up to the level 3 using db04 wavelet. Ninety-six statistical features were extracted from the wavelet packet coefficients and analyzed using linear and non-linear statistical methods. The results suggested a variation in the cardiac electrophysiology due to the abuse of bhang. Artificial neural networks (ANNs), namely, radial basis function (RBF) and multilayer perceptron (MLP) were able to classify the ECG signals with an accuracy of ≥95%. This supported the hypothesis that abuse of bhang may alter the cardiac electrophysiology. The results of the study may be used to increase awareness among people to avoid the abuse of cannabis products.

DOI: 10.4018/978-1-5225-4969-7.ch012

INTRODUCTION

The abuse of *Cannabis sativa* based products for recreational purposes is common across the globe (Bachs & Mørland, 2001). Although severe restrictions have been imposed by the Government of India (GoI) on many of the cannabis products such as Marijuana, and Hashish, the restrictions on bhang (a recreational product made from the leaves of cannabis plant) is not so strong. It is widely abused by the common people (especially in villages) due to its low cost. Further, it is also used to make drinks by people belonging to Hindu religion during certain carnivals (Nayak et al., 2016). However, some recent studies have reported the onset of cardiovascular diseases in the people abusing cannabis, which may even lead to mortality (Menahem, 2013). Although the effect of cannabis products on human health has been much reviewed, not much work was found to analyze the effect of cannabis on the cardiac electrophysiology (Nayak et al., 2016). The physiology of the heart can be non-invasively analyzed using ECG signal analysis (Opie, 2004). Feature extraction is one of the important steps in the analysis of the ECG signals. The features should be extracted in such a way that they can contain the essential information about the original data in a reduced dimension. Thus, the features can be used, instead of the original signal, for performing desired signal processing operations. In some cases, the features have been reported to provide better interpretation than the original signals (Guyon & Elisseeff, 2006; Li & Zhou, 2016). In recent years, wavelet-based feature extraction methods such as discrete wavelet transform (DWT) and its recent extension WPD are gaining popularity among the researchers for the extraction of features from the ECG signals (Gokhale & Khanduja, 2010; Mahapatra, Mohanta, Mohanty, kumar Nayak, & kumar Behari, 2016; Rai, Trivedi, & Shukla, 2013). Amongst them, WPD has been reported to be superior as it decomposes not only the approximation coefficients (AC) but also the detailed coefficients (DCs) in contrast to the DWT, which decomposes only the ACs. As a result, both the DCs and the ACs can be used to extract features to provide more information (Li & Zhou, 2016). Numerous methods have been proposed for the classification of the ECG signals such as Fuzzy Logic (Kundu, Nasipuri, & Basu, 1998), Support Vector Machine (SVM) (Maldonado, Leija, Vera, & Alvarado, 2016), K-Nearest Neighbor (K-NN) method (Faziludeen & Sankaran, 2016) and Artificial Neural Network (ANN) (Gautam & Giri, 2016). Amongst them, the ANN-based algorithms are gaining popularity in recent years (Roza, de Almeida, & Postolache, 2017). This may be attributed to the fact that ANN provides the facility to improve the classification accuracy easily because of its multi-parametric nature (Alexakis et al., 2003). Taking the motivation from the above-mentioned discussion, we have attempted to investigate the effect of regular bhang abuse on the cardiac electrophysiology of Indian women working in the paddy fields. The ECG signals were acquired from the volunteers, and WPD analysis of the ECG signals was performed to extract features. Statistical significance of the features was analyzed using linear and non-linear statistical methods, and ANN classification was carried out using the statistically significant features.

BACKGROUND

The rhythmic electrical activity within the heart results in the rhythmic contraction of the heart muscles. Initially, the electrical impulse is generated at the sinoatrial node (SA node), located on the right atrium close to the superior vena cava (Boyett, Honjo, & Kodama, 2000). The SA node is 15 mm long, 3 mm wide and 1 mm thick. It is made up of specialized cardiac muscles. A connection exists between the SA node and the atrial muscle fibers allowing the transmission of the electrical impulse (Monfredi, Dobrzynski, Mondal, Boyett, & Morris, 2010). The impulse gets transmitted to the atrioventricular node (AV node) within an interval of 0.03 msec. A bundle of fibers called AV bundle is associated with the AV node. The bundle is capable of providing an unidirectional flow of the impulse i.e. from the atrium to the ventricles due to its property of restricting the backward flow of the impulse (Hall, 2015). The bundle adds a delay of 1.3 msec to the impulse that allows the proper contraction of the atria to finish the flow of blood to the ventricles (Burns, 2013). A specialized cardiac muscle called Purkinje fiber is present between AV node and ventricles, which helps in the instantaneous distribution of the impulse across the endocardial surfaces of the ventricle within a time interval of 0.03 msec (Rentschler et al., 2001). Then it is transmitted to the epicardial surface of the ventricle by the ventricular muscle fiber (Torrent-Guasp et al., 2001). The impulse passing through the heart spreads to the surrounding environment and small amplitude of it reaches the surface of the body. The impulse reaching the skin surface is detected by placing electrodes on the skin, and provides an indication of the cardiac electrophysiology (Barr & Van Oosterom, 2010). A graphical illustration of this cardiac electrophysiology is called the electrocardiogram (ECG) (Harland, Clark, Peters, Everitt, & Stiffell, 2005). A physiologically standard ECG wave is comprised of different types of waves, namely, the P wave, the QRS complex and the T wave (Hurst, 1998). The P wave is defined as the electrical potential resulting from the depolarization of atria. The QRS complex denotes the electrical potential resulting from the depolarization of the ventricles (Dilaveris & Gialafos, 2001). The T wave is caused by the electrical potential resulting from the repolarization of the ventricles (Wellens, Bär, & Lie, 1978). Thus, the P wave and the QRS complex are often called the depolarization waves, whereas the T wave is called the repolarization wave (Opthof et al., 2007). The amplitude of these ECG constituent waves depends on the locations of the electrodes, placed on the skin surface, and their closeness to the heart (Schijvenaars, Kors, van Herpen, Kornreich, & van Bemmel, 1997). The QRS complex amplitude of 3-4 mV has been reported in the cases where one electrode is placed directly over the left ventricle and the other electrode is placed anywhere else on the body, away from the heart. This amplitude is, however, very less as compared to the electrode potential measured directly from the heart membrane, i.e. 110 mV. For electrodes placed on forearms of the two hands or on one forearm and one leg as per the Einthoven's triangle, the QRS complex has been reported to vary from 1 to 1.5 mV (Bacharova, Selvester, Engblom, & Wagner, 2005). For the same arrangement of the electrodes, the amplitude of the P wave ranges between 0.1 and 0.3 mV and the amplitude of the T wave ranges from 0.2 to 0.3 mV. An important parameter of the ECG signal is the PQ interval, which is defined as the time interval between the inception of the P wave and the inception of the Q wave. Physiologically it represents the time gap between the beginning of the atrial contraction and the ventricular contraction, with an average value of 0.16 sec. In case, the Q wave is absent, the time interval between the beginning of the atrial contraction and the ventricular contraction is depicted by the PR interval (Gervais et al., 2009). The ventricles contract for about 0.35 sec, and in a standard ECG signal, it is represented by the time interval between the inception of the Q wave and the completion of the T wave, also called as the QT interval (Okin et al., 2000). ECG signals have been widely explored for the diagnosis of various cardiological diseases (Desai, Martis, Nayak, Sarika, & Seshikala, 2015) as well as for understanding the effect of various stimuli (e.g., music, smoking, and exercise) on the cardiac electrophysiology (Hajizadeh, Abbasi, & Goshvarpour, 2015). Elhaj *et al.* (2016) reported the recognition and classification of five types of beat classes of arrhythmia (as per the recommendation of the Association for Advancement of Medical Instrumentation), namely, non-ectopic beats, supraventricular ectopic beats, ventricular ectopic beats, fusion beats, and unclassifiable paced beats using linear and non-linear features of ECG signals (Elhaj, Salim, Harris, Swee, & Ahmed, 2016). The linear features included the outcomes of the principal component analysis of the discrete wavelet transform coefficients, whereas the non-linear features included the higher order statistics and cumulants. The different classes of arrhythmia could be classified with a maximum classification accuracy of 98.91% using a composite method employing both SVM and ANN. Abedi *et al.* (2017) performed ECG signal analysis to understand the effect of a Persian music on the heart of young women. In their study, the ECG signals were acquired from 22 healthy females in resting condition and while listening to music (Abedi, Abbasi, & Goshvarpour, 2017). The ECG signals were processed to extract 20 morphological and DWT-based features. These features were subjected to classification using ANN and probabilistic neural network (PNN) by dividing the whole data into training and testing datasets. The training data set could be classified with the accuracy of 88% and 97% using ANN and PNN, respectively. On the other hand, the testing data set was classified with the accuracy of 84% and 93% using ANN and PNN, respectively. Fujita *et al.* (2017) reported the use of WPD analysis of ECG signals for the diagnosis of coronary artery disease, myocardial infarction, and congestive heart failure. The ECG signals were decomposed into 30 WPD coefficients and 12 nonlinear features were extracted from each coefficient. The KNN classifier was used to provide the classification accuracy of 97.98%, sensitivity of 99.61% and specificity of 94.84% using 8 ReliefF ranked features as the input.

The abuse of cannabis-based products (e.g., Marijuana, and Hashish) for recreational purposes is growing day-by-day (Bachs & Mørland, 2001), although the abuse of most of these products is strictly abandoned by the Government of India. Bhang is a recreational product made from the leaves of cannabis plant. It is widely abused by the people residing in the villages apart from people following Hindu religion. In the last few decades, many researchers have reported the incidence of cardiovascular diseases or even death in people abusing cannabis products (Menahem, 2013; Wolff, Rouyer, & Gény, 2013). However, not much research has been performed on understanding the cardiac physiology in people abusing cannabis regularly (Nayak et al., 2016). Based on the facts mentioned above, the present work aims at identifying the changes in the cardiac electrophysiology due to the cannabis abuse using WPD analysis of the ECG signals.

MAIN FOCUS OF THE CHAPTER

The main focus of this study is to analyze the effect of the abuse of cannabis-based products such as bhang on the cardiac electrophysiology of Indian women in a non-invasive manner using ECG signal analysis. The study was motivated by the fact that most of the Indian women, working in the paddy fields, abuse cannabis. The understanding of the effect of cannabis abuse on the electrical activity of the heart can be used enhance the awareness of these women regarding the negative impact of cannabis products on the cardiac health.

METHODOLOGY

Acquisition of ECG Signals

This study involved ECG signal acquisition from Indian women (volunteers), who have been working in the paddy field for at least last 5 years. 30 volunteers were invited for the study. The details of the study was explained to them, and they were requested to sign an informed consent form if they generated interested to take part in the study. Out of the 30 volunteers, 25 volunteers provided their consent to participate in this study. They belonged to the age group of 20 to 50 years. Amongst the 25 volunteers, 15 volunteers never abused bhang and were categorized under the Category-A. The rest 10 volunteers regularly abused bhang and were put under the Category-B. The ECG signals were acquired from the volunteers for 6 min using ECG clamp electrodes placed in the lead-1 configuration. The ECG signals were amplified using a commercially available ECG amplifier (Vernier EKG, Vernier Software & Technology, USA). The amplified ECG signals were then digitized using a data acquisition device (NI USB 6009, National Instruments, USA) and recorded into a computer using a LabVIEW (V13.0, National instruments, USA) program. The sampling frequency of the data acquisition device was set at 1000 Hz.

Wavelet Packet Analysis

In this study, the 6 min ECG signal was processed using a LabVIEW program to extract a 5 sec portion. This signal was band-limited using a low-pass filter of cut-off frequency 50 Hz and resampled at 360 Hz using a Spline interpolation function prior to WPD (Li & Zhou, 2016). The resampled ECG signals were subjected to WPD up to level 3 with Daubechies (db04) as the mother wavelet. The reason for choosing Daubechies wavelet may be attributed to its similarity with the shape of the QRS complex of the ECG wave (Ray, Nayak, Champaty, Tibarewala, & Pal, 2016). The WPD analysis resulted in the formation of 8 wavelet packet coefficients, representing the frequency sub-bands. Each of these 8 wavelet packet coefficients was used to extract 12 statistical parameters. As a result, 96 statistical parameters were extracted from each ECG signal. The entire wavelet packet analysis was implemented using in-lab designed LabVIEW programs.

Statistical Analysis and ANN Classification

These 96 wavelet-based statistical parameters were subjected to statistical analysis for identification of the important predictors, having significantly different values in Category-A and Category-B. The linear method t-test (p-value ≤ 0.05) and the decision tree-based non-linear methods (predictor importance ≥ 0.95), namely, Classification And Regression Tree (CART), Boosted Tree (BT) and Random Forest (RF) were employed for this purpose using Statistica software (trial V13.2, Dell Inc., USA). The statistically significant parameters obtained from the afore-mentioned statistical analysis were used as input for further analysis using ANN. The conventional ANN networks, namely, RBF and MLP were implemented using Statistical Data Miner toolkit to classify the ECG signals into Category-A and Category-B.

RESULTS AND DISCUSSION

The 3 level WPD analysis of each ECG signal resulted in the formation 8 wavelet packet coefficients (Figure 1). These coefficients were named as 000, 001, 010, 011, 100, 101, 110 and 111. The 12 parameters extracted from each wavelet packet coefficient include Arithmetic Mean (AM), Mode (MOD), Median (MED), Summation (SUM), Standard Deviation (SD), Variance, Root Mean Square value (RMS), Kurtosis, Skewness (SKNS), Energy Density (ED), Log Energy (LE), and Shannon Entropy (SE). Thus, the finally extracted 96 parameters were named as P-E, where P stands for the name of the

Figure 1. WPD of an ECG signal into level-3 using db04 wavelet

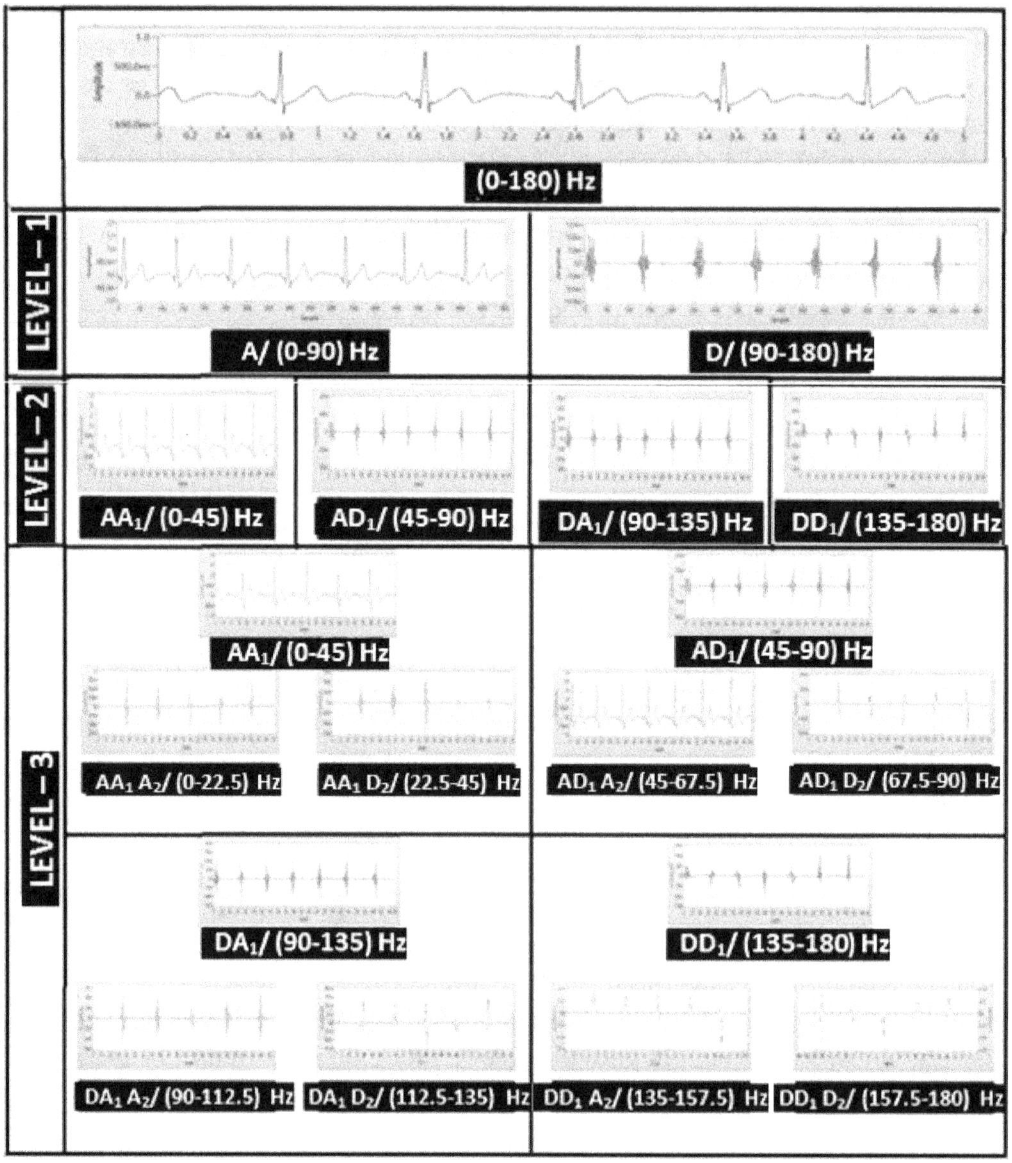

statistical parameter and E represents the name of the wavelet packet coefficient. Out of the statistical parameters, none was found to be statistically significant from the t-test analysis. The t-test is a linear statistical method that can be used to detect the occurrence of any significant variation in the mean values of the parameters of two populations (Ray et al., 2016). CART is a decision tree algorithm mainly used to design models for prediction from a given set of data (Lewis, 2000). In this method, the dataset is broken down into segments, and a prediction model is fitted for each segment. The problems which involve discrete values for the target variable would prefer a classification tree, whereas a regression tree would be useful for the problems involving continuous target variable. The misclassification cost is used to derive the classification error in the classification trees (Lemon, Roy, Clark, Friedmann, &

Rakowski, 2003). However, in the case of regression trees, the prediction error is calculated as the square of the difference between predicted and measured values (Harrell Jr, 2015). The CART analysis suggested that Skewness of the 1st wavelet packet coefficient (SKNS000) is an important predictor, having a higher value in Category-B as compared to Category-A (Table 1). Skewness measures the asymmetry of the frequency distribution curve of a variable with respect to its mean. This suggested that the frequency distribution curve of the first wavelet packet coefficient was more deviated from its mean value in Category-B as compared to Category-A. Boosted tree is considered as one of the most robust and efficient data mining tools for making predictions. It is used both for regression and classification problems, depending on whether the target variable is continuous or discrete (Windeatt & Ardeshir, 2002). The idea of boosted trees originated from the application of boosting methods to regression trees (Elith, Leathwick, & Hastie, 2008). This method involves the generation of a sequence of binary trees, and each successive tree is generated based on the prediction residuals of the previous tree. Mode of the 4th wavelet packet coefficient (MOD011) was found to be the only important predictor from BT analysis. RF is also a powerful decision tree algorithm, used for both classification and regression problems. It was first introduced by Breiman (Svetnik et al., 2003). It involves some simple tree predictors (Strobl, Malley, & Tutz, 2009), in which each tree predictor generates an outcome when a group of predictor variables is provided. The group of predictor variables is chosen independently and is responsible for the outcome of the tree predictor. The Median of the 4th wavelet packet coefficient (MED011) was identified as the important predictor from RF analysis. The occurrence of these important predictors suggested that the properties of the ECG signals acquired from the volunteers belonging to Category-A and Category-B varied significantly.

To further ascertain the variation in the characteristics of the ECG signals of the volunteers belonging to Category-A and Category-B, ANN classification was performed. ANN is a non-linear, supervised, computational method inspired by the working of the biological neural networks (Jain, Mao, & Mohiuddin, 1996). It consists of nodes (neurons), which are connected to each other. ANN uses multiple inputs with weights acting upon them, a threshold function and an activation function for finding the output. The weights are calculated during training, thus, generating the model (Agatonovic-Kustrin & Beresford, 2000). In our study, the important predictors, in various combinations, were used as the input for the widely used neural networks, namely, MLP and RBF. The MLP network is regarded as one of the best-known class of neural network. It is characterized by one or more hidden layer of neurons and does not generate closed class boundaries (Markou & Singh, 2003). On the other hand, the RBF network represents another important class of neural network containing only a single layer of hidden neurons. In a RBF network, the distance between an input vector and prototype vector determines the activation of the hidden unit. The MLP 2-8-2 network was able to classify the important predictors with an overall

Table 1. Important predictors obtained from statistical analysis of the wavelet packet coefficient parameters

Methods	Features	Mean ± SD		Predictor Importance
		Category-A	Category-B	
CART	SKNS000	1.862 ± 0.715	2.184 ± 0.568	1.000
BT	MOD011	0.000 ± 0.001	-0.0003 ± 0.002	1.000
RF	MED011	0.000 ± 0.0003	-0.0001 ± 0.0003	1.000

classification efficiency of 100% when SKNS000 and MED011 were used as the inputs (Table 2). The network used BFGS 50 algorithm for its training and Entropy was used as the error function. The hidden activation function and the output activation function were logistic function and Softmax function, respectively. On the other hand, the RBF 2-20-2 network was able to provide a classification efficiency of 95% with the same variables as the inputs and RBFT as the training algorithm. Gaussian function was used as the hidden activation function. The error function and the output activation function were same as that of the MLP 2-8-2 network. The classification summary of the MLP 2-8-2 and the RBF 2-20-2 networks has been tabulated in Table 3 and 4.

The Association for the Advancement of Medical Instrumentation (AAMI) recommends the evaluation of the performance of the neural networks using four benchmark statistical indices, i.e., sensitivity (SE), positive predictivity (+P), false positive rate (FPR) and accuracy (ACC) (Li & Zhou, 2016). These performance indices can be computed from the analysis of the true positive (TP), false negative (FN), true negative (TN) and false positive (FP) results of the test as given Equation 1-4 (Li & Zhou, 2016). TP indicates the number of cases of a particular class correctly classified, whereas, FN signifies the number of cases of a particular class incorrectly classified, respectively. TN is used to identify the number of

Table 2. Architecture details of MLP 2-8-2 and RBF 2-20-2 networks

Networks	Features Used	Classification Efficiency (%)	Training Performance (%)	Testing Performance (%)	Algorithm	Error Function	Hidden Activation Function	Output Activation Function
MLP 2-8-2	SKNS000, MED011	100	100	100	BFGS 50	Entropy	Logistic	Softmax
RBF 2-20-2	SKNS000, MED011	95	100	80	RBFT	Entropy	Gaussian	Softmax

Table 3. Classification summary of MLP 2-8-2 network

	Category-A	Category-B	Overall
Total	15.000	10.000	25.000
Correct	15.000	10.000	25.000
Incorrect	0.000	0.000	0.000
Correct (%)	100.000	100.000	100.000
Incorrect (%)	0.000	0.000	0.000

Table 4. Classification summary of RBF 2-20-2 network

	Category-A	Category-B	Overall
Total	15.000	10.000	25.000
Correct	15.000	9.000	24.000
Incorrect	0.0000	1.000	1.000
Correct (%)	100.0000	90.000	95.000
Incorrect (%)	0.000	10.000	5.000

cases, which do not belong to a particular class and are classified as not belonging to the considered class and FP represents the number of the cases incorrectly classified as belonging to a particular class, which in actuality do not belong that class (Luz, Nunes, De Albuquerque, Papa, & Menotti, 2013). The values of SE, +P, FPR and ACC were calculated for both the MLP 2-8-2 and RBF 2-20-2 networks and have been tabulated in Table 5. In summary, both the MLP and RBF ANN networks were able to classify the important ECG predictors with an accuracy ≥95%. This, in turn, supported the inference drawn from the statistical analysis of the wavelet packet based ECG parameters that significant variation has occurred in the ECG signals (i.e., cardiac electrophysiology) due to the abuse of bhang.

$$SE = \frac{TP}{TP + FN} \times 100\ \% \tag{1}$$

$$+P = \frac{TP}{TP + FP} \times 100\ \% \tag{2}$$

$$FPR = \frac{FP}{TN + FP} \times 100\ \% \tag{3}$$

$$ACC = \frac{TP + TN}{TP + TN + FP + FN} \times 100\ \% \tag{4}$$

FUTURE RESEARCH DIRECTIONS

The present research was devoted to the detection of the alteration in the cardiac electrophysiology in Indian women due to cannabis abuse using WPD-based analysis of ECG signals. Future studies may be performed using other ECG signal analysis techniques (e.g., empirical mode decomposition (EMD), recurrence quantification analysis (RQA), and autoregression moving average (ARMA) modeling) to identify the most suitable method. The RR intervals can be extracted from the ECG signals to perform heart rate variability (HRV) analysis, which can divulge information about the autonomic nervous system in a non-invasive manner.

Table 5. Performance evaluation of the RBF AND MLP networks

Networks Used	Sensitivity (SE)	Positive Predictivity (+P)	False Positive Rate (FPR)	Accuracy (ACC)
MLP 5-8-2	100%	100%	0%	100%
RBF 5-7-2	95%	95%	5%	95%

CONCLUSION

ECG signals were acquired for 6 min from 25 female volunteers belonging to Category-A (volunteers not abusing bhang) and Category-B (volunteers abusing bhang). 5 sec portion of the ECG signals were extracted and preprocessed before subjecting to WPD analysis. WPD of the ECG signals was performed up to level 3 using db04 wavelet, resulting in the formation of 8 wavelet packet coefficients from each ECG signal. A total of 96 statistical parameters were computed from these 8 wavelet packet coefficients. Linear and non-linear statistical methods indicated 3 parameters (i.e., SKNS000, MOD011, and MED011) as statistically important. These parameters suggested a variation in the cardiac electrophysiology due to the abuse of bhang. However, ANN classification was performed to further ascertain the variation. Both MLP and RBF ANN networks were able to provide a classification accuracy of ≥95%. This confirmed the variation the cardiac electrophysiology because of bhang abuse. An in-depth analysis can be performed in future to identify the exact changes in the cardiac electrophysiology.

REFERENCES

Abedi, B., Abbasi, A., & Goshvarpour, A. (2017). Investigating the effect of traditional Persian music on ECG signals in young women using wavelet transform and neural networks. *Anatolian Journal of Cardiology. Anadolu Kardiyoloji Dergisi*, *17*(5).

Agatonovic-Kustrin, S., & Beresford, R. (2000). Basic concepts of artificial neural network (ANN) modeling and its application in pharmaceutical research. *Journal of Pharmaceutical and Biomedical Analysis*, *22*(5), 717–727. doi:10.1016/S0731-7085(99)00272-1 PMID:10815714

Alexakis, C., Nyongesa, H., Saatchi, R., Harris, N., Davies, C., & Emery, C. (2003). *Feature extraction and classification of electrocardiogram (ECG) signals related to hypoglycaemia*. Paper presented at the Computers in Cardiology.

Bacharova, L., Selvester, R. H., Engblom, H., & Wagner, G. S. (2005). Where is the central terminal located?: In search of understanding the use of the Wilson central terminal for production of 9 of the standard 12 electrocardiogram leads. *Journal of Electrocardiology*, *38*(2), 119–127. doi:10.1016/j.jelectrocard.2005.01.002 PMID:15892021

Bachs, L., & Mørland, H. (2001). Acute cardiovascular fatalities following cannabis use. *Forensic Science International*, *124*(2), 200–203. doi:10.1016/S0379-0738(01)00609-0 PMID:11792512

Barr, R. C., & Van Oosterom, A. (2010). Genesis of the electrocardiogram. In *Comprehensive electrocardiology* (pp. 167–190). Springer. doi:10.1007/978-1-84882-046-3_5

Boyett, M. R., Honjo, H., & Kodama, I. (2000). The sinoatrial node, a heterogeneous pacemaker structure. *Cardiovascular Research*, *47*(4), 658–687. doi:10.1016/S0008-6363(00)00135-8 PMID:10974216

Burns, N. (2013). Cardiovascular Physiology. School of Medicine, Trinity College.

Camm, A. J., Malik, M., Bigger, J., Breithardt, G., Cerutti, S., & Cohen, R. J. (1996). Heart rate variability: Standards of measurement, physiological interpretation and clinical use. Task Force of the European Society of Cardiology and the North American Society of Pacing and Electrophysiology. *Circulation*, *93*(5), 1043–1065. doi:10.1161/01.CIR.93.5.1043 PMID:8598068

Desai, U., Martis, R. J., Nayak, C. G., Sarika, K., & Seshikala, G. (2015). *Machine intelligent diagnosis of ECG for arrhythmia classification using DWT, ICA and SVM techniques.* Paper presented at the India Conference (INDICON), 2015 Annual IEEE. 10.1109/INDICON.2015.7443220

Dilaveris, P. E., & Gialafos, J. E. (2001). P-wave dispersion: A novel predictor of paroxysmal atrial fibrillation. *Annals of Noninvasive Electrocardiology*, *6*(2), 159–165. doi:10.1111/j.1542-474X.2001.tb00101.x PMID:11333174

Elhaj, F. A., Salim, N., Harris, A. R., Swee, T. T., & Ahmed, T. (2016). Arrhythmia recognition and classification using combined linear and nonlinear features of ECG signals. *Computer Methods and Programs in Biomedicine*, *127*, 52–63. doi:10.1016/j.cmpb.2015.12.024 PMID:27000289

Elith, J., Leathwick, J. R., & Hastie, T. (2008). A working guide to boosted regression trees. *Journal of Animal Ecology*, *77*(4), 802–813. doi:10.1111/j.1365-2656.2008.01390.x PMID:18397250

Faziludeen, S., & Sankaran, P. (2016). ECG Beat Classification Using Evidential K-Nearest Neighbours. *Procedia Computer Science*, *89*, 499–505. doi:10.1016/j.procs.2016.06.106

Gautam, M. K., & Giri, V. K. (2016). An Approach of Neural Network For Electrocardiogram Classification. *APTIKOM Journal on Computer Science and Information Technologies*, *1*(3), 115–123.

Gervais, R., Leclercq, C., Shankar, A., Jacobs, S., Eiskjaer, H., Johannessen, A., ... Daubert, C. (2009). Surface electrocardiogram to predict outcome in candidates for cardiac resynchronization therapy: A sub-analysis of the CARE-HF trial. *European Journal of Heart Failure*, *11*(7), 699–705. doi:10.1093/eurjhf/hfp074 PMID:19505883

Gokhale, M., & Khanduja, D. K. (2010). Time domain signal analysis using wavelet packet decomposition approach. *International Journal of Communications. Network and System Sciences*, *3*(03), 321–329. doi:10.4236/ijcns.2010.33041

Guyon, I., & Elisseeff, A. (2006). An introduction to feature extraction. *Feature Extraction*, 1-25.

Hajizadeh, S., Abbasi, A., & Goshvarpour, A. (2015). *Intelligent classification of ECG signals to distinguish between pre and on-music states.* Paper presented at the Information and Knowledge Technology (IKT), 2015 7th Conference on. 10.1109/IKT.2015.7288790

Hall, J. E. (2015). *Guyton and Hall Textbook of Medical Physiology E-Book*. Elsevier Health Sciences.

Harland, C., Clark, T., Peters, N., Everitt, M. J., & Stiffell, P. (2005). A compact electric potential sensor array for the acquisition and reconstruction of the 7-lead electrocardiogram without electrical charge contact with the skin. *Physiological Measurement*, *26*(6), 939–950. doi:10.1088/0967-3334/26/6/005 PMID:16311443

Harrell, F. E. Jr. (2015). *Regression modeling strategies: with applications to linear models, logistic and ordinal regression, and survival analysis*. Springer. doi:10.1007/978-3-319-19425-7

Hurst, J. W. (1998). Naming of the waves in the ECG, with a brief account of their genesis. *Circulation*, *98*(18), 1937–1942. doi:10.1161/01.CIR.98.18.1937 PMID:9799216

Jain, A. K., Mao, J., & Mohiuddin, K. M. (1996). Artificial neural networks: A tutorial. *Computer*, *29*(3), 31–44. doi:10.1109/2.485891

Kundu, M., Nasipuri, M., & Basu, D. K. (1998). A knowledge-based approach to ECG interpretation using fuzzy logic. *IEEE Transactions on Systems, Man, and Cybernetics. Part B, Cybernetics*, *28*(2), 237–243. doi:10.1109/3477.662764 PMID:18255941

Lemon, S. C., Roy, J., Clark, M. A., Friedmann, P. D., & Rakowski, W. (2003). Classification and regression tree analysis in public health: Methodological review and comparison with logistic regression. *Annals of Behavioral Medicine*, *26*(3), 172–181. doi:10.1207/S15324796ABM2603_02 PMID:14644693

Lewis, R. J. (2000). *An Introduction to Classification and Regression Tree (CART) Analysis*. Paper presented at the Annual Meeting of the Society of Academic Emergency Medicine in.

Li, T., & Zhou, M. (2016). ECG classification using wavelet packet entropy and random forests. *Entropy (Basel, Switzerland)*, *18*(8), 285. doi:10.3390/e18080285

Luz, E. J. D. S., Nunes, T. M., De Albuquerque, V. H. C., Papa, J. P., & Menotti, D. (2013). ECG arrhythmia classification based on optimum-path forest. *Expert Systems with Applications*, *40*(9), 3561–3573. doi:10.1016/j.eswa.2012.12.063

Mahapatra, S., Mohanta, D., Mohanty, P., Nayak, S., & Behari, P. (2016). A Neuro-fuzzy Based Model for Analysis of an ECG Signal Using Wavelet Packet Tree. *Procedia Computer Science*, *92*, 175–180. doi:10.1016/j.procs.2016.07.343

Maldonado, H., Leija, L., Vera, A., & Alvarado, C. (2016). *Post myocardial infarct detection with support vector machine and ECG intervals ratios JTp/JT, Tpe/JTp and Tpe/JT.* Paper presented at the Medical Engineering Physics Exchanges/Pan American Health Care Exchanges (GMEPE/PAHCE), 2016 Global.

Markou, M., & Singh, S. (2003). Novelty detection: a review—part 2: neural network based approaches. *Signal Processing*, *83*(12), 2499–2521. doi:10.1016/j.sigpro.2003.07.019

Menahem, S. (2013). Cardiac asystole following cannabis (marijuana) usage–Additional mechanism for sudden death? *Forensic Science International*, *233*(1), e3–e5. doi:10.1016/j.forsciint.2013.10.007 PMID:24200372

Monfredi, O., Dobrzynski, H., Mondal, T., Boyett, M. R., & Morris, G. M. (2010). The anatomy and physiology of the sinoatrial node—a contemporary review. *Pacing and Clinical Electrophysiology*, *33*(11), 1392–1406. doi:10.1111/j.1540-8159.2010.02838.x PMID:20946278

Nayak, S. K., Suman, S., Nayak, B. M., Banerjee, I., Pal, K., & Champaty, B. (2016). *Effect of Cannabis consumption on ANS and conduction pathway of heart of Indian paddy field workers.* Paper presented at the India Conference (INDICON), 2016 IEEE Annual. 10.1109/INDICON.2016.7839018

Okin, P. M., Devereux, R. B., Howard, B. V., Fabsitz, R. R., Lee, E. T., & Welty, T. K. (2000). Assessment of QT interval and QT dispersion for prediction of all-cause and cardiovascular mortality in American Indians. *Circulation*, *101*(1), 61–66. doi:10.1161/01.CIR.101.1.61 PMID:10618305

Opie, L. H. (2004). *Heart physiology: from cell to circulation*. Lippincott Williams & Wilkins.

Opthof, T., Coronel, R., Wilms-Schopman, F. J., Plotnikov, A. N., Shlapakova, I. N., Danilo, P. Jr, ... Janse, M. J. (2007). Dispersion of repolarization in canine ventricle and the electrocardiographic T wave: T pe interval does not reflect transmural dispersion. *Heart Rhythm*, *4*(3), 341–348. doi:10.1016/j.hrthm.2006.11.022 PMID:17341400

Pal, K., Goel, R., Champaty, B., Samantray, S., & Tibarewala, D. (2013). Heart rate variability and wavelet-based studies on ECG signals from smokers and non-smokers. *Journal of The Institution of Engineers (India): Series B, 94*(4), 275-283.

Rai, H. M., Trivedi, A., & Shukla, S. (2013). ECG signal processing for abnormalities detection using multi-resolution wavelet transform and Artificial Neural Network classifier. *Measurement*, *46*(9), 3238–3246. doi:10.1016/j.measurement.2013.05.021

Ray, A., Nayak, S. K., Champaty, B., Tibarewala, D., & Pal, K. (2016). Non-Linear Analysis of Heart Rate Variability and ECG Signal Features of Swimmers from NIT-Rourkela: A Case Study. *Computational Tools and Techniques for Biomedical Signal Processing*, 56.

Rentschler, S., Vaidya, D. M., Tamaddon, H., Degenhardt, K., Sassoon, D., & Morley, G. E. (2001). Visualization and functional characterization of the developing murine cardiac conduction system. *Development*, *128*(10), 1785–1792. PMID:11311159

Roza, V. C. C., de Almeida, A. M., & Postolache, O. A. (2017). *Design of an artificial neural network and feature extraction to identify arrhythmias from ECG*. Paper presented at the Medical Measurements and Applications (MeMeA), 2017 IEEE International Symposium on.

Schijvenaars, B. J., Kors, J. A., van Herpen, G., Kornreich, F., & van Bemmel, J. H. (1997). Effect of electrode positioning on ECG interpretation by computer. *Journal of Electrocardiology*, *30*(3), 247–256. doi:10.1016/S0022-0736(97)80010-6 PMID:9261733

Strobl, C., Malley, J., & Tutz, G. (2009). An introduction to recursive partitioning: Rationale, application, and characteristics of classification and regression trees, bagging, and random forests. *Psychological Methods*, *14*(4), 323–348. doi:10.1037/a0016973 PMID:19968396

Svetnik, V., Liaw, A., Tong, C., Culberson, J. C., Sheridan, R. P., & Feuston, B. P. (2003). Random forest: A classification and regression tool for compound classification and QSAR modeling. *Journal of Chemical Information and Computer Sciences*, *43*(6), 1947–1958. doi:10.1021/ci034160g PMID:14632445

Torrent-Guasp, F., Ballester, M., Buckberg, G. D., Carreras, F., Flotats, A., Carrió, I., ... Narula, J. (2001). Spatial orientation of the ventricular muscle band: Physiologic contribution and surgical implications. *The Journal of Thoracic and Cardiovascular Surgery*, *122*(2), 389–392. doi:10.1067/mtc.2001.113745 PMID:11479518

Wellens, H. J., Bär, F. W., & Lie, K. (1978). The value of the electrocardiogram in the differential diagnosis of a tachycardia with a widened QRS complex. *The American Journal of Medicine*, *64*(1), 27–33. doi:10.1016/0002-9343(78)90176-6 PMID:623134

Windeatt, T., & Ardeshir, G. (2002). Boosted tree ensembles for solving multiclass problems. *Multiple Classifier Systems*, 179-182.

Wolff, V., Rouyer, O., & Gény, B. (2013). Response to letter regarding article,"cannabis-related stroke: Myth or reality? *Stroke*, *44*(5), e57–e57. doi:10.1161/STROKEAHA.113.001094 PMID:23741740

ADDITIONAL READING

Abo-Zahhad, M., Ahmed, S. M., & Abbas, S. N. (2015). *A new biometric authentication system using heart sounds based on wavelet packet features.* Paper presented at the Electronics, Circuits, and Systems (ICECS), 2015 IEEE International Conference on. 10.1109/ICECS.2015.7440238

Acharya, U. R., Sudarshan, V. K., Rong, S. Q., Tan, Z., Lim, C. M., Koh, J. E., ... Bhandary, S. V. (2017). Automated detection of premature delivery using empirical mode and wavelet packet decomposition techniques with uterine electromyogram signals. *Computers in Biology and Medicine*, *85*, 33–42. doi:10.1016/j.compbiomed.2017.04.013 PMID:28433870

Ai, D., Yang, J., Wang, Z., Fan, J., Ai, C., & Wang, Y. (2015). Fast multi-scale feature fusion for ECG heartbeat classification. *EURASIP Journal on Advances in Signal Processing*, *2015*(1), 46. doi:10.118613634-015-0231-0

Akar, S. A., Kara, S., & Bilgiç, V. (2016). Investigation of heart rate variability in major depression patients using wavelet packet transform. *Psychiatry Research*, *238*, 326–332. doi:10.1016/j.psychres.2016.02.058 PMID:27086252

Alickovic, E., Kevric, J., & Subasi, A. (2018). Performance evaluation of empirical mode decomposition, discrete wavelet transform, and wavelet packed decomposition for automated epileptic seizure detection and prediction. *Biomedical Signal Processing and Control*, *39*, 94–102. doi:10.1016/j.bspc.2017.07.022

Arvanaghi, R., Daneshvar, S., Seyedarabi, H., & Goshvarpour, A. (2017). Fusion of ECG and ABP signals based on wavelet transform for cardiac arrhythmias classification. *Computer Methods and Programs in Biomedicine*, *151*, 71–78. doi:10.1016/j.cmpb.2017.08.013 PMID:28947007

Bensafia, K., Mansour, A., & Haddab, S. (2017). Blind Source Subspace Separation and Classification of ECG Signals. 5th Internationale Confernce en Automatique & Traitement de Signal, Sousse, Tunisia.

Chandra, S., & Sharma, A. (2017). *A computationally efficient approach for ECG signal denoising and data compression.* Paper presented at the Control and System Graduate Research Colloquium (ICSGRC), 2017 IEEE 8th. 10.1109/ICSGRC.2017.8070561

Desai, U., Martis, R. J., Nayak, C. G., Sarika, K., & Seshikala, G. (2015). *Machine intelligent diagnosis of ECG for arrhythmia classification using DWT, ICA and SVM techniques.* Paper presented at the India Conference (INDICON), 2015 Annual IEEE. 10.1109/INDICON.2015.7443220

Deshmukh, S. V., & Dehzangi, O. (2017). *ECG-Based Driver Distraction Identification Using Wavelet Packet Transform and Discriminative Kernel-Based Features*. Paper presented at the Smart Computing (SMARTCOMP), 2017 IEEE International Conference on. 10.1109/SMARTCOMP.2017.7947003

Ergin, S., Uysal, A. K., Gunal, E. S., Gunal, S., & Gulmezoglu, M. B. (2014). *ECG based biometric authentication using ensemble of features*. Paper presented at the Information Systems and Technologies (CISTI), 2014 9th Iberian Conference on. 10.1109/CISTI.2014.6877089

Fraiwan, L. (2016). Predicting Preterm Delivery Based on Wavelet Packet Analysis of a Single Electrohysterography Channel. *Journal of Medical Imaging and Health Informatics*, *6*(6), 1419–1425. doi:10.1166/jmihi.2016.1821

Gayani, K., Jacob, V., & Nair, K. N. (2014). Automation of ECG heart beat detection using Morphological filtering and Daubechies wavelet transform. *IOSR Journal of Engineering*, *4*, 53–58. doi:10.9790/3021-041215358

Hassan, Z., Gilani, S. O., & Jamil, M. (2016). Improvement in ECG based biometric systems using Wavelet Packet Decomposition (WPD) algorithm. *Indian Journal of Science and Technology*, *9*(30). doi:10.17485/ijst/2016/v9i30/97958

He, H., Tan, Y., & Liu, X. (2013). *Feature extraction of ECG signals in meridian systems using wavelet packet transform and clustering algorithms*. Paper presented at the Networking, Sensing and Control (ICNSC), 2013 10th IEEE International Conference on.

Jegan, R., Anusuya, K., & George, E. M. (2015). Real-time ECG peak detection for heart rate measurement using wavelet packet transform. *International Journal of Biomedical Engineering and Technology*, *19*(3), 244–254. doi:10.1504/IJBET.2015.072994

Kearley, K., Selwood, M., Van den Bruel, A., Thompson, M., Mant, D., Hobbs, F. R., ... Heneghan, C. (2014). Triage tests for identifying atrial fibrillation in primary care: A diagnostic accuracy study comparing single-lead ECG and modified BP monitors. *BMJ Open*, *4*(5), e004565. doi:10.1136/bmjopen-2013-004565 PMID:24793250

Li, H., Feng, X., Cao, L., Li, E., Liang, H., & Chen, X. (2016). A new ECG signal classification based on WPD and ApEn feature extraction. *Circuits, Systems, and Signal Processing*, *35*(1), 339–352. doi:10.100700034-015-0068-7

Li, H., Yuan, D., Ma, X., Cui, D., & Cao, L. (2017). Genetic algorithm for the optimization of features and neural networks in ECG signals classification. *Scientific Reports*, *7*, 41011. doi:10.1038rep41011 PMID:28139677

Lin, C.-Y., Chang, S.-L., Lin, Y.-J., Lo, L.-W., Chung, F.-P., Chen, Y.-Y., ... Chen, S.-A. (2015). Long-term outcome of multiform premature ventricular complexes in structurally normal heart. *International Journal of Cardiology*, *180*, 80–85. doi:10.1016/j.ijcard.2014.11.110 PMID:25438221

Lowres, N., Freedman, S. B., Gallagher, R., Kirkness, A., Marshman, D., Orchard, J., & Neubeck, L. (2015). Identifying postoperative atrial fibrillation in cardiac surgical patients posthospital discharge, using iPhone ECG: A study protocol. *BMJ Open*, *5*(1), e006849. doi:10.1136/bmjopen-2014-006849 PMID:25586373

Maharaj, E. A., & Alonso, A. M. (2014). Discriminant analysis of multivariate time series: Application to diagnosis based on ECG signals. *Computational Statistics & Data Analysis*, *70*, 67–87. doi:10.1016/j.csda.2013.09.006

Raj, A. A. S., Dheetsith, N., Nair, S. S., & Ghosh, D. (2014). *Auto analysis of ECG signals using artificial neural network*. Paper presented at the Science Engineering and Management Research (ICSEMR), 2014 International Conference on. 10.1109/ICSEMR.2014.7043597

Raja, C., & Gangatharan, N. (2015). Appropriate sub-band selection in wavelet packet decomposition for automated glaucoma diagnoses. *Int. J. Autom. Comput.*.

Safara, F., Doraisamy, S., Azman, A., Jantan, A., & Ramaiah, A. R. A. (2013). Multi-level basis selection of wavelet packet decomposition tree for heart sound classification. *Computers in Biology and Medicine*, *43*(10), 1407–1414. doi:10.1016/j.compbiomed.2013.06.016 PMID:24034732

Shao, R., Hu, W., Wang, Y., & Qi, X. (2014). The fault feature extraction and classification of gear using principal component analysis and kernel principal component analysis based on the wavelet packet transform. *Measurement*, *54*, 118–132. doi:10.1016/j.measurement.2014.04.016

Singh, O., & Sunkaria, R. K. (2015). *The utility of wavelet packet transform in QRS complex detection-a comparative study of different mother wavelets*. Paper presented at the Computing for Sustainable Global Development (INDIACom), 2015 2nd International Conference on.

Singh, T., & Misal, A. (2015). Detection of Cardiac Abnormality from PCG Signal Using Wavelet Packet. *i-Manager's Journal on Digital Signal Processing, 3*(1), 12.

Wang, X., Gui, Q., Liu, B., Jin, Z., & Chen, Y. (2014). Enabling smart personalized healthcare: A hybrid mobile-cloud approach for ECG telemonitoring. *IEEE Journal of Biomedical and Health Informatics*, *18*(3), 739–745. doi:10.1109/JBHI.2013.2286157 PMID:24144678

Wess, M., Manoj, P. S., & Jantsch, A. (2017). *Neural network based ECG anomaly detection on FPGA and trade-off analysis*. Paper presented at the Circuits and Systems (ISCAS), 2017 IEEE International Symposium on. 10.1109/ISCAS.2017.8050805

Yan, J., & Lu, L. (2014). Improved Hilbert–Huang transform based weak signal detection methodology and its application on incipient fault diagnosis and ECG signal analysis. *Signal Processing*, *98*, 74–87. doi:10.1016/j.sigpro.2013.11.012

KEY TERMS AND DEFINITIONS

Artificial Neural Network (ANN): ANN is an electronic computational model that tries to mimic the functionalities of the biological neural networks.

Boosted Tree (BT): BT is one of the most robust and efficient decision tree method that uses a sequence of binary trees in which every new tree is generated based on the prediction residuals of the previous tree.

***Cannabis Sativa*:** *Cannabis sativa* is a flowering plant of the Cannabaceae family. It is used to develop a diverse group of products including industrial fiber, medicine, oil and recreational products.

Classification and Regression Tree (CART): CART is a conventional decision tree method used to design models for prediction from a given set of data.

Random Forest (RF): RF is a powerful ensemble learning method that can be used for both classification and regression problems.

Sinoatrial (SA) Node: SA node is a part of the heart, located in the upper side of the right atrium that is responsible for the generation of electrical impulse within it.

Wavelet Packet Decomposition (WPD): WPD is a special case of DWT that decomposes both the approximation coefficients and the detailed coefficients at each level of decomposition.

Chapter 13

Analysis of the Changes in the RR Interval Signals of Smokers (Before and After Smoking) Using Recurrence Analysis and ANN Classification

Prerana Talukdar
JIS College of Engineering, India

Karabi Ganguli
JIS College of Engineering, India

Gitika Yadu
National Institute of Technology Rourkela, India

Sandip Bag
JIS College of Engineering, India

Suraj Kumar Nayak
National Institute of Technology Rourkela, India

Anilesh Dey
Kaziranga University, India

Kunal Pal
National Institute of Technology Rourkela, India

ABSTRACT

This chapter has been inspired by the need to find an efficient method to study the changes in the cardiac autonomic regulation before and after smoking in young smokers. Appropriate processing and analysis of the RR intervals, extracted from the electrocardiogram (ECG) signals, is an important non-invasive tool to determine the autonomic nervous system (ANS)-based alteration of the cardiac physiology. The authors propose to analyze the RR interval signals by recurrence analysis and extracting the features thereof. In total, 17 young volunteers (smokers) participated in the study. The ECG signals were acquired before and after smoking. The statistical features obtained from the recurrence analysis were used as the input to artificial neural network (ANN)-based classification so as to classify the basal state from the post-stimulus state. A classification efficiency of 100% could be achieved using the recurrence features of the RR interval signals. Thus, the results evince that the proposed method is an efficient method to study the changes in the RR interval signal due to smoking.

DOI: 10.4018/978-1-5225-4969-7.ch013

INTRODUCTION

In the recent decade, the percentage of the abuse of tobacco-based products by the college and the university going students in the age group of 11-17 years has reached its peak. This has been due to the fact that smoking has evolved as a sign of higher social status (Sharma, 2007). Nearly 17% of the smokers worldwide have been concentrated in India (John, 2005). Tobacco smoking is a major risk factor for a number of diseases including the cardiovascular system, which is markedly affected. Cigarette smoking has been reported to increase the plasma catecholamine level. This has an immediate tachycardia effect, which is detrimental to the cardiac physiology, and on a long-term increases the risk factor towards cardiac mortality. Further, the baroreflex sensitivity is impaired due to smoking, thereby, increasing the blood pressure and the heart rate. A chronic smoker is at a higher risk of the down regulation of the beta-adrenergic receptors in regard to the autonomic neurohumoral response (Laustiola, 1988). An understanding of the alteration in the cardiac autonomic regulation can be useful for early detection of numerous potential cardiovascular diseases (Glos, Fietze, Blau, Baumann, & Penzel, 2014; Sharif, Millar, Incognito, & Ditor, 2016). The RR interval variability or heart rate variability (HRV) provides an easy and non-invasive means to analyse the ANS-based regulation of the cardiac physiology. Many studies have been carried out on the analysis of the HRV in smokers (Verplaetse, Smith, Smith, Oberleitner, & McKee, 2017). Various studies have revealed that the RR interval signals are non-stationary signals and may be analyzed via non-linear techniques like empirical mode decomposition and recurrence analysis (Pachori, Avinash, Shashank, Sharma, & Acharya, 2015; Turianikova et al., 2014). In the last few decades, recurrence plot-based methods have been widely studied for the classification of RR interval signals to detect various pathological conditions (Mohebbi, Ghassemian, & Asl, 2011; Nguyen, Wilkins, Cheng, & Benjamin, 2014). Bookmarking this in mind, it was decided to analyze the RR interval signals using recurrence analysis, which is a powerful tool for the analysis of the non-stationary signals. The important statistical features from the recurrence analysis of the signals were subjected to ANN classification.

BACKGROUND

Over the years, recurrence analysis has found numerous applications in the analysis of cardiovascular signals like ECG and RR interval signals (Zbilut, Thomasson, & Webber, 2002). This may be attributed to the fact that some changes in the ECG signals, which are not recognisable by the conventional methods, can be detected by analyzing the recurrence features. Marwan *et al.* (2002) proposed that the vertical structures in the recurrence plot analysis of a complex, non-linear data can be used as a measure of complexity to describe the transition between regular, laminar or chaotic behaviour (Marwan, Wessel, Meyerfeldt, Schirdewan, & Kurths, 2002). The authors were able to identify the occurrence of the laminar states before the occurrence of a life-threatening cardiac arrhythmia from the vertical structures in the recurrence plot of HRV data (Marwan et al., 2002). Based on their findings, the authors suggested that the proposed method can be useful for the therapy of malignant cardiac arrhythmia. Peng *et al.* (2011) investigated the non-linear dynamic properties of the fluctuations in ventricular repolarization, heart rate and their correlation during acute myocardial ischemia using recurrence quantification analysis (RQA) (Peng & Sun, 2011). 170 ischemic episodes from 13 ECG records were selected immediately before and after each ischemic episode. RQA was performed on the QT interval and the RR interval signals. RQA was noted to be a very efficient method in detecting the weakened coupling between the QT interval and the RR interval, suggesting decreased influence of the sinoatrial node on the QT interval modulation during ischemia. Acharya *et al.* (2013) used RQA along with other non-linear measures, namely, Largest Lyapunov Exponent (LLE), Approximate Entropy (ApEn) and Detrended Fluctuation Analysis (DFA) for the automated identification of normal and diabetes heart rate signals. The proposed system examined how diabetes affects the cardiac health by analyzing heart rate (HR) time series data, which were extracted from the ECG signals. Clinically significant features were selected based on the t-test results and these features were ranked using Bhattacharya distance method. The classification of the clinically relevant features was performed using six supervised learning algorithms, namely, probabilistic neural network, support vector machine, decision tree, AdaBoost, fuzzy sugeno classifier and k-nearest neighbour. The AdaBoost method provided the highest average classification accuracy of 90%, sensitivity of 92.5% and specificity of 88.7% as compared to the other methods (Chapman, 1931). Nguyen *et al.* (2014) introduced an online sleep apnea detection method based on heart rate complexity analysis using RQA of RR interval data (Nguyen et al., 2014). It was reported that the RQA statistic captured the non-linear dynamics of a complex cardiorespiratory system during obstructive sleep apnea. The most informative RQA parameters were selected using the conditional mutual information. The classification was performed using SVM and ANN algorithms. Finally, a soft decision fusion rule was implemented to combine the results of the individual classifiers for the improvement in the classification performance of the proposed system. Based on the experimental results, the authors suggested that the designed system can be a potential candidate for automatic sleep apnea detection. Tallapragada *et al.* (2014) performed RQA analysis of HRV signals for the diagnosis of different cardiac diseases (Tallapragada, Singavarapu, & Pradhan, 2014). 13 parameters were extracted from the RQA of the HRV signals and were used as input for radial basis probabilistic neural network-based classification of the various cardiac diseases. The proposed system was able to classify the different types of cardiac disorders with an accuracy of 94.2%. Considering this result, the authors recommended that their proposed methodology can be useful for the development of the automated diagnostic devices for myocardial dysfunctions (Tallapragada et al., 2014). Takakura *et al.* (2017) utilized recurrence plot-derived parameters, namely, percentage of determinism, percentage of recurrence, average diagonal length, Shannon entropy, and sample entropy for assessing the cardiac autonomic nervous system recovery after heart transplantation (Takakura et al., 2017). It was found that the heart re-innervation begins nearly 18 months after the heart transplantation and improves slowly.

MAIN FOCUS OF THE CHAPTER

This study focuses on investigating the instantaneous effect of smoking on the cardiac autonomic regulation by analyzing the RR interval signals. The RR interval signals have been reported to be non-invasive markers of the ANS activity (Camm et al., 1996), and were extracted from the 5 min ECG signals acquired before and after smoking in this study. Recurrence analysis was performed to extract the features from the RR interval signals. The statistically significant recurrence-based features were identified and used for classification using ANN.

METHODOLOGY

The ECG signals were acquired in the supine position from 17 young male volunteers (20-22 years of age), who happened to be smokers, for a period of 5 min, after explaining them about the study and receiving a written consent from them. Acquisition of the ECG signals was performed using an ECG amplifier at a sampling frequency of 1000 Hz. The volunteers were the undergraduate students of Narula Institute of Technology, India. None of the volunteers had any medical condition, which might have affected the results of the study. Thereafter, the volunteers were asked to smoke a cigarette. After a gap of 30 sec, the ECG was again acquired for a period of 5 min. R-R interval signal was extracted from the ECG signals using a MATLAB® (R2014a, MathWorks, Inc., USA) program. The signals were then processed using the software Bios Analyzer (a free ware from Inverudio Inc, USA) (H Sabelli et al., 2005). Recurrence plot of the R-R interval signals before and after smoking were plotted using an embedding dimension and cut-off radius (% of range of the time series) of 10 each. 300 points of the R-R interval signal were used for the plotting of the recurrence plot. Apart from the recurrence plot, the Bios Analyzer software provided a set of 837 statistical features. Out of these statistical features, a set of 125 features were selected for further study. Important features were estimated from the previously selected statistical features, which were extracted from the recurrence analysis of the R-R interval signal. t-test, Classification and Regression Tree (CART), Boosted Tree (BT) and Random Forest (RF) classifiers based statistical methods were used for the estimation of the important features using Statistica software (trial version, Dell Inc., USA). The important parameters were classified using Automated Neural Network based classification.

RESULTS AND DISCUSSION

Recurrence Plot

Recurrence is an elementary characteristic of the dynamical systems. It is used to characterise the behaviour of the systems in the phase space. Recurrence in the time series of a dynamical system was first explained by Poincare in 1890 (Nguyen et al., 2014; Poincaré, 1890). Recurrence plot, introduced by Eckmann et al. (1987) is a potential method for the visualisation of the trends present within the time series derived from a dynamical system (Eckmann, Kamphorst, & Ruelle, 1987). In this method, the time series data (say u(t)) is incorporated into the phase space using the Takens' time delay theorem. As per the theorem, whenever the dynamics of a system depends on a number of variables and the information about only one variable (say x) is available, the values of the measured variable can be plotted against themselves several times at a specific time delay to reconstruct the complete dynamics of the system (Takens, 1981; Wallot, Roepstorff, & Mønster, 2016). Recurrence plots are useful to describe the variation in the RRI patterns with time (Hector Sabelli & Lawandow, 2010). It has been reported earlier that the recurrence-rich regions represent a stable heart rate, whereas, the recurrence-free regions indicate the acceleration or deceleration of the heart rate (Hector Sabelli & Lawandow, 2010). In this study, recurrence plot was drawn for each volunteer in both the pre- and the post-stimulus conditions. The recurrence plots of a representative volunteer in the pre- and the post-stimulus conditions have been shown in Figure 1. A significant variation in the recurrence patterns were observed among the pre- and the post-stimulus conditions, with the post-stimulus condition exhibiting more recurrent regions. This suggested that the heart rate is more stable in the post-stimulus than the pre-stimulus condition, i.e., the variability in the

Figure 1. Recurrence plots of RR interval signal in (a) pre-stimulus condition, and (b) post-stimulus condition

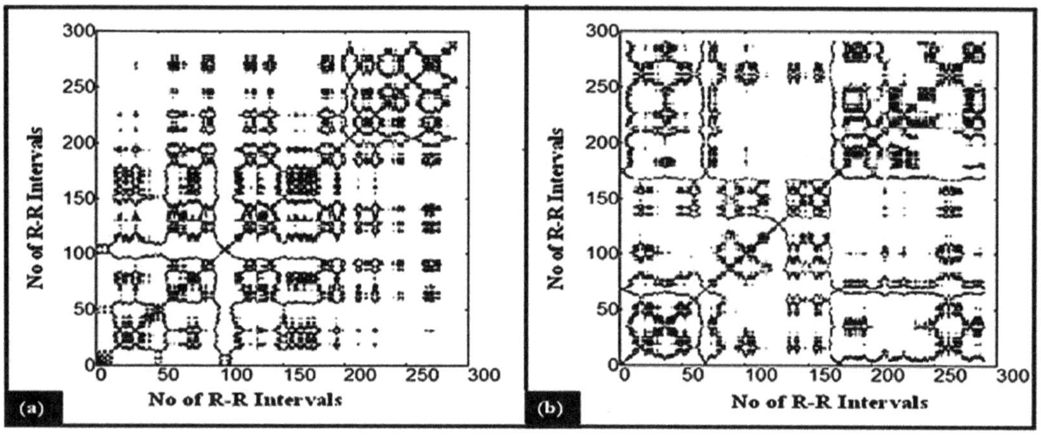

heart rate has reduced (H Sabelli, Messer, Kovacevic, & Walthall, 2011). As per the literature related to heart rate variability, a reduction in heart rate variability (HRV) has also been reported in many of the pathological conditions (Camm et al., 1996). An increase in the isometry recurrence rate of the R-R interval signals was also reported by Sabelli et al. (2011) in case of persons suffering from depression and psychosis as compared to healthy individuals (H Sabelli et al., 2011). However, the result obtained from recurrence plot is qualitative in nature. To quantitatively identify the variation the R-R interval signals in the pre- and the post-stimulus signals, recurrence related parameters were computed using the Bios Analyzer software and ANN classification was performed using the statistically significant parameters as discussed in the succeeding section

ANN Classification Using Recurrence Parameters

In the recurrence analysis, a sequence of points of the time series data (i.e., a vector) is used to represent a single point in the phase space. The number of the time series data points in this vector is regarded as the embedding (Hector Sabelli & Lawandow, 2010). Isometry is the recurrence of the vectors, the difference of whose Euclidean norms are below a cut-off radius (H Sabelli et al., 2005). It is measured as %isometry, which refers to the number of isometric recurrences expressed as a percentage of the total number of pairs of vectors compared in the time series data (H Sabelli et al., 2011). The recurrence-based parameters of the R-R intervals were calculated using Bios Analyser (H Sabelli et al., 2005). The important parameters were predicted using t-test, CART, BT and RF (Table 1) (Nayak et al., 2015). The t-test indicated that out of chosen 125 variables; the difference between the original series %Isometry and the shuffled series %isometry (SIS(%)) at embedding 1 (SIS(%)1), 20 (SIS(%)20), and 30 (SIS(%)30) were significantly different during the basal and the post-stimuli conditions. The negative value of SIS(%) can be regarded as an indicator of creativity (H Sabelli et al., 2005). Thus, the SIS(%)1 suggested that the RR interval signal was creative in the pre-stimulus condition, whereas the signal was not a creative signal during post-stimulus condition. A signal is said to be creative if it exhibits simple and complex components of variation and characterized by the properties, namely, diversification, novelty, complexes, and non- random complexity (H Sabelli et al., 2005). This further suggested that there was a reduction the R-R interval variation in the post-stimulus condition similar to that indicated by the recurrence plot.

Table 1. Predictor importance chart of RR interval parameters

Methods	Parameters	Mean ± SD		Predictor Importance	p-Value
		Category-N	Category-S		
t-test	SIS(%)1	-0.21±0.35	0.08±0.31	--	0.01
	SIS(%)20	-18.97±6.83	-13.69±7.95	--	0.04
	SIS(%)30	-20.13±8.67	-13.8768±9.12	--	0.04
	L:M	1.81±6.01	1.03±0.03	--	0.02
	Time	2.33±0.11	5.75±0.57	--	0.01
CART	Time	2.32±0.11	5.75±0.57	1.00	--
BT	Time	2.32±0.11	5.75±0.57	1.00	--
RF	SIS (%) 1	-0.21±0.35	0.080±0.31	1.00	--
	Time	2.32±0.11	5.75±057	0.97	--

Ratio of the last and the middle embedding (L:M), and Time were also found to be significant variables. SIS(%)1, SIS(%)20, SIS(%)30 were lower, while L:M and Time were higher during post-stimulus condition. The feature "Time" was also found to be important during decision tree based classifications, namely, CART and BT. "Time" was higher during post-stimulus condition. The features SIS(%)1 and "Time" were classified as important predictors in the RF based decision tree classifier.

In the present study multi-layered perceptron (MLP) and radial basis function (RBF) based ANN networks were employed for the classification of the important features, as estimated from the afore-mentioned classifiers. From the classification analysis, it was found that in both types of ANNs, an overall classification efficiency of 100% could be achieved using MLP 5-8-2 and RBF 5-7-2 ANN architectures. The confusion matrices for the afore-said ANN architectures have been summarized in Table 2 and 3. The performance of the classification algorithms was further evaluated using four standard statistical indices, namely, sensitivity (SE), positive predictivity (+P), false positive rate (FPR) and accuracy (ACC).

These performance indices were obtained by analysing true positive (TP), false negative (FN), true negative (TN) and false positive (FP) results of the neural networks as per Equation 1-4 following the recommendations of the Association for the Advancement of Medical Instrumentation (AAMI) (Li & Zhou, 2016). TP and FN represent the number of data points of a given class correctly and incorrectly classified, respectively. Similarly, TN represents the number of the data points not belonging to the considered class which are classified as not belonging to the considered class and FP denotes the number

Table 2. Confusion matrix of RBF 5-7-2 network

	Category-N	Category-S	Overall
Total	17.00	17.00	34.00
Correct	17.00	17.00	34.00
Incorrect	0.00	0.00	0.00
Correct (%)	100.00	100.00	100.00
Incorrect (%)	0.00	0.00	0.00

Table 3. Confusion matrix of MLP 5-8-2 network

	Category-N	Category-S	Overall
Total	17.00	17.00	34.00
Correct	17.00	17.00	34.00
Incorrect	0.00	0.00	0.00
Correct (%)	100.00	100.00	100.00
Incorrect (%)	0.00	0.00	0.00

of the data points incorrectly classified as belonging to a given class (Luz, Nunes, De Albuquerque, Papa, & Menotti, 2013).

$$SE = \frac{TP}{TP + FN} \times 100\ \% \quad (1)$$

$$+P = \frac{TP}{TP + FP} \times 100\ \% \quad (2)$$

$$FPR = \frac{FP}{TN + FP} \times 100\ \% \quad (3)$$

$$ACC = \frac{TP + TN}{TP + TN + FP + FN} \times 100\ \% \quad (4)$$

The values of SE, +P, FPR and ACC were 100%,100%,0% and 100%, respectively, for both the MLP 5-8-2 and RBF 5-7-2 (Table 5).

Table 4. Details of the RBF and MLP networks

Networks	Features Used	Classification Efficiency	Training Performance	Testing Performance	Algorithm	Error Function	Hidden Activation Function	Output Activation Function
MLP 5-8-2	SIS (%) 1 SIS (%) 20 SIS (%) 30 L:M Time	100.00	100.00	100.00	BFGS 5	Entropy	Exponential	Softmax
RBF 5-7-2	SIS (%) 1 SIS (%) 20 SIS (%) 30 L:M Time	100.00	100.00	100.00	RBFT	Entropy	Gaussian	Softmax

Table 5. Performance evaluation of the RBF and MLP networks

Networks Used	Sensitivity (SE)	Positive Predictivity (+P)	False Positive Rate (FPR)	Accuracy (ACC)
MLP 5-8-2	100%	100%	0%	100%
RBF 5-7-2	100%	100%	0%	100%

FUTURE RESEARCH DIRECTIONS

The present study used recurrence analysis of the RR interval signals to investigate the immediate effect of smoking on cardiac autonomic regulation. Future studies may be performed on the RR interval signals using other methods like Poincare plot, decomposition (wavelet packet decomposition or empirical mode decomposition), and modelling (e.g., autoregressive and autoregressive moving average). This can help to establish the most efficient method for the analysis of the RR intervals. The RR interval variability (or HRV) analysis can be performed to identify the exact changes in the ANS activity.

CONCLUSION

In the present study, the changes in the R-R interval signals, obtained from the ECG signals of the young male volunteers, before and after smoking were analyzed to determine the possibility of their changes in the cardiac physiology during smoking. The recurrence plot qualitatively suggested an increase in the recurrence of the R-R intervals due to smoking and a corresponding decrease in its variability. Recurrence parameters were calculated and the statistically important recurrence parameters were used for ANN classification. The SIS(%)1 suggested that the signal was creative in the pre-stimulus condition, whereas it lost its creativity during post-stimulus condition. An overall classification efficiency of 100% was achieved in both MLP and RBF networks. Thus, the results show that the recurrence analysis can be used as an effective feature extraction method to study the changes in the R-R intervals due to any stimulus

REFERENCES

Camm, A. J., Malik, M., Bigger, J., Breithardt, G., Cerutti, S., & Cohen, R. J. (1996). Heart rate variability: Standards of measurement, physiological interpretation and clinical use. Task Force of the European Society of Cardiology and the North American Society of Pacing and Electrophysiology. *Circulation*, *93*(5), 1043–1065. doi:10.1161/01.CIR.93.5.1043 PMID:8598068

Chapman, S. (1931). The absorption and dissociative or ionizing effect of monochromatic radiation in an atmosphere on a rotating earth. *Proceedings of the Physical Society*, *43*(1), 26–45. doi:10.1088/0959-5309/43/1/305

Eckmann, J.-P., Kamphorst, S. O., & Ruelle, D. (1987). Recurrence plots of dynamical systems. *EPL*, *4*(9), 973–977. doi:10.1209/0295-5075/4/9/004

Glos, M., Fietze, I., Blau, A., Baumann, G., & Penzel, T. (2014). Cardiac autonomic modulation and sleepiness: Physiological consequences of sleep deprivation due to 40h of prolonged wakefulness. *Physiology & Behavior*, *125*, 45–53. doi:10.1016/j.physbeh.2013.11.011 PMID:24291386

John, R. M. (2005). Tobacco consumption patterns and its health implications in India. *Health Policy (Amsterdam)*, *71*(2), 213–222. doi:10.1016/j.healthpol.2004.08.008 PMID:15607383

Laustiola, K. (1988). A study of monozygotic twin pairs discordant for smoking. *American Heart Association Journal, 78*, 1234-1240.

Li, T., & Zhou, M. (2016). ECG classification using wavelet packet entropy and random forests. *Entropy (Basel, Switzerland)*, *18*(8), 285. doi:10.3390/e18080285

Luz, E. J. D. S., Nunes, T. M., De Albuquerque, V. H. C., Papa, J. P., & Menotti, D. (2013). ECG arrhythmia classification based on optimum-path forest. *Expert Systems with Applications*, *40*(9), 3561–3573. doi:10.1016/j.eswa.2012.12.063

Marwan, N., Wessel, N., Meyerfeldt, U., Schirdewan, A., & Kurths, J. (2002). Recurrence-plot-based measures of complexity and their application to heart-rate-variability data. *Physical Review. E*, *66*(2), 026702. doi:10.1103/PhysRevE.66.026702 PMID:12241313

Mohebbi, M., Ghassemian, H., & Asl, B. M. (2011). Structures of the recurrence plot of heart rate variability signal as a tool for predicting the onset of paroxysmal atrial fibrillation. *Journal of Medical Signals and Sensors*, *1*(2), 113. PMID:22606666

Nayak, S. K., Panda, I., Champaty, B., Bagh, N., Pal, K., & Tibarewala, D. (2015). Automated Neural Network Based Classification of HRV and ECG Signals of Smokers: A Preliminary Study. In Advancements of Medical Electronics (pp. 271-279). Springer. doi:10.1007/978-81-322-2256-9_25

Nguyen, H. D., Wilkins, B. A., Cheng, Q., & Benjamin, B. A. (2014). An online sleep apnea detection method based on recurrence quantification analysis. *IEEE Journal of Biomedical and Health Informatics*, *18*(4), 1285–1293. doi:10.1109/JBHI.2013.2292928 PMID:25014935

Pachori, R. B., Avinash, P., Shashank, K., Sharma, R., & Acharya, U. R. (2015). Application of empirical mode decomposition for analysis of normal and diabetic RR-interval signals. *Expert Systems with Applications*, *42*(9), 4567–4581. doi:10.1016/j.eswa.2015.01.051

Peng, Y., & Sun, Z. (2011). Characterization of QT and RR interval series during acute myocardial ischemia by means of recurrence quantification analysis. *Medical & Biological Engineering & Computing*, *49*(1), 25–31. doi:10.100711517-010-0671-5 PMID:20725861

Poincaré, H. (1890). Sur le problème des trois corps et les équations de la dynamique. *Acta Mathematica*, *13*(1), A3–A270.

Sabelli, H., & Lawandow, A. (2010). Homeobios: The pattern of heartbeats in newborns, adults, and elderly patients. *Nonlinear Dynamics Psychology and Life Sciences*, *14*(4), 381. PMID:20887687

Sabelli, H., Messer, J., Kovacevic, L., & Walthall, K. (2011). Biotic patterns of heart rate variation in depressed and psychotic subjects. *Nonlinear Dynamics Psychology and Life Sciences*, *15*(1), 11–28. PMID:21176437

Sabelli, H., Sugerman, A., Kovacevic, L., Kauffman, L., Carlson-Sabelli, L., & Patel, M. (2005). Bios data analyzer. *Nonlinear Dynamics Psychology and Life Sciences*, *9*(4), 505–538. PMID:16194304

Sharif, H., Millar, P., Incognito, A., & Ditor, D. (2016). Non-invasive electrocardiographic assessments of cardiac autonomic modulation in individuals with spinal cord injury. *Spinal Cord*, *54*(3), 166–171. doi:10.1038c.2015.207 PMID:26597693

Sharma, S. (2007). New approaches in smoking cessation. *Indian Heart Journal*, *60*(2Suppl B), B34–B37. PMID:19359762

Takakura, I. T., Hoshi, R. A., Santos, M. A., Pivatelli, F. C., Nóbrega, J. H., & Guedes, D. L. (2017). Recurrence Plots: A New Tool for Quantification of Cardiac Autonomic Nervous System Recovery after Transplant. *Revista Brasileira de Cirurgia Cardiovascular; Orgao Oficial da Sociedade Brasileira de Cirurgia Cardiovascular*, *32*(4), 245–252. PMID:28977195

Takens, F. (1981). Detecting strange attractors in turbulence. *Lecture Notes in Mathematics*, *898*(1), 366–381. doi:10.1007/BFb0091924

Tallapragada, K., Singavarapu, S., & Pradhan, N. (2014). Understanding the dynamics of heart rate variability in cardiovascular disorders using recurrence quantification analysis and radial basis function neural network. *Intl J Sci Eng Res*, *4*, 863–873.

Turianikova, Z., Tonhajzerova, I., Czippelova, B., Javorka, K., Lazarova, Z., & Javorka, M. (2014). *Recurrence Quantification Analysis of heart rate and blood pressure variability in obese children and adolescents.* Paper presented at the Computing in Cardiology Conference (CinC), 2014.

Verplaetse, T. L., Smith, P. H., Smith, K. M., Oberleitner, L. M., & McKee, S. A. (2017). Guanfacine alters the effect of stress and smoking on heart rate variability in regular daily smokers. *Psychopharmacology*, *234*(5), 805–813. doi:10.100700213-016-4517-1 PMID:28028603

Wallot, S., Roepstorff, A., & Mønster, D. (2016). Multidimensional Recurrence Quantification Analysis (MdRQA) for the analysis of multidimensional time-series: A software implementation in MATLAB and its application to group-level data in joint action. *Frontiers in Psychology*, 7. PMID:27920748

Zbilut, J. P., Thomasson, N., & Webber, C. L. (2002). Recurrence quantification analysis as a tool for nonlinear exploration of nonstationary cardiac signals. *Medical Engineering & Physics*, *24*(1), 53–60. doi:10.1016/S1350-4533(01)00112-6 PMID:11891140

ADDITIONAL READING

Acharya, R., Kannathal, N., & Krishnan, S. (2004). Comprehensive analysis of cardiac health using heart rate signals. *Physiological Measurement*, *25*(5), 1139–1151. doi:10.1088/0967-3334/25/5/005 PMID:15535180

Alcaraz, R., Hornero, F., & Rieta, J. J. (2011). Noninvasive Time and Frequency Predictors of Long-Standing Atrial Fibrillation Early Recurrence after Electrical Cardioversion. *Pacing and Clinical Electrophysiology*, *34*(10), 1241–1250. doi:10.1111/j.1540-8159.2011.03125.x PMID:21605132

Alcaraz, R., & Rieta, J. J. (2010). A review on sample entropy applications for the non-invasive analysis of atrial fibrillation electrocardiograms. *Biomedical Signal Processing and Control*, *5*(1), 1–14. doi:10.1016/j.bspc.2009.11.001

Begum, R., & Ramesh, M. (2016). Detection of cardiomyopathy using support vector machine and artificial neural network. *International Journal of Computers and Applications*, *133*(14), 29–34. doi:10.5120/ijca2016908178

Cassileth, B. R., Walsh, W. P., & Lusk, E. J. (1988). Psychosocial correlates of cancer survival: A subsequent report 3 to 8 years after cancer diagnosis. *Journal of Clinical Oncology*, *6*(11), 1753–1759. doi:10.1200/JCO.1988.6.11.1753 PMID:3183705

Cauwenbergh, D., Nijs, J., Kos, D., Weijnen, L., Struyf, F., & Meeus, M. (2014). Malfunctioning of the autonomic nervous system in patients with chronic fatigue syndrome: A systematic literature review. *European Journal of Clinical Investigation*, *44*(5), 516–526. doi:10.1111/eci.12256 PMID:24601948

Cavalcanti, S., Chiari, L., Severi, S., Avanzolini, G., Enzmann, G., & Lamberti, C. (1996). Parametric analysis of heart rate variability during hemodialysis. *International Journal of Bio-Medical Computing*, *42*(3), 215–224. doi:10.1016/0020-7101(96)01205-6 PMID:8894777

Censi, F., Barbaro, V., Bartolini, P., Calcagnini, G., Michelucci, A., Gensini, G., & Cerutti, S. (2000). Recurrent patterns of atrial depolarization during atrial fibrillation assessed by recurrence plot quantification. *Annals of Biomedical Engineering*, *28*(1), 61–70. doi:10.1114/1.248 PMID:10645789

Chua, K., Chandran, V., Acharya, U., & Lim, C. (2008). Computer-based analysis of cardiac state using entropies, recurrence plots and Poincare geometry. *Journal of Medical Engineering & Technology*, *32*(4), 263–272. doi:10.1080/03091900600863794 PMID:18666006

Claudia, L., Oscar, I., Héctor, P. G., & Marco, V. J. (2003). Poincaré plot indexes of heart rate variability capture dynamic adaptations after haemodialysis in chronic renal failure patients. *Clinical Physiology and Functional Imaging*, *23*(2), 72–80. doi:10.1046/j.1475-097X.2003.00466.x PMID:12641600

Eckmann, J.-P., Kamphorst, S. O., & Ruelle, D. (1987). Recurrence plots of dynamical systems. [Europhysics Letters]. *EPL*, *4*(9), 973–977. doi:10.1209/0295-5075/4/9/004

González, H., Infante, O., Pérez-Grovas, H., Jose, M. V., & Lerma, C. (2013). Nonlinear dynamics of heart rate variability in response to orthostatism and hemodialysis in chronic renal failure patients: Recurrence analysis approach. *Medical Engineering & Physics*, *35*(2), 178–187. doi:10.1016/j.medengphy.2012.04.013 PMID:22647839

González, J. J., Cordero, J. J., Feria, M., & Pereda, E. (2000). Detection and sources of nonlinearity in the variability of cardiac RR intervals and blood pressure in rats. *American Journal of Physiology. Heart and Circulatory Physiology*, *279*(6), H3040–H3046. doi:10.1152/ajpheart.2000.279.6.H3040 PMID:11087262

Hartati, S., Wardoyo, R., & Setianto, B. Y. (2017). The Feature Extraction to Determine the Wave's Peaks in the Electrocardiogram Graphic Image. *International Journal of Image, Graphics &. Signal Processing*, *9*(6).

Javorka, M., Turianikova, Z., Tonhajzerova, I., Javorka, K., & Baumert, M. (2008). The effect of orthostasis on recurrence quantification analysis of heart rate and blood pressure dynamics. *Physiological Measurement*, *30*(1), 29–41. doi:10.1088/0967-3334/30/1/003 PMID:19039163

Kaur, M., & Singh, G. (2017). Classification of Seizure Prone EEG Signal Using Amplitude and Frequency Based Parameters of Intrinsic Mode Functions. *Journal of Medical and Biological Engineering*, *37*(4), 540–553. doi:10.100740846-017-0275-8

Kaya, C., Erkaymaz, O., Ayar, O., & Özer, M. (2017). Multi-Layer Perceptron and Radial Basis Function Neural Network Models for Classification of Diabetic Retinopathy Disease Using Video-Oculography Signals. *World Academy of Science, Engineering and Technology, International Journal of Medical, Health, Biomedical. Bioengineering and Pharmaceutical Engineering*, *11*(11), 562–567.

Koçer, S., & Tümer, A. E. (2016). Classifying neuromuscular diseases using artificial neural networks with applied Autoregressive and Cepstral analysis. *Neural Computing & Applications*, 1–8.

Li, Y., Liu, Q., Tan, S.-R., & Chan, R. H. (2016). High-resolution time-frequency analysis of EEG signals using multiscale radial basis functions. *Neurocomputing*, *195*, 96–103. doi:10.1016/j.neucom.2015.04.128

Logothetis, N. K., Pauls, J., Augath, M., Trinath, T., & Oeltermann, A. (2001). Neurophysiological investigation of the basis of the fMRI signal. *Nature*, *412*(6843), 150–157. doi:10.1038/35084005 PMID:11449264

Marwan, N., Kurths, J., & Saparin, P. (2007). Generalised recurrence plot analysis for spatial data. *Physics Letters. [Part A]*, *360*(4), 545–551. doi:10.1016/j.physleta.2006.08.058

Marwan, N., Thiel, M., & Nowaczyk, N. R. (2002). Cross recurrence plot based synchronization of time series. *arXiv preprint physics/0201062*.

Melillo, P., Bracale, M., & Pecchia, L. (2011). Nonlinear Heart Rate Variability features for real-life stress detection. Case study: Students under stress due to university examination. *Biomedical Engineering Online*, *10*(1), 96. doi:10.1186/1475-925X-10-96 PMID:22059697

Mohebbi, M., & Ghassemian, H. (2011). Prediction of paroxysmal atrial fibrillation using recurrence plot-based features of the RR-interval signal. *Physiological Measurement*, *32*(8), 1147–1162. doi:10.1088/0967-3334/32/8/010 PMID:21709338

Mohebbi, M., Ghassemian, H., & Asl, B. M. (2011). Structures of the recurrence plot of heart rate variability signal as a tool for predicting the onset of paroxysmal atrial fibrillation. *Journal of Medical Signals and Sensors*, *1*(2), 113. PMID:22606666

Moreira, M. W., Rodrigues, J. J., Oliveira, A. M., Saleem, K., & Neto, A. J. V. (2017). *Predicting hypertensive disorders in high-risk pregnancy using the random forest approach.* Paper presented at the Communications (ICC), 2017 IEEE International Conference on. 10.1109/ICC.2017.7996964

Nalband, S., Sundar, A., Prince, A. A., & Agarwal, A. (2016). Feature selection and classification methodology for the detection of knee-joint disorders. *Computer Methods and Programs in Biomedicine*, *127*, 94–104. doi:10.1016/j.cmpb.2016.01.020 PMID:27000292

Nayak, S., Sahoo, S., Champaty, B., & Pal, K. (2014). *Effect of horror clips on the physiology of ANS & heart using ECG signal classification.* Paper presented at the Control, Instrumentation, Communication and Computational Technologies (ICCICCT), 2014 International Conference on. 10.1109/ICCICCT.2014.6993010

Nayak, S. K., Srivastava, U., Tibarewala, D., Thakur, G., Mohapatra, B., & Pal, K. (2017). Effect of Odia and Tamil Music on the ANS and the Conduction Pathway of Heart of Odia Volunteers. In *Pattern and Data Analysis in Healthcare Settings* (pp. 240–263). IGI Global. doi:10.4018/978-1-5225-0536-5.ch012

Nguyen, H. D., Wilkins, B. A., Cheng, Q., & Benjamin, B. A. (2014). An online sleep apnea detection method based on recurrence quantification analysis. *IEEE Journal of Biomedical and Health Informatics*, *18*(4), 1285–1293. doi:10.1109/JBHI.2013.2292928 PMID:25014935

Pachori, R. B., Kumar, M., Avinash, P., Shashank, K., & Acharya, U. R. (2016). An improved online paradigm for screening of diabetic patients using RR-interval signals. *Journal of Mechanics in Medicine and Biology*, *16*(01), 1640003. doi:10.1142/S0219519416400030

Peng, Y., & Sun, Z. (2011). Characterization of QT and RR interval series during acute myocardial ischemia by means of recurrence quantification analysis. *Medical & Biological Engineering & Computing*, *49*(1), 25–31. doi:10.100711517-010-0671-5 PMID:20725861

Pérez, C. J., Naranjo, L., Martín, J., & Campos-Roca, Y. (2014). *A latent variable-based Bayesian regression to address recording replications in Parkinson's Disease.* Paper presented at the Signal Processing Conference (EUSIPCO), 2014 Proceedings of the 22nd European.

Sultana, N., Kamatham, Y., & Kinnara, B. (2016). *Performance Analysis of Artificial Neural Networks for Cardiac Arrhythmia Detection.* Paper presented at the Advanced Computing (IACC), 2016 IEEE 6th International Conference on. 10.1109/IACC.2016.84

Tarvainen, M. P., Niskanen, J.-P., Lipponen, J. A., Ranta-Aho, P. O., & Karjalainen, P. A. (2014). Kubios HRV–heart rate variability analysis software. *Computer Methods and Programs in Biomedicine*, *113*(1), 210–220. doi:10.1016/j.cmpb.2013.07.024 PMID:24054542

Thiel, M., Romano, M. C., & Kurths, J. (2004). How much information is contained in a recurrence plot? *Physics Letters. [Part A]*, *330*(5), 343–349. doi:10.1016/j.physleta.2004.07.050

Timothy, L. T., Krishna, B. M., & Nair, U. (2017). Classification of mild cognitive impairment EEG using combined recurrence and cross recurrence quantification analysis. *International Journal of Psychophysiology*, *120*, 86–95. doi:10.1016/j.ijpsycho.2017.07.006 PMID:28711698

Tripathy, R. K., Acharya, A., & Choudhary, S. K. (2012). Gender classification from ECG signal analysis using least square support vector machine. *American Journal of Signal Processing*, *2*(5), 145–149. doi:10.5923/j.ajsp.20120205.08

Vernekar, S., Nair, S., Vijaysenan, D., & Ranjan, R. (2016). *A novel approach for classification of normal/abnormal phonocardiogram recordings using temporal signal analysis and machine learning.* Paper presented at the Computing in Cardiology Conference (CinC), 2016.

Wallot, S., Fusaroli, R., Tylén, K., & Jegindø, E.-M. (2013). Using complexity metrics with RR intervals and BPM heart rate measures. *Frontiers in Physiology*, 4. PMID:23964244

Webber, C. L. Jr, & Marwan, N. (2015). *Recurrence quantification analysis*. Springer. doi:10.1007/978-3-319-07155-8

Webber, C. L. Jr, & Zbilut, J. P. (1994). Dynamical assessment of physiological systems and states using recurrence plot strategies. *Journal of Applied Physiology*, *76*(2), 965–973. doi:10.1152/jappl.1994.76.2.965 PMID:8175612

Wessel, N., Marwan, N., Meyerfeldt, U., Schirdewan, A., & Kurths, J. (2001). Recurrence quantification analysis to characterise the heart rate variability before the onset of ventricular tachycardia. *Medical Data Analysis*, 295-301.

Zbilut, J. P., & Webber, C. L. (2006). Recurrence quantification analysis. *Wiley encyclopedia of biomedical engineering*.

Zhang, X., Yao, L., Zhang, D., Wang, X., Sheng, Q. Z., & Gu, T. (2017). Multi-person brain activity recognition via comprehensive eeg signal analysis. *arXiv preprint arXiv:1709.09077*.

Zhang, Y., Liu, B., Ji, X., & Huang, D. (2017). Classification of EEG signals based on autoregressive model and wavelet packet decomposition. *Neural Processing Letters*, *45*(2), 365–378. doi:10.100711063-016-9530-1

KEY TERMS AND DEFINITIONS

Autonomic Nervous System (ANS): The ANS is a part of the peripheral nervous system that controls the functionality of most of the visceral organs of the body.

Artificial Neural Network (ANN): ANN is a supervised machine learning method that is inspired by the biological neural networks and tries to imitate some of their functionalities.

Classification and Regression Tree (CART): CART is a traditional decision tree used for both classification and regression problems.

Multilayer Perceptron (MLP): MLP is a class of feed-forward ANN, which consists of at least three layers of neurons.

Recurrence: Recurrence is an elementary characteristic of the dynamical systems that can be used to describe the behavior of the systems in the phase space.

Recurrence Plot: A recurrence plot is a non-linear method of data analysis that measures the recurrence of the states of a dynamical system in the phase space.

T-Test: The t-test is a statistical method that determines whether there is a significant difference between the means of the parameters belonging to two populations.

Chapter 14
Remote Monitoring via EEG of Persons in Severe Depression

Sudip Paul
North Eastern Hill University, India

Tapas Kumar Sinha
North Eastern Hill University, India

ABSTRACT

Mental illness in the form of depression or suicidal tendencies is found in one out of every four Indians. Severe depression usually leads to suicides. The numbers of well trained professionals, brilliant students at premier institutes who have committed suicide due to depression are on the rise. Recently the pilot of a major German airline, suffering from severe depression, deliberately plunged the aircraft into the Swiss Alps killing both himself and all the passengers in the plane. It is therefore important to develop a technique via which one can identify unambiguously who is suffering from depression. There are no general behavioral characteristics via which one can identify such people. However, analysis of the EEG spectra can accurately estimate the mental health of the patient. By making it mandatory for students/ employees of an organization to have their EEG done periodically, one can isolate the people who are suffering from this disease.

INTRODUCTION

Depression

Depression is thus a mental state characterized by specific (strange) brain attractors and unusual neuronal activity. This state of the brain can easily be identified using lyapunov exponents, correlation dimension analysis and PSD (Power Spectral Density) analysis of EEG spectra.*Our chapter is to first classify these attractors by taking the EEG spectra from patients known to be in a depression and severe depression.* The ideal next step would be to couple this with non invasive EEG monitoring.

DOI: 10.4018/978-1-5225-4969-7.ch014

Depression, especially manic depression is a disease much worse than cancer. Their entire internal biochemistry has changed. They look normal, act normal yet they are not normal. At any moment they can act in such a way that will bring great harm to themselves and to people around them. *The Armed Forces of our country will be very much interested in the outcome of this research.* A pilot who is severely depressed should not be flying a multi-billion dollar jet similarly depressed soldiers should not be going to mission critical engagements. In all these cases non invasive EEG diagnostic process is required. Electroencephalographic measurements are commonly used in medical and research areas.

EEG and Its Significance

The electroencephalography (EEG) is defined as electrical activity of an alternating type recorded from the scalp surface after being picked up by metal electrodes and conductive media. Thus electroencephalographic reading is a completely non-invasive procedure. When brain cells (neurons) are activated, local current flows are produced. EEG measures mostly the currents that flow during synaptic excitations of the dendrites of many pyramidal neurons in the cerebral cortex. Differences of electrical potentials are caused by summed postsynaptic graded potentials from pyramidal cells that create electrical dipoles between soma and apical dendrites (neural branches). Brain electrical current consists mostly of Na+, K+, Ca++, and Cl- ions that are pumped through channels in neuron membranes in the direction governed by membrane potential. Only large populations of active neurons can generate electrical activity recordable on the head surface.

Attractors

The mammalian brain exists in a number of attractors, which is a set that evolves to itself under the dynamics. Attractors may contain invariant sets. A limit set is a set of points such that there exists some initial state that ends up arbitrarily close to the limit set (i.e. to each point of the set) as time goes to infinity. Attractors are limit sets, but not all limit sets are attractors: It is possible to have some points of a system converge to a limit set, but different points when perturbed slightly off the limit set may get knocked off and never return to the vicinity of the limit set. In order to characterize these attractors generally the time series can be obtained by recording of signals from the frontoparietal, occipital and temporal regions of the brain.

Mathematical modeling like- Discrete Wavelet Transformation, Fast Fourier Transformation, Neural networks, Lyapunov exponents, Correlation dimensions, was formulated to correlate the prevalent condition with the normal condition and mathematical models which were help for determining the degree of depression cases via remote EEG.

MAIN FOCUS OF THE CHAPTER

The central aim of this chapter is to study the tools based on remote EEG parameters which characterize EEG spectra for accurate and rapid classification. These tools may lead to a comprehensive basis for analysis and characterization of human brain based on EEG signals for depression patient.

SOLUTIONS AND RECOMMENDATIONS

EEG Signal Analysis Techniques

The human brain is obviously a complex system and exhibits rich spatiotemporal dynamics. Among the noninvasive techniques for probing human brain dynamics, Electroencephalography (EEG) provides a direct measure of cortical activity with millisecond temporal resolution. Electroencephalographic measurements are commonly used in medical and research areas. It is a medical recording technique that reads scalp electrical activity generated by brain structures. The EEG is defined as electrical activity of an alternating type recorded from the scalp surface after being picked up by metal electrodes and conductive media. Thus electroencephalographic reading is a completely non-invasive procedure. When brain cells (neurons) are activated, local current flows are produced. EEG measures mostly the currents that flow during synaptic excitations of the dendrites of many pyramidal neurons in the cerebral cortex. Differences of electrical potentials are caused by summed postsynaptic graded potentials from pyramidal cells that create electrical dipoles between soma and apical dendrites (neural branches). Only large populations of active neurons can generate electrical activity recordable on the head surface. EEG is a recording of the electrical potentials generated by the cerebral cortex neurons. There are two different types of EEG depending on where the signals are taken on the head: scalp or intracranial. For scalp EEG, the focus of this research, small metal discs, also known as electrodes, are placed on the scalp with good mechanical and electrical contact. Intracranial EEG is obtained by special electrodes implanted in the brain during a surgery. In order to provide an accurate detection of the voltage of the brain neuron current, the electrodes are of low impedance (<5k). The changes in the voltage difference between electrodes are sensed and amplified before being transmitted to a computer program to display the tracing of the voltage potential recordings. The recorded EEG provides a continuous graphic exhibition of the spatial distribution of the changing voltage fields over time.EEG signals involve a great deal of information about the function of the brain. *But classification and evaluation of these signals are limited.* Since there is no definite criterion evaluated by the experts, visual analysis of EEG signals in time domain may be insufficient. Routine clinical diagnosis needs to analysis of EEG signals. Therefore, some automation and computer techniques have been used for this aim. EEG spectrum contains some characteristic waveforms that fall primarily within four frequency bands: delta (<4 Hz), theta (4-8 Hz), alpha (8-13 Hz) and beta (13-30 Hz). Such methods have proved beneficial for various EEG characterizations, but fast Fourier transform (FFT), suffer from large noise sensitivity. Parametric power spectrum estimation methods such as autoregressive (AR), reduces the spectral loss problems and gives better frequency resolution. But, since the EEG signals are non-stationary, the parametric methods are not suitable for frequency decomposition of these signals (Guler et al., 2001; Adeli et al., 2003). Bio signal analysis is one of the most important topics that researchers have tried to develop during the last century to understand numerous human diseases. Electroencephalograms (EEGs) are one of the techniques which provide an electrical representation of bio signals that reflect changes in the activity of the human brain. Electroencephalography (EEG) is the neurophysiologic measurement of the electrical activity of the brain. Normally, this signal is a function of time and is described in terms of amplitude, frequency, and phase. The neurons communicate through electrical impulses and generate a bio-electromagnetic field that propagates through the brain tissues, skull, and scalp. The detectors are placed on the scalp to monitor signals from different locations at a time; these signals describe the brain activity. Many other methods are used for data acquisition, such as functional magnetic resonance imaging (fMRI) and positron emission tomography (PET), but EEG is the most popular method for assessing brain activity because of its simplicity, high temporal resolution, and low cost (Hinterbergeret al., 2004; Jarchiet al., 2009). The first approaches to correlation measurements between two simultaneously measured EEG signals were made more than fifty years ago (Brazier and Barlow, 1956; Brazier and Casby, 1952). Before the possibilities of the computation of coherence spectra in early 1960s, most of the studies investigated the similarity and the time delay between two EEG signals recorded from two separate regions of the brain by the linear cross-correlation (Gevins and Schaffer, 1980; Shaw and Ongley, 1972). After the availability of the fast Fourier transform (FFT) algorithm in 1965, frequency based measures like coherence and phase spectra of neurophysiological signals such as EEG/MEG became increasingly popular.Most of these criteria were originally proposed for univariate AR modeling, so special care should be taken to look for consistent results by comparing the performances of different criteria on a same data window. Further, if there are several data epochs from the same experiment, it is suggested to fix a common model order for all the available epochs to be analyzed even if the optimal model orders may vary between epochs. A powerful method was proposed in the late 1980s to perform time-scale analysis of signals: the wavelet transforms (WT). This method provides a unified framework for different techniques that have been developed for various applications (Adeliet al., 2003; Ercelebiet al., 2004). Since the WT is appropriate for analysis of non-stationary signals and this represents a major advantage over spectral analysis, it is well suited to locating transient events, which may occur during epileptic seizures.The EEG is a result of the temporal and spatial summation of synaptic currents that arise on the dendrites and cell bodies of billions of cortical pyramidal cells that are primarily located a few centimeters below the scalp surface. The synaptic currents involve neurotransmitter storage and release which are dependent on the integrity of the sodium/potassium and calcium ionic pumps located in the membranes of each neuron. They have clearly documented that EEG have significantly changed in several brain regions following cerebral ischemia in animal model (Bhattacharya et al., 2013). The relationship between the global oscillatory EEG theta activity and the highlyindividuated activity of the place cells has been problematic for the spatial theory of hippocampal function since its initial proposal. On the one hand, the theta signal was similar across large areas of the hippocampal formation (Bullock et al., 1990; Fox et al., 1986) and clearly involved the synchronized activity of thousands ofcells; it was not difficult to imagine it served the function of tying together distant parts ofthe hippocampus into a single unified processor.

Univariate nonlinear time series analysis methods started to be applied to neurophysiological data about two decades ago (Babloyantz et al., 1985). As an example, the EEG has been characterized in terms of its correlation dimension, a nonlinear index that has been roughly interpreted as a measure of the irregularity or complexity of a signal (Kantz and Schreiber, 2004). This index has been shown useful in sleep-wake research (Pereda et al., 1998; Pradhan et al., 1995), *mental load research Multivariate time series analysis is extensively used in neurophysiology with the aim of studying the relationship between simultaneously recorded signals*. Recently, advances on information theory and nonlinear dynamical systems theory have allowed the study of various types of synchronization from time series (Pereda et al., 2005). EEG wave classification is achieved using the Discrete Wavelet Transform (DWT) with Fast Fourier Transform (FFT) by adopting the normalized EEG data. The DWT is used as a classifier of the EEG wave's frequencies, while FFT is implemented to visualize the EEG waves in multi-resolution of DWT (Maan M. Shaker, 2007).

Neural network detection systems have been proposed by a number of researchers (Peters et al., 2001; Qu et. al., 1997). Pradhan et al., 1996 used the raw EEG as an input to a neural network while Weng et al., 1996 used the features proposed by Gotman et al., 2007 with an adaptive structure neural network, but his results show a poor false detection rate. The ability of specifically designed and trained recurrent neural networks (RNN) combined with wavelet preprocessing, to predict the onset of epileptic seizures both on scalp and intracranial recordings only one channel of electroencephalogram (Petrosian et al., 2000). In order to provide faster and efficient algorithm, proposed a versatile signal processing and analysis framework for bioelectrical data and in particular for neural recordings and 128 channels EEG (Folkers et al., 2003).

CONCLUSION

Since the brain exists in a number of attractors and attractors are characterized by Lyapunov exponents and correlation dimensions. We can use the parameters to characterize the state of the brain. Hence via a non-invasive technique such as remote EEG coupled with neural networks one can determine/classify the state of the brain. Determining the stability of the attractor in depression casesare also important as it will tells about the stability of the brain. We developed tools which will characterize the stability of the attractors of the brain. This implies that we develop techniques for comprehensive characterization of the brain based on Lyapunov exponents and correlation dimensions. There are no parameter sets at present for proper characterization of EEG data. *For this reason we developed an approach analogous to characterization of attractors in nonlinear dynamics.* Accordingly, a rapid neural network based diagnostic tool was developed to characterize the EEG of the depressed brain. It is important to assess the state of the EEG rapidly and this is done by the neural network software. The utility of the software can be understood from the following scenario. Suppose an unconscious patient has been brought to the hospital. *The doctors do not know whether he/she is unconscious due to drugs or alcohol.* However the EEG of the patient can be matched with similar EEG of patients with substance or alcohol abuse and one can come to a definite conclusion.

REFERENCES

Brazier, M. A., & Casby, J. U. (1952). Cross-correlation and autocorrelation studies of electroencephalographic potentials. *Electroencephalography and Clinical Neurophysiology. Supplement*, *4*(2), 201–211. doi:10.1016/0013-4694(52)90010-2 PMID:13033798

Bullock, T. H., Buzsaki, G., & McClune, M. C. (1990). Coherence of compound field potentials reveals discontinuities in the CA1-subiculum of the hippocampus in freely-moving rats. *Neuroscience*, *38*(3), 609–619. doi:10.1016/0306-4522(90)90055-9 PMID:2270136

Callaway, J. K., Knight, M. J., Watkins, D. J., & Beart, P. M. (1999). Delayed Treatment With AM-36, a Novel Neuroprotective Agent, ReducesNeuronal Damage After Endothelin-1–Induced Middle Cerebral ArteryOcclusion in Conscious Rats. *Stroke*, *30*, 2704–2712. doi:10.1161/01.STR.30.12.2704 PMID:10583001

Cao, Y., D'Olhaberriague, L., Vikingstad, E. M., Levine, S. R., & Welch, K. M. (1998). Pilot study of functional MRI to assess cerebral activation of motor function after poststroke hemiparesis. *Stroke*, *29*(1), 112–122. doi:10.1161/01.STR.29.1.112 PMID:9445338

Cendelin, J., Korelusova, I., & Vozeh, F. (2008). The Effect of Repeated Rota Rod Training on motor skills and spatial learning ability in Lurcher Mutant mice. *Behavioural Brain Research*, *189*(1), 65–74. doi:10.1016/j.bbr.2007.12.013 PMID:18243354

Chan, P. H. (1996). Role of oxidants in ischemic brain damage. *Stroke*, *27*(6), 1124–1129. doi:10.1161/01.STR.27.6.1124 PMID:8650725

Corbett, D., & Nurse, S. (1998). The problem of assessing effective neuroprotection in experimental cerebral ischemia. *Progress in Neurobiology*, *54*(5), 531–548. doi:10.1016/S0301-0082(97)00078-6 PMID:9550190

Crack, P. J., & Taylor, J. M. (2005). Reactive oxygen species and the modulation of stroke. *Free Radical Biology & Medicine*, *38*(11), pp1433–pp1444. doi:10.1016/j.freeradbiomed.2005.01.019 PMID:15890617

Cramer, S. C., Nelles, G., Benson, R. R., Kaplan, J. D., Parker, R. A., Kwong, K. K., ... Rosen, B. R. (1997). A functional MRI study of subjects recovered from hemiparetic stroke. *Stroke*, *28*(12), 2518–2527. doi:10.1161/01.STR.28.12.2518 PMID:9412643

Crisostomo, E. A., Duncan, P. W., Propst, M., Dawson, D. V., & Davis, J. N. (1988). Evidence that amphetamine with physical therapy promotes recovery of motor function in stroke patients. *Annals of Neurology*, *23*(1), 94–97. doi:10.1002/ana.410230117 PMID:3345072

Danton, H. G., & Dietrich, D. (2004). The search for neuroprotective strategies in stroke. *AJNR. American Journal of Neuroradiology*, *25*, 181–194. PMID:14970016

Del Zoppo, G. J., & Hallenbeck, J. M. (2000). Advances in the vascular pathophysiology of ischemic stroke. *Thrombosis Research*, *98*(3), 73–81. doi:10.1016/S0049-3848(00)00218-8 PMID:10812160

Dirangle, U., Iadecola, C., & Moskowitz, M. A. (1999). 'Pathobiology of ischemic stroke: An integrated view'. *Trends in Neurosciences*, *22*(9), 391–397. doi:10.1016/S0166-2236(99)01401-0 PMID:10441299

Donnan, G. A., Bladin, P. F., Berkovic, S. F., Longley, W. A., & Saling, M. M. (1991). The stroke syndrome of striatocapsular infarction. *Brain*, *114*(Pt 1A), 51–70. PMID:1998890

Donnan, G. A., Fisher, M., Macleod, M., & Davis, S. M. (2008). Stroke. *Lancet*, *371*(9624), 1612–1623. doi:10.1016/S0140-6736(08)60694-7 PMID:18468545

Duff, J. (2004). The usefulness of quantitative EEG (QEEG) and neurotherapy in the assessment and treatment of post-concussion syndrome. *Clinical EEG and Neuroscience*, *35*(4), 198–209. doi:10.1177/155005940403500410 PMID:15493535

Dunham, N. W., & Miya, T. S. (1957). A note on a simple apparatus for detecting neurological deficit in rats and mice. *J Am Pharm Assoc Am Pharm Assoc (Baltim)*, *46*(3), 208–209. doi:10.1002/jps.3030460322 PMID:13502156

Ercelebi, E. (2004). Electrocardiogram signals de-noising using lifting-based discrete wavelet transform. *Computers in Biology and Medicine*, *34*(6), 479–493. doi:10.1016/S0010-4825(03)00090-8 PMID:15265720

Folkers, A., Mosch, F., Malina, T., & Hofmann, U. G. (2003). Realtime bioelectrical data acquisition and processing from 128 channels utilizing the wavelet-transformation. *Neurocomputing*, *52-54*, 247–254. doi:10.1016/S0925-2312(02)00763-4

Fox, S. E., Wolfson, S., & Ranck, J. B. Jr. (1986). Hippocampal theta rhythm and the firing of neurons in walking and urethane anesthetized rats. *Experimental Brain Research*, *62*(3), 495–508. doi:10.1007/BF00236028 PMID:3720881

Frigola, C.J., Colombo, P.A., & Pares, C.J. (1987). Eur. Pat., EP 242, 289, pp 6.

Geets, W., & Louette, N. (1985). Early EEG in 300 cerebral concussions. *EEG and Clinical Neurophysiology*, *14*(4), 333–338. PMID:4023359

Gevins, A. S., & Schaffer, R. E. (1980). A critical-review of electroencephalographic (EEG) correlates of higher cortical functions. *CRC Critical Reviews in Bioengineering*, *4*, 113–164. PMID:7004774

Gilligan, A. K., Thrift, A. G., Sturm, J. W., Dewey, H. M., Macdonell, R. A., & Donnan, G. A. (2005). Stroke units, tissue plasminogen activator, aspirin and neuroprotection: Which stroke intervention could provide the greatest community benefit? *Cerebrovascular Diseases (Basel, Switzerland)*, *20*(4), 239–244. doi:10.1159/000087705 PMID:16123543

Ginsberg, M. D. (2008). Neuroprotection for ischemic stroke: Past, present and future. *Neuropharmacology*, *55*(3), 363–389. doi:10.1016/j.neuropharm.2007.12.007 PMID:18308347

Grassberger, P., & Procaccia, I. (1983). Characterization of Strange Attractors. *Physical Review Letters*, *50*(5), 346–349. doi:10.1103/PhysRevLett.50.346

Guler, I., Kiymik, M. K., Akin, M., & Alkan, A. (2001). AR spectral analysis of EEG signals by using maximum likelihood estimation. *Computers in Biology and Medicine*, *31*(6), 441–450. doi:10.1016/S0010-4825(01)00022-1 PMID:11604150

Gu¨ler, N. F., Kiymik, M. K., & Güler, İ. (1995). Comparison of FFT and AR-based sonogram outputs of 20 MHz pulsed Doppler Data in real Time. *J. Computers Biol. Med*, *25*(4), 383–391. doi:10.1016/0010-4825(95)00024-X PMID:7497700

Guyot, L. L., Diaz, F. G., O'Regan, M. H., Mcleod, S., Park, H., & Phillis, J. W. (2001). Real-time measurement of glutamate release from the ischemic penumbra of the rat cerebral cortex using a focal middle cerebral artery occlusion mode. *Neuroscience Letters*, *299*(1-2), 37–40. doi:10.1016/S0304-3940(01)01510-5 PMID:11166932

Haselsteiner, E., & Pfurtscheller, G. (2000). Using time-dependent neural Networks for EEG classification. *IEEE Transactions on Rehabilitation Engineering*, *8*(4), 457–463. doi:10.1109/86.895948 PMID:11204036

Hinterberger, T., Weiskopf, N., Veit, R., Wilhelm, B., Betta, E., & Birbaumer, N. (2004). An EEG-driven brain-computer interface combined with functional magnetic resonance imaging (fMRI). *IEEE Transactions on Biomedical Engineering*, *51*(6), 971–974. doi:10.1109/TBME.2004.827069 PMID:15188866

Hong, J. T., Ryu, S. R., Kim, H. J., Lee, J. K., Lee, S. H., Kim, D. B., ... Kim, P. Y. (2000). Neuroprotective effect of green tea extract in experimental ischemia-reperfusion brain injury. *Brain Research Bulletin*, *53*(6), 743–749. doi:10.1016/S0361-9230(00)00348-8 PMID:11179838

Hong, J. T., Ryu, S. R., Kim, H. J., Lee, J. K., Lee, S. H., Yun, Y. P., ... Kim, P. Y. (2001). Protective effect of green tea extract on ischemia/reperfusion-induced brain injury in Mongolian gerbils. *Brain Research*, *888*(1), 11–18. doi:10.1016/S0006-8993(00)02935-8 PMID:11146047

Horn, J., & Limburg, M. (2001a). Calcium antagonists for ischemic stroke: A systematic review. *Stroke*, *32*(2), 570–576. doi:10.1161/01.STR.32.2.570 PMID:11157199

Ikeda, M., Suzuki, C., Umegaki, K., Saito, K., Tabuchi, M., & Tomita, T. (2007). Preventive effects of green tea catechins on spontaneous stroke in rats. *Medical Science Monitor*, *13*, BR40–BR45. PMID:17261979

Jarchi, D., Boostani, R., Taheri, M., & Sanei, S. (2009). Seizure source localization using a hybrid second order blind identification and extended rival penalized competitive learning algorithm. *Biomedical Signal Processing and Control*, *4*(2), 108–117. doi:10.1016/j.bspc.2009.01.004

Jasper, H. H. (1958). The ten-twenty electrode system of the International Federation. *EEG Clinical Neurophysiology*, *10*, 371–375.

Kumar, Y., Dewal, M. L., & Anand, R. S. (2012). Epileptic seizures detection in EEG using DWT-based ApEn and artificial neural network. *SIViP*. DOI 10.1007/s11760-012-0362-9

Kwon, S. K., Park, M. S., Sin, Y. S., & Nam, Y. J. (1996). Korean Pat., KR 9,C 04,829.

Laban, G., Guenther, W., & Lohmann, D. (1987). Ger. Pat., DD 247,674, pp4.

Lee, R. G., & van Donkelaar, P. (1995). Mechanisms underlying functional recovery following stroke. *The Canadian Journal of Neurological Sciences*, *22*(04), 257–263. doi:10.1017/S0317167100039445 PMID:8599767

Lipton, P. (1999). Ischemic cell death in brain neurons. *Physiological Reviews*, *79*(4), 1431–1568. doi:10.1152/physrev.1999.79.4.1431 PMID:10508238

Liu, C. H., Ma, X., Song, L. P., Fan, J., Wang, W. D., Lv, X. Y., ... Wang, C. Y. (2015). 'Abnormal spontaneous neural activity in the anterior insular and anterior cingulate cortices in anxious depression'. *Behavioural Brain Research*, *281*, 339–347. doi:10.1016/j.bbr.2014.11.047 PMID:25513974

Lloyd-Jones, D., Adams, R., & Carnethon, M. (2006). Diazepam to improve acute stroke outcome: Results of the early GABA-Ergic activation study in stroke trial. a randomized double-blind placebo-controlled trial. *Cerebrovascular Diseases (Basel, Switzerland)*, *21*(1-2), 120–127. doi:10.1159/000090210 PMID:16340187

Longa, E. Z., Weinstein, P. R., Carlson, S., & Cummins, R. (1989). Reversible middle cerebral artery occlusion without craniectomy in rats. *Stroke*, *20*(1), 84–91. doi:10.1161/01.STR.20.1.84 PMID:2643202

Lopes da Silva, F. (1991). Neural mechanisms underlying brain waves: From neural membranes to networks. *Electroencephalography and Clinical Neurophysiology*, *79*(2), 81–93. doi:10.1016/0013-4694(91)90044-5 PMID:1713832

Lutzenberger, W., Elbert, T., & Rockstroh, B. (1987). A brief tutorial on the implications of volume conduction for the interpretation of the EEG. *Journal of Psychophysiology*, *1*, 81–89.

Maan, M. S. (2007). EEG Waves Classifier using Wavelet Transform and Fourier Transform. *International Journal of Medical, Pharmaceutical Science and Engineering, 1*(3), 166-171.

Mergenthaler, P., Dirnagl, U., & Meisel, A. (2004). Pathophysiology of stroke: Lessons from animal models. *Metabolic Brain Disease*, *19*(3-4), 151–167. doi:10.1023/B:MEBR.0000043966.46964.e6 PMID:15554412

Mohanasundari, M., Srinivasan, M. S., Sethupathy, S., & Sabesan, M. (2006). Enhanced neuroprotective effect by combination of bromocriptine and Hypericumperforatumextract against MPTP-induced neurotoxicity in mice. *Journal of the Neurological Sciences*, *249*(2), 140–144. doi:10.1016/j.jns.2006.06.018 PMID:16876826

Muir, K. W., & Grosset, D. G. (1999). Neuroprotection for acute stroke: Making clinical trials work. *Stroke*, *30*(1), 180–182. doi:10.1161/01.STR.30.1.180 PMID:9880407

Murray, C. J., & Lopez, A. D. (1997). Mortality by cause for eight regions of the world: Global Burden of Disease Study. *Lancet*, *349*(9061), 1269–1276. doi:10.1016/S0140-6736(96)07493-4 PMID:9142060

Nagata, K. (1988). Topographic EEG in brain ischemia: Correlation with blood flow and metabolism. *Brain Topography*, *1*(2), 97–106. doi:10.1007/BF01129174 PMID:3079309

Nuwer, M., & Novda, D. (2005). Routine and quantitative EEG in mild traumatic brain injury. *Clinical Neurophysiology*, *116*(9), 2001–2025. doi:10.1016/j.clinph.2005.05.008 PMID:16029958

O'Keefe, J., & Burgess, N. (2005). Dual phase and rate coding in hippocampal place cells: Theoretical significance and relationship to entorhinal grid cells. *Hippocampus*, *15*(7), 853–866. doi:10.1002/hipo.20115 PMID:16145693

Ocak, H. (2009). Automatic detection of epileptic seizures in EEG using discrete wavelet transform and approximate entropy. *Expert Systems with Applications*, *36*(2), 2027–2036. doi:10.1016/j.eswa.2007.12.065

Orhan, H., & Sahin, G. (2001). In vitro effects of NSAIDS and paracetamolon oxidative stress-related parameters of human erythrocytes. *Experimental and Toxicologic Pathology*, *53*(2-3), 133–140. doi:10.1078/0940-2993-00179 PMID:11484831

Page, C. P., Curtis, M. J., Sutter, M., Walker, M., & Hoffman, B. (1998). *Farmacologíaintegrada*. Published by ElsevierEspaña. (in Spanish)

Pandit, S. M., & Wu, S.-M. (1983). *Time Series and System Analysis with Applications*. John Wiley & Sons.

Paul, S., Bhattacharya, P., Pandey, A. K., & Patnaik, R. (2014). Application of mathematical modeling as a tool to analyze the EEG signals in rat model of focal cerebral ischemia. *Journal of the Institution of Engineers. Springer, 95*(1), 23-27.

Paul, S., Bhattacharya, P., Pandey, A. K., Sharma, N., Tiwari, J. P., & Patnaik, R. (2012). A Strategic Application of Fast Fourier Transform as a Novel Tool to Evaluate the Extent of Neuronal Insult in Rat Model of Focal Cerebral Ischemia. *Bangladesh Journal of Medical Physics*, *5*(1), 29–36.

Paul, S., Sinha, T. K., Bhattacharya, P., & Patnaik, R. (2014). Neural Network based classification of EEG Signal in induced focal cerebral ischemic rat brain. *International Journal of Advanced Information Science and Technology*, *32*(32), 49–54.

Paul, S., Sinha, T. K., & Patnaik, R. (2015). EEG Time Series data analysis in Focal Cerebral ischemic rat model. *International Journal of Biomedical Engineering and Science, 2*(1), 1-10.

Percival, D. B., & Walden, A. T. (1993). *Spectral Analysis for Physical Applications*. Cambridge University Press. doi:10.1017/CBO9780511622762

Pereda, E., Quiroga, R. Q., & Bhattacharya, J. (2005). Nonlinear Multivariate Analysis of Neurophysiological Signals. *Progress in Neurobiology*, *77*(1–2), 1–37. doi:10.1016/j.pneurobio.2005.10.003 PMID:16289760

Peters, B. O., Pfurtscheller, G., & Flyvbjerg, H. (2001). Automatic differentiation of multichannel EEG signals. *IEEE Transactions on Biomedical Engineering*, *48*(1), 111–116. doi:10.1109/10.900270 PMID:11235582

Petrosian, A., Prokhorov, D., Homan, R., Dashei, R., & Wunsch, D. (2000). Recurrent neural network based prediction of epileptic seizures in intra- and extracranial EEG. *Neurocomputing*, *30*(1-4), 201–218. doi:10.1016/S0925-2312(99)00126-5

Pignataro, G., Tortiglione, A., Scorziello, A., Giaccio, L., Secondo, A., Severino, B., ... Annunziato, L. (2004b). Evidence for a protective role played by the Na+/Ca2+ exchanger in cerebral ischemia induced by middle cerebral artery occlusion in male rats. *Neuropharmacology*, *46*(3), 439–448. doi:10.1016/j.neuropharm.2003.09.015 PMID:14975699

Pointinger, H., Sarahrudi, K., Poeschl, G., & Munk, P. (2002). Electroencephalography in primary diagnosis of mild head trauma. *Brain Injury*, *16*(9), 799–805. doi:10.1080/02699050210131911 PMID:12217205

Pradhan, N., Sadasivan, P. K., & Arunodaya, G. R. (1996). Detection of seizure activity in EEG by an artificial neural network: A preliminary study. *Computers and Biomedical Research, an International Journal*, *29*(4), 303–313. doi:10.1006/cbmr.1996.0022 PMID:8812076

Proakis, J., & Manolakis, D. (1996). *Digital Signal Processing Principles, Algorithms, and Applications*. Prentice Hall.

Qu, H., & Gotman, J. (1997). A Patient-specific algorithm for the detection of seizure onset in long-term EEG monitoring: Possible use as a warning device. *IEEE Transactions on Biomedical Engineering*, *44*(2), 115–122. doi:10.1109/10.552241 PMID:9214791

Rafael, F.A., & Ortiz, H. (1982). J. Span Pat., ES 508,671, pp 10.

Rosamond, W., Flegal, K., Friday, G., Furie, K., Go, A., & Hong, Y. (2007). Heart disease and stroke statistics--2007 update: A report from the American Heart Association Statistics Committee and Stroke Statistics Subcommittee. *Circulation*, *115*(5), 69–171. doi:10.1161/CIRCULATIONAHA.106.179918 PMID:17194875

Ross, R. (1999). Atherosclerosis-an inflammatory disease. *Review New Engl. J. Med*, *340*(2), 115–126. doi:10.1056/NEJM199901143400207 PMID:9887164

Satoskar, R. S., Bhandarkar, S. D., & Ainapure, S. S. (2003). *Pharmacology and Pharmacotherapeutics* (18th ed.). Mumbai: Popular Prakashan.

Schacter, D. L. (1977). EEG theta waves and psychological phenomena: A review and analysis. *Biological Psychology*, *5*(1), 47–82. doi:10.1016/0301-0511(77)90028-X PMID:193587

Schallert, T. (1988). Aging-dependent emergence of sensorimotor dysfunction in rats recovered from dopamine depletion sustained early in life. *Annals of the New York Academy of Sciences*, *515*(1), 108–120. doi:10.1111/j.1749-6632.1988.tb32972.x PMID:3364880

Schallert, T., Hernandez, T. D., & Barth, T. M. (1986). Recovery of function after brain damage: Severe and chronic disruption by diazepam. *Brain Research*, *379*(1), 104–111. doi:10.1016/0006-8993(86)90261-1 PMID:3742206

Shafrir, E. (1993). Paul Ehrlich--pioneer in chemotherapy, histology and immunology. *Israel Journal of Medical Sciences*, *29*(5), 327. PMID:8314701

Sharma, V. N. (1999). *Essentials of pharmacology*. CBS Pub. &Distbrs.

Shaw, J. C., & Ongley, C. (1972). The measurement of synchronization. In H. Petsche & M. A. B. Brazier (Eds.), *Synchronization of EEG activity in epilepsies* (pp. 204–216). Springer-Verlag. doi:10.1007/978-3-7091-8306-9_13

Shin, H. S., Park, M. S., & Kwon, S. K. (2000). YakhakHoechi. *EJP*, *44*(3), 272–278.

Shin, S. C., Shin, E. Y., & Cho, C. W. (2000). Enhancing effects of fatty acids on permeation through rat skins. *Drug Development and Industrial Pharmacy*, *26*(5), 563–566. doi:10.1081/DDC-100101269 PMID:10789070

Suffczynski, Lopes da Silva, Parra, Velis, Bouwman, van Rijn, … Kalitzin. (2006). Dynamics of Epileptic Phenomena Determined From Statistics of Ictal Transitions. IEEE Transactions on Biomedical Engineering, 53.

Tye & Deisseroth. (2012). Optogenetic investigation of neural circuits underlying brain disease in animal models. *Nature Reviews, 13*, 251-266.

Wang, C. P. (2007). 'Dynamic covariation of symptoms of anxiety and depression among newly-diagnosed patients with major depressive episode, panic disorder, and controls'. *Nonlinear Dynamics Psychology and Life Sciences*, *11*(3), 349–365.

Chapter 15
Effect of a Motivational Song on the Autonomic Nervous System and the Heart of Indian Male Volunteers

Gitika Yadu
National Institute of Technology Rourkela, India

Suraj Kumar Nayak
National Institute of Technology Rourkela, India

Debasisha Panigrahi
National Institute of Technology Rourkela, India

Sirsendu Sekhar Ray
National Institute of Technology Rourkela, India

Kunal Pal
National Institute of Technology Rourkela, India

ABSTRACT

This chapter investigates the effect of a motivational song (stimulus) on the physiology of the autonomic nervous system and the electrical activity of the heart. Five min electrocardiogram (ECG) signals were acquired from 19 volunteers during the resting and the post-stimulus conditions. The RR intervals (RRIs) were extracted. Recurrence analysis of the RRI time series indicated a higher alteration (acceleration or deceleration) in the heart rate along with the reduction of the causality and patterned behavior of the RRIs. The exact alteration in the ANS physiology was examined using heart rate variability (HRV) analysis. The results of the HRV analysis suggested an increase in the parasympathetic activity in the post-stimulus condition. The alteration in the cardiac activity was analyzed using time domain and joint time-frequency domain analyses of ECG signals. The results suggested an alteration in the cardiac electrical activity of the heart in the post-stimulus condition.

DOI: 10.4018/978-1-5225-4969-7.ch015

INTRODUCTION

Music has been reported to evoke the emotion of the persons (Pannese, Rappaz, & Grandjean, 2016). In fact, it acts as a stimulus, which can initiate emotional memories in the person (Becker, 2004; Schulkind, Hennis, & Rubin, 1999). Recent studies have suggested that the alteration in the emotions while listening to music is also associated with a change in the physical state of the person (Schneck & Berger, 2005). Briefly, we can say that while listening to music, there is a temporary change in the physiological and psychological state of the person (Kemp & Quintana, 2013). Listening to music has been reported to alter the physiological processes like promoting sleep, reduce anxiety, increase positive post-task attitude towards exercise and/or increase brain activities (Elliott, Carr, & Orme, 2005; Lin et al., 2008). The afore-mentioned day-to-day activities are being controlled by the functioning of the Autonomic Nervous System. The analysis of the ANS can be achieved in a non-invasive manner by studying HRV (Dodds, Miller, Kyle, Marshall, & Gordon, 2017). HRV analysis deals with the study of the beat-to-beat interval variation of the heart (Kleiger, Stein, & Bigger, 2005). The beat-to-beat interval variation mainly occurs due to the intervention of the ANS on the cardiac activity (Tavernier & Jeanne, 2014). HRV is studied by recording ECG signals from the human volunteers and computing the RRIs. Recurrence analysis provides information about the temporal variation in a time series (H Sabelli et al., 2005). Numerous studies have revealed that recurrence analysis of the RRIs can also be used to identify changes in the cardiovascular activity due to any stimulus or pathological condition (Chen, Chou, & Tseng, 2014). Taking the motivation from the facts mentioned above, this study attempts to understand the effect of listening to a motivational song on the ANS and the cardiac electrophysiology. In this study, we have selected a new generation motivational song from the Bollywood movie "Marry Kom". This was intentionally done as the volunteers participating in our group are of the current generation, having age in the range of 21 and 23 years. The parameters of recurrence analysis were analysed to identify the variations in the RRIs of the pre- and the post-stimulus conditions. The HRV and the ECG (either original or wavelet processed) signal statistical parameters were used to classify the pre- and the post-stimulus conditions. In our study, we found that there are significant differences in both the ANS activity and cardiac physiology.

BACKGROUND

In the last few decades, the effect of music on the different human physiological systems has been extensively studied. Elliot *et al.* (2005) have reported that the exercise intensity, in-task effect and positive attitude towards exercise can be improved if the volunteers are made to listen to motivational music (Elliot, 2005). Recurrence analysis has evolved as an important non-linear tool for the analysis of different time series including the cardiovascular signals like the RRI series and the ECG signals (H Sabelli et al., 2005). Sun *et al.* (2008) have used recurrence analysis of RRIs for predicting the termination of atrial fibrillation, which can be useful to understand the mechanisms of arrhythmia (Sun & Wang, 2008). Sabelli *et al.* (2011) reported recurrence analysis-based estimation of distinct creative patterns in RRIs of depressed and psychotic persons (H Sabelli, Messer, Kovacevic, & Walthall, 2011). Chen *et al.* (2014) have proposed the use of recurrence analysis of HRV signals for quantifying the variation in the cardiovascular activity when exposed to low-frequency noise of a range of intensities (Chen et al., 2014). HRV analysis is an important non-invasive method to understand the ANS activity. Xue *et al.*

(2015) have implied time domain analysis on RRIs to analyse the features of HRV. The statistical features frequently used for the RRIs were difference between the square root mean square, overall standard deviation and mean (Xue, Chen, Fang, & Xia, 2015).

Over the years, ECG signals have received special attention of the researchers for the diagnosis of the cardiac disorders and understanding the effects of different stimuli on the heart (Maron et al., 2014; Yen et al., 2010). Hedge *et al.* (2013) have summarized currently employed methods for the processing and analysis of the ECG signals that can enable the establishment of resilient cardiac health monitoring devices. They have reported that better information about the cardiac health can be obtained from the time frequency decomposition of the ECG signals, mainly during the post operation condition. A trained model such as the higher order spectra (HOS) of the ECG features can be appointed for the classification of diseases, which can enable the monitoring of the cardiac diseases in a proper manner (Hegde, Deekshit, & Satyanarayana, 2013). Shufni *et al.* (2015) transformed the ECG signals using Fourier transform and discrete wavelet transform so as to obtain the significant features. Features were also extracted from the time domain analysis of the ECG signals. The features obtained from the time domain, frequency domain and joint time-frequency domain methods were analyzed and compared in order to detect the heart diseases (Shufni & Mashor, 2015). Hajizadeh *et al.* (2015) studied the effect of music on heart by classifying the ECG signals acquired during the pre- and the on-music states (Hajizadeh, Abbasi, & Goshvarpour, 2015). Tan *et al.* (2015) investigated the effect of relaxing music on heart rate and HRV in coronary heart patients and cancer patients (Tan, Ozdemir, Temiz, & Celik, 2015). Nayak *et al.* (2016) analyzed the effect of a slow and a fast music on the ANS and the heart of young Indian male volunteers using ECG and HRV analysis (Suraj Kumar Nayak et al., 2016). The results suggested that both the types of music altered the conduction pathway of the heart. However, the slow and the fast music affected the sympathovagal balance in different proportions. A number of studies have been performed previously to understand the effect of different types of music on the physiology of the ANS and the heart using ECG and RRI signal analysis. However, the implementation of the nonlinear dynamical system analysis method, namely, recurrence analysis distinguishes this study from the similar literature reported previously.

MAIN FOCUS OF THE CHAPTER

The main focus of present study is to analyse the effect of a motivational song (stimulus) on the physiology of ANS and cardiac electrophysiology. ECG signals were acquired from 19 volunteers for 5 min duration before and after exposing them to the motivational song and the RRIs were extracted. Recurrence analysis and HRV analysis were performed using the RRI time series to investigate the alteration in the ANS activity due to the stimulus. The time domain and joint time-frequency domain analyses of the ECG signals were performed to detect the change in the cardiac electrophysiology.

METHODOLOGY

In our study, healthy male volunteers within the age group of 21 and 23 years were invited for participation. The volunteers, who did not have any previous clinical conditions and were non-smokers, were selected for the participation. All the volunteers could be categorised as sedentary volunteers as they were not involved in any kind of regular physical activities. Out of the 30 volunteers, who showed interest to participate in the study, 19 volunteers were shortlisted based on the aforementioned criteria.

The volunteers were advised to report at the ECG recording station at 7.00 pm. They were advised not to take food prior to 1 h of reporting. They were made to sit comfortably on a chair. The ECG of the volunteers were recorded in the lead-I configuration (sampling frequency of the recording device was 1000 Hz). The ECG was recorded for 5 min, which was used as the pre-stimulus signal (Category-N). Thereafter, the volunteers were asked to relax for 30 min. After the resting stage, the volunteers were made to listen to the motivational song. At the end of the music, the ECG was recorded for 5 min, which was used as the post-stimulus signal (Category-S). The 5 min ECG data (both pre- and post-stimulus) were analysed using Biomedical Workbench toolkit of LabVIEW (Version 13.0, National Instruments, USA) to extract the RRIs.

The RRIs were used as input for the recurrence as well as the HRV analysis. Recurrence analysis was performed using Bios Data Analyzer (Inverudio Inc., USA)(H Sabelli et al., 2005). Recurrence related parameters, namely, isometry, consecutive isometry, radial isometry, consecutive radial isometry, and novelty were calculated. The recurrence plot was generated for the pre- and the post-stimulus conditions. The HRV analysis was performed using HRV analyzer palette available in Biomedical Workbench toolkit of LabVIEW, which allowed the extraction of 29 HRV parameters. The HRV features were tabulated in an Excel worksheet.

Further, for the time-domain analysis, 5 sec of ECG data was extracted. 12 statistical features of the ECG data were calculated and tabulated in an Excel worksheet. The extracted ECG signal was subsequently processed using db6 wavelet at level 8. The signal was reconstructed using sub-bands of D7 and D8. The statistical features of the reconstructed signals were also calculated and were tabulated in an excel-sheet. The HRV and the ECG signal parameters were used for artificial intelligence based signal classification using artificial neural network (ANN). The important parameters, as estimated from the t-test, Classification and Regression Tree (CART), Boosted Tree (BT) and Random Forest (Mokashi et al.), were used as the categorical inputs for the ANN classification.

RESULTS AND DISCUSSIONS

Recurrence Analysis

Recurrence analysis is an important discriminatory method that can provide information about the degree of determinism and complexity apart from the state changes of a system (Zbilut, Thomasson, & Webber, 2002). In recent years, many researchers have explored the recurrence analysis of RRI time series to predict various heart-related diseases like paroxysmal atrial fibrillation (Mohebbi, Ghassemian, & Asl, 2011; Sun & Wang, 2008). Isometry (or recurrence isometry) is one of the widely used methods of defining and measuring recurrence (H Sabelli et al., 2005). The recurrence of the same length (i.e., equal Euclidean norm within the specified tolerance) vectors in the phase space diagram of a dynamic system divulges information about the isometry. It is measured as the number of recurrence isometries expressed as a percentage of the entire number of pairs of vectors of the sample (Hector Sabelli & Lawandow, 2010).The plot of isometry or any of its derived parameters (expressed in %) with embedding (i.e., the dimensionality of vectors in the phase space diagram) is regarded as an embedding plot. In the current study, the embedding plots of isometry for the pre- and the post-stimulus conditions suggested that the isometry of the pre-stimulus condition was more than that of the post-stimulus condition (Figure 1a). This, in turn, meant that the pre-stimulus condition showed more patterned behaviour than that of the post-stimulus condition(Hector Sabelli & Lawandow, 2010).

Consecutive isometry, which is calculated as a percentage of isometry, can be defined as the number of recurrences that follow one another, i.e., if k_t is a vector recurrent with another vector k_{t+n} then vector k_{t+1} should be recurrent with vector k_{t+n+1} for k_t and k_{t+n} to be in consecutive isometry (H Sabelli et al., 2011). Numerous researchers have reported that consecutive isometry is an indicator of causality (Webber & Zbilut, 1994). In this study, the embedding plots of consecutive isometry obtained from the pre- and the post-stimulus conditions represented that the consecutive isometry of the pre-stimulus condition was more than that of the pre-stimulus condition (Figure 1b), suggesting a more causal behaviour in the pre-stimulus condition. The change in isometry due to the change in the cutoff radius is known as radial

Figure 1. (a) Embedding plot of isometry, (b) Embedding plot of consecutive isometry, (c) Bar graph of radial isometry versuscutoff radius and (d) Bar graph of consecutive radial isometry versuscutoff radius

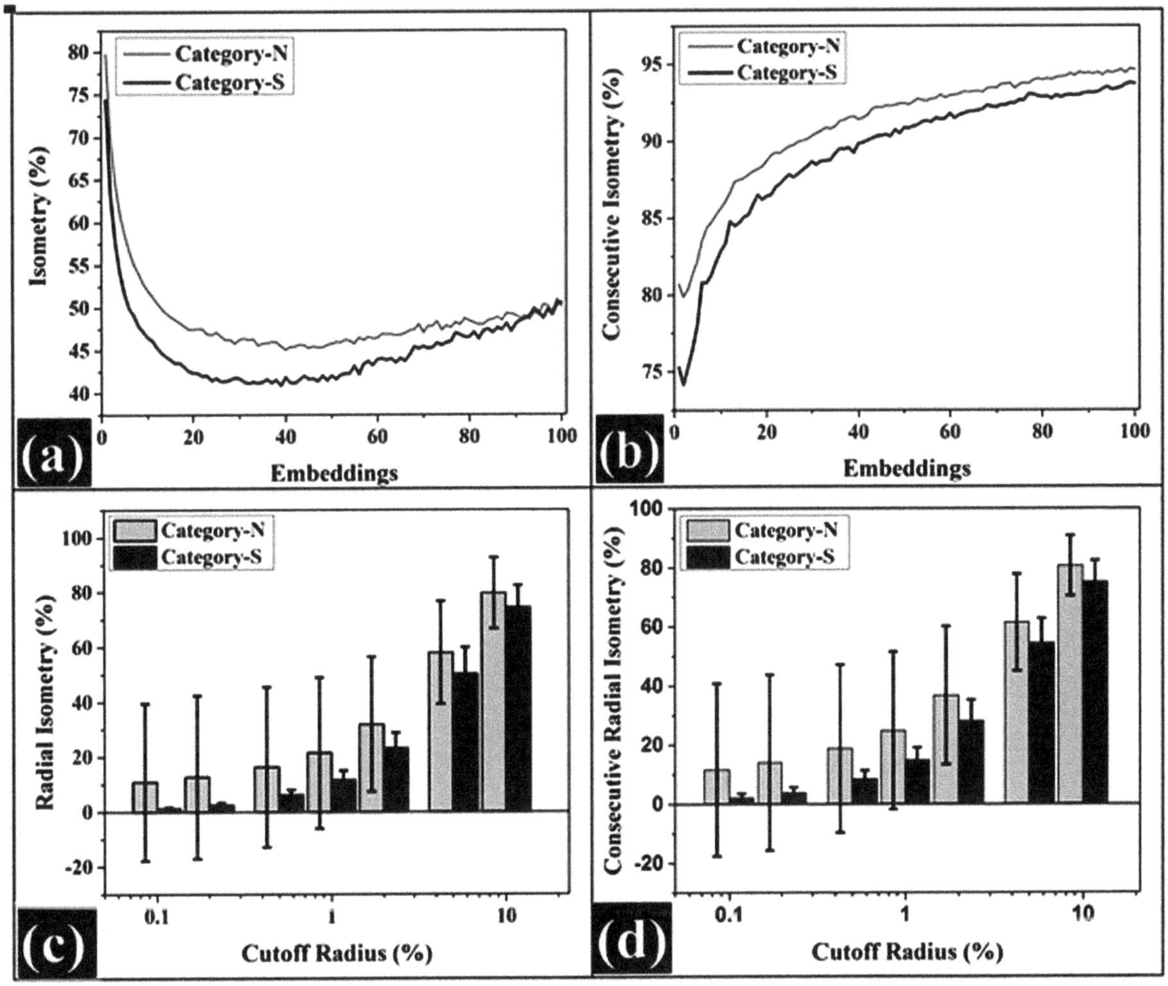

isometry, where the cutoff radius is expressed as a percentage of the range (maximum value - minimum value) of the time series data. Similarly, the change in the consecutive isometry due to the change in the cutoff radius is termed as consecutive radial isometry. As can be seen from Figure 1c and Figure 1d, both the radial isometry and consecutive radial isometry are more for the pre-stimulus condition than that of the post-stimulus condition. Novelty is another important parameter derived from isometry and is regarded as a measure of creativity in a time series (H Sabelli, 2001). It is measured as the ratio of isometry of the original time series data to the isometry obtained after shuffling to the original time series data (H Sabelli et al., 2011). If this ratio is greater than one, then the time series is said to be novel (H Sabelli et al., 2011). It is evident from the Figure 2 that novelty is exhibited by the RRI series of both the pre- and the post-stimulus conditions. However, none of them exhibited consistently higher novelty for the entire embedding range. The novelty of the pre-stimulus condition was higher in the mid region of the embedding plot, whereas, the post-stimulus condition exhibited higher novelty in the starting and the ending regions of the embedding plot. Recurrence plot is the graph of the isometry as a function of time that represents the temporal variations in the pattern. The diagonal line (from the lower left corner to the upper right corner) represents the time (Hector Sabelli & Lawandow, 2010). Sabelli *et al.* (2010) have investigated that the acceleration and deceleration of cardiac rate are depicted by recurrence-free regions, while the stable cardiac rate is represented by recurrence-rich regions in the recurrence plot of RRI time series (Hector Sabelli & Lawandow, 2010). As shown in Figure 3, the recurrence plots were drawn for the pre- and the post-stimulus conditions with 10 embedding and 10% cutoff radius. It is evident from the recurrence plots that more number of recurrence-free regions are present in the recurrence plot of the post-stimulus condition as compared to that of the pre-stimulus condition. This suggested more variation (acceleration or deceleration) of heart rate in the post-stimulus condition as compared to the pre-stimulus condition.

Figure 2. Embedding plot of novelty

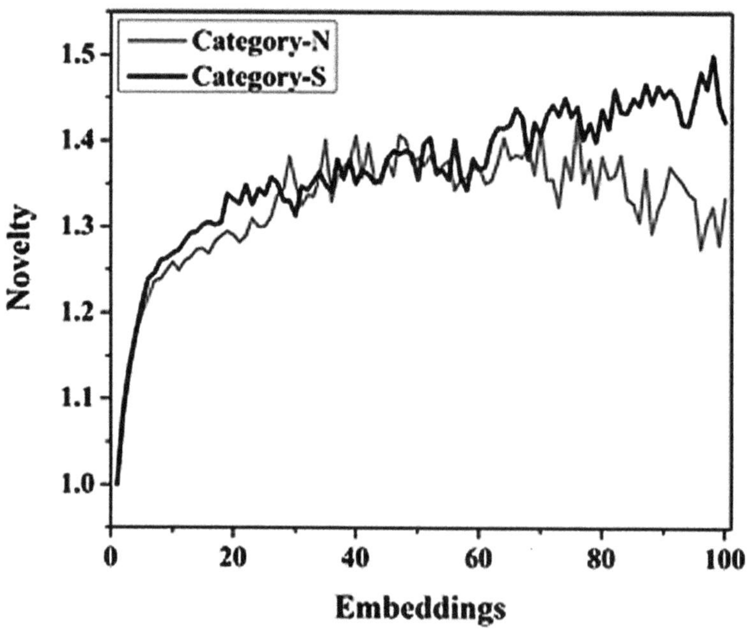

Figure 3. Recurrence plot: (a) pre-stimulus condition and (b) post-stimulus condition

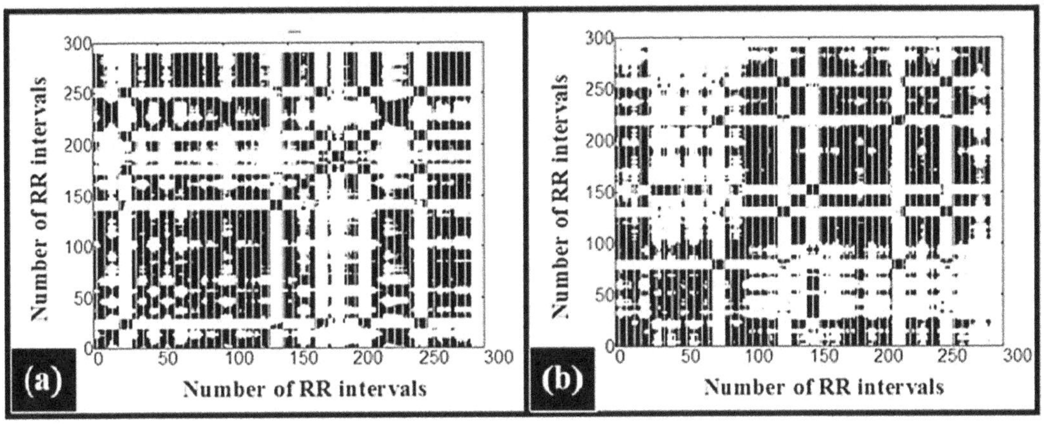

HRV Analysis

In the last few decades, HRV analysis has received special attention of the researchers. This can be attributed to the fact that HRV has emerged as a potential non-invasive marker of the ANS activity. HRV analysis is regarded as short-term if the ECG signal of 2-5 min is used. On the other hand, HRV analysis is called long-term, if it involves the use of 24 h ECG signals (Malik et al., 1996). In the current study, short-term HRV analysis was performed for the pre- and the post-stimulus conditions using 5 min ECG signals. The extraction of the QRS complexes (using a band-pass filter of 10-25 Hz) and the detection of R peaks were performed using Biomedical Workbench toolkit of LabVIEW to obtain the RR intervals. The Biomedical Workbench toolkit was further used to analyse the RR intervals, and 29 HRV parameters were obtained. The HRV parameters included the time domain statistical and geometric parameters, the frequency domain parameters (obtained using fast Fourier transform (FFT) and autoregression (AR) modeling) and the parameters derived from Poincare plot.

All parameters were initially subjected to t-test (with critical p-value ≤ 0.05) to identify the statistically significant parameters. The t-test is a linear statistical method, useful to identify the statistical significance (i.e. the existence of significant difference) of the parameters between two groups of data. HF norm (FFT) was found to be the only significant parameter from t-test (Table 1). The t-test was followed by the implementation of the non-linear decision tree-based methods, namely, CART, BT and RF (with critical predictor importance ≥ 0.95) to find out the parameters, which could be used as the important predictors to classify the HRV data into Category-N and Category-S, respectively. CART analysis resulted in LF power (FFT) as the important predictor, whereas, VLF% (AR) and HF norm (AR) were obtained as important predictors from BT analysis. RF analysis suggested HF % (AR), HF norm (FFT) and HF power (AR) as the important predictors. However, the mean heart rate was not found to be statistically significant from any of the afore-mentioned statistical analysis methods.

It is clear from Table 1 that all the important predictors belonged to the frequency domain parameters. The frequency-domain HRV parameters for short-term HRV analysis comprise of the components of the power spectral density (PSD) of the RR interval data, namely, very low frequency (VLF) power, low frequency (Reyes del Paso, Langewitz, Mulder, Roon, & Duschek) power, and high frequency (HF) power. These power components are expressed as a percentage of the total power (i.e., VLF%, LF% and

Table 1. Important predictors obtained from HRV analysis

Methods	HRV Features	Mean ± SD		Predictor Importance	p-Value
		Category-N	Category-S		
t-test	HF norm (FFT)	43.62±5.39	44.89±9.11		0.0319
CART	LF power(FFT)	2020.53±1460.91	1802.63±1196.51	1.00	----
BT	VLF % (AR)	10.21±2.61	11.06±3.94	1.00	----
	HF norm (AR)	50.18±6.21	50.94±6.86	0.97	----
RF	HF % (AR)	43.26±4.61	44.73±6.66	1.00	----
	HF norm (FFT)	43.61 ±5.39	44.89±9.10	0.95	----
	HF power (AR)	2424.31±1878.92	2790.21±1814.02	0.96	----

HF%) apart from being expressed in absolute units (msec^2) (Suraj K Nayak et al., 2016). LF and HF powers are also represented in normalised form (i.e. LF norm and HF norm) as given below in Equation 1 and 2 (Tarvainen, Niskanen, Lipponen, Ranta-Aho, & Karjalainen, 2014).

$$LF\ norm = \frac{LF\ power(m\sec^2)}{Total\ power(m\sec^2) - VLF\ power(m\sec^2)} \quad (1)$$

$$HF\ norm = \frac{HF\ power(m\sec^2)}{Total\ power(m\sec^2) - VLF\ power(m\sec^2)} \quad (2)$$

The important predictor HF power, calculated using both FFT and AR methods (and represented in absolute unit, in normalised unit and as a percentage of total power), exhibited an increased value in the post-stimulus condition. It has been reported by many researchers that HF power is an indicator of parasympathetic activity (Nijjar et al., 2014). Hence, the HF power suggested an increase in the parasympathetic activity during the post-stimulus condition. Apart from the HF power, VLF power has also been reported to be a marker of the parasympathetic activity (Kleiger et al., 2005). In our study, VLF power (expressed as VLF% and calculated using AR method) showed an increased value in the post-stimulus condition than the pre-stimulus condition. This further suggested an increase in the parasympathetic activity during the post-stimulus condition. Finally, LF power (expressed in the absolute unit and calculated using FFT method) was found to decrease in the post-stimulus condition than the pre-stimulus condition. It has been reported that LF power is related to the sympathetic and parasympathetic activity (Franco, Chabanski, Szliwowski, Dramaix, & Kahn, 2000). Hence, the ratio of the LF and the HF power components (i.e. LF/HF ratio) has been used as a marker of the sympathovagal interaction by many researchers (Billman, 2011; Reyes del Paso et al., 2013). An increase in the LF/HF ratio has been reported to indicate the sympathetic dominance, and the decrease in the LF/HF ratio has been proposed to indicate parasympathetic dominance (Billman, 2013). In our study, the LF/HF ratio computed using both FFT and AR methods showed a reduction in its value in the post-stimulus condition as compared to the pre-stimulus condition (Table 2). Hence, the decrease in the value of the LF power along with the LF/HF ratio further suggested parasympathetic dominance in the post-stimulus condition. In gist, an increase in the parasympathetic activity could be estimated in the post-stimulus condition.

The important predictors were used in various combinations as categorical inputs for the implementation of the ANN classification. Both RBF and MLP neural networks were designed using Statistica Automated Neural Network (SANN) feature of Statistica software (trial version 13.2, Statsoft Inc., USA). The highest classification accuracy of 94% was provided by RBF 2-11-2 network when VLF% (AR), HF% (AR) were used as the categorical inputs (Table 3). The MLP 5-12-2 network also provided the highest classification accuracy of 94% when HF norm (FFT), HF power (AR), HF norm (AR), VLF% (AR) and HF% (AR) were used as the categorical inputs (Table 4). The details of the RBF 2-11-2 and the MLP 5-12-2 networks have been tabulated in Table 5. The results of the ANN classification also confirmed that changes have occurred in the HRV data during the post-stimulus condition in comparison to the pre-stimulus condition.

Table 2. Values of LF/HF ratio during pre- and post-stimulus conditions

Parameter	Mean ± SD	
	Category-N	Category-S
LF/HF (FFT)	0.80 ± 0.26	0.78± 0.38
LF/HF (AR)	0.81 ± 0.23	0.78 ± 0.29

Table 3. Classification summary of RBF 2-11-2 network

	Category-N	Category-S	Overall
Total	19.00	19.00	38.00
Correct	18.00	18.00	36.00
Incorrect	1.00	1.00	2.00
Correct (%)	94.00	94.00	94.00
Incorrect (%)	6.00	6.00	6.00

Table 4. Classification summary of MLP 5-12-2 network

	Category-N	Category-S	Overall
Total	19.00	19.00	38.00
Correct	18.00	18.00	36.00
Incorrect	1.00	1.00	2.00
Correct (%)	94.00	94.00	94.00
Incorrect (%)	6.00	6.00	6.00

Table 5. Details of RBF 2-11-2 and the MLP 5-12-2 networks

Networks	Features Used	CA	Training Performance	Test Performance	Algorithm	Error Function	HAF	OAF
RBF 2-11-2	VLF% (AR), HF% (AR)	94.00	93.54	100.00	RBFT	Entropy	Gaussian	Softmax
MLP 5-12-2	HF norm (FFT), HF power (AR), HF norm (AR), VLF% (AR), HF% (AR)	94.00	96.77	85.71	BFGS 50	SOS	Tanh	Tanh

[CA=Classification accuracy, HAF = Hidden Activation Function, OAF=Output Activation Function]

Time Domain Analysis of ECG Signals

The time domain ECG analysis was performed using 5 sec recordings of the ECG signals, which were extracted from the 5 min ECG recordings. An in-lab developed LabVIEW program was used to calculate 12 statistical parameters from the ECG signals.

Afore-mentioned linear and non-linear analysis methods (i.e., t-test, CART, BT, and RF) were used to identify the important predictors, which could be used for classifying thc ECG signals. The results have been tabulated in Table 6. Although, none of the parameters was found to be statistically significant from t-test, the non-linear methods suggested energy density (Malik et al.), Shannon entropy (SE), log energy (LE), arithmetic mean (AM), summation (Suraj K Nayak et al.), and modeas the important predictors (with predictor importance ≥ 0.95) (Table 6). The existence of these important predictors suggested that the ECG signals acquired during the post-stimulus condition exhibited different characteristics than the ECG signals acquired during the pre-stimulus condition. The change in the characteristics might be non-linearly related as they could not be detected using the linear method (t-test). To further ascertain the occurrence of the changes in the ECG signals acquired during the post-stimulus condition, ANN classification of the ECG signals was performed using RBF and MLP networks. The RBF 2-18-2 network resulted in a classification accuracy of 91.5% (Table 7) with SUM and ED as the categorical inputs. However, the classification accuracy of 76% was achieved by the MLP 4-8-2 network (Table 8). The details of the RBF 2-18-2 and the MLP 4-8-2 networks are tabulated in Table 9.

Table 6. Important predictors obtained from time-domain analysis

Methods	Time Domain Features	Mean ± SD		Predictor Importance
		Category-N	Category-S	
CART	ED	0.01±0.02	0.01±0.03	1.00
	SE	0.04±0.07	0.04±0.06	1.00
	LE	-6.22±2.65	-6.51±3.06	1.00
BT	AM	0.0005±0.002	-0.0002±0.0011	1.00
	SUM	2.75±7.55	-1.16±5.50	1.00
RF	SE	0.04±0.07	0.04±0.06	1.00
	Mode	0.01±0.02	0.01±0.02	0.98

Table 7. Classification summary of RBF 2-18-2 network

	Category-N	Category-S	Overall
Total	19.00	19.00	38.00
Correct	18.00	17.00	35.00
Incorrect	1.00	2.00	3.00
Correct (%)	94.00	89.00	91.50
Incorrect (%)	6.00	11.00	8.50

Table 8. Classification summary of MLP 4-8-2 network

	Category-N	Category-S	Overall
Total	19.00	19.00	38.00
Correct	16.00	13.00	29.00
Incorrect	3.00	6.00	9.00
Correct (%)	84.00	68.00	76.00
Incorrect (%)	16.00	32.00	24.00

Table 9. Details of RBF 2-18-2 and the MLP 4-8-2 networks

Networks	Features Used	CA	Training Performance	Test Performance	Algorithm	Error Function	HAF	OAF
RBF 2-18-2	SUM and ED	91.50	93.54	85.71	RBFT	Entropy	Gaussian	Softmax
MLP 4-8-2	SUM, ED, SE, and LE	76.00	77.41	71.42	BFGS 24	Entropy	Exponential	Softmax

[CA = Classification Accuracy, HAF = Hidden Activation Function, OAF = Output Activation Function]

Joint Time-Frequency Analysis of ECG Signals

The joint time-frequency analysis of the 5 sec recordings of ECG signals was performed using wavelet transform. The decomposition of the ECG signals was done up to level 8 with Daubechies (db06) wavelet as the mother wavelet, followed by the reconstruction of the signal using D7+D8 sub-bands (Figure 4). Daubechies wavelet was chosen as the mother wavelet due to its similarity with the ECG signals (Mokashi et al., 2016). The wavelet processing resulted in the extraction of the R waves from the ECG signals.12 statistical parameters of these R waves were computed similarly to that of the ECG signals during time domain analysis. None of the parameters was found to be statistically significant from the t-test. On the other hand, the nonlinear methods (i.e., CART, BT, and RF) revealed skewness, mode, AM, SUM, median and SE as the important predictors (with predictor importance ≥ 0.95) (Table 10). This, in turn, suggested that the extracted R-waves (or in other way, the wavelet-processed ECG signals) exhibited significantly different and non-linearly related characteristics during post-stimulus condition than the pre-stimulus condition similar to the time domain analysis of the ECG signal. The ANN classification using RBF 3-14-2 network provided a classification accuracy of 91.5% (Table 11), which was

Figure 4. (a) Original ECG signal, (b) signal reconstructed using D7 sub-band, (c) signal reconstructed using D8 sub-band, and (d) signal reconstructed using D7+D8 sub-bands

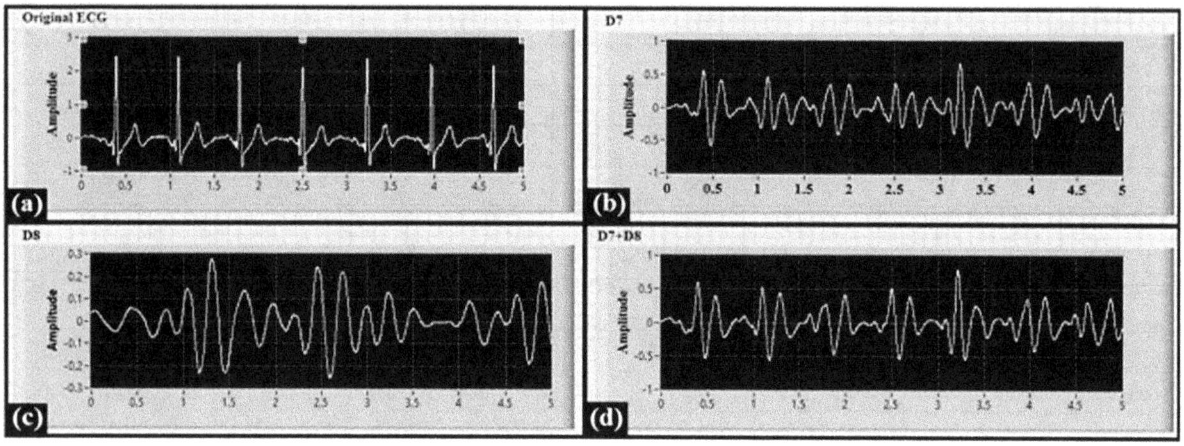

Table 10. Important predictors obtained from joint time-frequency analysis

Methods	Wavelet Domain Features	Mean ± SD		Predictor Importance
		Category-N	Category-S	
CART	Skewness	0.20±0.42	0.21±0.56	1.00
BT	Mode	-0.001±0.004	0.0008±0.0046	1.00
	AM	0.00±0.0001	0.00±0.0001	0.99
	SUM	0.17±0.74	0.03±0.83	0.99
	Median	-0.00±0.0001	-0.00±0.0002	0.96
RF	SE	0.02±0.08	0.01±0.06	1.00

Table 11. Classification summary of RBF 3-14-2 network

	Category-C	Category-N	Overall
Total	19.00	19.00	38.00
Correct	18.00	17.00	35.00
Incorrect	1.00	2.00	3.00
Correct (%)	94.00	89.00	91.50
Incorrect (%)	6.00	11.00	8.50

similar that of classification accuracy obtained from the RBF network (RBF 2-18-2) in the time domain analysis. Interestingly, the MLP 6-5-2network resulted in the classification accuracy of 89% (Table 12), which was significantly higher than that provided by the MLP network (MLP 4-8-2) in the time domain analysis. The details of the RBF 3-14-2 and the MLP 6-5-2 networks are tabulated in Table 13. This suggested that the joint time-frequency analysis may be used for obtaining higher classification accuracy than the time domain analysis of the ECG signals.

Table 12. Classification summary of MLP 6-5-2 network

	Category-C	Category-N	Overall
Total	19.00	19.00	38.00
Correct	17.00	17.00	34.00
Incorrect	2.00	2.00	4.00
Correct (%)	89.00	89.00	89.00
Incorrect (%)	11.00	11.00	11.00

Table 13. Details of RBF 3-14-2 and MLP 6-5-2 networks

Networks	Features Used	CA	Training Performance	Test Performance	Algorithm	Error Function	HAF	OAF
RBF 3-14-2	Mode, SE, Skewness	91.50	93.54	85.71	RBFT	Entropy	Gaussian	Softmax
MLP 6-5-2	Arithmetic Mean, Median, Mode, Summation, SE, Skewness	89.00	90.32	85.71	BFGS 13	Entropy	Tanh	Softmax

[CA = Classification Accuracy, HAF = Hidden Activation Function, OAF = Output Activation Function]

FUTURE RESEARCH DIRECTIONS

The future studies can be performed using other types of music stimuli. Proper validation of the results obtained from this study can be performed by involving more number of volunteers in each category. Decomposition based signal processing techniques such as wavelet packet decomposition and empirical mode decomposition can be employed for analysing the ECG signals. The statistically important features can be investigated using ranking based methods and other decision tree methods for more effective classification.

CONCLUSION

ECG signals were acquired from 19 healthy male volunteers for 5 min during resting condition as well as after listening to a motivational song (stimulus). These ECG signals were categorised as Category-N and Category-S, respectively. These ECG signals were processed to extract the RRIs. The RRIs were used for the recurrence analysis. The parameters of the recurrence analysis suggested a reduction in the patterned behaviour and causality of the RRIs, respectively, in the post-stimulus condition. The recurrence plot suggested an increase in the variation (either acceleration or deceleration) of heart rate in the post-stimulus condition. The HRV analysis was performed to understand the effect of the stimulus on the ANS activity. Linear and non-linear methods were used to find out the important predictors among the parameters obtained from HRV analysis. An in-depth analysis of the important predictors suggested an increase in the parasympathetic activity. The alteration in the ANS activity during post-stimulus condition was also evident from the ANN classification (accuracy of $\geq$ 90%) of the HRV data. The time-domain and the joint time-frequency domain analyses were performed using 5 sec ECG signals. Both the analyses suggested an alteration in the characteristics of the ECG signals acquired during the post-stimulus condition in comparison to those acquired during the pre-stimulus condition. This, in turn, indicated that an alteration in the cardiac electrical activity might have happened in the post-stimulus condition. However, an in-depth analysis is required to find out the exact change in the cardiac electrophysiology.

REFERENCES

Becker, J. O. (2004). *Deep listeners: Music, emotion, and trancing*. Indiana University Press.

Billman, G. E. (2011). Heart rate variability–a historical perspective. *Frontiers in Physiology*, 2. PMID:22144961

Billman, G. E. (2013). The LF/HF ratio does not accurately measure cardiac sympatho-vagal balance. *Frontiers in Physiology*, 4. PMID:23431279

Chen, S.-T., Chou, C.-Y., & Tseng, L.-H. (2014). Recurrence plot analysis of HRV for exposure to low-frequency noise. *Advanced Materials Research*.

Dodds, K. L., Miller, C. B., Kyle, S. D., Marshall, N. S., & Gordon, C. J. (2017). Heart rate variability in insomnia patients: A critical review of the literature. *Sleep Medicine Reviews*, *33*, 88–100. doi:10.1016/j.smrv.2016.06.004 PMID:28187954

Elliot, A. J. (2005). *A Conceptual History of the Achievement Goal Construct*. Academic Press.

Elliott, D., Carr, S., & Orme, D. (2005). The effect of motivational music on sub-maximal exercise. *European Journal of Sport Science*, *5*(2), 97–106. doi:10.1080/17461390500171310

Franco, P., Chabanski, S., Szliwowski, H., Dramaix, M., & Kahn, A. (2000). Influence of maternal smoking on autonomic nervous system in healthy infants. *Pediatric Research*, *47*(2), 215–215. doi:10.1203/00006450-200002000-00011 PMID:10674349

Hajizadeh, S., Abbasi, A., & Goshvarpour, A. (2015). *Intelligent classification of ECG signals to distinguish between pre and on-music states*. Paper presented at the Information and Knowledge Technology (IKT), 2015 7th Conference on. 10.1109/IKT.2015.7288790

Hegde, V. N., Deekshit, R., & Satyanarayana, P. (2013). A review on ECG signal processing and HRV analysis. *Journal of Medical Imaging and Health Informatics*, *3*(2), 270–279. doi:10.1166/jmihi.2013.1163

Kemp, A. H., & Quintana, D. S. (2013). The relationship between mental and physical health: Insights from the study of heart rate variability. *International Journal of Psychophysiology*, *89*(3), 288–296. doi:10.1016/j.ijpsycho.2013.06.018 PMID:23797149

Kleiger, R. E., Stein, P. K., & Bigger, J. T. (2005). Heart rate variability: Measurement and clinical utility. *Annals of Noninvasive Electrocardiology*, *10*(1), 88–101. doi:10.1111/j.1542-474X.2005.10101.x PMID:15649244

Lin, S.-H., Huang, Y.-C., Chien, C.-Y., Chen, Y.-C., Chou, L.-C., & Huang, S.-C. (2008). *A study of the relationship between two musical rhythm characteristics and heart rate variability (HRV).* Paper presented at the BioMedical Engineering and Informatics, 2008. BMEI 2008. International Conference on.

Malik, M., Camm, A., Bigger, J., Breithardt, G., Cerutti, S., & Cohen, R. (1996). Heart rate variability. Standards of measurement, physiological interpretation, and clinical use. *European Heart Journal*, *17*(3), 354–381. doi:10.1093/oxfordjournals.eurheartj.a014868 PMID:8737210

Maron, B. J., Friedman, R. A., Kligfield, P., Levine, B. D., Viskin, S., Chaitman, B. R., ... Thompson, P. D. (2014). Assessment of the 12-Lead ECG as a Screening Test for Detection of Cardiovascular Disease in Healthy General Populations of Young People (12–25 Years of Age). *Circulation*, *130*(15), 1303–1334. doi:10.1161/CIR.0000000000000025 PMID:25223981

Mohebbi, M., Ghassemian, H., & Asl, B. M. (2011). Structures of the recurrence plot of heart rate variability signal as a tool for predicting the onset of paroxysmal atrial fibrillation. *Journal of Medical Signals and Sensors*, *1*(2), 113. PMID:22606666

Mokashi, C., Nayak, S. K., Pradhan, A., Rout, S. K., Pal, K., & Champaty, B. (2016). *Effect of sound in a horror movie clip on the physiology of the ANS and the conduction pathway of the heart.* Paper presented at the India Conference (INDICON), 2016 IEEE Annual. 10.1109/INDICON.2016.7839020

Nayak, S. K., Shukla, R. D., Panda, I., Champaty, B., Thakur, G., Mohapatra, B. (2016). Effect of Slow and Fast Music on the Autonomic Nervous System and Cardiac Health: A Preliminary Investigation. *Classification and Clustering in Biomedical Signal Processing*, 198.

Nayak, S. K., Suman, S., Nayak, B. M., Banerjee, I., Pal, K., & Champaty, B. (2016). *Effect of Cannabis consumption on ANS and conduction pathway of heart of Indian paddy field workers.* Paper presented at the India Conference (INDICON), 2016 IEEE Annual. 10.1109/INDICON.2016.7839018

Nijjar, P. S., Puppala, V. K., Dickinson, O., Duval, S., Duprez, D., Kreitzer, M. J., & Benditt, D. G. (2014). Modulation of the autonomic nervous system assessed through heart rate variability by a mindfulness based stress reduction program. *International Journal of Cardiology*, *177*(2), 557–559. doi:10.1016/j.ijcard.2014.08.116 PMID:25179555

Pannese, A., Rappaz, M.-A., & Grandjean, D. (2016). Metaphor and music emotion: Ancient views and future directions. *Consciousness and Cognition*, *44*, 61–71. doi:10.1016/j.concog.2016.06.015 PMID:27362475

Reyes del Paso, G. A., Langewitz, W., Mulder, L. J., Roon, A., & Duschek, S. (2013). The utility of low frequency heart rate variability as an index of sympathetic cardiac tone: A review with emphasis on a re-analysis of previous studies. *Psychophysiology*, *50*(5), 477–487. doi:10.1111/psyp.12027 PMID:23445494

Sabelli, H. (2001). Novelty, a measure of creative organization in natural and mathematical time series. *Nonlinear Dynamics Psychology and Life Sciences*, *5*(2), 89–113. doi:10.1023/A:1026478316970

Sabelli, H., & Lawandow, A. (2010). Homeobios: The pattern of heartbeats in newborns, adults, and elderly patients. *Nonlinear Dynamics Psychology and Life Sciences*, *14*(4), 381. PMID:20887687

Sabelli, H., Messer, J., Kovacevic, L., & Walthall, K. (2011). Biotic patterns of heart rate variation in depressed and psychotic subjects. *Nonlinear Dynamics Psychology and Life Sciences*, *15*(1), 11–28. PMID:21176437

Sabelli, H., Sugerman, A., Kovacevic, L., Kauffman, L., Carlson-Sabelli, L., & Patel, M. (2005). Bios data analyzer. *Nonlinear Dynamics Psychology and Life Sciences*, *9*(4), 505–538. PMID:16194304

Schneck, D. J., & Berger, D. S. (2005). *The music effect: Music physiology and clinical applications*. Jessica Kingsley Publishers.

Schulkind, M. D., Hennis, L. K., & Rubin, D. C. (1999). Music, emotion, and autobiographical memory: They're playing your song. *Memory & Cognition*, *27*(6), 948–955. doi:10.3758/BF03201225 PMID:10586571

Shufni, S. A., & Mashor, M. Y. (2015). *ECG signals classification based on discrete wavelet transform, time domain and frequency domain features*. Paper presented at the Biomedical Engineering (ICoBE), 2015 2nd International Conference on. 10.1109/ICoBE.2015.7235914

Sun, R., & Wang, Y. (2008). Predicting termination of atrial fibrillation based on the structure and quantification of the recurrence plot. *Medical Engineering & Physics*, *30*(9), 1105–1111. doi:10.1016/j.medengphy.2008.01.008 PMID:18343707

Tan, Y. Z., Ozdemir, S., Temiz, A., & Celik, F. (2015). The effect of relaxing music on heart rate and heart rate variability during ECG GATED-myocardial perfusion scintigraphy. *Complementary Therapies in Clinical Practice*, *21*(2), 137–140. doi:10.1016/j.ctcp.2014.12.003 PMID:25747187

Tarvainen, M. P., Niskanen, J.-P., Lipponen, J. A., Ranta-Aho, P. O., & Karjalainen, P. A. (2014). Kubios HRV–heart rate variability analysis software. *Computer Methods and Programs in Biomedicine*, *113*(1), 210–220. doi:10.1016/j.cmpb.2013.07.024 PMID:24054542

Tavernier, B., & Jeanne, M. (2014). Heart Rate Variability. In *Monitoring Technologies in Acute Care Environments* (pp. 109–115). Springer. doi:10.1007/978-1-4614-8557-5_13

Webber, C. L. Jr, & Zbilut, J. P. (1994). Dynamical assessment of physiological systems and states using recurrence plot strategies. *Journal of Applied Physiology*, *76*(2), 965–973. doi:10.1152/jappl.1994.76.2.965 PMID:8175612

Xue, S., Chen, X., Fang, Z., & Xia, S. (2015). *An ECG arrhythmia classification and heart rate variability analysis system based on android platform*. Paper presented at the Future Information and Communication Technologies for Ubiquitous HealthCare (Ubi-HealthTech), 2015 2nd International Symposium on. 10.1109/Ubi-HealthTech.2015.7203323

Yen, B. S., Wang, H.-M., Hou, M. C., Tcm, D., Huang, S.-C., & Chou, L.-C. (2010). The relationship between music processing and electrocardiogram (ECG) in vegetative state (VS). *Circuits and Systems (ISCAS), Proceedings of 2010 IEEE International Symposium on*. 10.1109/ISCAS.2010.5537211

Zbilut, J. P., Thomasson, N., & Webber, C. L. (2002). Recurrence quantification analysis as a tool for nonlinear exploration of nonstationary cardiac signals. *Medical Engineering & Physics*, *24*(1), 53–60. doi:10.1016/S1350-4533(01)00112-6 PMID:11891140

ADDITIONAL READING

Acharya, U. R., Bhat, P. S., Iyengar, S. S., Rao, A., & Dua, S. (2003). Classification of heart rate data using artificial neural network and fuzzy equivalence relation. *Pattern Recognition*, *36*(1), 61–68. doi:10.1016/S0031-3203(02)00063-8

Alexakis, C., Nyongesa, H., Saatchi, R., Harris, N., Davies, C., Emery, C., ... (2003). *Feature extraction and classification of electrocardiogram (ECG) signals related to hypoglycaemia.* Paper presented at the Computers in Cardiology, 2003.

Anuradha, B., & Reddy, V. V. (2008). ANN for classification of cardiac arrhythmias. *Journal of Engineering and Applied Sciences (Asian Research Publishing Network)*, *3*(3), 1–6.

Aytemir, K., Aksoyek, S., Yildirir, A., Ozer, N., & Oto, A. (1999). Prediction of atrial fibrillation recurrence after cardioversion by P wave signal-averaged electrocardiography. *International Journal of Cardiology*, *70*(1), 15–21. doi:10.1016/S0167-5273(99)00038-8 PMID:10402041

Bentley, P. M., & McDonnell, J. (1994). Wavelet transforms: an introduction. *Electronics & communication engineering journal, 6*(4), 175-186.

Boashah, B., & Mesbah, M. (2001). A time-frequency approach for newborn seizure detection. *IEEE Engineering in Medicine and Biology Magazine*, *20*(5), 54–64. doi:10.1109/51.956820 PMID:11668897

Boashash, B. (2015). *Time-frequency signal analysis and processing: a comprehensive reference*. Academic Press.

Breithardt, G., Wichter, T., Fetsch, T., Seifert, T., Borggrefe, M., Shenasa, M., et al. (1993). The signal-averaged ECG: Time–domain analysis. *European heart journal, 14*(suppl_E), 27-32.

Budeus, M., Hennersdorf, M., Perings, C., Wieneke, H., Erbel, R., & Sack, S. (2005). Prediction of the recurrence of atrial fibrillation after successful cardioversion with P wave signal-averaged ECG. *Annals of Noninvasive Electrocardiology*, *10*(4), 414–419. doi:10.1111/j.1542-474X.2005.00059.x PMID:16255751

Chang, F., Chang, C., Chiu, C., Hsu, S., & Lin, Y. (2007). *Variations of HRV analysis in different approaches.* Paper presented at the Computers in Cardiology, 2007. cheol JEONG, I., & Finkelstein, J. (2015). Real-Time Classification of Exercise Exertion Levels Using Discriminant Analysis of HRV Data. *Enabling Health Informatics Applications, 213*, 171. 10.1109/CIC.2007.4745410

Chou, C.-C., Tseng, S.-Y., Chua, E., Lee, Y.-C., Fang, W.-C., & Huang, H.-C. (2011). *Advanced ECG processor with HRV analysis for real-time portable health monitoring.* Paper presented at the Consumer Electronics-Berlin (ICCE-Berlin), 2011 IEEE International Conference on. 10.1109/ICCE-Berlin.2011.6031850

Falcone, C., Colonna, A., Bozzini, S., Matrone, B., Guasti, L., Paganini, E., & ... . (2014). Cardiovascular risk factors and Sympatho-Vagal balance: Importance of time-domain heart rate variability. *Journal of Clinical & Experimental Cardiology*, *5*(2).

Haberl, R., Jilge, G., Pulter, R., & Steinbeck, G. (1988). Comparison of frequency and time domain analysis of the signal-averaged electrocardiogram in patients with ventricular tachycardia and coronary artery disease: Methodologic validation and clinical relevance. *Journal of the American College of Cardiology*, *12*(1), 150–158. doi:10.1016/0735-1097(88)90368-3 PMID:3379200

Hejjel, L., & Roth, E. (2004). What is the adequate sampling interval of the ECG signal for heart rate variability analysis in the time domain? *Physiological Measurement*, *25*(6), 1405–1411. doi:10.1088/0967-3334/25/6/006 PMID:15712719

Hier, D., Foulkes, M., Swiontoniowski, M., Sacco, R., Gorelick, P., Mohr, J., ... Wolf, P. A. (1991). Stroke recurrence within 2 years after ischemic infarction. *Stroke*, *22*(2), 155–161. doi:10.1161/01.STR.22.2.155 PMID:2003278

Hlawatsch, F., & Boudreaux-Bartels, G. F. (1992). Linear and quadratic time-frequency signal representations. *IEEE Signal Processing Magazine*, *9*(2), 21–67. doi:10.1109/79.127284

Jasper, J., & Othman, K. R. (2010). *Feature extraction for human identification based on envelogram signal analysis of cardiac sounds in time-frequency domain.* Paper presented at the Electronics and Information Engineering (ICEIE), 2010 International Conference On. 10.1109/ICEIE.2010.5559770

Jeyhani, V., Mahdiani, S., Peltokangas, M., & Vehkaoja, A. (2015). *Comparison of HRV parameters derived from photoplethysmography and electrocardiography signals.* Paper presented at the Engineering in Medicine and Biology Society (EMBC), 2015 37th Annual International Conference of the IEEE. 10.1109/EMBC.2015.7319747

Kanagala, R., Murali, N. S., Friedman, P. A., Ammash, N. M., Gersh, B. J., Ballman, K. V., et al. (2003). Obstructive sleep apnea and the recurrence of atrial fibrillation. *circulation, 107*(20), 2589-2594.

Khandoker, A. H., Palaniswami, M., & Karmakar, C. K. (2009). Support vector machines for automated recognition of obstructive sleep apnea syndrome from ECG recordings. *IEEE Transactions on Information Technology in Biomedicine*, *13*(1), 37–48. doi:10.1109/TITB.2008.2004495 PMID:19129022

Kinoshita, O., Fontaine, G., Rosas, F., Elias, J., Iwa, T., Tonet, J., et al. (1995). Time-and frequency-domain analyses of the signal-averaged ECG in patients with arrhythmogenic right ventricular dysplasia. *circulation, 91*(3), 715-721.

Kleiger, R., Stein, P., Bosner, M., & Rottman, J. (1992). Time domain measurements of heart rate variability. *Cardiology Clinics*, *10*(3), 487–498. PMID:1504980

Lai, S. M., Alter, M., Friday, G., & Sobel, E. (1994). A multifactorial analysis of risk factors for recurrence of ischemic stroke. *Stroke*, *25*(5), 958–962. doi:10.1161/01.STR.25.5.958 PMID:8165690

Musialik-Łydka, A., Średniawa, B., & Pasyk, S. (2003). Heart rate variability in heart failure. [Polish Heart Journal]. *Kardiologia Polska*, *58*(1), 14–16. PMID:14502297

Mustafa, M., RTaid, M., Murat, Z. H., & Sulaiman, N. (2012). Comparison between KNN and ANN classification in brain balancing application via spectrogram image. *JCSCM, 2*(4), 17-22.

Tarvainen, M. P., Niskanen, J.-P., Lipponen, J. A., Ranta-Aho, P. O., & Karjalainen, P. A. (2014). Kubios HRV–heart rate variability analysis software. *Computer Methods and Programs in Biomedicine*, *113*(1), 210–220. doi:10.1016/j.cmpb.2013.07.024 PMID:24054542

Tarvainen, M. P., Ranta-Aho, P. O., & Karjalainen, P. A. (2002). An advanced detrending method with application to HRV analysis. *IEEE Transactions on Biomedical Engineering*, *49*(2), 172–175. doi:10.1109/10.979357 PMID:12066885

Tirtom, H., Engin, M., & Engin, E. Z. (2008). Enhancement of time-frequency properties of ECG for detecting micropotentials by wavelet transform based method. *Expert Systems with Applications*, *34*(1), 746–753. doi:10.1016/j.eswa.2006.10.009

Vijaya, G., Kumar, V., & Verma, H. (1998). ANN-based QRS-complex analysis of ECG. *Journal of Medical Engineering & Technology*, *22*(4), 160–167. doi:10.3109/03091909809032534 PMID:9680599

Weinschenk, S. W., Beise, R. D., & Lorenz, J. (2016). Heart rate variability (HRV) in deep breathing tests and 5-min short-term recordings: Agreement of ear photoplethysmography with ECG measurements, in 343 subjects. *European Journal of Applied Physiology*, *116*(8), 1527–1535. doi:10.100700421-016-3401-3 PMID:27278521

Zbilut, J. P., Koebbe, M., Loeb, H., & Mayer-Kress, G. (1990). *Use of recurrence plots in the analysis of heart beat intervals.* Paper presented at the Computers in Cardiology 1990, Proceedings.

Zhang, D. (2005). *Wavelet approach for ECG baseline wander correction and noise reduction.* Paper presented at the Engineering in Medicine and Biology Society, 2005. IEEE-EMBS 2005. 27th Annual International Conference of the.

KEY TERMS AND DEFINITIONS

Artificial Neural Network (ANN): Artificial neural networks are the efficient computing systems that try to mimic the structure and the function of the human nervous system.

Boosted Trees (BT): An ensemble classifier that iteratively re-weights training examples based on errors. This method is slow to train but fast to predict.

Classification and Regression Tree (CART): A decision tree that uses binary partitioning method. It is designed for both classification and regression problems. It can handle the missing values.

Electrocardiogram (ECG): The transthoracic interpretation of the electrical events of the cardiac cycle over time is termed as ECG.

Heart Rate Variability (HRV): Heart rate variability can be regarded as the study of the beat-to-beat intervals that vary with time.

Random Forest (RF): An ensemble classifier that employs many decision tree models. It is a collection of unpruned CART-like trees that follows certain rules for tree combination, self-testing, post-processing, and tree growing.

Recurrence Analysis: Recurrence analysis is a computational method that is useful to detect and quantify deterministic temporal patterns in a time series, which are not detectable by the conventional time series analysis methods.

Chapter 16
Applications of Machine Learning Techniques in Disease Classification From Medical Images:
Recent Practices and Future Challenges

Bikesh Kumar Singh
National Institute of Technology Raipur, India

Satya Eswari Jujjavarapu
National Institute of Technology Raipur, India

ABSTRACT

Machine learning techniques such as artificial neural network (ANN), support vector machine (SVM), radial basis function network (RBFN), random forest (RF), naive Bayes classifier, etc. have gained much attention in recent years due to their widespread applications in diverse fields. This chapter is focused on providing a comprehensive insight of various techniques employed for key areas of medical image processing and analysis. Different applications covered in this chapter include feature extraction, feature selection, and cancer classification in medical images. The authors present current practices and evaluation measures used for objective evaluation of different machine learning methods in context to above-mentioned applications. Various factors associated with acceptance/rejection of such automated systems by medical research community are discussed. The authors also discuss how the interaction between automated analysis systems and medical professionals can be improved for its acceptance in clinical practice. They conclude the chapter by presenting research gaps and future challenges.

DOI: 10.4018/978-1-5225-4969-7.ch016

CANCER DETECTION AND CLASSIFICATION BASED ON MEDICAL IMAGES: INTRODUCTION TO COMPUTER AIDED DIAGNOSIS (CAD) SYSTEM

In order to reduce the number of unnecessary biopsies by automatic detection and diagnosis of cancer, several researchers have investigated computer aided diagnosis (CAD) systems. CAD systems can be an effective tool for diagnosis of cancer due to following reasons:

1. It can assist the physicians in decreasing observational oversights (i.e. decreasing the false negative rate), in the detection and classification of breast cancer in early stages and thus reducing death rates due to cancer.
2. Interpretation of medical images varies from expert to expert and is subject to expert's variability. CAD systems can improve inter-reader and intra-reader variability by providing more objective evidences for diagnosing cancer.
3. It can provide a second opinion to the physicians by detecting and classifying masses automatically.
4. It is less time consuming and less expensive compared to conventional methods used to classify cancer.
5. It can be used to extract and select most appropriate features suitable for classification of cancer.

Figure 1 shows the general layout of methodology used in CAD systems. Various stages of the CAD system are summarized below:

Data Collection

The first step in development of CAD systems for medical image analysis is to collect reliable and authentic image data in consultation of expert medical professionals. Subjects involved in the experiments must be made aware of the experimental protocol and side effects of the data acquisition process. Informed consent of the participants is usually obtained before acquiring data. Approval of institute ethical committee/international review board should be obtained in prior. To develop a reliable CAD system the images collected should be accompanied by patient's demographics, criterions adopted for

Figure 1. A general layout of CAD system

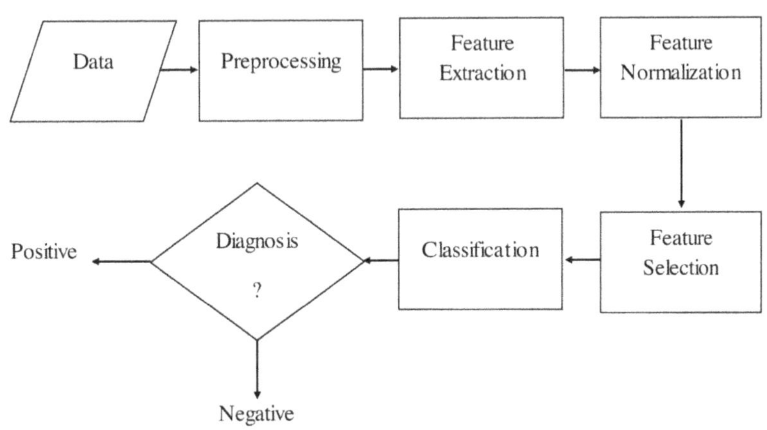

inclusion/rejection of the participants, ground truth validations and pathology reports. Ground truth can be generated by experts in case of segmentation problems wherein the radiologists can manually plot the contours of the lesion. The manual delineations thus provided by the expert radiologists can be used as reference for performance evaluation of segmentation techniques. On the other hand, for classification problems, ground truth is required to confirm whether the detected lesion is benign (low risk) or malignant (high risk). This information can be obtained from expert radiologists, biopsy reports and other pathology reports.

Some of the application areas of CAD systems which can be applied to different types of medical images are: classification of lesions into malignant or benign in medical imaging modalities such as breast mammography, breast ultrasound, lung computed tomography images, chest radiographs, brain computed tomography images, brain magnetic resonance imaging, detecting calcifications in mammogram, hairline fractures in x-ray images etc.

Pre-Processing

The acquired/collected images may be subjected to poor resolution, artifacts and noises. For example, ultrasound images are subjected to artifacts such as speckle noise, shadowing effects and acoustic enhancement as illustrated in Figure 2. Thus, image denoising is carried out to lessen the ill effects of speckle noise thereby improving the image resolution. However, appropriate choice of denoising filter is critical as most of the denoising filters not only smoothen the noise but also blurs the sharp features of the image which may carry diagnostic information. Thus appropriate filter which maintains trade off between smoothening and preservation of sharp features should be adopted. Linear filtering techniques like Gaussian filtering for removal of speckle noise results in blurring of edges and boundaries. Linear filters sometimes also dislocate some important image features such as edges resulting in poor resolution.

To deal with the drawbacks of linear filtering techniques Perona and Malik (1990) introduced the concept and formulation of anisotropic diffusion filtering which are one of the most popular in this area. In (Yu, acton, 2002) anisotropic diffusion was combined with local statistics filters such as Lee (1986) and frost (1982). Relation between local directional variance and local geometry of image was reported in (Krissian, Westin, Kikinis, Vosbourg, 2007) in which matrix anisotropic diffusion for filtering across the image contours and in principal curvature directions was proposed. In (Han, Min, Sohn, 2013) relation between anisotropic diffusion and adaptive smoothening was studied. An improved anisotropic diffusion method in which smallest univalue segment assimilating nucleus (SUSAN) edge detector is used to determine image statistics using local information is reported in (Yu, Tan, Wang, 2010). Wavelet based approaches have been successfully used for removal of speckle noise in ultrasound images (Gupta, Chauhan, Sexana, 2004; Mateo, Caballero, Rabbani, Vafadust, Abolmaesumi, Gazor, 2008; Sudha, Suresh, Sukanesh, 2009). In (Singh, Verma, Thoke, 2015) Daubechies complex wavelet transform is employed for speckle removal in ultrasound images. A detailed review and comparative evaluation of various image denoising techniques can be found in (Sing, et al, 2015; Singh, Verma and Thoke, 2015; Deng, Wang, Shen, 2011; Zhang, Cheng, Tian, Huang, Tang, 2010).

Lesion Segmentation

After pre-processing, the next step is to segment lesion/tumour area or suspicious tissues from the medical images. Several techniques have been proposed in literature for lesion detection in medical images.

Some of the traditional ones include threshold based, region based and edge based. The threshold based segmentation techniques involves determining an appropriate threshold to separate the desired region of interest (ROI) from the undesired ones. The region based techniques attempts to determine similarity or dissimilarity between certain pixels/regions of the image based on some pre-defined criterion. Some of the traditional region based segmentation methods are region growing, region splitting and region merging. Edge based segmentation techniques involves determining edges in an image followed by edge linking for boundary detection. We now discuss some of the recently proposed breast ultrasound segmentation techniques in literature. Shi et al. (2010) employed Markov Random field (MRF) for detecting breast lesions in ultrasound images. The authors extract features from segmented images followed by classification using fuzzy support vector machine (FSVM). Though robust and effective, their study was limited to a very small data size comprising of 36 malignant and 51 benign cases. Further, ground truth validation of tumor contours was not available. Liu et al. (2010) reported an automatic segmentation and classification methods using local texture features of breast ultrasound images. They used data size consisting of 60 malignant and 52 benign cases to evaluate the proposed approach. The authors declared that this method can accurately segment the lesion area without human intervention. However, their technique incurred high computational complexity due to large training time of the classifier adopted.

Huang et al. (2012) proposed a novel graph based technique for segmenting breast lesions in ultrasound. They used an enhanced neighborhood model to determine homogeneous sub regions represented by sub graphs. Drukker et al. (2014) presented an automated breast cancer detection method for women with dense breast. Initially, they applied adaptive thresholding and k-means clustering to detect tumor candidate regions. Lo et al. (2014) proposed a topographic watershed technique for segmentation and abnormality extraction in breast ultrasound images. Firstly, they used watershed transform to segment homogeneous regions of identical tissues. Next, they determined the possibility of segmented region being tumor region using features related to morphology, texture and intensity. However, this method may not be suited to images corrupted by noises such as speckle noise, acoustic shadowing, acoustic enhancement etc., since these noises may distort the local texture of the lesions. Further, this method may not perform well on all kinds of breast cancers due to their varying texture. Zhou et al. (2014) presented a combination of mean shift filtering and graph cuts for detecting breast lesions in ultrasound images. The ultrasound images were initially subjected to shrinking, smoothening using Gaussian filter and enhancement using histogram equalization. Further, mean shift filtering is used for improving the homogeneity followed by graph cuts for segmentation. Though computationally faster, their technique was sensitive to noise or blur resulting in unclear tumor contour. Further, the data size used for evaluation was also limited in this study.

Zhou et al. (2015) employed thresholding and disk expansion method for segmentation of breast lesions in ultrasound. Their technique extracted half contour features for classification of breast tumors. Their main objective was to classify images with acoustic shadowing. The performance of this method is highly dependent on correct extraction of half contour. Further, manual omission may be needed to detect half contour in case the original image is very noisy. Prabusankarlal et al. (2015) proposed multi resolution analysis for detecting breast tumors in ultrasound images. They calculated the undecimated discrete wavelet transform of the image followed by feature extraction and dimensionality reduction using principal component analysis. Lastly, they used Fuzzy c-means clustering for segmentation. The performance of this approach is highly dependent on the quality of features used for clustering. Guo et al. (2016) transformed the image into neutrosophic domain followed by computation of neutrosophic similarity score (NSS). NSS was used as measure of belongingness to the true tumor. Then they used level set method for segmenting the breast lesions based on NSS. Though promising, this approach needs further investigation due to the small data size used in this study.

Having discussed some of the recent studies, it is apparent that several techniques have been reported for segmentation of breast lesions in ultrasound images. However, these approaches have some limitations. The data size used in most of the studies is limited. Thus, it is difficult to evaluate the generalization ability of these segmentation techniques. Except Zhou et al. (2015), none of the reported studies included images with artifacts such as acoustic shadowing, acoustic enhancement etc. None of these studies evaluated the impact of pre-processing techniques such as noise removal, enhancement etc. on performance of segmentation and classifier techniques. New techniques are needed to address the above-mentioned research gaps.

Feature Extraction

Given a medical image, the objective of feature extraction is to extract suitable features which are useful in characterization of an object to be recognized. The values of features should be very similar for objects in the same category and different for objects in different categories. In most of the cases, benign tumors often have round or ellipsoid shapes, smooth borders and homogenous internal echoes; whereas malignant tumors often have branch patterns, irregular/angular boundary and heterogeneous internal echoes. Thus, for classifying the breast masses into benign or malignant, texture and shape features may be useful. Furthermore, in practice the extracted features are normalized to approximately equalize the range of features and make them have approximately the same effect in the computation of similarity. Some popular texture and shape feature extraction techniques includes:

1. **First Order Statistic Features:** First-order statistics measures the likelihood of observing a gray value at a randomly-chosen location in the image. They are calculated from the original image values without considering neighbourhood pixel relationships (Srinivassan, Shobha, 2008). Initially, first order gray level histogram is derived, then features such as mean, variance, standard deviation, skewness, kurtosis, measures of uniformity, smoothness and entropy are calculated. Though simple to compute, texture analysis based exclusively on the gray level histogram suffers from the drawback that it does not provide any information about the relative position of various gray levels within the image (Theodoridis, Koutroumbas, 2009; Haralick, 1979)
2. **Gray Level Co-Occurrence Matrices:** First order statistics wholly ignores the relative position of pixel intensities within the image. The information regarding relative position of pixel intensities can be obtained using gray level co-occurrence texture features proposed in (Haralick, 1997; Haralick, Shanmugam, Dinstein, 2973; Eeszka, Dyer, Rosenfeld, 1976; Wu, Chen, 1992) The Gray level co-occurrence matrix (GLCM) (also called as spatial gray-level dependence matrices (SGLDM)) are based on estimation of second order joint probability density function $f(i, j; d, \theta)$. Each entry in GLCM indicates the relative frequency with which two neighbouring resolution cells with intensities i and j respectively are separated by distance d and orientation θ. The orientation θ is quantized into four directions: horizontal, diagonal, vertical, and antidiagonal (0^0, 45^0, 90^0, and 135^0) as shown in figure 2. After deriving the GLCM, several texture features such as angular second moment, contrast, correlation, sum of squares variance, inverse difference moment, sum average, sum variance, sum entropy, entropy, difference variance, difference entropy, information measures of correlation 1 and 2.

Figure 2. The four orientations used to construct co-occurrence matrices

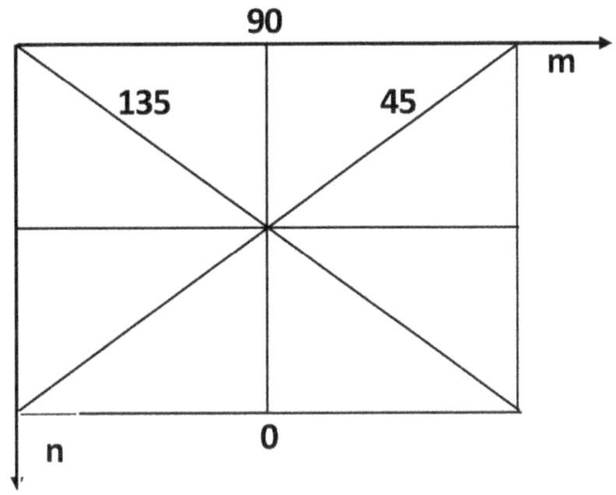

3. **Gray Level Difference Statistics:** The gray level difference statistics are obtained from statistics of local property values proposed in (Weszka et al, 1976). In this technique, local properties such as mean, contrast, etc. based on absolute differences between pairs of gray levels or average gray levels are computed.
4. **Neighbourhood Gray Tone Difference Matrix:** The texture features corresponding to visual properties of texture are highly desirable due to their applicability to all kinds of texture (Amadasun, King, 1989). For each segmented region of interest (ROI), information about spatial changes in intensity can be obtained by looking at the difference between each pixel and the gray tones of its surrounding neighbours. A one-dimensional (1-D) matrix can be estimated for each ROI, in which the ith entry corresponds to the summation of the differences between the gray levels of all pixels with gray level i and the average gray level of their surrounding neighbours. This matrix is called neighbourhood gray tone difference matrix (NGTDM). Features such as coarseness, complexity, busyness, contrast, texture strength are computed from NGTDM.
5. **Statistical Feature Matrix:** A method to analyze texture using statistical feature matrix (SFM) was proposed in (Wu, Chen, 1992). A SFM, M_{sf} is an $(L_r +1) \times (2L_c +1)$ matrix whose (i, j) element is the d statistical feature of the image, where $d = (j - L_c, i)$ is an inter-sample spacing distance vector for $i=0, 1, 2, \ldots\ldots, L_r, j = 0, 1, 2, \ldots\ldots, 2L_c$ and L_r, L_c are the constants which determine the maximum inter-sample spacing distance. Four texture features, namely coarseness, contrast, periodicity and roughness, are calculated from SFM.
6. **Laws Texture Energy Measures:** Laws (1980) developed a texture energy approach to measure variations in a fixed size window. These texture energy measures are considered as one of the first filtering approaches to texture analysis (Zie, Mirmehdi, 2008). A set of nine 7×7 convolution masks is used to compute texture energy, which is then represented by vector of nine numbers for each pixel of the image being analyzed. In this work masks are computed from the following vectors:

$$L7\ (level) = [1\ 6\ 15\ 20\ 15\ 6\ 1] \tag{1}$$

$$E7\ (edge) = [-1\ -4\ -5\ 0\ 5\ 4\ 1] \tag{2}$$

$S7\ (spot) = [-1\ -2\ 1\ 4\ 1\ -2\ -1]$ (3)

The *L7* vector gives a center weighted local average while *E7* detects edges and *S7* detects spots. A *3×3* or *5×5* mask may also be used resulting in *3×3* or *5×5* convolution masks respectively (Laws, 1980; Xie et al, 2008; Shapiro, Stockman, 2000) The 2D convolution masks are obtained by computing product of pair of vectors. A total of nine such masks namely *L7L7, E7E7, S7S7, L7E7, E7L7, E7S7, S7E7, L7S7, S7L7* are computed. Each of the nine *7×7* masks are applied to preprocessed images resulting in nine filtered images. Let $F_k\ [i, j]$ be the result of filtering with the kth mask at pixel *[i, j]* then the texture energy map E_k for filter k and window size *15×15* is defined as-

$$E_k[r,c] = \sum_{j=c-7}^{c+7} \sum_{i=r-7}^{r+7} \left|F_k[i,j]\right| \tag{4}$$

After generating nine energy maps, symmetric pairs are averaged out to produce six final maps. For example, *L7E7* measures the vertical edge gradient and *E7L7* measures the horizontal edge gradient. The average of two maps measures the total edge content. The final six energy maps are *L7L7, E7E7, S7S7, L7E7/ E7L7, E7S7/ S7E7, L7S7/ S7L7* resulting in a single vector consisting of six texture attributes.

7. **Fractal Dimension Texture Analysis:** The fractional Brownian motion model is used to describe the roughness of natural surfaces. It regards naturally occurring surfaces at the end result of random walks. The most important parameter to represent a fractal surface is the fractal dimension. The detailed procedure to find fractal dimensions texture features based on multiple resolution feature extraction can be found in (Wu, 1992).
8. **Spectral Measures of Texture:** Texture feature based on Fourier transform have been extensively used for texture depiction and discrimination (Eszka et al, 1976; Wu et al, 1992; Gonzalez, Woods, 2010; Dyer et al, 1976; Stomberg, Farr, 1986; Shou, Feng, Shi, 2001). Spectral texture is useful for discriminating periodic and non-periodic texture patterns. Furthermore, it is also useful for quantifying differences between periodic patterns (Shapiro et al, 2015)
9. **Run Length Texture Features:** The run length method (Galloway, 1975; Chu, Shegal, Greenleaf, 1990; Dasarathy, Holder, 1991; Tang, 1998) to classify texture is very popular and widespread in the analysis of biomedical images. A run is a sequence in a straight scan direction of pixels with identical image value. The length of the run is number of pixels in the run. Run length features encode textural information related to the number of times each gray level appears by itself, the number of times it appears as pairs and so on. Let p(i, j) be the (i, j)th entry in the given run length matrix, N_g be the number of gray levels in the image, N_r be the number of different run lengths that occur, p be the number of points in the image, then eleven texture features namely, short run emphasis, long run emphasis, gray level non uniformity, run length non uniformity, run percentage, low gray level run emphasis, high gray level run emphasis, short run low gray level emphasis, short run high gray level emphasis, long run high gray level emphasis and long run low gray level emphasis can be extracted from run length matrices.
10. **Regional Properties:** In applications concerned with pattern recognition from medical images, shape and size of tumors/lesions, calcifications, bone fractures etc. within the image carries important diagnostic information. For instance, in ultrasound imaging of breast the shape, size, margin and

orientation of the tumor are key criteria in classifying normal and abnormal tissues. Tumors with irregular and angular margins have a high likelihood of being malignant and those with regular boundary are more likely to be benign. Some of the popular regional features are area, perimeter, major axis, minor axis, compactness etc. These regional properties are based on gray level intensities (Gonzalez and Woods, 2010).

11. **Moment Invariants:** Geometric moments provide rich information about the image and are popular features for pattern recognition. Each moment coefficient conveys a certain amount of information residing in an image (Theodoridis, Koutroumbas, 2009). Let *f(x, y)* is the digital image; its 2-D moment of order (p+q) [37] is defined as-

$$m_{pq} = \sum_x \sum_y x^p y^q f(x,y), \text{for p, q} = 0, 1, 2, \dots\dots\dots \quad (5)$$

where the summations are over the values of the spatial coordinates x and y spanning the image. The corresponding central moment is defined as-

$$\mu_{pq} = \sum_x \sum_y (x-\overline{x})^p (y-\overline{y})^q f(x,y) \quad (6)$$

where, $\overline{x} = \frac{m_{10}}{m_{00}}$ and $\overline{y} = \frac{m_{01}}{m_{00}}$. The normalized central moment of order (p+q) is defined as-

$$\eta_{pq} = \frac{\mu_{pq}}{\mu_{00}^{\gamma}}, \text{for p, q} = 0, 1, 2, \dots\dots\dots \quad (7)$$

where,

$$\gamma = \frac{p+q}{2} + 1, \text{for p + q} = 2, 3, \dots\dots\dots \quad (8)$$

An essential issue in the field of pattern analysis is the recognition of objects and characters regardless of their position, size and orientation (Mercimek, Gulez, Mumcu, 2005). The solution to this is proposed by set of seven moments that are invariant under the actions of translation, rotation, mirroring and scaling, defined by Hu (1962).

12. **Frequency Domain Features:** All the feature selection techniques discussed previously are spatial domain techniques. The second method is to extract features from frequency domain representation of an image. Some popular techniques include texture feature extraction using spatial-frequency image transforms, viz. discrete wavelet transform, discrete Gabor wavelets, dual-tree complex wavelet and contourlet transform etc. Further, combination of spatial domain features with frequency domain features can also be adopted for detection and classification of abnormal tissues in medical images.

Feature Selection

Large number of extracted features at the input of classifier model results in computational complexity and redundant information. Although few features may carry good classification information when treated separately, there is little gain if they are combined into a feature vector consisting of a large number of features (Theodoridis et al, 2009). Thus to enhance the performance of classifier model, feature selection is usually performed after feature extraction.

Figure 3 shows various steps of feature selection process in general (Zhao, Morstatter, Sharma, Alelyani, Anand, Liu, nd). It includes two parts. In the initial phase, a subset of features is generated based on definite pre-defined strategy and then he generated subset is evaluated using evaluation criterion. The performance of recent feature subset is compared with the last best one with respect to the evaluation measure and the better one is retained. This process is repeated until the given stopping criterion is met. In second phase, the finally selected subset is validated using learning and classification models.

Feature selection techniques are broadly classified into three categories, namely filter method, wrapper method and embedded method. Further, combination of these approaches has recently gained attention by many researchers.

1. **Filter Methods:** Filter based feature selection methods ranks filter using principal ranking criteria such as criteria are information gain, symmetrical uncertainty, gain ratio, chi-square, 1-R, relief-F, T-test, Fisher score etc (Chandrashekar, Sahin, 2014). Algorithm 1 gives the basic layout of filter method.
2. **Wrapper Methods:** Wrapper methods use the predictor as a black box and predictor performance as objective function to evaluate the variable subset (Chandrashekar et al, 2014). The subset of features is selected by first defining a search process in the possible feature subset space, followed

Figure 3. The general layout of feature selection process
Zhao et al, 2014.

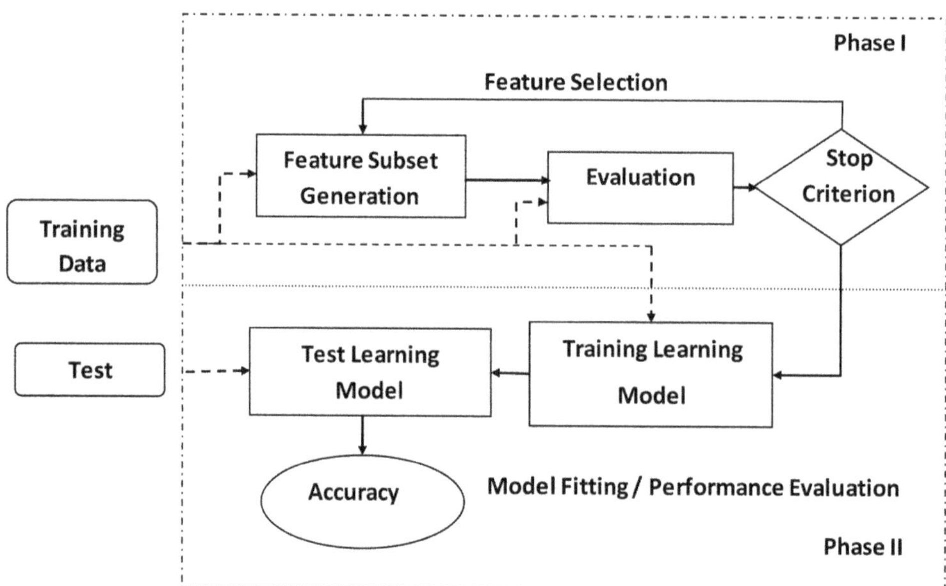

Algorithm 1. Filter method using variable ranking

```
Input: S ← set of features
Output: N ← Top n ranked features
Method
Features ← Evaluation_criteria(D)
Rank_features ← sort_descending(Features)
Return (top n ranked features)
```

by generating and evaluating various subsets of features. The subsets of features are evaluated by using a specific classification model thus making wrappers method specific (Khan, Quadri, 2013). Further, evaluating 2^n subsets become a non deterministic polynomial time (NP) hard problem and suffer from high computational complexity (Blachnik, 2009). Algorithm 2 gives the basic layout of wrapper method.

3. **Embedded Methods:** In embedded methods, the process of searching an optimal subset of features is included within the classifier construction. Like wrapper methods, embedded methods are also specific to learning algorithm under consideration (Khan et al, 2013). Examples of such approaches include decision trees, artificial neural networks, support vector machines, etc. Some examples, advantages and disadvantages of various feature selection methods are summarized in Table 1.

Algorithm 2. Subset feature selection

```
Input: S ← All subsets {}
Output: Subset
Method
For each subset s ∈ S
Evaluate (s)
Return {subset}
```

Table 1. Examples and characteristics of feature selection methods

Feature Selection Approach	Examples	Advantages	Disadvantages
Filter	Mutual information, gain ratio, symmetrical uncertainty, chi-square, one-R, relief-F, T-test, Fisher score etc.	Computationally fastest method, independent of particular algorithm, avoids over fitting and simple implementation.	Does not take in to account the feature dependencies, selected subset may not be optimal, finding suitable learning algorithm may be hard and no ideal method for choosing the dimension of feature space.
Wrapper	Sequential search algorithms like forward, backward, floating forward selection, adaptive sequential forward floating selection, heuristic search algorithms like genetic algorithms, particle swarm optimization etc.	Includes classifier interaction, considers feature dependencies, easy and straight forward implementation in supervised learning.	Computationally expensive, over-fitting may occur if the classifier model learns the data too well, poor generalization capability.
Embedded	Decision trees, Naive Bayes, SVM, ANN etc.	Less computational complexity.	Classifier specific and dependent.

4. **Hybrid Methods:** In last few years, combination of the above mentioned feature selection methods have gained considerable attention by researchers. For example, a new multi-criterion attribute selection technique is recently proposed in (Singh, Verma, & Thoke, 2017). In this method, ten different filter and wrapper methods were jointly used to assess the significance of a particular feature using majority voting rule. Another approach called robust rank aggregation is an ensemble method in which ranking outcomes of various filter based feature selection modules are aggregated to decide an overall improved rank of an individual feature (Sarkar, Cooley and Srivastava, 2014). Rank aggregation further combine with genetic algorithm for feature selection is proposed in (Onan and Korukoglu, 2017) for text sentiment classification.

Classification/Risk Stratification

After extraction and choice of appropriate set of features, the next stage is to employ these features for categorizing the breast ultrasound images into benign (low risk) or malignant class (high risk). Soft computing approaches have been extensively applied in computer aided design and diagnostic systems. According to Prof. Zadeh, it is a rising approach to computing, which parallels the outstanding capability of the human brain to explain and learn in an environment of ambiguity and vagueness (Shukla, Tiwari, Kala, 2010). Its guiding principle is to make use of the tolerance for uncertainty to achieve tractability, sturdiness and low solution cost (Zadeh, 1994). Artificial neural network (ANN) and support vector machine (SVM based classifiers have been the most popular in the researcher's community to classify images with cancer. These methods have confirmed excellent performance in detecting cancer (Hafizah, Ubaidillah, Sallehuddin, Ali, 2013).

1. **Artificial Neural Network:** An ANN is a simplified model which replicates the structure and functioning of a biological neural network. ANN can be defined as a massively parallel distributed processor, which can store input-output experiential knowledge and makes it available for use whenever required. It consists of a large number of neurons called processing units which are interconnected in accordance with a certain topology to accomplish a given specific pattern classification and recognition task. The inputs to a processing unit are derived from the outputs of other processing units and/or from external sources. Depending on the type of application the inputs and/or the outputs can contain discrete or continuous data values.

Figure 4 shows the structure of the simplest ANN consisting of single neuron. The summation unit receives a number of input values (xi) with weights (wi) attached to each of them and computes a weighted sum (y1). The weighted sum of the input is acted by a function (f(.)), commonly referred to as activation function to produce the final output (y) from the output function unit. The learning process,

Figure 4. Block diagram representation of single layer ANN

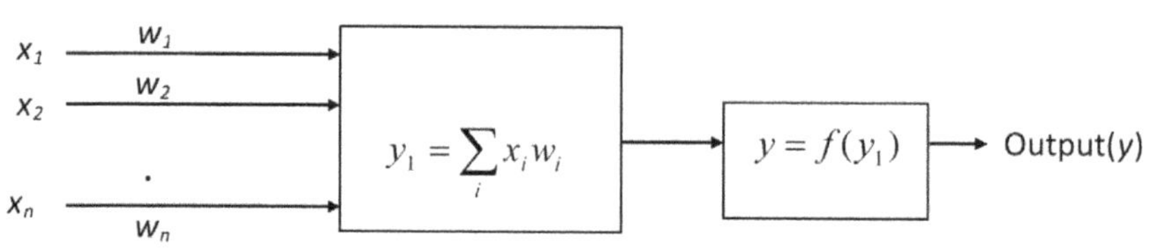

also referred to as training involves altering the weights between the interconnecting neurons as per a given criterion with the aim of mapping a given set of input-output data. The type of learning paradigm depends on the manner in which the weights are adapted. Learning algorithms are broadly classified into two groups. In supervised learning, a data set comprising of input vectors and a target(s) (desired output) associated with each input vector is provided to the network. The supervised learning aims to reduce the error between the actual output and the desired output of the network by adjusting the weights and bias. In unsupervised learning, no target (desired output) is provided to the input data set. This learning tries to find similar patterns or features to form clusters in the input data. In brief, an ANN is characterized by its architecture or topology, the processing algorithm and the learning algorithm employed to update its weight and bias.

Among the various models of neural network, Back-propagation neural networks (BPNN) are the most popular models in the neural network research field (Hafizah et al, 2013). The back-propagation training method is simple, even for complex models having hundreds or thousands of parameters (Duda, 2006). In back-propagation algorithm initially the network is presented with training examples {(x(n), d(n)}, where n = 1 to N, N being the total number of samples. The input vector x(n) is applied to the input layer of sensory nodes and the desired response vector d(n) is presented to the output layer of computation nodes. Two computations namely forward and backward are then performed (Haykin, 2009). In forward computation the induced local fields and function signals of the network are computed by proceeding forward through the network, layer by layer. While, in Backward computation, the error computed at the output side is back-propagated from the output layer, to the hidden layer and finally to the input layer, recursively computing the local gradient for each neuron. An illustrative topology of BPNN is shown in Figure 5. It consists of an input layer, two hidden layers and an output layer. The number of hidden neurons is fixed at 20 and 10 respectively. Transfer functions used are hyperbolic tangent segment at the output of the first hidden layer and linear at the output of second hidden layer as well as the output layer respectively.

2. **Support Vector Machine (SVM):** SVM is based on statistical learning theory, introduced in 1992, has proven to be a powerful tool in classification and regression problems (Shi, Cheng, Hu, Ju, Tian, 2010). SVMs evolved from sound theory to implementations and experiments, while, the ANNs followed a more heuristic path, from applications and extensive experimentations to theory (Soman, Loganthan, Ajay, 2009) SVM is a supervised learning technique that seeks an optimal hyperplane to separate two classes of samples (Cheng, Shan, Ju, Guo, Zhang, 2010). There may be multiple hyperplanes separating the data, however the one with maximum distance from members to nonmembers is selected. The two planes parallel to the classifier and which pass through one or more points in the data set are called bounding planes. The distance between these bounding

Figure 5. A general ANN topology

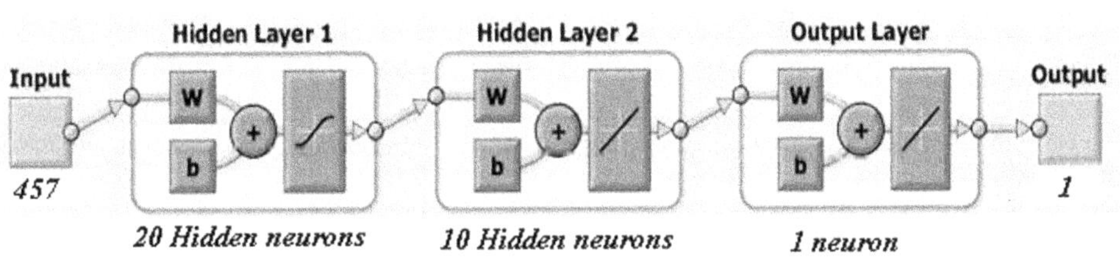

planes are called margin (Soman, et al, 2009). The points in the data set falling on the boundary planes are called support vectors. When the data set is not linearly separable, SVM transforms the data into higher dimensional space called feature space, where a maximal separating hyperplane is constructed (Subashini, Ramlingam, Palanivel, 2009). The mapping of data into a feature space can be performed using kernel functions. If training samples are nonlinearly separable, nonlinear kernel functions are better choice (Ren, 2012). Some of the commonly used kernel functions are-

a. **Linear Kernel:** $x_i^T \cdot x_j$

b. **Polynomial Kernel:** $\left(x_i^T \cdot x_j + 1\right)^d$, where *d* is the degree of kernel.

c. **Radial Basis Function (RBF):** $e^{-\gamma\|x_i - x_j\|2}, \gamma = \left(2\sigma^2\right)^{-1}$, where σ is the parameter controlling the width of the kernel.

Table 2 presents some advantages and drawbacks of ANN and SVM based classification techniques. Both these techniques possess some desirable characteristics. However, in order to improve the performance of the classifier, these techniques can be combined with each other or other supervised/unsupervised learning algorithms so as to achieve an overall improved performance (Haykin, 2009; Cheng et al, 2010; Shi, He, Nakamura, Suzuki, Itoh, 2009).

3. **Naïve Bayes Classifier:** Naive Bayes algorithm learns the probability of an object with certain features belonging to a particular group or class. It is a kind of probabilistic classifier (Karabatak, 2015). Naïve Bayes classifier assumes that each feature is statistically independent to that of other features. For example, if one is trying to identify a fruit based on its color, shape, and taste then an orange colored, spherical shaped, and tangy fruit would most likely be an orange. Even if these features depend on each other, a Naive Bayes classifier considers each of these features to contribute independently to the probability that the fruit is an orange. An advantage of naive Bayes is that it requires small number of training data to estimate the class of an object. The Naive Bayes classifier algorithm based upon Bayes' theorem. In this the conditional probability is calculated which is the probability of an event based on previous knowledge available on the events (Duda, 1973). Mathematically:

$$P(A / B) = \frac{P\left(B / A\right)P\left(A\right)}{P\left(B\right)} \tag{9}$$

Table 2. Advantages and disadvantages of ANN and SVM

Classifier	Advantages	Disadvantages
ANN	Robustness, no rule or explicit expression is needed and widely applicable.	Long training time, non-repeatability, requires large training data and initial value dependent.
SVM	Training process is faster than ANN, repeatable training process, good generalization performance, relative ease of use, rigorous theoretical foundations and robust performance.	Fast increase in their computing and storage requirements with respect to number of training examples.

A is called the proposition and B is called the evidence. P(A) is called the prior probability of proposition and P(B) is called the prior probability of evidence. P(A/B) is called the posterior. P(B/A) is the likelihood. This represents the Bayes' theorem equation as-

$$Posterior = \frac{\left(Likelihood\right)\left(Proposition\ prior\ probability\right)}{Evidence\ prior\ probability} \tag{10}$$

4. **Deep Learning Classifier:** Deep learning (deep structured learning or hierarchical learning) is part of a family of Artificial Intelligence and machine learning. It directly learns the data representations or feature values from the set of data. It can be used in supervised, semi supervised and unsupervised learning of class of the object(s). The feature learning or representation learning is a set of techniques through which a system automatically finds the representations needed for feature detection and classification from the set of data, hence replaces manual feature detection and selection process. It is a cascading of multiple layers of usually nonlinear processing units performs feature extraction (Fei-Fei, Karapathy, Leung, Shetty, Sukthankar, Toderici, 2014)

The structure of deep neural network (DNN) involves multiple hidden layers between the input and output layers. Similar to shallow ANNs, DNNs can also be used for modeling complex non-linear relationships. In DNN object is expressed as a layered composition of primitives. DNNs are typically feed forward networks in which data flows from the input layer to the output layer without looping back. Since it has many hidden layers, DNN is complex to train. Some of the research has been reported to make the training process convenient (Kaiming, Xiangyu, Zhang, Ren, Sun, 2016).

5. **Combining Classifiers:** One can achieve better performance and greater degree of accuracy by combining the individual advantages of different classifiers (Duda, 1973). The different classifiers complement each other's weaker section hence suitable for all kind of pattern recognition problems as there is not a single classifier that can be considered optimal for all problems. The sum rule, average rule and majority voting rule are among the techniques most popularly used for combining the classifiers. The individual classifiers are separately trained and then their outputs are used for designing the combiner (Theodoridis, Koutoumbas, 2009). Some other techniques rely on optimizing the combiner independently or jointly with individual classifiers (Yaxin, Guan, Bell, 20008). But in general this requires a very complex procedure which sometimes leads to impracticality of the procedure.

Performance Evaluation

The performance of the classifiers is quantified based on how accurate the classifier could classify the normal and diseased tissues in medical images correctly. Several measuring tools are available in literature to evaluate the performance of classifiers. Most of these measures are built from a confusion matrix which is a record of correctly and incorrectly classified samples from negative and positive class. The layout of confusion matrix for two class problem is given in Table 3. Here TP, FP, FN and TN are true positive, false positive, false negative and true negative respectively. TP represents the number of malignant samples correctly classified as malignant while FN represents the number of malignant

Table 3. Layout of confusion matrix for two class problem

Actual Class	Recognized Class as Positive (1)	Recognized Class as Negative (0)
Positive(1, e. g. Malignant)	TP	FN
Negative(0, e. g. Benign)	FP	TN

samples wrongly classified as benign. Similarly, TN represents the number of benign samples correctly classified as benign while FP represents the number of benign samples wrongly classified as malignant. From these values performance measures like sensitivity, specificity, accuracy and area under receiver operating characteristics etc. are calculated (Sing, Verma, 2016; Sing, Verma, 2017).

RESEARCH GAPS AND FUTURE CHALLENGES

Applications of machine learning techniques in classification and risk stratification of medical images have gained much attention in last few years. However, there are some limitations common in these studies. Some of the challenges and possible solutions are as follows:

- The performance of proposed algorithms in different reported works cannot be compared with each other due to non-availability of the dataset used in these studies. The solution to this is that the dataset used should be available in public domain so as to compare and evaluate different algorithms on a common platform.
- The techniques developed are far away from the requirements of real time use to limitations posed by quality of images, different protocols of data recording, lack of trust of medical professionals on CAD systems, incomplete datasets and un availability of supporting information like pathology reports, biopsy reports etc. thus, development of CAD systems should include data from different centers, different machines and different modalities. In future, evaluation of machine learning techniques in clinical practice and on enlarged multi-center data set can be explored.
- Experts from medical domain may have varying thoughts about the image quality and diagnostic evidence. To address this issue, inter- and intra- observer differences to evaluate the expert opinion can be conducted in future. Further, the performance of automated systems must be compared with that of manual approach.
- Feature extraction and selection plays important role in classification of medical images. Mapping of pathological features with image features can be worked out in future.
- Real world data tend to be noisy and may contain errors and artifacts. Fault tolerant classification techniques can be developed in future. Opinion of medical professionals can be integrated in development of different phases of CAD systems.

REFERENCES

Amadasun, M., & King, R. (1989). Texture features corresponding to textural properties. *IEEE Transactions on Systems, Man, and Cybernetics*, *19*(5), 1264–1274. doi:10.1109/21.44046

Bi, Y., Guan, J., & Bell, D. (2008). The combination of multiple classifiers using an evidential reasoning approach. *Artificial Intelligence*, *172*(15), 1731–1751. doi:10.1016/j.artint.2008.06.002

Blachnik, M. (2009). Comparison of various feature selection methods in application to prototype best rules, Computer Recognition Systems 3. *Advances in Intelligent and Soft Computing*, *57*, 257–264. doi:10.1007/978-3-540-93905-4_31

Chandrashekar, G., & Sahin, F. (2014). A survey of feature selection methods. *Computers & Electrical Engineering*, *40*(1), 16–28. doi:10.1016/j.compeleceng.2013.11.024

Cheng, H. D., Shan, J., Ju, W., Guo, Y., & Zhang, L. (2010). Automated breast cancer detection and classification using ultrasound images: A survey. *Pattern Recognition*, *43*(1), 299–317. doi:10.1016/j.patcog.2009.05.012

Chu, A., Sehgal, C. M., & Greenleaf, J. F. (1990). Use of gray value distribution of run lengths for texture analysis. *Pattern Recognition Letters*, *11*(6), 415–420. doi:10.1016/0167-8655(90)90112-F

Dasarathy, B. V., & Holder, E. B. (1991). Image characterizations based on joint gray level run length distributions. *Pattern Recognition Letters*, *12*(8), 497–502. doi:10.1016/0167-8655(91)80014-2

Deng, Y., Wang, Y., & Shen, Y. (2011). Speckle reduction in ultrasound images based on Rayleigh-trimmed anisotropic diffusion filter. *Pattern Recognition Letters*, *32*(13), 1516–1525. doi:10.1016/j.patrec.2011.06.007

Drukker, K., Sennett, C. A., & Giger, M. L. (2014). Computerized detection of breast cancer on automated breast ultrasound imaging of women with dense breast. *Medical Physics*, *41*(1), 1– 19. PMID:24718570

Duda, R. O., & Hart, P. E. (1973). *Pattern Classification and Scene Analysis* (Vol. 3). New York: Wiley.

Duda, R. O., Hart, P. E., & Stork, D. G. (2006). *Pattern classification* (2nd ed.). Wiley India.

Dyer, C. R., & Rosenfeld, A. (1976). Fourier texture features: Suppression of aperture effects. *IEEE Transactions on Systems, Man, and Cybernetics*, *SMC-6*(10), 703–705. doi:10.1109/TSMC.1976.4309422

Fei-Fei, L., Karpathy, A., Leung, T., Shetty, S., Sukthankar, R., & Toderici, G. (2014). Large-Scale Video Classification with Convolutional Neural Networks. *IEEE Conference on Computer Vision and Pattern Recognition*.

Frost, V. S., Stiles, J. A., Shanmugam, K. S., & Holtzman, J. C. (1982). A model for radar images and its application to adaptive digital filtering of multiplicative noise. *IEEE Transactions on Pattern Analysis and Machine Intelligence*, *PAMI-4*(2), 157–165. doi:10.1109/TPAMI.1982.4767223 PMID:21869022

Galloway, M. M. (1975). Texture analysis using gray level run lengths. *Computer Graphics and Image Processing*, *4*(2), 172–179. doi:10.1016/S0146-664X(75)80008-6

Gonzalez, R. C., & Woods, R. E. (2010). *Digital Image Processing Using MATLAB* (2nd ed.). Pearson Prentice Hall.

Guo, Y., Sengur, A., & Tian, J. W. (2016). A novel breast ultrasoundimage segmentation algorithm based on neutrosophic similarity score and level set. *Computer Methods and Programs in Biomedicine*, *123*, 43–53. doi:10.1016/j.cmpb.2015.09.007 PMID:26483304

Gupta, S., Chauhan, R. C., & Sexana, S. C. (2004). Wavelet-based statistical approach for speckle reduction in medical ultrasound images. *Medical & Biological Engineering & Computing*, *42*(2), 189–192. doi:10.1007/BF02344630 PMID:15125148

Hafizah, S., Ubaidillah, S. A., Sallehuddin, R., & Ali, N. A. (2013). Cancer detection using artificial neural network and support vector machine: A comparative study. *Jurnal Teknologi*, *65*(1), 73–81.

Ham, B., Min, D., & Sohn, K. (2013). Revisiting the relationship between adaptive smoothing and anisotropic diffusion with modified filters. *IEEE Transactions on Image Processing*, *22*(3), 1096–1107. doi:10.1109/TIP.2012.2226904 PMID:23193236

Haralick, R. M. (1979). Statistical and structural approaches to texture. *Proceedings of the IEEE*, *67*(5), 786–804. doi:10.1109/PROC.1979.11328

Haralick, R. M., Shanmugam, K., & Dinstein, I. (1973). Textural features for image classification. *IEEE Transactions on Systems, Man, and Cybernetics*, *SMC-3*(6), 610–621. doi:10.1109/TSMC.1973.4309314

Haykin, S. (2009). *Neural Network and Learning Machines* (3rd ed.). Pearson Education.

He, K., Zhang, X., Ren, S., & Sun, J. (2016). *Deep Residual Learning for Image Recognition, Computer Vision Foundation, Open access*. IEEE Xplore.

Hu, M. K. (1962). Visual pattern recognition by moment invariants. *I.R.E. Transactions on Information Theory*, *8*(2), 179–187. doi:10.1109/TIT.1962.1057692

Huang, Q. H., Lee, S. Y., Liu, L. Z., Lu, M.-H., Jin, L.-W., & Li, A.-H. (2012). A robust graph based segmentation method for breast tumors in ultrasound images. *Ultrasonics*, *52*(2), 266–275. doi:10.1016/j.ultras.2011.08.011 PMID:21925692

Karabatak, M. (2015). A new classifier for breast cancer detection based on Naïve Bayesian. *Measurement*, *72*, 32–36. doi:10.1016/j.measurement.2015.04.028

Khan, M., & Quadri, S. M. K. (2013). Effect of using filter based feature selection on performance of machine learners using different datasets. *BVICAM's International Journal of Information Technology*, *5*(2), 597–603.

Khare, A., Khare, M., Jeong, Y., Kim, H., & Jeon, M. (2010). Despeckling of medical ultrasound images using Daubechies complex wavelet transform. *Signal Processing*, *90*(2), 428–439. doi:10.1016/j.sigpro.2009.07.008

Krissian, K., Westin, C. F., Kikinis, R., & Vosburgh, K. G. (2007). Oriented speckle reducing anisotropic diffusion. *IEEE Transactions on Image Processing*, *16*(5), 1412–1424. doi:10.1109/TIP.2007.891803 PMID:17491469

Kumar Singh. (2015). Investigations on edge preservation and smoothening of frequency domain filters for speckle removal in breast ultrasound images. *International Journal of Biomedical Engineering and Technology*.

Kumar Singh, Verma, & Thoke. (2015). Objective and Optical Evaluation of Despeckle Filters in Breast Ultrasound Images. *IETE Technical Review*. DOI: 10.1080/02564602.2015.1019943

Laws, K. I. (1980). Rapid texture identification. *Proceedings of SPIE Image Processing for Missile Guidance*, 238, 376-380. 10.1117/12.959169

Lee, J. S. (1986). Speckle suppression and analysis for synthetic aperture radar. *Optical Engineering (Redondo Beach, Calif.)*, *25*(5), 636–643. doi:10.1117/12.7973877

Liu, B., Cheng, H. D., Huang, J., Tian, J., Tang, X., & Liu, J. (2010). Fully automatic and segmentation-robust classification of breast tumors based on local texture analysis of ultrasound images. *Pattern Recognition*, *43*(1), 280–298. doi:10.1016/j.patcog.2009.06.002

Lo, C. M., Chen, R. T., Chang, Y. C., Yang, Y. W., Hung, M. J., Huang, C. S., & Chang, R. F. (2014). Multi-dimensional tumor detection in automated whole breast ultrasound using topographic watershed. *IEEE Transactions on Medical Imaging*, *33*(7), 1503–1511. doi:10.1109/TMI.2014.2315206 PMID:24718570

Mateo, J. L., & Caballero, A. F. (2009). Finding out general tendencies in speckle noise reduction in ultrasound images. *Expert Systems with Applications*, *36*(4), 7786–7797. doi:10.1016/j.eswa.2008.11.029

Mercimek, M., Gulez, K., & Mumcu, T. V. (2005). Real object recognition using moment invariants. *Sadhana*, *30*(6), 765–775. doi:10.1007/BF02716709

Onan, A., Hasan, B., & Korukoglu, S. (2017). An improved ant algorithm with LDA-based representation for text document clustering. *Journal of Information Science, 43*(2), 275-292.

Perona, P., & Malik, J. (1990). Scale space and edge detection using anisotropic diffusion. *IEEE Transactions on Pattern Analysis and Machine Intelligence*, *12*(7), 629–639. doi:10.1109/34.56205

Plagianakos, V. P., Magoulas, G. D., & Vrahatis, M. N. (2001). Learning rate adaptation in stochastic gradient descent, Proc. Advances Convex Anal. Global Optimization. *Noncovex Optimization Applicat.*, *54*, 433–444. doi:10.1007/978-1-4613-0279-7_27

Prabusankarlal, K. M., Thirumoorthy, P., & Manavalan, R. (2015). Segmentation of breast lesions in ultrasound images through multiresolution analysis using undecimated discrete wavelet transform. *Ultrasonic Imaging*, *38*(6), 384–402. doi:10.1177/0161734615615838 PMID:26586725

Rabbani, H., Vafadust, M., Abolmaesumi, P., & Gazor, S. (2008). Speckle noise reduction of medical ultrasound images in complex wavelet domain using mixture priors. *IEEE Transactions on Biomedical Engineering*, *55*(9), 2152–2160. doi:10.1109/TBME.2008.923140 PMID:18713684

Ren, J. (2012). ANN vs. SVM: Which one performs better in classification of MCCs in mammogram imaging. *Knowledge-Based Systems*, *26*(February), 144–153. doi:10.1016/j.knosys.2011.07.016

Sarkar, C., Cooley, S., & Srivastava, J. (2014, January 1). Robust Feature Selection Technique using Rank Aggregation. *Applied Artificial Intelligence*, *28*(3), 243–257. doi:10.1080/08839514.2014.883903 PMID:24839351

Shapiro, L. G., & Stockman, G. C. (n.d.). *Texture, Chapter 7, Computer Vision, 2000*. Available online from https://courses.cs.washington.edu/courses/cse576 /book/ch7.pdf

Shi, X., Cheng, H. D., Hu, L., Ju, W., & Tian, J. (2010). Detection and classification of masses in breast ultrasound images. *Digital Signal Processing*, *20*(3), 824–836. doi:10.1016/j.dsp.2009.10.010

Shi, Z., He, L., Nakamura, T., Suzuki, K., & Itoh, H. (2009). Survey on neural networks used for medical image processing. *International Journal of Computational Science*, *3*(1), 86–100. PMID:26740861

Shukla, Tiwari, & Kala. (2010). *Real life applications of soft computing*. CRC Press.

Singh, B. K., Verma, K., Panigrahi, L., & Thoke, A. S. (2017). A.S. Thoke, Integrating radiologist feedback with computer aided diagnostic systems for breast cancer risk prediction in ultrasonic images: An experimental investigation in machine learning paradigm. *Expert Systems with Applications*, *90*, 209–223. doi:10.1016/j.eswa.2017.08.020

Singh, B. K., Verma, K., & Thoke, A. S. (2016). Fuzzy cluster based neural network classifier for classifying breast tumors in ultrasound images. *Expert Systems with Applications*, *66*, 114–123. doi:10.1016/j.eswa.2016.09.006

Singh, B. K., Verma, K., Thoke, A. S., & Suri, J. S. (2017). Risk stratification of 2D ultrasound-based breast lesions using hybrid feature selection in machine learning paradigm. *Measurement*, *105*, 146–157. doi:10.1016/j.measurement.2017.01.016

Soman, K. P., Loganathan, R., & Ajay, V. (2009). *Machine learning with SVM and other kernel methods*. PHI Learning Private Limited.

Srinivasan, G. N., & Shobha, G. (2008). Statistical texture analysis. Proceedings of World Academy of Science, Engineering and Technology, 36, 1264-1269.

Stromberg, W. D., & Farr, T. G. (1986). A Fourier based textural feature extraction procedure. *IEEE Transactions on Geoscience and Remote Sensing*, *GE-24*(5), 722–731. doi:10.1109/TGRS.1986.289620

Subashini, T. S., Ramalingam, V., & Palanivel, S. (2009). Breast mass classification based on cytological patterns using RBFNN and SVM. *Expert Systems with Applications*, *36*(3), 5284–5290. doi:10.1016/j.eswa.2008.06.127

Sudha, S., Suresh, G. R., & Sukanesh, R. (2009). Speckle noise reduction in ultrasound images by wavelet thresholding based on weighted variance. *International Journal of Computer Theory and Engineering*, *1*, 1793–8201.

Tang, X. (1998). Texture information in run length matrices. *IEEE Transactions on Image Processing*, *7*(11), 1602–1609. doi:10.1109/83.725367 PMID:18276225

Theodoridis, S., & Koutroumbas, K. (2009). *Pattern Recognition* (4th ed.). Elsevier.

Theodoridis, S., & Koutroumbas, K. (2009). *Pattern Recognition*. Academic Press, Elsevier.

Weszka, J. S., Dyer, C. R., & Rosenfeld, A. (1976). A comparative study of texture measures for terrain classification. *IEEE Transactions on Systems, Man, and Cybernetics*, *SMC-6*(4), 269–285. doi:10.1109/TSMC.1976.5408777

Wu, C. M., & Chen, Y. C. (1992). Statistical feature matrix for texture analysis. *CVGIP. Graphical Models and Image Processing*, *54*(5), 407–419. doi:10.1016/1049-9652(92)90025-S

Wu, C. M., Chen, Y. C., & Hsieh, K. S. (1992). Texture features for classification of ultrasonic liver images. *IEEE Transactions on Medical Imaging*, *11*(2), 141–152. doi:10.1109/42.141636 PMID:18218367

Xie, X., & Mirmehdi, M. (2008). A galaxy of texture features. In Handbook of Texture Analysis (pp. 347–406). Imperial College Press.

Xu, L., Krzyzak, A., & Suen, C. Y. (1992, May-June). Methods of Combining Multiple Classifiers and Their Applications to Handwriting Recognition. *IEEE Transactions on Systems, Man, and Cybernetics*, *22*(3), 418–435. doi:10.1109/21.155943

Yu, J., Tan, J., & Wang, Y. (2010). Ultrasound speckle reduction by SUSAN-controlled anisotropic diffusion method. *Pattern Recognition*, *43*(9), 3083–3092. doi:10.1016/j.patcog.2010.04.006

Yu, Y., & Acton, S. (2002). Speckle reducing anisotropic diffusion. *IEEE Transactions on Image Processing*, *11*(11), 1260–1270. doi:10.1109/TIP.2002.804276 PMID:18249696

Zadeh, L. A. (1994). Soft computing and fuzzy logic. *IEEE Software*, *11*(6), 48–56. doi:10.1109/52.329401

Zhang, Y., Cheng, H. D., Tian, J., Huang, J., & Tang, X. (2010). Fractional subpixel diffusion and fuzzy logic approach for ultrasound speckle reduction. *Pattern Recognition*, *43*(8), 2962–2970. doi:10.1016/j.patcog.2010.02.014

Zhao, Z., Morstatter, F., Sharma, S., Alelyani, S., Anand, A., & Liu, H. (n.d.). *Advancing feature selection research – ASU feature selection repository*. Available online at http://featureselection.asu.edu/index.php

Zhou, F., Feng, J. F., & Shi, Q. Y. (2001). Texture feature based on local Fourier transform. *Proceedings - International Conference on Image Processing*, *2*, 610–613.

Zhou, Z., Wu, S., Chang, K. J., Chen, W. R., Chen, Y. S., Kuo, W. H., ... Tsui, P. H. (2015). Classification of benign and malignant breast tumors in ultrasound images with posterior acoustic shadowing using half-contour features. *Journal of Medical and Biological Engineering*, *35*(2), 178–187. doi:10.100740846-015-0031-x PMID:25960706

Zhou, Z., Wu, W., Wu, S., Tsui, P. H., Lin, C. C., Zhang, L., & Wang, T. (2014). Semi-automatic breast ultrasound image segmentation based on mean shift and graph cuts. *Ultrasonic Imaging*, 1–21. PMID:24759696

Compilation of References

Abbate, S., Avvenuti, M., & Light, J. (2012). MIMS: A Minimally Invasive Monitoring Sensor Platform. *IEEE Sensors Journal*, *12*(3), 677–684. doi:10.1109/JSEN.2011.2149515

Abedi, B., Abbasi, A., & Goshvarpour, A. (2017). Investigating the effect of traditional Persian music on ECG signals in young women using wavelet transform and neural networks. *Anatolian Journal of Cardiology. Anadolu Kardiyoloji Dergisi*, *17*(5).

Adams, L., Krybus, W., Ebrecht, D. M., & Rueger, R. (1990). Computer-assisted surgery. *IEEE Computer Graphics and Applications*, *10*(3), 43–52. doi:10.1109/38.55152

Ades & Brookhart. (1949). The central auditory pathway. *Neurophysiology*, *13*(1), 1–2. PMID:15415767

Agatonovic-Kustrin, S., & Beresford, R. (2000). Basic concepts of artificial neural network (ANN) modeling and its application in pharmaceutical research. *Journal of Pharmaceutical and Biomedical Analysis*, *22*(5), 717–727. doi:10.1016/S0731-7085(99)00272-1 PMID:10815714

Ahmad, K. (2007). Pakistan struggles to eradicate polio. *The Lancet Infectious Diseases*, *7*(4), 247. doi:10.1016/S1473-3099(07)70066-X PMID:17419137

Akhlagi, N. N., Lonn, F., & Wittrup, P. (2003). *Reading pen*. Google Patents.

Al-Dowaihi, D., Al-Ajlan, M., Al-Zahrani, N., Al-Quwayfili, N., Al-Jwiser, N., & Kanjo, E. (2013). mBreath: Asthma monitoring system on the go. In *Proceedings of the International Conference on Computer Medical Applications (ICCMA)* (pp. 5–8). Sousse, Tunisia: Academic Press. 10.1109/ICCMA.2013.6506169

Alemdar, H., & Ersoy, C. (2010). Wireless sensor networks for healthcare: A survey. *Computer Networks*, *54*(15), 2688–2710. doi:10.1016/j.comnet.2010.05.003

Alexakis, C., Nyongesa, H., Saatchi, R., Harris, N., Davies, C., & Emery, C. (2003). *Feature extraction and classification of electrocardiogram (ECG) signals related to hypoglycaemia.* Paper presented at the Computers in Cardiology.

Ali, H. (2014). *Bionic Exoskeleton: History, Development and the Future.* Paper presented at the IOSR Journal of Mechanical and Civil Engineering (IOSR-JMCE), International Conference on Advances in Engineering & Technology.

Allen, G. S., & Coates, N. E. (1996). Pulmonary contusion: A collective review. *The American Surgeon*, *62*(11), 895–900. PMID:8895709

Amadasun, M., & King, R. (1989). Texture features corresponding to textural properties. *IEEE Transactions on Systems, Man, and Cybernetics*, *19*(5), 1264–1274. doi:10.1109/21.44046

Amir, O., Weinstein, D., Zilberman, S., Less, M., Perl-Treves, D., Primack, H., ... Karasik, A. (2007). Continuous Noninvasive Glucose Monitoring Technology Based on "Occlusion Spectroscopy.". *Journal of Diabetes Science and Technology*, *1*(4), 463–469. doi:10.1177/193229680700100403

Anatomy and Function of the Liver. (n.d.). Retrieved 2017 from http://www.stanfordchildrens.org/en/topic/default?id=anatomy-and-function-of-the-liver-90-P03069.(2017).

Arif, M. (2016, January 4). Health cards will not end Pakistan's Healthcare nightmare. *DAWN*. Retrieved from http://www.dawn.com/news/1230294

Ashfaq, Y. (2016, January 12). Pakistan, Afghanistan need extra efforts to eradicate polio. *DAWN*. Retrieved from https://www.dawn.com/news/1232373

Aström, K. J., & Murray, R. M. (2010). *Feedback systems: An introduction for scientists and engineers*. Princeton, NJ: Princeton university press.

Australian Institute of Health and Welfare. (n.d.). Retrieved from http://www.aihw.gov.au/

Bacharova, L., Selvester, R. H., Engblom, H., & Wagner, G. S. (2005). Where is the central terminal located?: In search of understanding the use of the Wilson central terminal for production of 9 of the standard 12 electrocardiogram leads. *Journal of Electrocardiology*, *38*(2), 119–127. doi:10.1016/j.jelectrocard.2005.01.002 PMID:15892021

Bachir, A., Dohler, M., Watteyne, T., & Leung, K. K. (2010). Article. *MAC Essentials for Wireless Sensor Networks*, *12*(2), 222–248.

Bachs, L., & Mørland, H. (2001). Acute cardiovascular fatalities following cannabis use. *Forensic Science International*, *124*(2), 200–203. doi:10.1016/S0379-0738(01)00609-0 PMID:11792512

Ballard, F. J., & Oliver, I. T. (1965). Carbohydrate metabolism in liver from foetal and neonatal sheep. *The Biochemical Journal*, *95*(1), 191–200. doi:10.1042/bj0950191 PMID:14333556

Bardoli, A. D., Taylor, W. S. J., & Mahmalji, W. (2017). Can the UroLift prostatic implant device treat the symptoms of benign prostatic hypertrophy, avoid sexual dysfunction and reduce hospital TURP waiting times? A single centre, single surgeon experience and review of the literature. *The Aging Male*, 1–6. doi:10.1080/13685538.2017.1336531 PMID:28609136

Barmpalexis, P., Kachrimanis, K., & Georgarakis, E. (2011a). Solid dispersions in the development of animodipine floating tablet formulation and optimization by artificial neural networks and genetic programming. *European Journal of Pharmaceutics and Biopharmaceutics*, *77*(1), 122–131. doi:10.1016/j.ejpb.2010.09.017 PMID:20934511

Barmpalexis, P., Kachrimanis, K., Tsakonas, A., & Georgarakis, E. (2011b). Symbolic regression via genetic programming in the optimization of a controlled release pharmaceutical formulation. *Chemometrics and Intelligent Laboratory Systems*, *107*(1), 75–82. doi:10.1016/j.chemolab.2011.01.012

Barnard, K. D., Lloyd, C. E., & Skinner, T. C. (2007). Systematic literature review: Quality of life associated with insulin pump use in Type 1 diabetes. *Diabetic Medicine*, *24*(6), 607–617. doi:10.1111/j.1464-5491.2007.02120.x PMID:17367304

Barnes, P. J., Rodger, I. W., & Thomson, N. C. (Eds.). (1998). *Asthma: basic mechanisms and clinical management*. Academic Press.

Barreto, A. B., Scargle, S. D., & Adjouadi, M. A. (2000). practical EMG-based human–computer interface for users with motor disabilities. *Journal of Rehabilitation Research and Development*, *37*, 53–63. PMID:10847572

Barr, R. C., & Van Oosterom, A. (2010). Genesis of the electrocardiogram. In *Comprehensive electrocardiology* (pp. 167–190). Springer. doi:10.1007/978-1-84882-046-3_5

Baselli, G., Bolis, D., Cerutti, S., & Freschi, C. (1985). Autoregressive modeling and power spectral estimate of RR interval time series in arrhythmic patients. *Computers and Biomedical Research, an International Journal, 18*(6), 510–530. doi:10.1016/0010-4809(85)90027-8 PMID:4075786

Becker, J. O. (2004). *Deep listeners: Music, emotion, and trancing*. Indiana University Press.

Beebe, D. J., Hsieh, A. S., Denton, D. D., & Radwin, R. G. (1995). A Silicon Force Sensor for Robotics and Medicine. *Sensors and Actuators. A, Physical, 50*(1-2), 55–65. doi:10.1016/0924-4247(96)80085-9

Benard, Kahm, Heuer, & Huff. (1998). Thin-Film Shape-Memory Alloy Actuated Micropumps. *Journal of Microelectromechanical Systems, 7*(2), 245-251.

Bharathan, R., Dexter, S., & Hanson, M. (2009). Laparoscopic retrieval of retained Redivac drain fragment. *Journal of Obstetrics & Gynaecology, 29*(3), 263–264. doi:10.1080/01443610902754000 PMID:19358050

Bhattacharya, A. (2014). Costs of occupational musculoskeletal disorders (MSDs) in the United States. *International Journal of Industrial Ergonomics, 44*(3), 448–454. doi:10.1016/j.ergon.2014.01.008

Biggs, A. (2013). *Health in Australia: A quick guide*. Parliamentary Library.

Billman, G. E. (2011). Heart rate variability–a historical perspective. *Frontiers in Physiology*, 2. PMID:22144961

Billman, G. E. (2013). The LF/HF ratio does not accurately measure cardiac sympatho-vagal balance. *Frontiers in Physiology*, 4. PMID:23431279

Bi, Y., Guan, J., & Bell, D. (2008). The combination of multiple classifiers using an evidential reasoning approach. *Artificial Intelligence, 172*(15), 1731–1751. doi:10.1016/j.artint.2008.06.002

Blachnik, M. (2009). Comparison of various feature selection methods in application to prototype best rules, Computer Recognition Systems 3. *Advances in Intelligent and Soft Computing, 57*, 257–264. doi:10.1007/978-3-540-93905-4_31

Bohm, S., Timmer, B., Olthuis, W., & Bergveld, P. (2000). A closed-loop controlled electrochemically actuated micro-dosing system. *Journal of Micromechanics and Microengineering, 10*(4), 498–504. doi:10.1088/0960-1317/10/4/303

Bojwani, D. (2017). *Cervical Di 3 level cer* [Online image]. Retrieved 2017 from. http://www.dheerajbojwani.com/computer-assisted-surgery-India-low-cost-benefits.html

Bønaa, K. H., Mannsverk, J., Wiseth, R., Aaberge, L., Myreng, Y., Nygård, O., ... Bendz, B. (2016). Drug-eluting or bare-metal stents for coronary artery disease. *The New England Journal of Medicine, 375*(13), 1242–1252. doi:10.1056/NEJMoa1607991 PMID:27572953

Bonfils-Roberts, E. (1972). The Rib Spreader: A Chapter in the History of Thoracic Surgery. Chest, 61(5), 469–474.

Bonfils-Roberts, E. (2008). The Rib Spreader: A Chapter in the History of Thoracic Surgery. *Chest, 61*(5), 469–474. doi:10.1378/chest.61.5.469 PMID:4558402

Bong, S. Z., Murugappan, M., & Yaacob, S. (2012). *Analysis of electrocardiogram (ecg) signals for human emotional stress classification.* Paper presented at the First International Conference on Trends in Intelligent Robotics, Automation, and Manufacturing, Kuala Lumpur, Malaysia. 10.1007/978-3-642-35197-6_22

Bourke, T. (2001). *Development of a robotic wheelchair*. University or Wollongong.

Boyett, M. R., Honjo, H., & Kodama, I. (2000). The sinoatrial node, a heterogeneous pacemaker structure. *Cardiovascular Research*, *47*(4), 658–687. doi:10.1016/S0008-6363(00)00135-8 PMID:10974216

Braat, H., Rottiers, P., Hommes, D. W., Huyghebaert, N., Remaut, E., Remon, J. P., ... Steidler, L. (2006). A phase I trial with transgenic bacteria expressing interleukin-10 in Crohn's disease. *Clinical Gastroenterology and Hepatology*, *4*(6), 754–759. doi:10.1016/j.cgh.2006.03.028 PMID:16716759

Brazier, M. A., & Casby, J. U. (1952). Cross-correlation and autocorrelation studies of electroencephalographic potentials. *Electroencephalography and Clinical Neurophysiology. Supplement*, *4*(2), 201–211. doi:10.1016/0013-4694(52)90010-2 PMID:13033798

Brier, E., Zurada, J. M., & Aronoff, G. R. (1995). Neural network predicted peak and trough of gentamicin concentrations. *Pharmaceutical Research*, *12*(3), 406–412. doi:10.1023/A:1016260720218 PMID:7617529

Brocchini, S., James, K., Tangpasuthadol, V., & Kohn, J. (1998). Structure–property correlations in a combinatorial library of degradable biomaterials. *Journal of Biomedical Materials Research. Part A*, *42*(1), 66–75. doi: PMID:9740008

Bronzino, J. D., & Peterson, D. R. (2014). *Biomedical engineering fundamentals*. CRC press.

Bruen, D., Delaney, C., Florea, L., & Diamond, D. (2017). Glucose sensing for diabetes monitoring: Recent developments. *Sensors (Basel)*, *17*(8), 1866. doi:10.339017081866

Brundage, Jurkovich, Hoyt, Patel, Ross, Marburger, ... Maier. (2001). Stapled versus Sutured Gastrointestinal Anastomoses in the Trauma Patient: A Multicenter Trial. *The Journal of Trauma Injury Infection and Critical Care*, *51*(6), 1054–1061.

Bullock, T. H., Buzsaki, G., & McClune, M. C. (1990). Coherence of compound field potentials reveals discontinuities in the CA1-subiculum of the hippocampus in freely-moving rats. *Neuroscience*, *38*(3), 609–619. doi:10.1016/0306-4522(90)90055-9 PMID:2270136

Burns, N. (2013). Cardiovascular Physiology. School of Medicine, Trinity College.

Bwititi, P., Angel, L., & Day, S. (2008). Self-monitoring of Blood Glucose Levels Using Glucometers in Riverina NSW: Patients' Perspectives. *Australian Journal of Medical Science*, *29*(1), 3.

Cabuz, C., Herb, W. R., Cabuz, E. I., & Lu, S. T. (2001)The dual diaphragm pump. In *Proceedings of the 14th IEEE International Conference on Micro Electro Mechanical Systems* (pp. 519–522). Interlaken, Switzerland: IEEE.

Callaway, J. K., Knight, M. J., Watkins, D. J., & Beart, P. M. (1999). Delayed Treatment With AM-36, a Novel Neuroprotective Agent, ReducesNeuronal Damage After Endothelin-1–Induced Middle Cerebral ArteryOcclusion in Conscious Rats. *Stroke*, *30*, 2704–2712. doi:10.1161/01.STR.30.12.2704 PMID:10583001

Cameron, B. D., & Cote, G. L. (1997). Noninvasive glucose sensing utilizing a digital closed-loop polarimetric approach. *IEEE Transactions on Biomedical Engineering*, *44*(12), 1221–1227. doi:10.1109/10.649993

Camm, A. J., Malik, M., Bigger, J., Breithardt, G., Cerutti, S., & Cohen, R. J. (1996). Heart rate variability: Standards of measurement, physiological interpretation and clinical use. Task Force of the European Society of Cardiology and the North American Society of Pacing and Electrophysiology. *Circulation*, *93*(5), 1043–1065. doi:10.1161/01.CIR.93.5.1043 PMID:8598068

Campadelli, P., Casiraghi, E., Campadelli, P., & Casiraghi, E. (2009). Liver Segmentation from CT Scans : A Survey Liver Segmentation from CT Scans : A Survey. *Artificial Intelligence in Medicine*, *45*, 185–196. doi:10.1016/j.artmed.2008.07.020 PMID:19059767

Cao, Y., D'Olhaberriague, L., Vikingstad, E. M., Levine, S. R., & Welch, K. M. (1998). Pilot study of functional MRI to assess cerebral activation of motor function after poststroke hemiparesis. *Stroke*, *29*(1), 112–122. doi:10.1161/01.STR.29.1.112 PMID:9445338

Capodanno, D., Gori, T., Nef, H., Latib, A., Mehilli, J., Lesiak, M., ... Colombo, A. (2015). Percutaneous coronary intervention with everolimus-eluting bioresorbable vascular scaffolds in routine clinical practice: Early and midterm outcomes from the European multicentre GHOST-EU registry. *EuroIntervention*, *10*(10), 1144–1153. doi:10.4244/EIJY14M07_11 PMID:25042421

Cartensen, J. T. (1996). *Modeling and data treatment in the pharmaceutical sciences*. New York: Technomic Publishing Co. Inc.

Carter, P. (1993). Perforation of the bowel by suction drains. *British Journal of Surgery*, *80*, 129. PMID:8428277

Casciaro, S. (2012). Fully Automatic Segmentations of Liver and Hepatic Tumors From 3-DComputed Tomography Abdominal Images. *Comparative Evaluation of Two Automatic Methods.*, *12*, 464–473.

Castelein, B., Cagnie, B., Parlevliet, T., Danneels, L., & Cools, A. (2015). Optimal normalization tests for muscle activation of the levator scapulae, pectoralis minor, and rhomboid major: An electromyography study using maximum voluntary isometric contractions. *Archives of Physical Medicine and Rehabilitation*, *96*(10), 1820–1827. doi:10.1016/j.apmr.2015.06.004 PMID:26119465

Cendelin, J., Korelusova, I., & Vozeh, F. (2008). The Effect of Repeated Rota Rod Training on motor skills and spatial learning ability in Lurcher Mutant mice. *Behavioural Brain Research*, *189*(1), 65–74. doi:10.1016/j.bbr.2007.12.013 PMID:18243354

Chai, T., & Draxler, R. R. (2014). *Root mean square error (RMSE) or mean absolute error (MAE)? –Arguments against avoiding RMSE in the literature*. Copernicus Publications.

Chaichanasiri, E., & Puangumpan, T. (2011). *A prototype of a stair-climbing system for a wheelchair.* Paper presented at the The Second TSME International Conference on Mechanical Engineering.

Chambers, W. M., Bicsak, M., Lamparelli, M., & Dixon, A. R. (2011). Single-incision laparoscopic surgery (SILS) in complex colorectal surgery: A technique offering potential and not just cosmesis. *Colorectal Disease*, *13*(4), 393–398. doi:10.1111/j.1463-1318.2009.02158.x PMID:20002691

Chandrashekar, G., & Sahin, F. (2014). A survey of feature selection methods. *Computers & Electrical Engineering*, *40*(1), 16–28. doi:10.1016/j.compeleceng.2013.11.024

Chankong, V., & Haimes, Y. Y. (1983). *Multiobjective Decision making theory & methodology*. New York: Elsevier.

Chan, M., Estève, D., Fourniols, J., Escriba, C., & Campo, E. (2012). Artificial Intelligence in Medicine Smart wearable systems : Current status and future challenges. *Artificial Intelligence in Medicine*, *56*(3), 137–156. doi:10.1016/j.artmed.2012.09.003

Chan, P. H. (1996). Role of oxidants in ischemic brain damage. *Stroke*, *27*(6), 1124–1129. doi:10.1161/01.STR.27.6.1124 PMID:8650725

Chansanroj, K., Petrović, J., Ibrić, S., & Betz, G. (2011). Drug release control and system understanding of sucrose esters matrix tablets by artificial neural networks. *European Journal of Pharmaceutical Sciences*, *44*(3), 321–331. doi:10.1016/j.ejps.2011.08.012 PMID:21878388

Chao, E. Y. (2003). Graphic-based musculoskeletal model for biomechanical analyses and animation. *Medical Engineering & Physics*, *25*(3), 201–212. doi:10.1016/S1350-4533(02)00181-9 PMID:12589718

Chapman, S. (1931). The absorption and dissociative or ionizing effect of monochromatic radiation in an atmosphere on a rotating earth. *Proceedings of the Physical Society*, *43*(1), 26–45. doi:10.1088/0959-5309/43/1/305

Cheng, H. D., Shan, J., Ju, W., Guo, Y., & Zhang, L. (2010). Automated breast cancer detection and classification using ultrasound images: A survey. *Pattern Recognition*, *43*(1), 299–317. doi:10.1016/j.patcog.2009.05.012

Cheng, K. K., Wu, J., Lin, Z. N., & Zhang, J. A. (2014). Aerobic and sequential anaerobic fermentation to produce xylitol and ethanol using non-detoxified acid pretreated corncob. *Biotechnology for Biofuels*, *7*(1), 166. doi:10.118613068-014-0166-y PMID:25431622

Chen, M., Gonzalez, S., Vasilakos, A., Cao, H., & Leung, V. C. M. (2011). Body Area Networks: A Survey. *Mobile Networks and Applications*, *16*(2), 171–193. doi:10.100711036-010-0260-8

Chen, S.-T., Chou, C.-Y., & Tseng, L.-H. (2014). Recurrence plot analysis of HRV for exposure to low-frequency noise. *Advanced Materials Research*.

Chen, Z., Kwon, K., & Tan, X. (2008). Integrated IMPC/PVDF sensory actuator and its validation in feedback control. *Sensors and Actuators. A, Physical*, *144*(2), 231–241. doi:10.1016/j.sna.2008.01.023

Cheung, C. S., & Cheung, V. Y. (2016). Response to "Uterine perforation in an adolescent using an intrauterine device with memory function: A case report and review of the published work". *Journal of Obstetrics and Gynaecology Research*, *42*(2), 228–229. doi:10.1111/jog.12836 PMID:26461807

Chiarini, G., Ray, P., Akter, S., Masella, C., & Ganz, A. (2013). mHealth technologies for chronic diseases and elders : A systematic review. *IEEE Journal on Selected Areas in Communications*, *31*(9), 6–18. doi:10.1109/JSAC.2013.SUP.0513001

Choi, B., Loh, X. J., Tan, A., Loh, C. K., Ye, E., Joo, M. K., & Jeong, B. (2015). Introduction to in situ forming hydrogels for biomedical applications. In *In-Situ Gelling Polymers* (pp. 5–35). Springer Singapore. doi:10.1007/978-981-287-152-7_2

Christini, D. J., Bennett, F., Lutchen, K., Ahmed, H., Hausdorff, J., & Oriol, N. (1995). Application of linear and nonlinear time series modeling to heart rate dynamics analysis. *IEEE Transactions on Biomedical Engineering*, *42*(4), 411–415. doi:10.1109/10.376135 PMID:7729840

Chu, A., Sehgal, C. M., & Greenleaf, J. F. (1990). Use of gray value distribution of run lengths for texture analysis. *Pattern Recognition Letters*, *11*(6), 415–420. doi:10.1016/0167-8655(90)90112-F

Cifrek, M., Medved, V., Tonković, S., & Ostojić, S. (2009). Surface EMG based muscle fatigue evaluation in biomechanics. *Clinical Biomechanics (Bristol, Avon)*, *24*(4), 327–340. doi:10.1016/j.clinbiomech.2009.01.010 PMID:19285766

Cirrhosis (Liver). (n.d.). Retrieved 2017 from http://www.medicinenet.com/cirrhosis/article.htm

Cline, G. B., & Luiz, J. M. (2013). Information technology systems in public sector health facilities in developing countries: The case of South Africa. *BMC Medical Informatics and Decision Making*, *13*(1), 13. doi:10.1186/1472-6947-13-13 PMID:23347433

Cooney, C. G., & Towe, B. C. (2004). A thermopneumatic dispensing micropump. Sens. Actuators A, 116, 519–524.

Corbett, D., & Nurse, S. (1998). The problem of assessing effective neuroprotection in experimental cerebral ischemia. *Progress in Neurobiology*, *54*(5), 531–548. doi:10.1016/S0301-0082(97)00078-6 PMID:9550190

Coupland, R. M., & Koever, A. (1991). Injuries from antipersonnel mines: The experience of the International Committee of the Red Cross. *BMJ (Clinical Research Ed.)*, *330*(6816), 1509–1512. doi:10.1136/bmj.303.6816.1509 PMID:1838290

Crack, P. J., & Taylor, J. M. (2005). Reactive oxygen species and the modulation of stroke. *Free Radical Biology & Medicine*, *38*(11), pp1433–pp1444. doi:10.1016/j.freeradbiomed.2005.01.019 PMID:15890617

Cramer, S. C., Nelles, G., Benson, R. R., Kaplan, J. D., Parker, R. A., Kwong, K. K., ... Rosen, B. R. (1997). A functional MRI study of subjects recovered from hemiparetic stroke. *Stroke*, *28*(12), 2518–2527. doi:10.1161/01.STR.28.12.2518 PMID:9412643

Crisostomo, E. A., Duncan, P. W., Propst, M., Dawson, D. V., & Davis, J. N. (1988). Evidence that amphetamine with physical therapy promotes recovery of motor function in stroke patients. *Annals of Neurology*, *23*(1), 94–97. doi:10.1002/ana.410230117 PMID:3345072

Csapó, Á., Wersényi, G., Nagy, H., & Stockman, T. (2015). A survey of assistive technologies and applications for blind users on mobile platforms: A review and foundation for research. *Journal on Multimodal User Interfaces*, *9*(4), 275–286. doi:10.100712193-015-0182-7

CT Scan or CAT Scan: How Does It Work? What is a CT scan? When is a CT scan used? (2017). [Online image]. Retrieved 2017 from http://www.lumen.luc.edu/lumen/MedEd/Radio/curriculum/Surgery/Hepatic_mass.htm

Cutkosky, M. R., & Kao, I. (1989). Computing and controlling the compliance of a robotic hand. *IEEE Transactions on Robotics and Automation*, *5*(2), 151–165. doi:10.1109/70.88036

da Costa, J. C., Ortigueira, M. D., Batista, A., & Paiva, T. (2013). *ARMA modelling for sleep disorders diagnose*. Paper presented at the Doctoral Conference on Computing, Electrical and Industrial Systems.

Dale, A. M., Addison, L., Lester, J., Kaskutas, V., & Evanoff, B. (2014). Weak grip strength does not predict upper extremity musculoskeletal symptoms or injuries among new workers. *Journal of Occupational Rehabilitation*, *24*(2), 325–331. doi:10.100710926-013-9460-y PMID:23857165

Danton, H. G., & Dietrich, D. (2004). The search for neuroprotective strategies in stroke. *AJNR. American Journal of Neuroradiology*, *25*, 181–194. PMID:14970016

Darabi, J., Ohadi, M. M., & DeVoe, D. (2001). An Electrohydrodynamic polarization micropump for electronic cooling. *Journal of Microelectromechanical Systems*, *10*(1), 98–106. doi:10.1109/84.911097

Dasarathy, B. V., & Holder, E. B. (1991). Image characterizations based on joint gray level run length distributions. *Pattern Recognition Letters*, *12*(8), 497–502. doi:10.1016/0167-8655(91)80014-2

Dash, S., Murthy, P. N., Nath, L., & Chowdhury, P. (2010). Kinetic modelling on drug release from controlled drug delivery systems. *Acta Poloniae Pharmaceutica-Drug Research*, *67*(3), 217–223. PMID:20524422

Deb, K. (2001). *Multi-objective optimization using evolutionary algorithms*. New York: John Wiley & Sons Limited.

Del Zoppo, G. J., & Hallenbeck, J. M. (2000). Advances in the vascular pathophysiology of ischemic stroke. *Thrombosis Research*, *98*(3), 73–81. doi:10.1016/S0049-3848(00)00218-8 PMID:10812160

Deng, Y., Wang, Y., & Shen, Y. (2011). Speckle reduction in ultrasound images based on Rayleigh-trimmed anisotropic diffusion filter. *Pattern Recognition Letters*, *32*(13), 1516–1525. doi:10.1016/j.patrec.2011.06.007

Deros, B., Daruis, B., & Ismail, A. (2010). Work-related musculoskeletal disorders among workers' performing manual material handling work in an automotive manufacturing company. *American Journal of Applied Sciences*, *7*(8), 1087–1092. doi:10.3844/ajassp.2010.1087.1092

Desai, U., Martis, R. J., Nayak, C. G., Sarika, K., & Seshikala, G. (2015). *Machine intelligent diagnosis of ECG for arrhythmia classification using DWT, ICA and SVM techniques*. Paper presented at the India Conference (INDICON), 2015 Annual IEEE. 10.1109/INDICON.2015.7443220

Di, J., Yao, S., Ye, Y., Cui, Z., Yu, J., Ghosh, T. K., ... Gu, Z. (2015). Stretch-triggered drug delivery from wearable elastomer films containing therapeutic depots. *ACS Nano*, *9*(9), 9407–9415. doi:10.1021/acsnano.5b03975 PMID:26258579

Dilaveris, P. E., & Gialafos, J. E. (2001). P-wave dispersion: A novel predictor of paroxysmal atrial fibrillation. *Annals of Noninvasive Electrocardiology*, *6*(2), 159–165. doi:10.1111/j.1542-474X.2001.tb00101.x PMID:11333174

Dirangle, U., Iadecola, C., & Moskowitz, M. A. (1999). 'Pathobiology of ischemic stroke: An integrated view'. *Trends in Neurosciences*, *22*(9), 391–397. doi:10.1016/S0166-2236(99)01401-0 PMID:10441299

Djupesland, P. G. (2013). Nasal drug delivery devices: Characteristics and performance in a clinical perspective—a review. *Drug Delivery and Translational Research*, 1–21. PMID:23316447

Dodds, K. L., Miller, C. B., Kyle, S. D., Marshall, N. S., & Gordon, C. J. (2017). Heart rate variability in insomnia patients: A critical review of the literature. *Sleep Medicine Reviews*, *33*, 88–100. doi:10.1016/j.smrv.2016.06.004 PMID:28187954

Donnan, G. A., Bladin, P. F., Berkovic, S. F., Longley, W. A., & Saling, M. M. (1991). The stroke syndrome of striatocapsular infarction. *Brain*, *114*(Pt 1A), 51–70. PMID:1998890

Donnan, G. A., Fisher, M., Macleod, M., & Davis, S. M. (2008). Stroke. *Lancet*, *371*(9624), 1612–1623. doi:10.1016/S0140-6736(08)60694-7 PMID:18468545

Dressman, J. B., & Fleisher, D. (1986). Mixing-tank model for predicting dissolution rate control or oral absorption. *Journal of Pharmaceutical Sciences*, *75*(2), 109–116. doi:10.1002/jps.2600750202 PMID:3958917

Drukker, K., Sennett, C. A., & Giger, M. L. (2014). Computerized detection of breast cancer on automated breast ultrasound imaging of women with dense breast. *Medical Physics, 41*(1), 1– 19. PMID:24718570

Duda, R. O., & Hart, P. E. (1973). *Pattern Classification and Scene Analysis* (Vol. 3). New York: Wiley.

Duda, R. O., Hart, P. E., & Stork, D. G. (2006). *Pattern classification* (2nd ed.). Wiley India.

Duff, J. (2004). The usefulness of quantitative EEG (QEEG) and neurotherapy in the assessment and treatment of post-concussion syndrome. *Clinical EEG and Neuroscience*, *35*(4), 198–209. doi:10.1177/155005940403500410 PMID:15493535

Du, J., & O'Reilly, R. K. (2009). Advances and challenges in smart and functional polymer vesicles. *Soft Matter*, *5*(19), 3544–3561. doi:10.1039/b905635a

Dunham, N. W., & Miya, T. S. (1957). A note on a simple apparatus for detecting neurological deficit in rats and mice. *J Am Pharm Assoc Am Pharm Assoc (Baltim)*, *46*(3), 208–209. doi:10.1002/jps.3030460322 PMID:13502156

Durai, R., Mownah, A., & Ng, P. C. (2009). Use of drains in surgery: A review. *Journal of Perioperative Practice*, *19*(6), 180–186. doi:10.1177/175045890901900603 PMID:19591322

Dyer, C. R., & Rosenfeld, A. (1976). Fourier texture features: Suppression of aperture effects. *IEEE Transactions on Systems, Man, and Cybernetics*, *SMC-6*(10), 703–705. doi:10.1109/TSMC.1976.4309422

Eadie, M., & Steele, R. J. (2017). Non-invasive Blood Glucose Monitoring and Data Analytics. In *Proceedings of the International Conference on Compute and Data Analysis* (pp. 138–142). Lakeland, FL: ACM. 10.1145/3093241.3093283

Eckmann, J.-P., Kamphorst, S. O., & Ruelle, D. (1987). Recurrence plots of dynamical systems. *EPL*, *4*(9), 973–977. doi:10.1209/0295-5075/4/9/004

Ekroos, H. (2008). *Exhaled nitric oxide: Variability and association with bronchial hyperresponsiveness and atopy.* Academic Press.

El-gayar, O., Timsina, P., Nawar, N., & Eid, W. (2013). Mobile Applications for Diabetes Self-Management. *Status and Potential*, *7*(1), 247–262.

Elhaj, F. A., Salim, N., Harris, A. R., Swee, T. T., & Ahmed, T. (2016). Arrhythmia recognition and classification using combined linear and nonlinear features of ECG signals. *Computer Methods and Programs in Biomedicine*, *127*, 52–63. doi:10.1016/j.cmpb.2015.12.024 PMID:27000289

Elith, J., Leathwick, J. R., & Hastie, T. (2008). A working guide to boosted regression trees. *Journal of Animal Ecology*, *77*(4), 802–813. doi:10.1111/j.1365-2656.2008.01390.x PMID:18397250

Elliot, A. J. (2005). *A Conceptual History of the Achievement Goal Construct*. Academic Press.

Elliott, D., Carr, S., & Orme, D. (2005). The effect of motivational music on sub-maximal exercise. *European Journal of Sport Science*, *5*(2), 97–106. doi:10.1080/17461390500171310

Ercelebi, E. (2004). Electrocardiogram signals de-noising using lifting-based discrete wavelet transform. *Computers in Biology and Medicine*, *34*(6), 479–493. doi:10.1016/S0010-4825(03)00090-8 PMID:15265720

Espinosa, H., Capito, R.M., & Lucas, L.A. (2000). *Microchip for Drug Delivery*. Academic Press.

Evans, D. A., & Whitsett, J. A. (1997). Surfactant Replacement Therapies in Children. In The Pediatric Lung (pp. 199-227). Birkhäuser Basel. doi:10.1007/978-3-0348-8960-5_9

Evarts, E. V. (1966). Pyramidal tract activity associated with a conditioned hand movement in the monkey. *Journal of Neurophysiology*, *29*(6), 1011–1027. doi:10.1152/jn.1966.29.6.1011 PMID:4961643

Fang, T., & Tan, X. (2010). A novel diaphragm micropump actuated by conjugated polymer petals: Fabrication, modeling, and experimental results. *Sensors and Actuators. A, Physical*, *158*(1), 121–131. doi:10.1016/j.sna.2009.12.012

Faziludeen, S., & Sankaran, P. (2016). ECG Beat Classification Using Evidential K-Nearest Neighbours. *Procedia Computer Science*, *89*, 499–505. doi:10.1016/j.procs.2016.06.106

Fei-Fei, L., Karpathy, A., Leung, T., Shetty, S., Sukthankar, R., & Toderici, G. (2014). Large-Scale Video Classification with Convolutional Neural Networks. *IEEE Conference on Computer Vision and Pattern Recognition.*

Fend, M. (2017). *Fleshing Out Surfaces: Skin in French Art and Medicine, 1650-1850*. Oxford University Press. doi:10.7228/manchester/9780719087967.001.0001

Fernandez, F., & Pallis, G. C. (2014, November). Opportunities and challenges of the Internet of Things for healthcare: Systems engineering perspective. In *Wireless Mobile Communication and Healthcare (Mobihealth), 2014 EAI 4th International Conference on* (pp. 263-266). IEEE.

Fernando, J. L. I. N., Wickramaratne, C. P., Dissanayake, R. S. B., Kolambage, S. H., Aminda, M. A. U., Cooray, N. H., ... Muthukudaarachchi, A. D. (2012). Studying current status of intensive care services in Sri Lanka. *International Journal of Critical Illness and Injury Science*, *2*(1), 11. doi:10.4103/2229-5151.94884 PMID:22624096

Ferrari, A., Benedetti, M. G., Pavan, E., Frigo, C., Bettinelli, D., Rabuffetti, M., ... Leardini, A. (2008). Quantitative comparison of five current protocols in gait analysis. *Gait & Posture*, *28*(2), 207–216. doi:10.1016/j.gaitpost.2007.11.009 PMID:18206374

Ferrari, M., & Torchilin, V. (2008). *Fundamental biomedical technologies-Multifunctional pharmaceutical nanocarriers. In Multifunctional polymeric nanosystems for tumor-targeted delivery* (pp. 33–66). New York: Springer Sicences.

Finkelstein, J., Eckersberger, E., Sadri, H., Taneja, S. S., Lepor, H., & Djavan, B. (2010). Open Versus Laparoscopic Versus Robot-Assisted Laparoscopic Prostatectomy: The European and US Experience. *Reviews in Urology*, *12*(1), 35–43. PMID:20428292

Flanagan, J. R., & Wing, A. M. (1993). Modulation of Grip Force with Load Force during point-to-point arm movements. *Experimental Brain Research*, *95*(1), 131–143. doi:10.1007/BF00229662 PMID:8405245

Florence, A. T., & Siepmann, J. (Eds.). (2009). *Modern Pharmaceutics: Applications and Advances* (Vol. 2). Informa Healthcare USA.

Folkers, A., Mosch, F., Malina, T., & Hofmann, U. G. (2003). Realtime bioelectrical data acquisition and processing from 128 channels utilizing the wavelet-transformation. *Neurocomputing*, *52-54*, 247–254. doi:10.1016/S0925-2312(02)00763-4

Foregut, D. (2017). *For other uses, see Liver (disambiguation)* [Online image]. Retrieved 2017 from https://wiki2.org/en/Liver

Foster, A., & Resnikoff, S. (2005). The impact of Vision 2020 on global blindness. *Eye (London, England)*, *19*(10), 1133–1135. doi:10.1038j.eye.6701973 PMID:16304595

Fox, S. E., Wolfson, S., & Ranck, J. B. Jr. (1986). Hippocampal theta rhythm and the firing of neurons in walking and urethane anesthetized rats. *Experimental Brain Research*, *62*(3), 495–508. doi:10.1007/BF00236028 PMID:3720881

Franco, P., Chabanski, S., Szliwowski, H., Dramaix, M., & Kahn, A. (2000). Influence of maternal smoking on autonomic nervous system in healthy infants. *Pediatric Research*, *47*(2), 215–215. doi:10.1203/00006450-200002000-00011 PMID:10674349

Freudenrich, C. C. (n.d.). *How Ultrasound Works*. Retrieved 2017 from https://www.physics.utoronto.ca/~jharlow/teaching /phy138_0708/lec04/ultrasoundx.htm

Frigola, C.J., Colombo, P.A., & Pares, C.J. (1987). Eur. Pat., EP 242, 289, pp 6.

Frontino, G., Meschi, F., Bonfanti, R., Rigamonti, A., Battaglino, R., Favalli, V., ... Chiumello, G. (2013). Future Perspectives in Glucose Monitoring Sensors. *European Endocrinology*, *9*(1), 21–26. doi:10.17925/EE.2013.09.01.21

Frost, V. S., Stiles, J. A., Shanmugam, K. S., & Holtzman, J. C. (1982). A model for radar images and its application to adaptive digital filtering of multiplicative noise. *IEEE Transactions on Pattern Analysis and Machine Intelligence*, *PAMI-4*(2), 157–165. doi:10.1109/TPAMI.1982.4767223 PMID:21869022

Fuhr, G., Hagedorn, R., Muller, T., Benecke, W., & Wagner, B. (1992). Pumping of Water Solutions in Microfabricated Electrohydrodynamic Systems. *Proceedings of IEEE Micro Electro Mechanical Systems. An Investigation of Micro Structures, Sensors, Actuators, Machines and Robots MEMS,Travemunde*, 25–30. 10.1109/MEMSYS.1992.187685

Furht, B. (2007). *Encyclopedia of Wireless and Mobile Communications-3 Volume Set*. Auerbach Publications. doi:10.1201/NOE1420043266

Galloway, M. M. (1975). Texture analysis using gray level run lengths. *Computer Graphics and Image Processing*, *4*(2), 172–179. doi:10.1016/S0146-664X(75)80008-6

Gao, L., Mantell, S., & Polla, D. (2000). Implantable medical drug delivery systems using micro-electro-mechanical systems technology. *First IEEE-EMBS Special Topic Conference on Microtechnologies in Medicine and Biology*, 487–490.

Garrick, R., Kliger, A., & Stefanchik, B. (2012). Patient and facility safety in hemodialysis: Opportunities and strategies to develop a culture of safety. *Clinical Journal of the American Society of Nephrology; CJASN*, *7*(4), 680–688. doi:10.2215/CJN.06530711 PMID:22282480

Gautam, M. K., & Giri, V. K. (2016). An Approach of Neural Network For Electrocardiogram Classification. *APTIKOM Journal on Computer Science and Information Technologies*, *1*(3), 115–123.

Ge, D., Srinivasan, N., & Krishnan, S. M. (2002). Cardiac arrhythmia classification using autoregressive modeling. *Biomedical Engineering Online*, *1*(1), 5. doi:10.1186/1475-925X-1-5 PMID:12473180

Geets, W., & Louette, N. (1985). Early EEG in 300 cerebral concussions. *EEG and Clinical Neurophysiology*, *14*(4), 333–338. PMID:4023359

Gerhardus, D. (2003). Robot-assisted surgery: The future is here. *Journal of Healthcare Management*, *48*(4), 242–251. doi:10.1097/00115514-200307000-00008 PMID:12908224

Gervais, R., Leclercq, C., Shankar, A., Jacobs, S., Eiskjaer, H., Johannessen, A., ... Daubert, C. (2009). Surface electrocardiogram to predict outcome in candidates for cardiac resynchronization therapy: A sub-analysis of the CARE-HF trial. *European Journal of Heart Failure*, *11*(7), 699–705. doi:10.1093/eurjhf/hfp074 PMID:19505883

Gevins, A. S., & Schaffer, R. E. (1980). A critical-review of electroencephalographic (EEG) correlates of higher cortical functions. *CRC Critical Reviews in Bioengineering*, *4*, 113–164. PMID:7004774

Ghamari, M., Arora, H., Sherratt, R. S., & Harwin, W. (2015). Comparison of low-power wireless communication technologies for wearable health-monitoring applications. In *2015 International Conference on Computer, Communications, and Control Technology (I4CT)* (pp. 1–6). Kuching, Malaysia: Academic Press. 10.1109/I4CT.2015.7219525

Gifford, H. S., III, & Reich, C. J. (2017). *Drug delivery treatment device*. U.S. Patent 9,668,917.

Gilligan, A. K., Thrift, A. G., Sturm, J. W., Dewey, H. M., Macdonell, R. A., & Donnan, G. A. (2005). Stroke units, tissue plasminogen activator, aspirin and neuroprotection: Which stroke intervention could provide the greatest community benefit? *Cerebrovascular Diseases (Basel, Switzerland)*, *20*(4), 239–244. doi:10.1159/000087705 PMID:16123543

Ginsberg, M. D. (2008). Neuroprotection for ischemic stroke: Past, present and future. *Neuropharmacology*, *55*(3), 363–389. doi:10.1016/j.neuropharm.2007.12.007 PMID:18308347

Giri, S., Trewyn, B. G., Stellmaker, M. P., & Lin, V. S. Y. (2005). Stimuli-responsive controlled-release delivery system based on mesoporous silica nanorods capped with magnetic nanoparticles. *Angewandte Chemie International Edition*, *44*(32), 5038–5044. doi:10.1002/anie.200501819 PMID:16038000

Gite, L. P., Majumder, J., Mehta, C. R., & Khadatkar, A. (2009). *Anthropometric and strength data of Indian agricultural workers for Farm equipment design*. Bhopal, India: Central Institute of Agricultural Engineering.

Glauche, F., Pilarek, M., Bournazou, M. N. C., Grunzel, P., & Neubauer, O. (2016). Design of experiments based high-throughput strategy for development and optimization of efficient cell disruption protocols. *Engineering in Life Sciences*, 1–7.

Glos, M., Fietze, I., Blau, A., Baumann, G., & Penzel, T. (2014). Cardiac autonomic modulation and sleepiness: Physiological consequences of sleep deprivation due to 40h of prolonged wakefulness. *Physiology & Behavior*, *125*, 45–53. doi:10.1016/j.physbeh.2013.11.011 PMID:24291386

Gokhale, M., & Khanduja, D. K. (2010). Time domain signal analysis using wavelet packet decomposition approach. *International Journal of Communications. Network and System Sciences*, *3*(03), 321–329. doi:10.4236/ijcns.2010.33041

Gomi, T., & Griffith, A. (1998). Developing intelligent wheelchairs for the handicapped. *Assistive Technology and Artificial Intelligence*, 150-178.

Gonzalez, R. C., & Woods, R. E. (2010). *Digital Image Processing Using MATLAB* (2nd ed.). Pearson Prentice Hall.

Göran, B. M. D. (1981). Natural history of patients with untreated liver metastases from colorectal cancer. *American Journal of Surgery*, *141*(5), 586–589. doi:10.1016/0002-9610(81)90057-X PMID:7223955

Govender, T., Choonara, Y. E., Kumar, P., Bijukumar, D., du Toit, L. C., Modi, G., ... Pillay, V. (2017). Implantable and transdermal polymeric drug delivery technologies for the treatment of central nervous system disorders. *Pharmaceutical Development and Technology*, *22*(4), 476–486. doi:10.1080/10837450.2016.1189937 PMID:27268737

Grassberger, P., & Procaccia, I. (1983). Characterization of Strange Attractors. *Physical Review Letters*, *50*(5), 346–349. doi:10.1103/PhysRevLett.50.346

Graupe, D., & Cline, W. K. (1975). Functional separation of EMG signals via ARMA identification methods for prosthesis control purposes. *IEEE Transactions on Systems, Man, and Cybernetics*, *SMC-5*(2), 252–259. doi:10.1109/TSMC.1975.5408479

Grayson, A. C. R., Choi, I. S., Tyler, B. M., Wang, P. P., Brem, H., Cima, M. J., & Langer, R. (2003). Multi-pulse drug delivery from a resorbable polymeric microchip device. *Nature Materials*, *2*(11), 767–772. doi:10.1038/nmat998 PMID:14619935

Grayson, A. R., Shawgo, R. S., Johnson, A. M., Flynn, N. T., Yawen, L., Cima, M. J., & Langer, R. (2004). A BioMEMS review: MEMS technology for physiologically integrated devices. *Proceedings of the IEEE*, *92*(1), 6–21. doi:10.1109/JPROC.2003.820534

Gu¨ler, N. F., Kiymik, M. K., & Güler, İ. (1995). Comparison of FFT and AR-based sonogram outputs of 20 MHz pulsed Doppler Data in real Time. *J. Computers Biol. Med*, *25*(4), 383–391. doi:10.1016/0010-4825(95)00024-X PMID:7497700

Guerreiro, J., & Gonçalves, D. (2015). Faster Text-to-Speeches: Enhancing Blind People's Information Scanning with Faster Concurrent Speech. *Proceedings of the 17th International ACM SIGACCESS Conference on Computers & Accessibility*. 10.1145/2700648.2809840

Guidoin, M. F., & Guidoin, R. G. (2004). Sélection des matériaux pour la conception et le développement du boîtier d'un cœur artificiel total implantable: Supériorité du titane et de ses alliages. *ITBM-RBM*, *25*(3), 126–138. doi:10.1016/j.rbmret.2004.05.003

Guler, I., Kiymik, M. K., Akin, M., & Alkan, A. (2001). AR spectral analysis of EEG signals by using maximum likelihood estimation. *Computers in Biology and Medicine*, *31*(6), 441–450. doi:10.1016/S0010-4825(01)00022-1 PMID:11604150

Guo, Y., Sengur, A., & Tian, J. W. (2016). A novel breast ultrasoundimage segmentation algorithm based on neutrosophic similarity score and level set. *Computer Methods and Programs in Biomedicine*, *123*, 43–53. doi:10.1016/j.cmpb.2015.09.007 PMID:26483304

Gupta, S., Chauhan, R. C., & Sexana, S. C. (2004). Wavelet-based statistical approach for speckle reduction in medical ultrasound images. *Medical & Biological Engineering & Computing*, *42*(2), 189–192. doi:10.1007/BF02344630 PMID:15125148

Guyon, I., & Elisseeff, A. (2006). An introduction to feature extraction. *Feature Extraction*, 1-25.

Guyot, L. L., Diaz, F. G., O'Regan, M. H., Mcleod, S., Park, H., & Phillis, J. W. (2001). Real-time measurement of glutamate release from the ischemic penumbra of the rat cerebral cortex using a focal middle cerebral artery occlusion mode. *Neuroscience Letters*, *299*(1-2), 37–40. doi:10.1016/S0304-3940(01)01510-5 PMID:11166932

Haciibrahimoglu, G., Solak, O., Olcmen, A., Bedirhan, M. A., Solmazer, N., & Gurses, A. (2004, February). Management of Traumatic Diaphragmatic Rupture. *Surgery Today*, *34*(2), 111–114. doi:10.100700595-003-2662-8 PMID:14745609

Hafeez, A., Mohamud, B. K., Shiekh, M. R., Shah, S. A. I., & Jooma, R. (2011). Lady health workers programme in Pakistan: Challenges, achievements and the way forward. *JPMA. The Journal of the Pakistan Medical Association, 61*(3), 210. PMID:21465929

Hafizah, S., Ubaidillah, S. A., Sallehuddin, R., & Ali, N. A. (2013). Cancer detection using artificial neural network and support vector machine: A comparative study. *Jurnal Teknologi, 65*(1), 73–81.

Hajizadeh, S., Abbasi, A., & Goshvarpour, A. (2015). *Intelligent classification of ECG signals to distinguish between pre and on-music states.* Paper presented at the Information and Knowledge Technology (IKT), 2015 7th Conference on. 10.1109/IKT.2015.7288790

Hall, G. F. (2007). Hepatitis A, B, C, D, E, G: an update. *Ethn Dis. Spring, 17*(2 Suppl 2), S2-40-5. Retrieved 2017 from http://www.hopkinsmedicine.org/healthlibrary/conditions/liver_biliary_and_pancreatic_disorders/liver_anatomy_and_functions_85,P00676/

Hall, J. E. (2015). *Guyton and Hall Textbook of Medical Physiology E-Book.* Elsevier Health Sciences.

Ham, B., Min, D., & Sohn, K. (2013). Revisiting the relationship between adaptive smoothing and anisotropic diffusion with modified filters. *IEEE Transactions on Image Processing, 22*(3), 1096–1107. doi:10.1109/TIP.2012.2226904 PMID:23193236

Hamiti, M., & Kastrati, R. (2014). Adapting eSpeak for converting text into speech in Albanian. *International Journal of Computer Science Issues, 11*(4), 21.

Hannan, A. (2010). Providing patients online access to their primary care computerised medical records: A case study of sharing and caring. *Journal of Innovation in Health Informatics, 18*(1), 41–49. doi:10.14236/jhi.v18i1.752 PMID:20429977

Haralick, R. M. (1979). Statistical and structural approaches to texture. *Proceedings of the IEEE, 67*(5), 786–804. doi:10.1109/PROC.1979.11328

Haralick, R. M., Shanmugam, K., & Dinstein, I. (1973). Textural features for image classification. *IEEE Transactions on Systems, Man, and Cybernetics, SMC-3*(6), 610–621. doi:10.1109/TSMC.1973.4309314

Harland, C., Clark, T., Peters, N., Everitt, M. J., & Stiffell, P. (2005). A compact electric potential sensor array for the acquisition and reconstruction of the 7-lead electrocardiogram without electrical charge contact with the skin. *Physiological Measurement, 26*(6), 939–950. doi:10.1088/0967-3334/26/6/005 PMID:16311443

Harrell, F. E. Jr. (2015). *Regression modeling strategies: with applications to linear models, logistic and ordinal regression, and survival analysis.* Springer. doi:10.1007/978-3-319-19425-7

Haselsteiner, E., & Pfurtscheller, G. (2000). Using time-dependent neural Networks for EEG classification. *IEEE Transactions on Rehabilitation Engineering, 8*(4), 457–463. doi:10.1109/86.895948 PMID:11204036

Hayashi, T., Mizuno-Matsumoto, Y., Okamoto, E., Ishii, R., Ukai, S., & Shinosaki, K. (2008). *Anterior brain activities related to emotional stress.* Paper presented at the Automation Congress, 2008. WAC 2008. World.

Haykin, S. (2009). *Neural Network and Learning Machines* (3rd ed.). Pearson Education.

Hegde, V. N., Deekshit, R., & Satyanarayana, P. (2013). A review on ECG signal processing and HRV analysis. *Journal of Medical Imaging and Health Informatics, 3*(2), 270–279. doi:10.1166/jmihi.2013.1163

Heidbuchel, H., Hindricks, G., Broadhurst, P., Van Erven, L., Fernandez-Lozano, I., Rivero-Ayerza, M., ... Beeton, I. (2015). EuroEco (European Health Economic Trial on Home Monitoring in ICD Patients): A provider perspective in five European countries on costs and net financial impact of follow-up with or without remote monitoring. *European Heart Journal*, *36*(3), 158–169. doi:10.1093/eurheartj/ehu339 PMID:25179766

He, K., Zhang, X., Ren, S., & Sun, J. (2016). *Deep Residual Learning for Image Recognition, Computer Vision Foundation, Open access*. IEEE Xplore.

Herman, D. C., Onate, J. A., Weinhold, P. S., Guskiewicz, K. M., Garrett, W. E., Yu, B., & Padua, D. A. (2009). The effects of feedback with and without strength training on lower extremity biomechanics. *The American Journal of Sports Medicine*, *37*(7), 1301–1308. doi:10.1177/0363546509332253 PMID:19299530

Herring, D. R., Burleson, M. H., Roberts, N. A., & Devine, M. J. (2011). Coherent with laughter: Subjective experience, behavior, and physiological responses during amusement and joy. *International Journal of Psychophysiology*, *79*(2), 211–218. doi:10.1016/j.ijpsycho.2010.10.007 PMID:21034782

Hersh, M. A., & Johnson, M. A. (2008). Disability and assistive technology systems. *Assistive technology for visually impaired and blind people*, 1-50.

Hibbs, A. E., Thompson, K. G., French, D. N., Hodgson, D., & Spears, I. R. (2011). Peak and average rectified EMG measures: Which method of data reduction should be used for assessing core training exercises? *Journal of Electromyography and Kinesiology*, *21*(1), 102–111. doi:10.1016/j.jelekin.2010.06.001 PMID:20655245

Hinterberger, T., Weiskopf, N., Veit, R., Wilhelm, B., Betta, E., & Birbaumer, N. (2004). An EEG-driven brain-computer interface combined with functional magnetic resonance imaging (fMRI). *IEEE Transactions on Biomedical Engineering*, *51*(6), 971–974. doi:10.1109/TBME.2004.827069 PMID:15188866

Hoerbst, A., & Ammenwerth, E. (2010). Electronic health records. *Methods of Information in Medicine*, *49*(4), 320–336. doi:10.3414/ME10-01-0038 PMID:20603687

Hofer, T., Schumacher, M., & Bromuri, S. (2015). COMPASS : an Interoperable Personal Health System to Monitor and Compress Signals in Chronic Obstructive Pulmonary Disease. In *Proceedings of the 9th International Conference on Pervasive Computing Technologies for Healthcare* (pp. 304 – 311). Istanbul, Turkey: Academic Press. 10.4108/icst.pervasivehealth.2015.259186

Hoffman, A. S. (2008). The origins and evolution of "controlled" drug delivery systems. *Journal of Controlled Release*, *132*(3), 153–163. doi:10.1016/j.jconrel.2008.08.012 PMID:18817820

Holan, S. H., Lund, R., & Davis, G. (2010). The ARMA alphabet soup: A tour of ARMA model variants. *Statistics Surveys*, *4*(0), 232–274. doi:10.1214/09-SS060

Hong, J. T., Ryu, S. R., Kim, H. J., Lee, J. K., Lee, S. H., Kim, D. B., ... Kim, P. Y. (2000). Neuroprotective effect of green tea extract in experimental ischemia-reperfusion brain injury. *Brain Research Bulletin*, *53*(6), 743–749. doi:10.1016/S0361-9230(00)00348-8 PMID:11179838

Hong, J. T., Ryu, S. R., Kim, H. J., Lee, J. K., Lee, S. H., Yun, Y. P., ... Kim, P. Y. (2001). Protective effect of green tea extract on ischemia/reperfusion-induced brain injury in Mongolian gerbils. *Brain Research*, *888*(1), 11–18. doi:10.1016/S0006-8993(00)02935-8 PMID:11146047

Horn, J., & Limburg, M. (2001a). Calcium antagonists for ischemic stroke: A systematic review. *Stroke*, *32*(2), 570–576. doi:10.1161/01.STR.32.2.570 PMID:11157199

Horta, E. T., Lopes, I. C., Rodrigues, J. J. P. C., & Proenca, M. L. (2013). A mobile health application for falls detection and biofeedback monitoring. In *2013 IEEE 15th International Conference on e-Health Networking, Applications and Services (Healthcom 2013)* (pp. 36–40). Lisbon, Portugal: IEEE. 10.1109/HealthCom.2013.6720634

Hovell, C. M., Sei, Y. J., & Kim, Y. (2015). Microengineered vascular systems for drug development. *Journal of Laboratory Automation*, *20*(3), 251–258. doi:10.1177/2211068214560767 PMID:25424383

How does text-to-speech work? (n.d.). Retrieved 08/07/2017, from http://www.acapela-group.com/voices/how-does-it-work/

Howell. (2016). *5 Ways Technology is Transforming Developing Nations*. Available: http://epics.ieee.org/582-2/

Hsu, H.-H., Chen, J.-S., Huang, P.-M., Lee, J.-M., & Lee, Y.-C. (2004, June). Comparison of manual and mechanical cervical esophagogastric anastomosis after esophageal resection for squamous cell carcinoma: A prospective randomized controlled trial. *European Journal of Cardio-Thoracic Surgery*, *25*(6), 1097–1101. doi:10.1016/j.ejcts.2004.02.026 PMID:15145015

Htay, T., & Liu, M. W. (2005). Drug-eluting stent: A review and update. *Vascular Health and Risk Management*, *1*(4), 263–276. doi:10.2147/vhrm.2005.1.4.263 PMID:17315599

Huang, L., Shi, Y., Wang, N., & Dong, Y. (2014). Anaerobic/aerobic conditions and biostimulation for enhanced chlorophenols degradation in biocathode microbial fuel cells. *Biodegradation*, *25*(4), 615–632. doi:10.100710532-014-9686-1 PMID:24902896

Huang, Q. H., Lee, S. Y., Liu, L. Z., Lu, M.-H., Jin, L.-W., & Li, A.-H. (2012). A robust graph based segmentation method for breast tumors in ultrasound images. *Ultrasonics*, *52*(2), 266–275. doi:10.1016/j.ultras.2011.08.011 PMID:21925692

Huizenga, T., Riyaz, F., & Ozog, D. M. (2017). Implantable Body Jewelry and Methods for Their Removal. *Dermatologic Surgery*, *43*(5), 761–764. doi:10.1097/DSS.0000000000000979 PMID:27984327

Hu, M. K. (1962). Visual pattern recognition by moment invariants. *I.R.E. Transactions on Information Theory*, *8*(2), 179–187. doi:10.1109/TIT.1962.1057692

Hunkeler, U., & Scotton, P. (2008). A Quality-of-Information-Aware Framework for Data Models in Wireless Sensor Networks. In *2008 5th IEEE International Conference on Mobile Ad Hoc and Sensor Systems* (pp. 742–747). Atlanta, GA: IEEE. 10.1109/MAHSS.2008.4660118

Hurst, J. W. (1998). Naming of the waves in the ECG, with a brief account of their genesis. *Circulation*, *98*(18), 1937–1942. doi:10.1161/01.CIR.98.18.1937 PMID:9799216

Huzooree, G., Khedo, K. K., & Joonas, N. (2017a). Glucose Prediction Data Analytics for Diabetic Patients Monitoring. In *2017 1st International Conference on Next Generation Computing Applications (NextComp)* (pp. 188–195). Academic Press. 10.1109/NEXTCOMP.2017.8016197

Huzooree, G., Khedo, K. K., & Joonas, N. (2017b). Pervasive mobile healthcare systems for chronic disease monitoring. *Health Informatics Journal*, 1 –25. 10.1177/1460458217704250

Huzooree, G., Khedo, K. K., & Joonas, N. (2016). Wireless Body Area Network System Architecture for Real-Time Diabetes Monitoring. In *Emerging Trends in Electrical* (pp. 262–271). Electronic and Communications Engineering. ELECOM.

IDF Diabetes Atlas. (2017). *IDF Diabetes Atlas*. 10.1017/CBO9781107415324.004

Igbokwe, O. (2004). *Wireless technology and healthcare*. Academic Press.

Ikeda, M., Suzuki, C., Umegaki, K., Saito, K., Tabuchi, M., & Tomita, T. (2007). Preventive effects of green tea catechins on spontaneous stroke in rats. *Medical Science Monitor*, *13*, BR40–BR45. PMID:17261979

Ikram, J. (2016, January 1). PM launches Health scheme for the poor. *DAWN*. Retrieved from https://www.dawn.com/news/1229970

InnerBody- Liver Anatomy Explorer. (n.d.). Retrieved 2017 from http://www.innerbody.com/image_digeov/card10-new2.html

Irfan, S. M., & Ijaz, A. (2011). Comparison of service quality between private and public hospitals: Empirical evidences from Pakistan. *Journal of Quality and Technology Management*, *7*(1), 1–22.

Islam, S. R., Kwak, D., Kabir, M. H., Hossain, M., & Kwak, K. S. (2015). The internet of things for health care: A comprehensive survey. *IEEE Access: Practical Innovations, Open Solutions*, *3*, 678–708. doi:10.1109/ACCESS.2015.2437951

Ivana, P., Jovana, G., Jelena, D., & Aleksandar, J. (2017). Applicaton of artificial neural networks in modelling and optimization of biofuels production. *Journal on Processing and Energy in Agriculture*, *21*(2), 66–70. doi:10.5937/JPEA1702066P

Jabnoun, N., & Chaker, M. (2003). Comparing the quality of private and public hospitals. *Managing Service Quality: An International Journal*, *13*(4), 290–299. doi:10.1108/09604520310484707

Jahanzeb, E. (2017, April 7). Those who can't afford to live are left to die - my experiences as a doctor in karachi. *Dawn*. Retrieved from https://www.dawn.com/news/1325471

Jain, A. K., Mao, J., & Mohiuddin, K. M. (1996). Artificial neural networks: A tutorial. *Computer*, *29*(3), 31–44. doi:10.1109/2.485891

Jantaro, S., Sayowan, W., Kotchabhakdi, N., Iamsupasit, S., Wankum, N., Hongsranagon, P., & … . (2014). Effect of Comedy Video Clip on Autonomic Response and Subjective Happiness of Thai Early Adults. *J Health Res-vol*, *28*(4).

Jarchi, D., Boostani, R., Taheri, M., & Sanei, S. (2009). Seizure source localization using a hybrid second order blind identification and extended rival penalized competitive learning algorithm. *Biomedical Signal Processing and Control*, *4*(2), 108–117. doi:10.1016/j.bspc.2009.01.004

Jasper, H. H. (1958). The ten-twenty electrode system of the International Federation. *EEG Clinical Neurophysiology*, *10*, 371–375.

Jenkins, N., Smith, G., Stewart, S., & Kamphuis, C. (2016). Pre-employment physical capacity testing as a predictor for musculoskeletal injury in paramedics: A review of the literature. *Work (Reading, Mass.)*, *55*(3), 565–575. doi:10.3233/WOR-162422 PMID:27792024

Jeong, O. C., & Yang, S. S. (2000). Fabrication and test of a thermopneumatic micropump with a corrugated p+ diaphragm. *Sensors and Actuators. A, Physical*, *83*(1-3), 249–255. doi:10.1016/S0924-4247(99)00392-1

Jewett, W. R., & Williams, R. C., III. (2001). *Metered dose inhaler pump*. U.S. Patent 6,223,746.

Jiang, W., Kim, B. Y., Rutka, J. T., & Chan, W. C. (2007). Advances and challenges of nanotechnology-based drug delivery systems. *Expert Opinion on Drug Delivery*, *4*(6), 621–633. doi:10.1517/17425247.4.6.621 PMID:17970665

Jin-kyu, B., Il-han, P., & Song-yop, H. (2002). Topology optimization of electrostatic actuator using design sensitivity. *Magnetics. IEEE Transactions*, *38*, 1053–1056.

Johari, J., Yunas, J., & Yeopmajlis, B. (2009). Piezoeletric Micropump for Drug Delivery System Fabricated Using Two Optical Masks. *Advanced Materials Research*, *74*, 279–282. doi:10.4028/www.scientific.net/AMR.74.279

John, G. W. (2006). Encyclopedia of Medical Devices and Instrumentation, 6 Volume Set. Wiley-Inter-science.

John, K. (2006). *The Evolution of Surgical Instruments – An Illustrated History from Ancient Times to the Twentieth Century*. Norman Publishing.

John, R. M. (2005). Tobacco consumption patterns and its health implications in India. *Health Policy (Amsterdam)*, *71*(2), 213–222. doi:10.1016/j.healthpol.2004.08.008 PMID:15607383

Johnson,, C.D., & Almen. (1993). Revison based on Functional Listening Evaluation: Curr. *Neurophysiology*, *21*(5), 45–78.

Jones, D. A. (1996). Principles and prevention of corrosion. Prentice Hall.

Joshua, J., Qian, C., & Bruce, S. (2015). A Natural Walking Monitor for Pulmonary Patients Using Mobile Phones. *IEEE Journal of Biomedical and Health Informatics*, *19*(4), 1399–1405. doi:10.1109/JBHI.2015.2427511

Kakria, P., Tripathi, N. K., & Kitipawang, P. (2015). A real-time health monitoring system for remote cardiac patients using smartphone and wearable sensors. *International Journal of Telemedicine and Applications*, 8.

Karabatak, M. (2015). A new classifier for breast cancer detection based on Naïve Bayesian. *Measurement*, *72*, 32–36. doi:10.1016/j.measurement.2015.04.028

Karman, S., Ibrahim, F., & Soin, N. (2007). A review of MEMS drug delivery in medical application, Biomed 06. *Proc. IFMBE* 15, 312–315. 10.1007/978-3-540-68017-8_80

Kemeny, M. E. (2003). The psychobiology of stress. *Current Directions in Psychological Science*, *12*(4), 124–129. doi:10.1111/1467-8721.01246

Kemp, A. H., & Quintana, D. S. (2013). The relationship between mental and physical health: Insights from the study of heart rate variability. *International Journal of Psychophysiology*, *89*(3), 288–296. doi:10.1016/j.ijpsycho.2013.06.018 PMID:23797149

Keyserling, W. M. (2000). Workplace risk factors and occupational musculoskeletal disorders, Part 2: A review of biomechanical and psychophysical research on risk factors associated with upper extremity disorders. *AIHAJ-American Industrial Hygiene Association*, *61*(2), 231–243. doi:10.1080/15298660008984532 PMID:10782195

Khan, M., & Quadri, S. M. K. (2013). Effect of using filter based feature selection on performance of machine learners using different datasets. *BVICAM's International Journal of Information Technology*, *5*(2), 597–603.

Khare, A., Khare, M., Jeong, Y., Kim, H., & Jeon, M. (2010). Despeckling of medical ultrasound images using Daubechies complex wavelet transform. *Signal Processing*, *90*(2), 428–439. doi:10.1016/j.sigpro.2009.07.008

Kheirati Roonizi, E. (2017). *Adaptive models-based cardiac signal analysis and feature extraction*. Università degli Studi di Milano.

Kim, J. H., Laua, K. T., Shepherd, R., Wu, Y., Wallace, G., & Diamond, D. (2008). Performance characteristics of a polypyrrole modified polydimethylsiloxane (PDMS) membrane based microfluidic pump. *Sensors and Actuators. A, Physical*, *148*(1), 239–244. doi:10.1016/j.sna.2008.07.029

Kjome, R. L. S., Granas, A. G., Nerhus, K., Roraas, T. H., & Sandberg, S. (2010). The Prevalence of Self-Monitoring of Blood Glucose and Costs of Glucometer Strips in a Nationwide Cohort. *Diabetes Technology & Therapeutics*, *12*(9), 701–705. doi:10.1089/dia.2010.0056

Kleiger, R. E., Stein, P. K., & Bigger, J. T. (2005). Heart rate variability: Measurement and clinical utility. *Annals of Noninvasive Electrocardiology*, *10*(1), 88–101. doi:10.1111/j.1542-474X.2005.10101.x PMID:15649244

Klonoff, D. C. (2012). Overview of Fluorescence Glucose Sensing: A Technology with a Bright Future. *Journal of Diabetes Science and Technology*, *6*(6), 1242–1250. doi:10.1177/193229681200600602

Kocher's Forceps. (2016). In *Merriam-Webster Medical Dictionary*. Retrieved from merriam-webster.com

Koch, M., Harris, N., Evans, A. G. R., White, N. M., & Brunnschweiler, A. (1998). Brunnschweiler, A. A novel micromachined pump based on thick film piezoelectric actuation. *Sensors and Actuators. A, Physical*, *70*(1-2), 98–103. doi:10.1016/S0924-4247(98)00120-4

Konstantinov, I. E. (2004). Circular vascular stapling in coronary surgery. *The Annals of Thoracic Surgery*, *78*(1), 369–373. doi:10.1016/j.athoracsur.2003.11.050 PMID:15223474

Kost, J., & Langer, R. (2012). Responsive polymeric delivery systems. *Advanced Drug Delivery Reviews*, *64*, 327–341. doi:10.1016/j.addr.2012.09.014 PMID:11259837

Kotadiya, S., Majumder, J., & Nag, A. (2013). *Muscular loading during manual material handling tasks*. National Institute of Occupational health, Annual Report 2012-13. Ahmedabad, India.

Kottayil, S., Crooks, P., Riggs, D., Murty, R., & Kottayil, S. (2001). *Thermal vaporizing device for drug delivery*. U.S. Patent Application 09/984,294.

Kozlovskaya, L., Abou-Kaoud, M., & Stepensky, D. (2014). Quantitative analysis of drug delivery to the brain via nasal route. *Journal of Controlled Release*, *189*, 133–140. doi:10.1016/j.jconrel.2014.06.053 PMID:24997277

Krissian, K., Westin, C. F., Kikinis, R., & Vosburgh, K. G. (2007). Oriented speckle reducing anisotropic diffusion. *IEEE Transactions on Image Processing*, *16*(5), 1412–1424. doi:10.1109/TIP.2007.891803 PMID:17491469

Kroh, M. (2015). *Essentials of robotic surgery*. Cham: Springer. doi:10.1007/978-3-319-09564-6

Kumar Singh, Verma, & Thoke. (2015). Objective and Optical Evaluation of Despeckle Filters in Breast Ultrasound Images. *IETE Technical Review*. DOI: 10.1080/02564602.2015.1019943

Kumar Singh. (2015). Investigations on edge preservation and smoothening of frequency domain filters for speckle removal in breast ultrasound images. *International Journal of Biomedical Engineering and Technology*.

Kumar, Y., Dewal, M. L., & Anand, R. S. (2012). Epileptic seizures detection in EEG using DWT-based ApEn and artificial neural network. *SIViP*. DOI 10.1007/s11760-012-0362-9

Kumaravelrajan, R. (2016). Development and Evaluation of Elementary Osmotic Pump for the Simultaneous Delivery of Nifedipine and Metoprolol Tartrate. *Asian Journal of Pharmaceutics (AJP)*, *10*(4).

Kumar, G. S., Kar, S. S., & Jain, A. (2011). Health and environmental sanitation in India: Issues for prioritizing control strategies. *Indian Journal of Occupational and Environmental Medicine*, *15*(3), 93. doi:10.4103/0019-5278.93196 PMID:22412284

Kumari, K., Prasad, K., & Kundu, P. P. (2009). Optimization of chlorpheniramine maleate (CPM) delivery by response surface methodology – four component modeling using various response times and concentrations of chitosan-alanine, glutaraldehyde and CPM. *Express Polymer Letters*, *3*(4), 207–218. doi:10.3144/expresspolymlett.2009.27

Kumar, T. S., & Ganesan, R. (2011). Sharon: Tension free mobile incorporated with health care system using Christina heart card. *3rd International Conference on Advanced Computing, ICoAC 2011*, 46–51. 10.1109/ICoAC.2011.6165217

Kundu, M., Nasipuri, M., & Basu, D. K. (1998). A knowledge-based approach to ECG interpretation using fuzzy logic. *IEEE Transactions on Systems, Man, and Cybernetics. Part B, Cybernetics*, *28*(2), 237–243. doi:10.1109/3477.662764 PMID:18255941

Ku, P. X., Osman, N. A., Yusof, A., & Abas, W. W. (2012). Biomechanical evaluation of the relationship between postural control and body mass index. *Journal of Biomechanics*, *45*(9), 1638–1642. doi:10.1016/j.jbiomech.2012.03.029 PMID:22507349

Kurji, Z., Premani, Z. S., & Mithani, Y. (2016). Analysis of the health care system of Pakistan: Lessons learnt and way forward. *Journal of Ayub Medical College, Abbottabad*, *28*(3), 601–604. PMID:28712245

Kwatra, S., Taneja, G., & Nasa, N. (2012). Alternatives routes of drug administration-transdermal, pulmonary & parenteral. *Indo Global Journal of Pharmaceutical Sciences*, 2(4), 409–426.

Kwon, S. K., Park, M. S., Sin, Y. S., & Nam, Y. J. (1996). Korean Pat., KR 9,C 04,829.

Kwon, G. S., & Okano, T. (1996). Polymeric micelles as new drug carriers. *Advanced Drug Delivery Reviews*, *21*(2), 107–116. doi:10.1016/S0169-409X(96)00401-2

Laban, G., Guenther, W., & Lohmann, D. (1987). Ger. Pat., DD 247,674, pp4.

Labiris, N. R., & Dolovich, M. B. (2003). Pulmonary drug delivery. Part II: The role of inhalant delivery devices and drug formulations in therapeutic effectiveness of aerosolized medications. *British Journal of Clinical Pharmacology*, *56*(6), 600–612. doi:10.1046/j.1365-2125.2003.01893.x PMID:14616419

LabVIEW. (2014). *Discrete Gabor Transform and Expansion (Advanced Signal Processing Toolkit) - LabVIEW 2014 Advanced Signal Processing Toolkit Help - National Instruments*. Retrieved 25 May, 2017, from http://zone.ni.com/reference/en-XX/help/372656C-01/lvasptconcepts/tfa_discrete_gabor_trans_exp/

Lakshmi, K., & Rao, M. T. C. S. (2016). Design and implementation of text to speech conversion using Raspberry Pi. *IJITR*, *4*(6), 4564–4567.

Langer, R. S., & Wise, D. L. (Eds.). (1984). *Medical Applications of Controlled Release, Applications and Evaluation* (Vols. 1-2). Boca Raton, FL: CRC Press.

Laparoscopic graspers. (n.d.). Retrieved from Laparoscopic.md

Latiff, N. A. A., Latiff, N. M. A., & Ahmad, R. B. (2011). Prolonging lifetime of wireless sensor networks with mobile base station using particle swarm optimization. In *2011 Fourth International Conference on Modeling, Simulation and Applied Optimization* (pp. 1–6). Kuala Lumpur, Malaysia: Academic Press. 10.1109/ICMSAO.2011.5775487

Laustiola, K. (1988). A study of monozygotic twin pairs discordant for smoking. *American Heart Association Journal, 78*, 1234-1240.

Laws, K. I. (1980). Rapid texture identification. *Proceedings of SPIE Image Processing for Missile Guidance*, 238, 376-380. 10.1117/12.959169

Lee, S., Yee, S. Y., Besharatian, A., Kim, H., Bernal, L. P., & Najafi, K. (2009). Adaptive gas pumping by ontrolled timing of active microvalves in peristaltic micropumps. In Proceedings of Transducers (pp. 21–25). Academic Press.

Lee, J. S. (1986). Speckle suppression and analysis for synthetic aperture radar. *Optical Engineering (Redondo Beach, Calif.)*, *25*(5), 636–643. doi:10.1117/12.7973877

Lee, J., Nam, Y., McManus, D. D., & Chon, K. H. (2013). Time-varying coherence function for atrial fibrillation detection. *IEEE Transactions on Biomedical Engineering*, *60*(10), 2783–2793. doi:10.1109/TBME.2013.2264721 PMID:23708769

Lee, R. G., & van Donkelaar, P. (1995). Mechanisms underlying functional recovery following stroke. *The Canadian Journal of Neurological Sciences*, *22*(04), 257–263. doi:10.1017/S0317167100039445 PMID:8599767

Lee, Y., & Lee, M. (2008). SMS application using EMG signal of clenching teeth for e-health communication. *Telemedicine Journal and e-Health, 14*(6), 593–597. doi:10.1089/tmj.2007.0098 PMID:18729760

Leite, C. R. M., Sizilio, G. R., Ribeiro, A. G., Valentim, R. A., Neto, P. F., & Guerreiro, A. M. (2012). Mobile Technologies Applied to Hospital Automation. In *Advances and Applications in Mobile Computing*. InTech. doi:10.5772/36478

Lemon, S. C., Roy, J., Clark, M. A., Friedmann, P. D., & Rakowski, W. (2003). Classification and regression tree analysis in public health: Methodological review and comparison with logistic regression. *Annals of Behavioral Medicine, 26*(3), 172–181. doi:10.1207/S15324796ABM2603_02 PMID:14644693

Lewis, R. J. (2000). *An Introduction to Classification and Regression Tree (CART) Analysis*. Paper presented at the Annual Meeting of the Society of Academic Emergency Medicine in.

Li, V. H. K., & Lee, V. H. L. (1987). Controlled drug delivery: Fundamentals and applications (2nd ed.). Marcel Dekker Inc.

Li, C., Li, H.-B., & Kohno, R. (2009). Performance Evaluation of IEEE 802.15.4 for Wireless Body Area Network (WBAN). In *IEEE International Conference on Communications (ICC) Workshops, 2009.* (pp. 1–5). Dresden, Germany: IEEE. 10.1109/ICCW.2009.5208087

Li, C., Wang, X., Li, J., Eberl, S., Fulham, M., Yin, Y., & Feng, D. D. (2013). Joint probabilistic model of shape and intensity for multiple abdominal organ segmentation from volumetric CT images. *IEEE Journal of Biomedical and Health Informatics, 17*(1), 92–102. doi:10.1109/TITB.2012.2227273 PMID:23193317

Lightstone, A. (2007). Eye health and sight loss: The UK Vision Strategy. *The Journal of Family Health Care, 18*(5), 162–164. PMID:18973088

Li, H., Yuan, D., Ma, X., Cui, D., & Cao, L. (2017). Genetic algorithm for the optimization of features and neural networks in ECG signals classification. *Scientific Reports*, 7. PMID:28139677

Lil, L., Zhu, R., Zhou, Z., & Ren, J. (2010). Modeling of a Micropump Membrane with Electrostatic Actuator. *Proceedings of 2nd International Conference on Advanced Computer Control (ICACC)*, 27–29.

Li, M., Lou, W., & Ren, K. (2010). Data Security and Privacy in Wireless Body Area Networks. *IEEE Wireless Communications, 17*(1), 51–58. doi:10.1109/MWC.2010.5416350

Lim, C. P., Quek, S. S., & Peh, K. K. (2003). Prediction of drug release profiles using an intelligent learning system: An experimental study in transdermal iontophoresis. *Journal of Pharmaceutical and Biomedical Analysis, 31*(1), 159–168. doi:10.1016/S0731-7085(02)00573-3 PMID:12560060

Lin, S.-H., Huang, Y.-C., Chien, C.-Y., Chen, Y.-C., Chou, L.-C., & Huang, S.-C. (2008). *A study of the relationship between two musical rhythm characteristics and heart rate variability (HRV)*. Paper presented at the BioMedical Engineering and Informatics, 2008. BMEI 2008. International Conference on.

Lindblad, S., Ernestam, S., Van Citters, A. D., Lind, C., Morgan, T. S., & Nelson, E. C. (2017). Creating a culture of health: Evolving healthcare systems and patient engagement. *QJM: An International Journal of Medicine, 110*(3), 125–129. PMID:27803364

Lipton, P. (1999). Ischemic cell death in brain neurons. *Physiological Reviews, 79*(4), 1431–1568. doi:10.1152/physrev.1999.79.4.1431 PMID:10508238

Li, T., & Zhou, M. (2016). ECG classification using wavelet packet entropy and random forests. *Entropy (Basel, Switzerland), 18*(8), 285. doi:10.3390/e18080285

Liu, B., Cheng, H. D., Huang, J., Tian, J., Tang, X., & Liu, J. (2010). Fully automatic and segmentation-robust classification of breast tumors based on local texture analysis of ultrasound images. *Pattern Recognition*, *43*(1), 280–298. doi:10.1016/j.patcog.2009.06.002

Liu, C. H., Ma, X., Song, L. P., Fan, J., Wang, W. D., Lv, X. Y., ... Wang, C. Y. (2015). 'Abnormal spontaneous neural activity in the anterior insular and anterior cingulate cortices in anxious depression'. *Behavioural Brain Research*, *281*, 339–347. doi:10.1016/j.bbr.2014.11.047 PMID:25513974

Liu, C. H., Wen, J., Yu, Q., Yang, B., & Wang, W. (2011). HealthKiosk: A family-based connected healthcare system for long-term monitoring. In *2011 IEEE Conference on Computer Communications Workshops (INFOCOM WKSHPS)* (pp. 241–246). Shanghai, China: IEEE. 10.1109/INFCOMW.2011.5928816

Liu, G., Shen, C., Yang, Z., Cai, X., & Zhang, H. (2010). A disposable piezoelectric micropump with high performance for closed-loop insulin therapy system. *Sensors and Actuators. A, Physical*, *163*(1), 291–296. doi:10.1016/j.sna.2010.06.030

Liu, W. (2010). Research on Electrostatic Micropump Pull-in Phenomena Based On Reduced Order Model. *Proceedings of International Conference on Intelligent Computation Technology and Automation*, 11–12. 10.1109/ICICTA.2010.99

Liu, X., Wang, S., Chai, L., Zhang, D., Sun, Y., Xu, L., & Sun, J. (2014). A two-step strategy to design high bioavailable controlled-release nimodipine tablets: The push–pull osmotic pump in combination with the micronization/solid dispersion techniques. *International Journal of Pharmaceutics*, *461*(1), 529–539. doi:10.1016/j.ijpharm.2013.12.023 PMID:24374219

Liver Anatomy and Functions Anatomy of the liver. (2017). [Online image]. Retrieved 2017 from http://www.hopkinsmedicine.org/healthlibrary/conditions/liver_biliary_and_pancreatic_disorders/liver_anatomy_and_functions_85,P00676/

Liver Cancer (Hepatocellular Carcinoma). (n.d.). Retrieved 2017 from http://www.medicinenet.com/liver_cancer_hepatocellular_carcinoma/article.htm

Liver fibrosis. (n.d.). [Online image]. Retrieved 2017 from http://www.meddean.luc.edu/lumen/meded/orfpath/fibrosis.htm

Li, W., & McLeod, A. (1981). Distribution of the residual autocorrelations in multivariate ARMA time series models. *Journal of the Royal Statistical Society. Series B. Methodological*, 231–239.

Li, Y., Shawgo, R. S., Tyler, B., Henderson, P. T., Vogel, J. S., Rosenberg, A., ... Cima, M. J. (2004). In vivo release from a drug delivery MEMS device. *Journal of Controlled Release*, *100*(2), 211–219. doi:10.1016/j.jconrel.2004.08.018 PMID:15544869

Llera, S. J., & Newman, M. G. (2010). Effects of worry on physiological and subjective reactivity to emotional stimuli in generalized anxiety disorder and nonanxious control participants. *Emotion (Washington, D.C.)*, *10*(5), 640–650. doi:10.1037/a0019351 PMID:21038947

Lloyd-Jones, D., Adams, R., & Carnethon, M. (2006). Diazepam to improve acute stroke outcome: Results of the early GABA-Ergic activation study in stroke trial. a randomized double-blind placebo-controlled trial. *Cerebrovascular Diseases (Basel, Switzerland)*, *21*(1-2), 120–127. doi:10.1159/000090210 PMID:16340187

Lo, C. M., Chen, R. T., Chang, Y. C., Yang, Y. W., Hung, M. J., Huang, C. S., & Chang, R. F. (2014). Multi-dimensional tumor detection in automated whole breast ultrasound using topographic watershed. *IEEE Transactions on Medical Imaging*, *33*(7), 1503–1511. doi:10.1109/TMI.2014.2315206 PMID:24718570

Longa, E. Z., Weinstein, P. R., Carlson, S., & Cummins, R. (1989). Reversible middle cerebral artery occlusion without craniectomy in rats. *Stroke*, *20*(1), 84–91. doi:10.1161/01.STR.20.1.84 PMID:2643202

Lopes da Silva, F. (1991). Neural mechanisms underlying brain waves: From neural membranes to networks. *Electroencephalography and Clinical Neurophysiology*, *79*(2), 81–93. doi:10.1016/0013-4694(91)90044-5 PMID:1713832

Luo, Z., Cai, K., Hu, Y., Zhao, L., Liu, P., Duan, L., & Yang, W. (2011). Mesoporous Silica Nanoparticles End-Capped with Collagen: Redox-Responsive Nanoreservoirs for Targeted Drug Delivery. *Angewandte Chemie International Edition*, *50*(3), 640–643. doi:10.1002/anie.201005061 PMID:21226142

Lutzenberger, W., Elbert, T., & Rockstroh, B. (1987). A brief tutorial on the implications of volume conduction for the interpretation of the EEG. *Journal of Psychophysiology*, *1*, 81–89.

Luz, E. J. D. S., Nunes, T. M., De Albuquerque, V. H. C., Papa, J. P., & Menotti, D. (2013). ECG arrhythmia classification based on optimum-path forest. *Expert Systems with Applications*, *40*(9), 3561–3573. doi:10.1016/j.eswa.2012.12.063

Maan, M. S. (2007). EEG Waves Classifier using Wavelet Transform and Fourier Transform. *International Journal of Medical, Pharmaceutical Science and Engineering, 1*(3), 166-171.

Maberley, D., Hollands, H., Chuo, J., Tam, G., Konkal, J., Roesch, M., ... Bassett, K. (2006). The prevalence of low vision and blindness in Canada. *Eye (London, England)*, *20*(3), 341–346. doi:10.1038j.eye.6701879 PMID:15905873

Machado, L., & Savi, M. (2003). Medical applications of shape memory alloys. *Brazilian Journal of Medical and Biological Research*, *36*(6), 683–691. doi:10.1590/S0100-879X2003000600001 PMID:12792695

Mahapatra, P., Srilatha, S., & Sridhar, P. (2001). A Patient Satisfaction Survey in Public Hospitals. *Journal Academy of Hospital Administration*, *13*(2).

Mahapatra, S., Mohanta, D., Mohanty, P., Nayak, S., & Behari, P. (2016). A Neuro-fuzzy Based Model for Analysis of an ECG Signal Using Wavelet Packet Tree. *Procedia Computer Science*, *92*, 175–180. doi:10.1016/j.procs.2016.07.343

Mahoto, N. A., Shaikh, F. K., & Chowdhry, B. S. (2014). Innovative Architecture to Enhance Quality of Service for Laboratory Management Information Systems. *Laboratory Management Information Systems: Current Requirements and Future Perspectives: Current Requirements and Future Perspectives, 237.*

Maillefer, D., Lintel, H. V., Mermet, G. R., & Hirschi, R. (1999). A high-performance silicon micropump for an implantable drug delivery system. *Proceedings of IEEE MEMS*, 212–215. 10.1109/MEMSYS.1999.746886

Mainardes, R. M., & Silva, L. P. (2004). Drug delivery systems: Past, present, and future. *Current Drug Targets*, *5*(5), 449–455. doi:10.2174/1389450043345407 PMID:15216911

Maisel, W. H., & Laskey, W. K. (2007). Drug-eluting stents. *Circulation*, *115*(17), e426–e427. doi:10.1161/CIRCULATIONAHA.107.688176 PMID:17470700

Maiti, R. (2008). Workload assessment in building construction related activities in India. *Applied Ergonomics*, *39*(6), 754–765. doi:10.1016/j.apergo.2007.11.010 PMID:18206852

Makino, E., Mitsuya, T., & Shibata, T. (2000). Micromachining of NiTi shape memory thin-film for fabrication of micropump. *Sensors and Actuators. A, Physical*, *79*(3), 251–259. doi:10.1016/S0924-4247(99)00290-3

Maldonado, H., Leija, L., Vera, A., & Alvarado, C. (2016). *Post myocardial infarct detection with support vector machine and ECG intervals ratios JTp/JT, Tpe/JTp and Tpe/JT.* Paper presented at the Medical Engineering Physics Exchanges/Pan American Health Care Exchanges (GMEPE/PAHCE), 2016 Global.

Malik, B. H., & Coté, G. L. (2010). Real-time, closed-loop dual-wavelength optical polarimetry for glucose monitoring. *Journal of Biomedical Optics*, *15*(1), 1–6. doi:10.1117/1.3290819

Malik, M., Camm, A., Bigger, J., Breithardt, G., Cerutti, S., & Cohen, R. (1996). Heart rate variability. Standards of measurement, physiological interpretation, and clinical use. *European Heart Journal*, *17*(3), 354–381. doi:10.1093/oxfordjournals.eurheartj.a014868 PMID:8737210

Mamykina, L., & Mynatt, E. (2008). MAHI: investigation of social scaffolding for reflective thinking in diabetes management. In *Proceedings of the SIGCHI Conference on Human Factors in Computing Systems* (pp. 477–486). Florence, Italy: ACM. 10.1145/1357054.1357131

Manelli, Gastaldo, Rinaldo, Luigi, & Zonta. (1990). A new vascular stapler for pulmonary artery anastomosis in experimental single lung transplantation. *Proceedings of the 4th Annual Meeting of The Association for Cardio-Thoracic Surgery*.

Marin, J., Blanco, T., & Marin, J. J. (2017). Research Lines to Improve Access to Health Instrumentation Design. *Procedia Computer Science*, *113*, 641–646. doi:10.1016/j.procs.2017.08.323

Markou, M., & Singh, S. (2003). Novelty detection: a review—part 2: neural network based approaches. *Signal Processing*, *83*(12), 2499–2521. doi:10.1016/j.sigpro.2003.07.019

Maron, B. J., Friedman, R. A., Kligfield, P., Levine, B. D., Viskin, S., Chaitman, B. R., ... Thompson, P. D. (2014). Assessment of the 12-Lead ECG as a Screening Test for Detection of Cardiovascular Disease in Healthy General Populations of Young People (12–25 Years of Age). *Circulation*, *130*(15), 1303–1334. doi:10.1161/CIR.0000000000000025 PMID:25223981

Marwan, N., Wessel, N., Meyerfeldt, U., Schirdewan, A., & Kurths, J. (2002). Recurrence-plot-based measures of complexity and their application to heart-rate-variability data. *Physical Review. E*, *66*(2), 026702. doi:10.1103/PhysRevE.66.026702 PMID:12241313

Ma, S., & Sood, N. (2008). *A comparison of the health systems in China and India* (Vol. 212). Rand Corporation.

Massof, R. W. (2003). *Auditory assistive devices for the blind*. Academic Press.

Mateo, J. L., & Caballero, A. F. (2009). Finding out general tendencies in speckle noise reduction in ultrasound images. *Expert Systems with Applications*, *36*(4), 7786–7797. doi:10.1016/j.eswa.2008.11.029

Mathur, M., & Mishra, R. (2016). A review on osmotic pump drug delivery system. *International Journal of Pharmaceutical Sciences and Research*, *7*(2), 453.

MathWorks. (n.d.). *Differences and Approximate Derivatives*. Retrieved 23 May, 2017, from https://in.mathworks.com/help/matlab/ref/diff.html?searchHighlight=diff&s_tid=doc_srchtitle

Matuleviciene, V., Joseph, J. I., Andelin, M., Hirsch, I. B., Attvall, S., Pivodic, A., ... Lind, M. (2014). A clinical trial of the accuracy and treatment experience of the Dexcom G4 sensor (Dexcom G4 system) and Enlite sensor (guardian REAL-time system) tested simultaneously in ambulatory patients with type 1 diabetes. *Diabetes Technology & Therapeutics*, *16*(11), 759–767. doi:10.1089/dia.2014.0238

McLeod, A. I., & Li, W. K. (1983). Diagnostic checking ARMA time series models using squared-residual autocorrelations. *Journal of Time Series Analysis*, *4*(4), 269–273. doi:10.1111/j.1467-9892.1983.tb00373.x

Mello, R., Oliveir, L., & Nada, J. (2007). Anticipation mechanism in body sway control and effect of muscle fatigue. *Journal of Electromyography and Kinesiology*, *17*(6), 739–746. doi:10.1016/j.jelekin.2006.08.011 PMID:17142060

Menahem, S. (2013). Cardiac asystole following cannabis (marijuana) usage–Additional mechanism for sudden death? *Forensic Science International*, *233*(1), e3–e5. doi:10.1016/j.forsciint.2013.10.007 PMID:24200372

Mercimek, M., Gulez, K., & Mumcu, T. V. (2005). Real object recognition using moment invariants. *Sadhana*, *30*(6), 765–775. doi:10.1007/BF02716709

Mergenthaler, P., Dirnagl, U., & Meisel, A. (2004). Pathophysiology of stroke: Lessons from animal models. *Metabolic Brain Disease*, *19*(3-4), 151–167. doi:10.1023/B:MEBR.0000043966.46964.e6 PMID:15554412

Michelle, A. (2014, March 24). FAQ: What are the penalties for not getting Health insurance? *PBS Newshour.* Retrieved from http://www.pbs.org/newshour/updates/faq-penalties-getting-health-insurance/

Michelle, H. (2016). *Clinical Medical Assisting: A professional.* Field Smart Approach to the Workplace.

Milenković, A., Otto, C., & Jovanov, E. (2006). Wireless sensor networks for personal health monitoring: Issues and an implementation. *Computer Communications*, *29*(13), 2521–2533. doi:10.1016/j.comcom.2006.02.011

Mills, A. (2014). Health care systems in low-and middle-income countries. *The New England Journal of Medicine*, *370*(6), 552–557. doi:10.1056/NEJMra1110897 PMID:24499213

Ministry of Finance. (n.d.). Retrieved from http://www.finance.gov.pk/

Ministry of Health. (n.d.). *Nutrition and Indigenous Online*. Retrieved from http://www.health.gov.lk/moh_final/english/

Mohan, P., Marin, D., Sultan, S., & Deen, A. (2008). MediNet: Personalizing the Self-Care Process for Patients with Diabetes and Cardiovascular Disease Using Mobile Telephony. In *2008 30th Annual International Conference of the IEEE Engineering in Medicine and Biology Society* (pp. 755–758). Vancouver, Canada: IEEE.

Mohanasundari, M., Srinivasan, M. S., Sethupathy, S., & Sabesan, M. (2006). Enhanced neuroprotective effect by combination of bromocriptine and Hypericumperforatumextract against MPTP-induced neurotoxicity in mice. *Journal of the Neurological Sciences*, *249*(2), 140–144. doi:10.1016/j.jns.2006.06.018 PMID:16876826

Mohebbi, M., Ghassemian, H., & Asl, B. M. (2011). Structures of the recurrence plot of heart rate variability signal as a tool for predicting the onset of paroxysmal atrial fibrillation. *Journal of Medical Signals and Sensors*, *1*(2), 113. PMID:22606666

Mokashi, C., Nayak, S. K., Pradhan, A., Rout, S. K., Pal, K., & Champaty, B. (2016). *Effect of sound in a horror movie clip on the physiology of the ANS and the conduction pathway of the heart.* Paper presented at the India Conference (INDICON), 2016 IEEE Annual. 10.1109/INDICON.2016.7839020

Monfredi, O., Dobrzynski, H., Mondal, T., Boyett, M. R., & Morris, G. M. (2010). The anatomy and physiology of the sinoatrial node—a contemporary review. *Pacing and Clinical Electrophysiology*, *33*(11), 1392–1406. doi:10.1111/j.1540-8159.2010.02838.x PMID:20946278

Mossialos, E., Wenzl, M., Osborn, R., & Anderson, C. (2016). *2015 International Profiles of Health Care Systems.* The Commonwealth Fund. doi:10.15868ocialsector.25100

MRI. A Guided Tour. (2003). [Online image]. Retrieved 2017 from http://www.medscape.org/viewarticle/488088

Muir, K. W., & Grosset, D. G. (1999). Neuroprotection for acute stroke: Making clinical trials work. *Stroke*, *30*(1), 180–182. doi:10.1161/01.STR.30.1.180 PMID:9880407

Mupela, E. N., Mustarde, P., & Jones, H. L. (2011). Telemedicine in primary health: The virtual doctor project Zambia. *Philosophy, Ethics, and Humanities in Medicine; PEHM*, *6*(1), 9. doi:10.1186/1747-5341-6-9 PMID:21569490

Mura, S., Nicolas, J., & Couvreur, P. (2013). Stimuli-responsive nanocarriers for drug delivery. *Nature Materials*, *12*(11), 991–1003. doi:10.1038/nmat3776 PMID:24150417

Murray, C. J., & Lopez, A. D. (1997). Mortality by cause for eight regions of the world: Global Burden of Disease Study. *Lancet*, *349*(9061), 1269–1276. doi:10.1016/S0140-6736(96)07493-4 PMID:9142060

Murthy, C. D., Sunkara, G., & Young, D. (Eds.). (2007). *Pharmaceutical product development: in vitro-in vivo correlation*. Taylor & Francis US.

Murugappan, M., Murugappan, S., & Zheng, B. S. (2013). Frequency band analysis of electrocardiogram (ECG) signals for human emotional state classification using discrete wavelet transform (DWT). *Journal of Physical Therapy Science*, *25*(7), 753–759. doi:10.1589/jpts.25.753 PMID:24259846

Nachman, L., Baxi, A., Bhattacharya, S., Darera, V., Deshpande, P., & Kodalapura, N., … Acharya, R. (2010). Jog Falls : A Pervasive Healthcare Platform for Diabetes Management. In *8th International Conference, Pervasive Computing* (pp. 94–111). Helsinki, Finland: Academic Press. 10.1007/978-3-642-12654-3_6

Nagata, K. (1988). Topographic EEG in brain ischemia: Correlation with blood flow and metabolism. *Brain Topography*, *1*(2), 97–106. doi:10.1007/BF01129174 PMID:3079309

Nag, P. K., Vyas, H., Nag, A., & Pal, S. (2013). Postural stability of sitting women. *International Journal of Occupational Safety and Ergonomics*, *19*(4), 583–595. doi:10.1080/10803548.2013.11077022 PMID:24321637

Nag, P., Nag, A., Vyas, H., & Shah, P. (2014). Occupation, participation, inclusion, work role postural control in different load handling tasks. *Work (Reading, Mass.)*, *49*(4), 577–584. PMID:24004795

Nair, G., Jungreuthmayer, C., & Zanghellini, J. (2017). Optimal knockout strategies in genome-scale metabolic networks using particle swarm optimization. *BMC Bioinformatics*, *18*(1), 78. doi:10.118612859-017-1483-5 PMID:28143607

Narasimhan, B., & Langer, R. (1997). Zero-order release of micro-and macromolecules from polymeric devices: The role of the burst effect. *Journal of Controlled Release*, *47*(1), 13–20. doi:10.1016/S0168-3659(96)01611-2

Nashner, L. M. (2014). Practical biomechanics and physiology of balance. In *Balance Function Assessment and Management* (pp. 431–449). San Diego, CA: Plural Publishing.

National Clinical Guideline Centre. (2015). *Type 1 diabetes in adults: diagnosis and management*. National Institute for Health and Care Excellence.

Nayak, S. K., Panda, I., Champaty, B., Bagh, N., Pal, K., & Tibarewala, D. (2015). Automated Neural Network Based Classification of HRV and ECG Signals of Smokers: A Preliminary Study. In Advancements of Medical Electronics (pp. 271-279). Springer. doi:10.1007/978-81-322-2256-9_25

Nayak, S. K., Shukla, R. D., Panda, I., Champaty, B., Thakur, G., & Mohapatra, B. (2016). Effect of Slow and Fast Music on the Autonomic Nervous System and Cardiac Health: A Preliminary Investigation. *Classification and Clustering in Biomedical Signal Processing*, 198.

Nayak, S. K., Shukla, R. D., Panda, I., Champaty, B., Thakur, G., Mohapatra, B. (2016). Effect of Slow and Fast Music on the Autonomic Nervous System and Cardiac Health: A Preliminary Investigation. *Classification and Clustering in Biomedical Signal Processing*, 198.

Nayak, S. K., Suman, S., Nayak, B. M., Banerjee, I., Pal, K., & Champaty, B. (2016). *Effect of Cannabis consumption on ANS and conduction pathway of heart of Indian paddy field workers*. Paper presented at the India Conference (INDICON), 2016 IEEE Annual. 10.1109/INDICON.2016.7839018

Nayak, S., Champaty, B., Ray, S. S., & Pal, K. (2014). *A study on the changes in the autonomic nervous system and cardio-electric physiology after viewing comedy movie clip: A case study.* Paper presented at the Control, Instrumentation, Communication and Computational Technologies (ICCICCT), 2014 International Conference on. 10.1109/ICCICCT.2014.6993113

Nerlich, M., & Kretschmer, R. (Eds.). (1999). *The impact of telemedicine on health care management* (Vol. 64). IOS Press.

Nguyen, H. D., Wilkins, B. A., Cheng, Q., & Benjamin, B. A. (2014). An online sleep apnea detection method based on recurrence quantification analysis. *IEEE Journal of Biomedical and Health Informatics*, *18*(4), 1285–1293. doi:10.1109/JBHI.2013.2292928 PMID:25014935

Nijjar, P. S., Puppala, V. K., Dickinson, O., Duval, S., Duprez, D., Kreitzer, M. J., & Benditt, D. G. (2014). Modulation of the autonomic nervous system assessed through heart rate variability by a mindfulness based stress reduction program. *International Journal of Cardiology*, *177*(2), 557–559. doi:10.1016/j.ijcard.2014.08.116 PMID:25179555

Nimitz, R. (2010). *Surgical Instrumentation: an Interactive Approach.* Saunders.

NIOSH. (1981). *Work practices guide for manual load lifting*. Cincinnati, OH: National Institute for Occupational Safety and Health.

Nolte, J., & Sundsten, J. (2002). *The human brain: an introduction to its functional anatomy* (Vol. 5). Mosby St. Louis.

Nuwer, M., & Novda, D. (2005). Routine and quantitative EEG in mild traumatic brain injury. *Clinical Neurophysiology*, *116*(9), 2001–2025. doi:10.1016/j.clinph.2005.05.008 PMID:16029958

O'Keefe, J., & Burgess, N. (2005). Dual phase and rate coding in hippocampal place cells: Theoretical significance and relationship to entorhinal grid cells. *Hippocampus*, *15*(7), 853–866. doi:10.1002/hipo.20115 PMID:16145693

Ocak, H. (2009). Automatic detection of epileptic seizures in EEG using discrete wavelet transform and approximate entropy. *Expert Systems with Applications*, *36*(2), 2027–2036. doi:10.1016/j.eswa.2007.12.065

Ochsner, J. (1999). The surgical knife. *Bulletin of the American College of Surgeons*, *84*(2), 27–37. PMID:10350986

OECD Online. (n.d.). Retrieved from http://www.oecd.org/

OECD. (2015). Retrieved from https://www.oecd.org/health/health-systems/Focus-Health-Spending-2015.pdf

OECD. (2016). Retrieved from http://www.oecd.org/

OECD. (2017). *Doctors (indicator)*. OECD. doi: 10.1787/4355e1ec-en

Oh, P. P., Rangaiah, G. P., & Ray, A. K. (2002). Simulation and multi-objective optimization of an industrial hydrogen plant based on refinery off-gas. *Industrial & Engineering Chemistry Research*, *41*(9), 248–2261. doi:10.1021/ie010277n

Okin, P. M., Devereux, R. B., Howard, B. V., Fabsitz, R. R., Lee, E. T., & Welty, T. K. (2000). Assessment of QT interval and QT dispersion for prediction of all-cause and cardiovascular mortality in American Indians. *Circulation*, *101*(1), 61–66. doi:10.1161/01.CIR.101.1.61 PMID:10618305

Oktayoğlu, P., Gür, A., Yardımeden, İ., Çağlayan, M., Çevik, F., Bozkurt, M., ... Nas, K. (2014). Comparison of the Efficacy of Phonophoresis and Conventional Ultrasound Therapy in Patients with Primary Knee Osteoarthritis. Erciyes Medical Journal. *Erciyes Tip Dergisi*, *36*(1), 11–18. doi:10.5152/etd.2013.64

Oliver, N. S., Toumazou, C., Cass, E. G., & Johnston, D. G. (2009). Glucose sensors: A review of current and emerging technology. *Diabetic Medicine*, *26*(3), 197–210. doi:10.1111/j.1464-5491.2008.02642.x

Olsson, A., Stemme, G., & Stemme, E. (1995). A valve-less planar fluid pump with two pump chambers. *Sensors and Actuators. A, Physical*, *47*(1-3), 549–556. doi:10.1016/0924-4247(94)00960-P

Olsson, L. (2007). *Biofuels*. Berlin, Germany: Springer-Verlag. doi:10.1007/978-3-540-73651-6

Onan, A., Hasan, B., & Korukoglu, S. (2017). An improved ant algorithm with LDA-based representation for text document clustering. *Journal of Information Science, 43*(2), 275-292.

Opie, L. H. (2004). *Heart physiology: from cell to circulation*. Lippincott Williams & Wilkins.

Opthof, T., Coronel, R., Wilms-Schopman, F. J., Plotnikov, A. N., Shlapakova, I. N., Danilo, P. Jr, ... Janse, M. J. (2007). Dispersion of repolarization in canine ventricle and the electrocardiographic T wave: T pe interval does not reflect transmural dispersion. *Heart Rhythm*, *4*(3), 341–348. doi:10.1016/j.hrthm.2006.11.022 PMID:17341400

Orhan, H., & Sahin, G. (2001). In vitro effects of NSAIDS and paracetamolon oxidative stress-related parameters of human erythrocytes. *Experimental and Toxicologic Pathology*, *53*(2-3), 133–140. doi:10.1078/0940-2993-00179 PMID:11484831

Orini, M., Bailón, R., Mainardi, L., & Laguna, P. (2012). Synthesis of HRV signals characterized by predetermined time-frequency structure by means of time-varying ARMA models. *Biomedical Signal Processing and Control*, *7*(2), 141–150. doi:10.1016/j.bspc.2011.05.003

Ozana, N., Arbel, N., Beiderman, Y., Mico, V., Sanz, M., Garcia, J., ... Zalevsky, Z. (2014). Improved noncontact optical sensor for detection of glucose concentration and indication of dehydration level. *Biomedical Optics Express*, *5*(6), 1926–1940. doi:10.1364/BOE.5.001926

Pachori, R. B., Avinash, P., Shashank, K., Sharma, R., & Acharya, U. R. (2015). Application of empirical mode decomposition for analysis of normal and diabetic RR-interval signals. *Expert Systems with Applications*, *42*(9), 4567–4581. doi:10.1016/j.eswa.2015.01.051

Page, C. P., Curtis, M. J., Sutter, M., Walker, M., & Hoffman, B. (1998). *Farmacologíaintegrada*. Published by ElsevierEspaña. (in Spanish)

Paillard, T. (2012). Effects of general and local fatigue on postural control: A review. *Neuroscience and Biobehavioral Reviews*, *36*(1), 162–176. doi:10.1016/j.neubiorev.2011.05.009 PMID:21645543

Pai, P. P., Sanki, P. K., & Banerjee, S. (2015). A Photoacoustics based Continuous Non-Invasive Blood Glucose Monitoring System. In *IEEE International Symposium on Medical Measurements and Applications* (pp. 106–111). Turin, Italy: IEEE. 10.1109/MeMeA.2015.7145181

Pakistan Bureau of Statistics. (n.d.). Retrieved from http://www.pbs.gov.pk/

Pakistan Federal budget spending for fiscal years 2016-2017. (n.d.). Retrieved from https://en.dailypakistan.com.pk/headline/live-finance-minister-unveils-budget-for-2016-2017/

Pal, K., Goel, R., Champaty, B., Samantray, S., & Tibarewala, D. (2013). Heart rate variability and wavelet-based studies on ECG signals from smokers and non-smokers. *Journal of The Institution of Engineers (India): Series B, 94*(4), 275-283.

Pandit, S. M., & Wu, S.-M. (1983). *Time Series and System Analysis with Applications*. John Wiley & Sons.

Pannese, A., Rappaz, M.-A., & Grandjean, D. (2016). Metaphor and music emotion: Ancient views and future directions. *Consciousness and Cognition*, *44*, 61–71. doi:10.1016/j.concog.2016.06.015 PMID:27362475

Pantelopoulos, A., & Bourbakis, N. G. (2010). A Survey on Wearable Sensor-Based Systems for Health Monitoring and Prognosis. *IEEE Transactions on Systems, Man and Cybernetics. Part C, Applications and Reviews*, *40*(1), 1–12. doi:10.1109/TSMCC.2009.2032660

Pardey, J., Roberts, S., & Tarassenko, L. (1996). A review of parametric modelling techniques for EEG analysis. *Medical Engineering & Physics, 18*(1), 2–11. doi:10.1016/1350-4533(95)00024-0 PMID:8771033

Park, S. (2008). *The Voice Stick.* Retrieved from http://www.yankodesign.com/2008/08/21/voice-stick/

Pascolini, D., & Mariotti, S. P. (2011). Global estimates of visual impairment: 2010. *British Journal of Ophthalmology.*

Patel, A., Dodiya, H., Shelate, P., Shastri, D., & Dave, D. (2016). Design, Characterization, and Optimization of Controlled Drug Delivery System Containing Antibiotic Drug/s. *Journal of Drug Delivery, 2016*, 9024173. doi:10.1155/2016/9024173 PMID:27610247

Patel, C., Patel, A., & Patel, D. (2012). Optical character recognition by open source OCR tool tesseract: A case study. *International Journal of Computers and Applications, 55*(10).

Paul, S., Bhattacharya, P., Pandey, A. K., & Patnaik, R. (2014). Application of mathematical modeling as a tool to analyze the EEG signals in rat model of focal cerebral ischemia. *Journal of the Institution of Engineers. Springer, 95*(1), 23-27.

Paul, S., Sinha, T. K., & Patnaik, R. (2015). EEG Time Series data analysis in Focal Cerebral ischemic rat model. *International Journal of Biomedical Engineering and Science, 2*(1), 1-10.

Paul, S., Bhattacharya, P., Pandey, A. K., Sharma, N., Tiwari, J. P., & Patnaik, R. (2012). A Strategic Application of Fast Fourier Transform as a Novel Tool to Evaluate the Extent of Neuronal Insult in Rat Model of Focal Cerebral Ischemia. *Bangladesh Journal of Medical Physics, 5*(1), 29–36.

Paul, S., Sinha, T. K., Bhattacharya, P., & Patnaik, R. (2014). Neural Network based classification of EEG Signal in induced focal cerebral ischemic rat brain. *International Journal of Advanced Information Science and Technology, 32*(32), 49–54.

Peng, Y., & Sun, Z. (2011). Characterization of QT and RR interval series during acute myocardial ischemia by means of recurrence quantification analysis. *Medical & Biological Engineering & Computing, 49*(1), 25–31. doi:10.100711517-010-0671-5 PMID:20725861

Peppas, N. A., Caldorera-Moore, M. E., & Steichen, S. D. (2015). *Historical Survey of Drug Delivery Devices.* Drug-device Combinations for Chronic Diseases.

Percival, D. B., & Walden, A. T. (1993). *Spectral Analysis for Physical Applications.* Cambridge University Press. doi:10.1017/CBO9780511622762

Pereda, E., Quiroga, R. Q., & Bhattacharya, J. (2005). Nonlinear Multivariate Analysis of Neurophysiological Signals. *Progress in Neurobiology, 77*(1–2), 1–37. doi:10.1016/j.pneurobio.2005.10.003 PMID:16289760

Perednia, D. A., & Allen, A. (1995). Telemedicine technology and clinical applications. *Journal of the American Medical Association, 273*(6), 483–488. doi:10.1001/jama.1995.03520300057037 PMID:7837367

Perona, P., & Malik, J. (1990). Scale space and edge detection using anisotropic diffusion. *IEEE Transactions on Pattern Analysis and Machine Intelligence, 12*(7), 629–639. doi:10.1109/34.56205

Pessoa, C. M., Ranzan, C., Trierweiler, L. F., & Trierweile, J. O. (2015). Development of Ant Colony Optimization (ACO) Algorithms Based on Statistical Analysis and Hypothesis Testing for Variable Selection. *IFAC-PapersOnLine, 48*(8), 900–905. doi:10.1016/j.ifacol.2015.09.084

Peters, B. O., Pfurtscheller, G., & Flyvbjerg, H. (2001). Automatic differentiation of multichannel EEG signals. *IEEE Transactions on Biomedical Engineering, 48*(1), 111–116. doi:10.1109/10.900270 PMID:11235582

Petrosian, A., Prokhorov, D., Homan, R., Dashei, R., & Wunsch, D. (2000). Recurrent neural network based prediction of epileptic seizures in intra- and extracranial EEG. *Neurocomputing, 30*(1-4), 201–218. doi:10.1016/S0925-2312(99)00126-5

Petrović, J., Ibrić, S., Betz, G., & Djurić, Z. (2012). Optimization of matrix tablets controlled drug release using Elman dynamic neural networks and decision trees. *International Journal of Pharmaceutics*, *428*(1-2), 57–67. doi:10.1016/j.ijpharm.2012.02.031 PMID:22402474

Pham, P., & Wang, J. (2017). *Understanding Emotional Responses to Mobile Video Advertisements via Physiological Signal Sensing and Facial Expression Analysis.* Paper presented at the Proceedings of the 22nd International Conference on Intelligent User Interfaces. 10.1145/3025171.3025186

Phil, G. (2015, July 21). 7.5 million Americans paid fine for having no health insurance in 2014. *PBS Newshour.* Retrieved from http://www.pbs.org/newshour/rundown/7-5-million-americans-paid-fine-health-insurance-2014/

Phinyomark, A., Phukpattaranont, P., & Limsakul, C. (2011). A review of control methods for electric power wheelchairs based on electromyography signals with special emphasis on pattern recognition. *IETE Technical Review*, *28*(4), 316–326. doi:10.4103/0256-4602.83552

Pickup, J. C., Hussain, F., Evans, N. D., Rolinski, O. J., & Birch, D. J. S. (2005). Fluorescence-based glucose sensors. *Biosensors & Bioelectronics*, *20*(12), 2555–2565. doi:10.1016/j.bios.2004.10.002

Pignataro, G., Tortiglione, A., Scorziello, A., Giaccio, L., Secondo, A., Severino, B., ... Annunziato, L. (2004b). Evidence for a protective role played by the Na+/Ca2+ exchanger in cerebral ischemia induced by middle cerebral artery occlusion in male rats. *Neuropharmacology*, *46*(3), 439–448. doi:10.1016/j.neuropharm.2003.09.015 PMID:14975699

Pirmoradi, F. N., Jackson, J. K., Burt, H. M., & Chiao, M. (2011). A magnetically controlled MEMS device for drug delivery: Design, fabrication, and testing. *Lab on a Chip*, *11*(18), 3072–3080. doi:10.1039/c1lc20438f PMID:21860883

Plagianakos, V. P., Magoulas, G. D., & Vrahatis, M. N. (2001). Learning rate adaptation in stochastic gradient descent, Proc. Advances Convex Anal. Global Optimization. *Noncovex Optimization Applicat.*, *54*, 433–444. doi:10.1007/978-1-4613-0279-7_27

Poincaré, H. (1890). Sur le problème des trois corps et les équations de la dynamique. *Acta Mathematica*, *13*(1), A3–A270.

Pointinger, H., Sarahrudi, K., Poeschl, G., & Munk, P. (2002). Electroencephalography in primary diagnosis of mild head trauma. *Brain Injury*, *16*(9), 799–805. doi:10.1080/02699050210131911 PMID:12217205

Pollak, A. N. (Ed.). (2011). Airway Management. Emergency Care and Transportation of the Sick and Injured. Jones and Bartlett Publishers.

Potts, R. O., Tamada, J., & Tierney, M. J. (2002). Glucose monitoring by reverse iontophoresis. *Diabetes/Metabolism Research and Reviews*, *18*(S1), 49–53. doi:10.1002/dmrr.210

Prabusankarlal, K. M., Thirumoorthy, P., & Manavalan, R. (2015). Segmentation of breast lesions in ultrasound images through multiresolution analysis using undecimated discrete wavelet transform. *Ultrasonic Imaging*, *38*(6), 384–402. doi:10.1177/0161734615615838 PMID:26586725

Pradhan, N., Sadasivan, P. K., & Arunodaya, G. R. (1996). Detection of seizure activity in EEG by an artificial neural network: A preliminary study. *Computers and Biomedical Research, an International Journal*, *29*(4), 303–313. doi:10.1006/cbmr.1996.0022 PMID:8812076

Preedy, E. C., & Prokopovich, P. (2013). *History of inhaler devices. In Inhaler devices-fundamentals, design and drug delivery* (p. 13). Cambridge, MA: Woodhead Publishing.

Preul, M, C. (2005). History of brain tumor surgery. *Neurosurgical Focus*, *18*(4), 1. doi:10.3171/foc.2005.18.4.1 PMID:15844868

Preuveneers, D., & Berbers, Y. (2008). Internet of things: A context-awareness perspective. In L. Yan, Y. Zhang, L. T. Yang, & H. Ning (Eds.), *The Internet of Things: From RFID to the Next-Generation Pervasive Networked Systems* (pp. 287–308). Auerbach. doi:10.1201/9781420052824.ch13

Proakis, J., & Manolakis, D. (1996). *Digital Signal Processing Principles, Algorithms, and Applications*. Prentice Hall.

Proverbio, A. M., Manfrin, L., Arcari, L. A., De Benedetto, F., Gazzola, M., Guardamagna, M., & ... . (2015). Non-expert listeners show decreased heart rate and increased blood pressure (fear bradycardia) in response to atonal music. *Frontiers in Psychology*, 6. PMID:26579029

Public hospitals become part of problem rather than solution. (2015, August 31). *International the news*. Retrieved from https://www.thenews.com.pk/print/59580-public-hospitals-become-part-of-problem-rather-than-solution

Qu, H., & Gotman, J. (1997). A Patient-specific algorithm for the detection of seizure onset in long-term EEG monitoring: Possible use as a warning device. *IEEE Transactions on Biomedical Engineering*, *44*(2), 115–122. doi:10.1109/10.552241 PMID:9214791

Rabbani, H., Vafadust, M., Abolmaesumi, P., & Gazor, S. (2008). Speckle noise reduction of medical ultrasound images in complex wavelet domain using mixture priors. *IEEE Transactions on Biomedical Engineering*, *55*(9), 2152–2160. doi:10.1109/TBME.2008.923140 PMID:18713684

Rafael, F.A., & Ortiz, H. (1982). J. Span Pat., ES 508,671, pp 10.

Rafieniaa, M., Amirib, M., Janmalekic, M., & Sadeghiand, A. (2010). Application of artificial neural networks in controlled drug delivery systems. *Applied Artificial Intelligence*, *24*(8), 807–820. doi:10.1080/08839514.2010.508606

Rai, H. M., Trivedi, A., & Shukla, S. (2013). ECG signal processing for abnormalities detection using multi-resolution wavelet transform and Artificial Neural Network classifier. *Measurement*, *46*(9), 3238–3246. doi:10.1016/j.measurement.2013.05.021

Rajagopal, R., & Subbaiah, P. (2015). a Survey on Liver Tumor Detection and Segmentation. *Journal of Engineering and Applied Sciences (Asian Research Publishing Network)*, *10*(6), 2681–2685.

Rajesh, J. K., Gupta, S. K., Rangaiah, G. P., & Ray, A. K. (2001). Multi-objective optimization of industrial hydrogen plants. *Chemical Engineering Science*, *56*(3), 999–1010. doi:10.1016/S0009-2509(00)00316-X

Ray, A., Nayak, S. K., Champaty, B., Tibarewala, D., & Pal, K. (2016). Non-Linear Analysis of Heart Rate Variability and ECG Signal Features of Swimmers from NIT-Rourkela: A Case Study. *Computational Tools and Techniques for Biomedical Signal Processing*, 56.

Rayatt, S. S., Dancey, A. L., & Jaffe, W. (2005). Soft fluted silicone drains: A prospective, randomized, patient-controlled study. *Plastic and Reconstructive Surgery*, *115*(6), 1605–1608. doi:10.1097/01.PRS.0000160696.19137.37 PMID:15861064

Ray, W. H. (1989). *Advanced Process Control*. New York: Butterworths.

Reinkensmeyer, D. J., & Dietz, V. (2016). *Neurorehabilitation technology*. Springer. doi:10.1007/978-3-319-28603-7

Ren, J. (2012). ANN vs. SVM: Which one performs better in classification of MCCs in mammogram imaging. *Knowledge-Based Systems*, *26*(February), 144–153. doi:10.1016/j.knosys.2011.07.016

Rentschler, S., Vaidya, D. M., Tamaddon, H., Degenhardt, K., Sassoon, D., & Morley, G. E. (2001). Visualization and functional characterization of the developing murine cardiac conduction system. *Development*, *128*(10), 1785–1792. PMID:11311159

Reyes del Paso, G. A., Langewitz, W., Mulder, L. J., Roon, A., & Duschek, S. (2013). The utility of low frequency heart rate variability as an index of sympathetic cardiac tone: A review with emphasis on a reanalysis of previous studies. *Psychophysiology, 50*(5), 477–487. doi:10.1111/psyp.12027 PMID:23445494

Reynaerts, D., Peirs, J., & Brussel, H. V. (1997). An implantable drug-delivery system based on shape memory alloy micro-actuation. *Sensors and Actuators. A, Physical*, 488–562.

Richter, A., & Sandmaier, H. (1990). An Electrohydrodynamic Micropump. *Proceedings of IEEE Microelectromechanical Systems,* 99–104.

Richterich, J. P., Heigl, A., Muff, B., Luchsinger, S., & Gutzwiller, J. P. (2008). Endo-SPONGE: A new endoscopic treatment option in colonoscopy. *Gastrointestinal Endoscopy, 68*(5), 1019–1022. doi:10.1016/j.gie.2008.02.038 PMID:18534581

Ritzmann, R., Gollhofer, A., & Freyler, K. (2017). Posture and Locomotion. In *Sensory Motor and Behavioral Research in Space* (pp. 1–35). Cham, Switzerland: Springer. doi:10.1007/978-3-319-68201-3_1

Robertson, G., Caldwell, G., Hamill, J., Kamen, G., & Whittlesey, S. (2004). *Research methods in biomechanics, 2E.* Champaign, IL: Human Kinetics.

Robertson, R., Gregory, S., & Jabbal, J. (2014). *The social care and health systems of nine countries.* The King's Fund.

Robitaille, S. (2010). *The Illustrated Guide to Assistive Technology and Devices.* Academic Press.

Rocha, M., Pinto, J. P., Rocha, I., & Ferreira, E. C. (2007). Evaluating Evolutionary Algorithms and Differential Evolution for the Online Optimization of Fermentation Processes. In E. Marchiori, J. H. Moore, & J. C. Rajapakse (Eds.), Lecture Notes in Computer Science: Vol. 4447. *Evolutionary Computation, Machine Learning and Data Mining in Bioinformatics. EvoBIO 2007.* Berlin: Springer. doi:10.1007/978-3-540-71783-6_23

Rohokale, V. M., Prasad, N. R., & Prasad, R. (2011, February). A cooperative Internet of Things (IoT) for rural healthcare monitoring and control. In *Wireless Communication, Vehicular Technology, Information Theory and Aerospace & Electronic Systems Technology (Wireless VITAE), 2011 2nd International Conference on* (pp. 1-6). IEEE.

Rosamond, W., Flegal, K., Friday, G., Furie, K., Go, A., & Hong, Y. (2007). Heart disease and stroke statistics--2007 update: A report from the American Heart Association Statistics Committee and Stroke Statistics Subcommittee. *Circulation, 115*(5), 69–171. doi:10.1161/CIRCULATIONAHA.106.179918 PMID:17194875

Rosenbaum, S. (2011). The Patient Protection and Affordable Care Act: Implications for public health policy and practice. *Public Health Reports, 126*(1), 130–135. doi:10.1177/003335491112600118 PMID:21337939

Ross, R. (1999). Atherosclerosis-an inflammatory disease. *Review New Engl. J. Med, 340*(2), 115–126. doi:10.1056/NEJM199901143400207 PMID:9887164

Roza, V. C. C., de Almeida, A. M., & Postolache, O. A. (2017). *Design of an artificial neural network and feature extraction to identify arrhythmias from ECG.* Paper presented at the Medical Measurements and Applications (MeMeA), 2017 IEEE International Symposium on.

Rumani, S. P. (2014). *Impact of Corruption in India's Healthcare Sector.* Retrieved from https://www.mapsofindia.com/my-india/india/impact-of-corruption-in-indias-healthcare-sector

Russotti, J., Shaw, R., & Spungin, S. J. (2004). *When you have a visually impaired student in your classroom: a guide for paraeducators.* American Foundation for the Blind.

Rutkowski, L. (2004). Generalized regression neural networks in time-varying environment. *IEEE Transactions on Neural Networks, 15*(3), 576–596. doi:10.1109/TNN.2004.826127 PMID:15384547

Sabelli, H. (2001). Novelty, a measure of creative organization in natural and mathematical time series. *Nonlinear Dynamics Psychology and Life Sciences*, *5*(2), 89–113. doi:10.1023/A:1026478316970

Sabelli, H., & Lawandow, A. (2010). Homeobios: The pattern of heartbeats in newborns, adults, and elderly patients. *Nonlinear Dynamics Psychology and Life Sciences*, *14*(4), 381. PMID:20887687

Sabelli, H., Messer, J., Kovacevic, L., & Walthall, K. (2011). Biotic patterns of heart rate variation in depressed and psychotic subjects. *Nonlinear Dynamics Psychology and Life Sciences*, *15*(1), 11–28. PMID:21176437

Sabelli, H., Sugerman, A., Kovacevic, L., Kauffman, L., Carlson-Sabelli, L., & Patel, M. (2005). Bios data analyzer. *Nonlinear Dynamics Psychology and Life Sciences*, *9*(4), 505–538. PMID:16194304

Sachan, V. K., Singh, A. K., Jahan, K., Kumbar, S. G., Nagarale, R. K., & Bhattacharya, P. K. (2014). Development of redox-conducting polymer electrodes for non-gassing electro-osmotic pumps: A novel approach. *Journal of the Electrochemical Society*, *161*(13), H3029–H3034. doi:10.1149/2.0071413jes

Sahu, U. (2016). *8 Major Differences Between Healthcare In The US And India.* Available: http://www.huffingtonpost.in/utkarsh-sahu/a-tale-of-two-nations-ind_b_9261892.html

Saito, A., Nawano, S., & Shimizu, A. (2016). Joint optimization of segmentation and shape prior from level-set-based statistical shape model, and its application to the automated segmentation of abdominal organs. *Medical Image Analysis*, *28*, 46–65. doi:10.1016/j.media.2015.11.003 PMID:26716720

Sakuragi, S., Sugiyama, Y., & Takeuchi, K. (2002). Effects of laughing and weeping on mood and heart rate variability. *Journal of Physiological Anthropology and Applied Human Science*, *21*(3), 159–165. doi:10.2114/jpa.21.159 PMID:12148458

Salam, N. A. B. A., bin Mohd Saad, W. H., Manap, Z. B., & Salehuddin, F. (2016). The Evolution of Non-invasive Blood Glucose Monitoring System for Personal Application. *Journal of Telecommunication Electronic and Computer Engineering*, *8*(1), 59–65.

Salunke, P., & Nerkar, R. (2017). IoT Driven Healthcare System for Remote Monitoring of Patients. *Journal for Modern Trends in Science and Technology*, *3*(06), 100–103.

Salvioli, B., Pellegatta, G., Malacarne, M., Pace, F., Malesci, A., Pagani, M., & Lucini, D. (2015). Autonomic nervous system dysregulation in irritable bowel syndrome. *Neurogastroenterology and Motility*, *27*(3), 423–430. doi:10.1111/nmo.12512 PMID:25581440

Sanidas, E. A., Golemati, S., & Dangas, G. D. (2015). Interventional Pharmacology: Stent Based Drug Delivery, Local Drug Delivery Management of Patients Before and After PCI. In PanVascular Medicine (pp. 993-1007). Springer Berlin Heidelberg.

Santini, J. T., Cima, M. J., & Langer, R. (1999). A controlled-release microchip. *Nature*, *397*(6717), 335–338. doi:10.1038/16898 PMID:9988626

Sara, M. (2016, June 27). Pakistan's Healthcare crisis. *DAWN.* Retrieved from https://www.dawn.com/news/1267410

Sarkar, C., Cooley, S., & Srivastava, J. (2014, January 1). Robust Feature Selection Technique using Rank Aggregation. *Applied Artificial Intelligence*, *28*(3), 243–257. doi:10.1080/08839514.2014.883903 PMID:24839351

Satoskar, R. S., Bhandarkar, S. D., & Ainapure, S. S. (2003). *Pharmacology and Pharmacotherapeutics* (18th ed.). Mumbai: Popular Prakashan.

Satya Eswari, J., & Mohan, A. (2013). Optimum Culture Medium Composition for Rhamnolipid Production by Pseudomonas Aeruginosa AT10 Using a Novel Multiobjective Optimization Method. *Journal of Chemical Technology and Biotechnology (Oxford, Oxfordshire)*, *88*(2), 271–279. doi:10.1002/jctb.3825

Satya, E. J., & Ch, V. (2012). Optimization of Culture Conditions for Chinese Hamster Ovary (CHO) Cells Production Using Differential Evolution. *International Journal of Pharmacy and Pharmaceutical Sciences*, *4*(1), 465–470.

Satya, E. J., & Ch, V. (2013). Evaluation of Kinetic Parameters of an Anaerobic Biofilm Reactor Treating Pharmaceutical Industry Wastewater by Ant Colony Optimization. [PubMed]. *Environmental Engineering Science*, *30*(9), 527–535. doi:10.1089/ees.2012.0158

Schacter, D. L. (1977). EEG theta waves and psychological phenomena: A review and analysis. *Biological Psychology*, *5*(1), 47–82. doi:10.1016/0301-0511(77)90028-X PMID:193587

Schallert, T. (1988). Aging-dependent emergence of sensorimotor dysfunction in rats recovered from dopamine depletion sustained early in life. *Annals of the New York Academy of Sciences*, *515*(1), 108–120. doi:10.1111/j.1749-6632.1988.tb32972.x PMID:3364880

Schallert, T., Hernandez, T. D., & Barth, T. M. (1986). Recovery of function after brain damage: Severe and chronic disruption by diazepam. *Brain Research*, *379*(1), 104–111. doi:10.1016/0006-8993(86)90261-1 PMID:3742206

Schijvenaars, B. J., Kors, J. A., van Herpen, G., Kornreich, F., & van Bemmel, J. H. (1997). Effect of electrode positioning on ECG interpretation by computer. *Journal of Electrocardiology*, *30*(3), 247–256. doi:10.1016/S0022-0736(97)80010-6 PMID:9261733

Schneck, D. J., & Berger, D. S. (2005). *The music effect: Music physiology and clinical applications*. Jessica Kingsley Publishers.

Schulkind, M. D., Hennis, L. K., & Rubin, D. C. (1999). Music, emotion, and autobiographical memory: They're playing your song. *Memory & Cognition*, *27*(6), 948–955. doi:10.3758/BF03201225 PMID:10586571

Science Education Computed Tomography (CT). (n.d.). Retrieved 2017 from https://www.nibib.nih.gov/science-education/science-topics/computed-tomography-ct

Scott, R. E., Mars, M., Scott, R. E., & Mars, M. (2015). Telehealth in the developing world: Current status and future prospects. *Smart Homecare Technology and TeleHealth*, *3*, 25–37. doi:10.2147/SHTT.S75184

Scrobotă, I., Băciuţ, G., Filip, A. G., Todor, B., Blaga, F., & Băciuţ, M. F. (2017). Application of Fuzzy Logic in Oral Cancer Risk Assessment. *Iranian Journal of Public Health*, *46*(5), 612–619. PMID:28560191

Selhorst, J. B., & Chen, Y. (2009). *The optic nerve*. Paper presented at the Seminars in neurology.

Selver, M. A. (2015). Exploring brushlet based 3d textures in transfer function specification for direct volume rendering of abdominal organs. *IEEE Transactions on Visualization and Computer Graphics*, *21*(2), 174–187. doi:10.1109/TVCG.2014.2359462 PMID:26357028

Sendrescu, D. (2013). Parameter Identification of Anaerobic Wastewater Treatment Bioprocesses Using Particle Swarm Optimization. *Mathematical Problems in Engineering*, *2013*, 103748. doi:10.1155/2013/103748

Sentul Medical Centre Kuala Lumpur. (2017). [Online image]. Retrieved 2017 from https://www.absolutemed.com/ultrasound-machines/

Sethi, P. K. (1972). A rubber foot for amputees in underdeveloped countries. *The Journal of Bone and Joint Surgery. British Volume*, *54-B*, 177–178.

Shadmand, S., & Mashoufi, B. (2016). Personalized ECG signal classification using block-based neural-network and particle swarm optimization. *Biomedical Signal Processing and Control*, *25*, 203–208. doi:10.1016/j.bspc.2015.10.008

Shafrir, E. (1993). Paul Ehrlich--pioneer in chemotherapy, histology and immunology. *Israel Journal of Medical Sciences*, *29*(5), 327. PMID:8314701

Shah. (2011). *Health Care Around the World*. Available: http://www.globalissues.org/article/774/health-care-around-the-world

Shapiro, L. G., & Stockman, G. C. (n.d.). *Texture, Chapter 7, Computer Vision, 2000*. Available online from https://courses.cs.washington.edu/courses/cse576 /book/ch7.pdf

Sharif, H., Millar, P., Incognito, A., & Ditor, D. (2016). Non-invasive electrocardiographic assessments of cardiac autonomic modulation in individuals with spinal cord injury. *Spinal Cord*, *54*(3), 166–171. doi:10.1038c.2015.207 PMID:26597693

Sharma, R. (Ed.). (2012). Epidemiology of Musculoskeletal Conditions in India. New Delhi, India: Indian Council of Medical Research (ICMR).

Sharma, S. (2007). New approaches in smoking cessation. *Indian Heart Journal*, *60*(2Suppl B), B34–B37. PMID:19359762

Sharma, S., Nijdam, A. J., Sinha, P. M., Walczak, R. J., Liu, X., Cheng, M. M., & Ferrari, M. (2006). Controlled-release microchips. *Expert Opinion on Drug Delivery*, *3*(3), 379–394. doi:10.1517/17425247.3.3.379 PMID:16640498

Sharma, V. N. (1999). *Essentials of pharmacology*. CBS Pub. &Distbrs.

Shaw, J. C., & Ongley, C. (1972). The measurement of synchronization. In H. Petsche & M. A. B. Brazier (Eds.), *Synchronization of EEG activity in epilepsies* (pp. 204–216). Springer-Verlag. doi:10.1007/978-3-7091-8306-9_13

Shaw, J. E., Sicree, R., & Zimmet, P. Z. (2010). Global estimates of the prevalence of diabetes for 2010 and 2030. *Diabetes Research and Clinical Practice*, *87*(1), 4–14. doi:10.1016/j.diabres.2009.10.007

Shehzad, S. (2005). *Alternative Resource Mobilization Strategies for Pakistan's Health Care*. Sustainable Development Policy Institute.

Shi, C., Cheng, Y., Liu, F., Wang, Y., Bai, J., & Tamura, S. (2016). A hierarchical local region-based sparse shape composition for liver segmentation in CT scans. *Pattern Recognition*, *50*, 88–106. doi:10.1016/j.patcog.2015.09.001

Shiffrin, E., Schwierz, E., Wassiljew, S., & Caggianos, C. (2007). Evaluation of an aortic stapler for an open aortic anastomosis. *The Journal of Cardiovascular Surgery*, *48*(5), 659–665. PMID:17989637

Shifrin, E. G., Moore, W. S., Bell, P. R. F., Kolvenbach, R., & Daniline, E. I. (2007). Intravascular Stapler for "Open Aortic Surgery: Preliminary Results". *European Journal of Vascular and Endovascular Surgery*, *33*(4), 408–411. doi:10.1016/j.ejvs.2006.10.019 PMID:17137806

Shilkrot, R., Huber, J., Liu, C., Maes, P., & Nanayakkara, S. C. (2014). *FingerReader: a wearable device to support text reading on the go.* Paper presented at the CHI'14 Extended Abstracts on Human Factors in Computing Systems. 10.1145/2559206.2581220

Shimizu, A., Nakagomi, K., Narihira, T., & Kobatake, H. (2010). Automated Segmentation of 3D CT Images Based on Statistical Atlas and Graph Cuts. In *International MICCAI Workshop on Medical Computer Vision*. Springer Berlin Heidelberg.

Shin, H. S., Park, M. S., & Kwon, S. K. (2000). YakhakHoechi. *EJP*, *44*(3), 272–278.

Shin, S. C., Shin, E. Y., & Cho, C. W. (2000). Enhancing effects of fatty acids on permeation through rat skins. *Drug Development and Industrial Pharmacy*, *26*(5), 563–566. doi:10.1081/DDC-100101269 PMID:10789070

Shi, X., Cheng, H. D., Hu, L., Ju, W., & Tian, J. (2010). Detection and classification of masses in breast ultrasound images. *Digital Signal Processing*, *20*(3), 824–836. doi:10.1016/j.dsp.2009.10.010

Shi, Z., He, L., Nakamura, T., Suzuki, K., & Itoh, H. (2009). Survey on neural networks used for medical image processing. *International Journal of Computational Science*, *3*(1), 86–100. PMID:26740861

Shufni, S. A., & Mashor, M. Y. (2015). *ECG signals classification based on discrete wavelet transform, time domain and frequency domain features.* Paper presented at the Biomedical Engineering (ICoBE), 2015 2nd International Conference on. 10.1109/ICoBE.2015.7235914

Shukla, Tiwari, & Kala. (2010). *Real life applications of soft computing*. CRC Press.

Singh, R. P., Batish, A. G., & Singh, T. P. (2015). *Ergonomic Investigations of Asymmetrical Manual Lifting Tasks on Indian Male Workers* (Doctoral dissertation).

Singhal, V., & Garimella, S. V. (2007). Induction electrohydrodynamics micropump for high heat flux cooling. *Sensors and Actuators. A, Physical*, *134*(2), 650–659. doi:10.1016/j.sna.2006.05.007

Singh, B. K., Verma, K., Panigrahi, L., & Thoke, A. S. (2017). A.S. Thoke, Integrating radiologist feedback with computer aided diagnostic systems for breast cancer risk prediction in ultrasonic images: An experimental investigation in machine learning paradigm. *Expert Systems with Applications*, *90*, 209–223. doi:10.1016/j.eswa.2017.08.020

Singh, B. K., Verma, K., & Thoke, A. S. (2016). Fuzzy cluster based neural network classifier for classifying breast tumors in ultrasound images. *Expert Systems with Applications*, *66*, 114–123. doi:10.1016/j.eswa.2016.09.006

Singh, B. K., Verma, K., Thoke, A. S., & Suri, J. S. (2017). Risk stratification of 2D ultrasound-based breast lesions using hybrid feature selection in machine learning paradigm. *Measurement*, *105*, 146–157. doi:10.1016/j.measurement.2017.01.016

Singh, I. (2015). A Study of Effective Segmentation Techniques for Liver Segmentation. *International Journal of Advanced Research in Computer Engineering & Technology*, *4*(4), 1661–1666.

Siqueira, J., de Melo Nunes, F. A. A., Silva, C. R. G., de Oliveira Berretta, L., Ferreira, C. B. R., Félix, I. M., & Luna, M. M. (2016). *BrailleÉcran: A Braille Approach to Text Entry on Smartphones.* Paper presented at the Computer Software and Applications Conference (COMPSAC), 2016 IEEE 40th Annual. 10.1109/COMPSAC.2016.5

Smith, C. (2017). *Nike FuelBand: The rise and fall of the wearable that started it all.* Retrieved from https://www.wareable.com/nike/not-so-happy-birthday-nike-fuelband-2351

Smith, J. L. (2017). *The Pursuit of Noninvasive Glucos : Hunting the Deceitful Turkey.* Retrieved December 8, 2017, from https://www.researchgate.net/publication/317267760_The_Pursuit_of_Noninvasive_Glucose_5th_Edition

Smith, R. (2007). *An overview of the Tesseract OCR engine.* Paper presented at the Document Analysis and Recognition, 2007. ICDAR 2007. Ninth International Conference on. 10.1109/ICDAR.2007.4376991

Smithuis, R., & Lange, E. E. (2015). *Anatomy of the Liver.* Retrieved 2017 from http://www.radiologyassistant.nl/en/p4375bb8dc241d/anatomy-of-the-liver-segments.html

So, C. F., Choi, K. S., Wong, T. K. S., & Chung, J. W. Y. (2012). Recent advances in noninvasive glucose monitoring. *Medical Devices: Evidence and Research*, *5*(1), 45–52. doi:10.2147/MDER.S28134

Soman, K. P., Loganathan, R., & Ajay, V. (2009). *Machine learning with SVM and other kernel methods*. PHI Learning Private Limited.

Sonalkar, S., & Kapp, N. (2015). Intrauterine device insertion in the postpartum period: A systematic review. *The European Journal of Contraception & Reproductive Health Care*, *20*(1), 4–18. doi:10.3109/13625187.2014.971454 PMID:25397890

Sparacino, G., Zanon, M., Facchinetti, A., Zecchin, C., Maran, A., & Cobelli, C. (2012). Italian contributions to the development of continuous glucose monitoring sensors for diabetes management. *Sensors (Basel)*, *12*(10), 13753–13780. doi:10.3390121013753

Srinivasan, G. N., & Shobha, G. (2008). Statistical texture analysis. Proceedings of World Academy of Science, Engineering and Technology, 36, 1264-1269.

Srinivasan, V., Stankovic, J., & Whitehouse, K. (2008). Protecting your Daily In-Home Activity Information from a Wireless Snooping Attack. In *Proceedings of the 10th International Conference on Ubiquitous Computing* (pp. 202–211). Seoul, South Korea: Academic Press. 10.1145/1409635.1409663

Staples, M., Daniel, K., Cima, M. J., & Langer, R. (2006). Application of micro and nano electromechanical devices to drug delivery. *Pharmaceutical Research*, *23*(5), 847–863. doi:10.100711095-006-9906-4 PMID:16715375

Steidler, L., & Rottiers, P. (2006). Therapeutic drug delivery by genetically modified Lactococcus lactis. *Annals of the New York Academy of Sciences*, *1072*(1), 176–186. doi:10.1196/annals.1326.031 PMID:17057198

Stockmann, C., Roberts, J. K., Yellepeddi, V. K., & Sherwin, C. M. (2015). Clinical pharmacokinetics of inhaled antimicrobials. *Clinical Pharmacokinetics*, *54*(5), 473–492. doi:10.100740262-015-0250-x PMID:25735634

Strasser, H. (2007). *Assessment of the ergonomic quality of handheld tools and computer input devices*. Amsterdam: IOS Press.

Strobl, C., Malley, J., & Tutz, G. (2009). An introduction to recursive partitioning: Rationale, application, and characteristics of classification and regression trees, bagging, and random forests. *Psychological Methods*, *14*(4), 323–348. doi:10.1037/a0016973 PMID:19968396

Stromberg, W. D., & Farr, T. G. (1986). A Fourier based textural feature extraction procedure. *IEEE Transactions on Geoscience and Remote Sensing*, *GE-24*(5), 722–731. doi:10.1109/TGRS.1986.289620

Stronks, H. C., Nau, A. C., Ibbotson, M. R., & Barnes, N. (2015). The role of visual deprivation and experience on the performance of sensory substitution devices. *Brain Research*, *1624*, 140–152. doi:10.1016/j.brainres.2015.06.033 PMID:26183014

Subashini, T. S., Ramalingam, V., & Palanivel, S. (2009). Breast mass classification based on cytological patterns using RBFNN and SVM. *Expert Systems with Applications*, *36*(3), 5284–5290. doi:10.1016/j.eswa.2008.06.127

Sudhamani, M. V., & Raju, G. T. (2014). Segmentation and Classification of Tumour in Computed Tomography Liver Images for Detection, Analysis and Preoperative Planning. *International Journal of Advanced Computer Research*, *4*(1), 166–171.

Sudha, S., Suresh, G. R., & Sukanesh, R. (2009). Speckle noise reduction in ultrasound images by wavelet thresholding based on weighted variance. *International Journal of Computer Theory and Engineering*, *1*, 1793–8201.

Suffczynski, Lopes da Silva, Parra, Velis, Bouwman, van Rijn, … Kalitzin. (2006). Dynamics of Epileptic Phenomena Determined From Statistics of Ictal Transitions. IEEE Transactions on Biomedical Engineering, 53.

Sun, R., & Wang, Y. (2008). Predicting termination of atrial fibrillation based on the structure and quantification of the recurrence plot. *Medical Engineering & Physics*, *30*(9), 1105–1111. doi:10.1016/j.medengphy.2008.01.008 PMID:18343707

Suparna, G. (2017). *Study Finds India Is Asia's Most Corrupt Country, While Japan Comes In Last.* Retrieved from https://www.forbes.com/sites/suparnagoswami/2017/03/08/study-finds-india-is-asias-most-corrupt-country-while-japan-comes-in-last/#7fea8d931201

Svetnik, V., Liaw, A., Tong, C., Culberson, J. C., Sheridan, R. P., & Feuston, B. P. (2003). Random forest: A classification and regression tool for compound classification and QSAR modeling. *Journal of Chemical Information and Computer Sciences*, *43*(6), 1947–1958. doi:10.1021/ci034160g PMID:14632445

Tadokoro, S., Yamagami, S., & Ozawa, M. (1999). Soft Micromanipulation Device with Multiple Degrees of Freedom Consisting of High Polymer Gel Actuators. In *Proceedings of IEEE International Conference on Microelectromechanical Systems* (pp. 37–42). Orlando, FL: IEEE. 10.1109/MEMSYS.1999.746748

Takakura, I. T., Hoshi, R. A., Santos, M. A., Pivatelli, F. C., Nóbrega, J. H., & Guedes, D. L. (2017). Recurrence Plots: A New Tool for Quantification of Cardiac Autonomic Nervous System Recovery after Transplant. *Revista Brasileira de Cirurgia Cardiovascular; Orgao Oficial da Sociedade Brasileira de Cirurgia Cardiovascular*, *32*(4), 245–252. PMID:28977195

Takens, F. (1981). Detecting strange attractors in turbulence. *Lecture Notes in Mathematics*, *898*(1), 366–381. doi:10.1007/BFb0091924

Tallapragada, K., Singavarapu, S., & Pradhan, N. (2014). Understanding the dynamics of heart rate variability in cardiovascular disorders using recurrence quantification analysis and radial basis function neural network. *Intl J Sci Eng Res*, *4*, 863–873.

Tanaka, Y., Tajima, T., & Seyama, M. (2017). Acoustic Modal Analysis of Resonant Photoacoustic Spectroscopy with Dual-Wavelength Differential Detection for Noninvasive Glucose Monitoring. *IEEE Sensors Letters*, *1*(3), 1–4. doi:10.1109/LSENS.2017.2698062

Tan, C., & Degim, I. T. (2012). Development of sustained release formulation of an antithrombotic drug and application of fuzzy logic. *Pharmaceutical Development and Technology*, *17*(2), 242–250. doi:10.3109/10837450.2010.531739 PMID:21062232

Tang, X. (1998). Texture information in run length matrices. *IEEE Transactions on Image Processing*, *7*(11), 1602–1609. doi:10.1109/83.725367 PMID:18276225

Tan, H. Y., Loke, W. K., & Nguyen, N. (2010). A reliable method for bonding polydimethylsiloxane (PDMS) to polymethylmethacrylate (PMMA) and its application in micropumps. *Sensors and Actuators. B, Chemical*, *151*(1), 133–139. doi:10.1016/j.snb.2010.09.035

Tan, L. T. H., & Ong, K. L. (2002). The impact of medical technology on healthcare today. *Hong Kong Journal of Emergency Medicine*, *9*(4), 231–236. doi:10.1177/102490790200900410

Tan, Y. Z., Ozdemir, S., Temiz, A., & Celik, F. (2015). The effect of relaxing music on heart rate and heart rate variability during ECG GATED-myocardial perfusion scintigraphy. *Complementary Therapies in Clinical Practice*, *21*(2), 137–140. doi:10.1016/j.ctcp.2014.12.003 PMID:25747187

Tao, Lubeley, & Desai. (2003). Bioadhesive poly(methyl methacrylate) microdevices for controlled drug delivery. *J. Control. Rel.*, 215–228.

Tarvainen, M. P., Niskanen, J.-P., Lipponen, J. A., Ranta-Aho, P. O., & Karjalainen, P. A. (2014). Kubios HRV–heart rate variability analysis software. *Computer Methods and Programs in Biomedicine*, *113*(1), 210–220. doi:10.1016/j.cmpb.2013.07.024 PMID:24054542

Tavernier, B., & Jeanne, M. (2014). Heart Rate Variability. In *Monitoring Technologies in Acute Care Environments* (pp. 109–115). Springer. doi:10.1007/978-1-4614-8557-5_13

Tayade, M. C., & Karandikar, P. M. (2013). Role of data mining techniques in healthcare sector in India. *Sch J App Med Sci*, *1*(3), 158–160.

Teoh, M. K., & Bird, D. A. (1987). Removal of skin staples in an emergency. *Annals of the Royal College of Surgeons of England*, *69*, 222–224. PMID:3314634

Thampi, G. K. (2002). *Corruption in South Asia: Insights and benchmarks from citizen feedback surveys in five countries*. Transparency International.

Thanuja, R., & Balakrishnan, R. (2013). Real Time Sleep Apnea Monitor Using ECG. In *2013 IEEE Conference on Information Communication Technologies* (pp. 973–976). IEEE. 10.1109/CICT.2013.6558237

The World Bank. (2016). Retrieved from http://www.worldbank.org/

Theodoridis, S., & Koutroumbas, K. (2009). *Pattern Recognition* (4th ed.). Elsevier.

Thomas, D. A., Myers, M. A., Wichert, B., Schreier, H., & Gonzalez-Rothi, R. J. (1991). Acute effects of liposome aerosol inhalation on pulmonary function in healthy human volunteers. *Chest*, *99*(5), 1268–1270. doi:10.1378/chest.99.5.1268 PMID:2019191

Thompson, V. (2017). *Cataract surgery*. Available: http://www.allaboutvision.com/conditions/cataract-surgery.htm

Tiwari, P. S., Gite, L. P., Majumder, J., Pharade, S. C., & Singh, V. V. (2010). Push/pull strength of agricultural workers in Central India. *International Journal of Industrial Ergonomics*, *40*(1), 1–7. doi:10.1016/j.ergon.2009.10.001

Tkaczyszyn, M., Olbrycht, T., Makowska, A., Soboń, K., Paleczny, B., Rydlewska, A., & Jankowska, E. A. (2013). The influence of the sounds of crying baby and the sounds of violence on haemodynamic parameters and autonomic status in young, healthy adults. *International Journal of Psychophysiology*, *87*(1), 52–59. doi:10.1016/j.ijpsycho.2012.10.017 PMID:23142485

Toh, K. L. (2008). Basic science review on circadian rhythm biology and circadian sleep disorders. *Annals of the Academy of Medicine, Singapore*, *37*(8), 662–668. PMID:18797559

Tomasi, E., Facchini, L. A., & Maia, M. D. F. S. (2004). Health information technology in primary health care in developing countries: A literature review. *Bulletin of the World Health Organization*, *82*(11), 867–874. PMID:15640923

Tomines, A., Readhead, H., Readhead, A., & Teutsch, S. (2013). Applications of electronic health information in public health: Uses, opportunities & barriers. *EGEMS (Washington, DC)*, *1*(2), 5. doi:10.13063/2327-9214.1019 PMID:25848571

Torrent-Guasp, F., Ballester, M., Buckberg, G. D., Carreras, F., Flotats, A., Carrió, I., ... Narula, J. (2001). Spatial orientation of the ventricular muscle band: Physiologic contribution and surgical implications. *The Journal of Thoracic and Cardiovascular Surgery*, *122*(2), 389–392. doi:10.1067/mtc.2001.113745 PMID:11479518

Touati, F., & Tabish, R. (2013). U-healthcare system: State-of-the-art review and challenges. *Journal of Medical Systems*, *37*(3), 9949. doi:10.100710916-013-9949-0

Trenkle, F., Haeberle, S., & Zengerle, R. (2009). Normally-closed peristaltic micropump with re-usable actuator and disposable fluidic chip. *Procedia Chemistry*, *1*(1), 1515–1518. doi:10.1016/j.proche.2009.07.378

Tsai, H.-H., & Yi, C.-W. (2015). *Wearable ECG for Tension Assessment in Movie Watching and Adventure Riding*. Paper presented at the Moile Ad-hoc and Sensor Networks (MSN), 2015 11th International Conference on. 10.1109/MSN.2015.45

Tsai, N. C., & Sue, C. Y. (2007). Review of MEMS based drug delivery and dosing systems. *Sensors and Actuators, 134*(2), 555–564. doi:10.1016/j.sna.2006.06.014

Tsals, I., Gross, J., & Lavi, G. (1999). *Cartridge-based drug delivery device*. U.S. Patent 5,858,001.

Tsuda, Y., Takemura, T., Shimamura, Y., & Iwasa, S. (2003). Usefulness of silicone Blake drains after cardiac surgery (in Japanese). *Kyobu Geka, 56*, 1017–1019. PMID:14608925

Tura, A. (2008). Noninvasive glycaemia monitoring: Background, traditional findings, and novelties in the recent clinical trials. *Current Opinion in Clinical Nutrition and Metabolic Care, 11*(5), 607–612. doi:10.1097/MCO.0b013e328309ec3a

Tura, A., Maran, A., & Pacini, G. (2007). Non-invasive glucose monitoring: Assessment of technologies and devices according to quantitative criteria. *Diabetes Research and Clinical Practice, 77*(1), 16–40. doi:10.1016/j.diabres.2006.10.027

Turianikova, Z., Tonhajzerova, I., Czippelova, B., Javorka, K., Lazarova, Z., & Javorka, M. (2014). *Recurrence Quantification Analysis of heart rate and blood pressure variability in obese children and adolescents*. Paper presented at the Computing in Cardiology Conference (CinC), 2014.

Turner, H. R. (2010). *Science in medieval Islam: an illustrated introduction*. University of Texas Press.

Tyagi, A., Hutton, G., & Sen, S. (2010). *The economic impacts of inadequate sanitation in India: Inadequate sanitation costs India Rs. 2.4 trillion (US $53.8 billion)*. Academic Press.

Tye & Deisseroth. (2012). Optogenetic investigation of neural circuits underlying brain disease in animal models. *Nature Reviews, 13*, 251-266.

Ultrasound Machines. (2017). [Online image]. Retrieved 2017 from http://site.sentulmedical.com.my/main/3138/index.asp?pageid=138470&t=ultrasound

Uniyal, D., & Raychoudhury, V. (2014). *Pervasive Healthcare-A Comprehensive Survey of Tools and Techniques, 48*. Retrieved from http://arxiv.org/abs/1411.1821

Untitled. (n.d.). [Online image]. Retrieved 2017 from https://en.wikipedia.org/ wiki/Liver#/media/ File:Liver_04_Couinaud_classification.svg.

USA FY16 Federal Budget Spending Estimates for Fiscal Years 2015 – 2020. (n.d.). Retrieved from http://www.usgovernmentspending.com/health_care_budget_2016_1.html

Vaghefi, F. (1999). *Dry powder inhaler*. U.S. Patent 5,875,776.

Valadka, A. B. (2004). Injury to the cranium. In E. J. Moore, D. V. Feliciano, & K. L. Mattox (Eds.), *Trauma* (pp. 385–406). New York: McGraw-Hill, Medical Pub. Division.

Valafar, H., & Valafar, F. (1999). Prediction of a patient's response to a specific drug treatment using artificial neural networks. IEEE, 3694–3697.

Van de Pol, F. C. M., & van Lintel, H. T. G. (1990). A thermopneumatic micropump based on microengineering techniques. *Sensors and Actuators. A, Physical, 21*, pp198–pp202. doi:10.1016/0924-4247(90)85038-6

van den Berg, A., & Lammerink, T. (1998). Micro total analysis systems: microfluidic aspects, integration concept and applications. In Microsystem technology in chemistry and life science (pp. 21-49). Springer.

Van Der Beek, A. J., Dennerlein, J. T., Huysmans, M. A., Mathiassen, S. E., Burdorf, A., Van Mechelen, W., ... Van Der Molen, H. F. (2017). A research framework for the development and implementation of interventions preventing work-related musculoskeletal disorders. *Scandinavian Journal of Work, Environment & Health*, *43*(6), 526–539. PMID:28945263

Van Lintel, H. T. G., Van de Pol, F. C. M., & Bouwstra, S. (1988). A piezoelectric micropump based on micromachining of silicon. *Sensors and Actuators. A, Physical*, *15*(2), 153–168. doi:10.1016/0250-6874(88)87005-7

van Weel, C., Kassai, R., Qidwai, W., Kumar, R., Bala, K., Gupta, P. P., ... Howe, A. (2016). Primary healthcare policy implementation in South Asia. *BMJ Global Health*, *1*(2), e000057. doi:10.1136/bmjgh-2016-000057 PMID:28588938

Vashist, S. K. (2012). Non-invasive glucose monitoring technology in diabetes management: A review. *Analytica Chimica Acta*, *750*, 16–27. doi:10.1016/j.aca.2012.03.043

Vasičkaninová, A., Bakošová, M., & Mészáros, A. (2017). Control of a biochemical process using fuzzy approach. *2017 21st International Conference on Process Control (PC)*, 173-178.

Veerapen, K., Wigley, R. D., & Valkenburg, H. (2007). Musculoskeletal pain in Malaysia: A COPCORD survey. *The Journal of Rheumatology*, *34*(1), 207–213. PMID:17216688

Ventola, C. L. (2014). Social media and health care professionals: Benefits, risks, and best practices. *P&T*, *39*(7), 491. PMID:25083128

Verplaetse, T. L., Smith, P. H., Smith, K. M., Oberleitner, L. M., & McKee, S. A. (2017). Guanfacine alters the effect of stress and smoking on heart rate variability in regular daily smokers. *Psychopharmacology*, *234*(5), 805–813. doi:10.100700213-016-4517-1 PMID:28028603

Vilensky, J. A., Robertson, W., & Suarez-Quian, C. A. (2015). *The Clinical Anatomy of the Cranial Nerves: The Nerves of" On Old Olympus Towering Top*. John Wiley & Sons. doi:10.1002/9781118491959

Visser, J. E., Carpenter, M. G., van der Kooij, H., & Bloem, B. R. (2008). The clinical utility of posturography. *Clinical Neurophysiology*, *119*(11), 2424–2436. doi:10.1016/j.clinph.2008.07.220 PMID:18789756

Wallot, S., Roepstorff, A., & Mønster, D. (2016). Multidimensional Recurrence Quantification Analysis (MdRQA) for the analysis of multidimensional time-series: A software implementation in MATLAB and its application to group-level data in joint action. *Frontiers in Psychology*, 7. PMID:27920748

Wang, C. P. (2007). 'Dynamic covariation of symptoms of anxiety and depression among newly-diagnosed patients with major depressive episode, panic disorder, and controls'. *Nonlinear Dynamics Psychology and Life Sciences*, *11*(3), 349–365.

Wardoyo, S., Hutajulu, P. T., & Togibasa, O. (2016). A Development of Force Plate for Biomechanics Analysis of Standing and Walking. *Journal of Physics: Conference Series*, *739*(1), 012118. doi:10.1088/1742-6596/739/1/012118

Weaver, C. A., Ball, M. J., Kim, G. R., & Kiel, J. M. (2016). *Healthcare information management systems*. Cham: Springer International Publishing. doi:10.1007/978-3-319-20765-0

Web, M. D. (n.d.). *Picture of the Liver*. Retrieved 2017 from http://www.webmd.com/digestive-disorders/picture-of-the-liver#2.(2005-2017)

Webber, C. L. Jr, & Zbilut, J. P. (1994). Dynamical assessment of physiological systems and states using recurrence plot strategies. *Journal of Applied Physiology*, *76*(2), 965–973. doi:10.1152/jappl.1994.76.2.965 PMID:8175612

Weinstein, L. A., Richards, F. M., Laun, D. A., & Middleton, D. T., Jr. (1999). *Metered dose inhaler spacer*. U.S. Patent D412, 979.

Weisstein, E. W. (2002). *CRC concise encyclopedia of mathematics*. CRC Press. doi:10.1201/9781420035223

Wellens, H. J., Bär, F. W., & Lie, K. (1978). The value of the electrocardiogram in the differential diagnosis of a tachycardia with a widened QRS complex. *The American Journal of Medicine*, *64*(1), 27–33. doi:10.1016/0002-9343(78)90176-6 PMID:623134

Weszka, J. S., Dyer, C. R., & Rosenfeld, A. (1976). A comparative study of texture measures for terrain classification. *IEEE Transactions on Systems, Man, and Cybernetics*, *SMC-6*(4), 269–285. doi:10.1109/TSMC.1976.5408777

Whitelock, J., & Melrose, J. (2006). *Wiley Encyclopaedia of Biomedical Engineering*. Wiley.

WHO. (n.d.). Retrieved from http://www.who.int/en/

Wickens, A. , P. (2014). *A History of the Brain: From Stone Age surgery to modern neuroscience*. Psychology Press.

Wicklund, E. (2014). *"Silo" one of healthcare's biggest flaws*. Available: http://www.healthcareitnews.com/news/silo-one-healthcares-biggest-flaws

Williams, O. E., Elghenzai, S., Subbe, C., Wyatt, J. C., & Williams, J. (2017). The use of telemedicine to enhance secondary care: Some lessons from the front line. *Future Hospital Journal*, *4*(2), 109–114.

Windeatt, T., & Ardeshir, G. (2002). Boosted tree ensembles for solving multiclass problems. *Multiple Classifier Systems*, 179-182.

Winter, D. A. (2009). *Biomechanics and Motor Control of Human Movement*. Hoboken, NJ: Wiley. doi:10.1002/9780470549148

Woias, P. (2001). *Micropumps: summarizing the first two decades*. Micromachining and Microfabrication.

Wolff, V., Rouyer, O., & Gény, B. (2013). Response to letter regarding article,"cannabis-related stroke: Myth or reality? *Stroke*, *44*(5), e57–e57. doi:10.1161/STROKEAHA.113.001094 PMID:23741740

Wolinsky, J. B., Colson, Y. L., & Grinstaff, M. W. (2012). Local drug delivery strategies for cancer treatment: Gels, nanoparticles, polymeric films, rods, and wafers. *Journal of Controlled Release*, *159*(1), 14–26. doi:10.1016/j.jconrel.2011.11.031 PMID:22154931

Wolz, R., Chu, C., Misawa, K., Fujiwara, M., Mori, K., & Rueckert, D. (2013). Automated abdominal multi-organ segmentation with subject-specific atlas generation. *IEEE Transactions on Medical Imaging*, *32*(9), 1723–1730. doi:10.1109/TMI.2013.2265805 PMID:23744670

Wong, C., Zhang, Z. Q., Lo, B., & Yang, G. Z. (2015). Wearable sensing for solid biomechanics: A review. *IEEE Sensors Journal*, *15*(5), 2747–2760.

Wood, K. C., Zacharia, N. S., Schmidt, D. J., Wrightman, S. N., Andaya, B. J., & Hammond, P. T. (2008). Electroactive controlled release thin films. *Proceedings of the National Academy of Sciences of the United States of America*, *105*(7), 2280–2285. doi:10.1073/pnas.0706994105 PMID:18272499

World Health Organization. (2008). *Change the definition of blindness*. Retrieved from http://www. who. int/blindness/ChangetheDefinitionofBlindness. pdf

World Report. (n.d.). Retrieved from https://www.hrw.org/world-report/2017

Worldometers. (n.d.). Retrieved from http://www.worldometers.info/world-population/pakistan-population/

Wu, S. Z., Harish, S., Sanders-Millare, D., & Guruwaiya, J. A. (2001). *Implantable medical device having protruding surface structures for drug delivery and cover attachment*. U.S. Patent 6,254,632.

Wu, C. M., & Chen, Y. C. (1992). Statistical feature matrix for texture analysis. *CVGIP. Graphical Models and Image Processing*, *54*(5), 407–419. doi:10.1016/1049-9652(92)90025-S

Wu, C. M., Chen, Y. C., & Hsieh, K. S. (1992). Texture features for classification of ultrasonic liver images. *IEEE Transactions on Medical Imaging*, *11*(2), 141–152. doi:10.1109/42.141636 PMID:18218367

Xia, F., Yang, L. T., Wang, L., & Vinel, A. (2012). Internet of things. *International Journal of Communication Systems*, *25*(9), 1101–1102. doi:10.1002/dac.2417

Xie, X., & Mirmehdi, M. (2008). A galaxy of texture features. In Handbook of Texture Analysis (pp. 347–406). Imperial College Press.

Xue, S., Chen, X., Fang, Z., & Xia, S. (2015). *An ECG arrhythmia classification and heart rate variability analysis system based on android platform.* Paper presented at the Future Information and Communication Technologies for Ubiquitous HealthCare (Ubi-HealthTech), 2015 2nd International Symposium on. 10.1109/Ubi-HealthTech.2015.7203323

Xu, L., Krzyzak, A., & Suen, C. Y. (1992, May-June). Methods of Combining Multiple Classifiers and Their Applications to Handwriting Recognition. *IEEE Transactions on Systems, Man, and Cybernetics*, *22*(3), 418–435. doi:10.1109/21.155943

Yadav, J., Rani, A., Singh, V., & Murari, B. M. (2015). Comparative Study of Different Measurement Sites Using NIR Based Non-invasive Glucose Measurement System. In *Proceedings of the 4th International Conference on Eco-friendly Computing and Communication Systems (ICECCS)* (*Vol. 70*, pp. 469–475). Academic Press. 10.1016/j.procs.2015.10.082

Yang, Y., Zhaoying, Z., Xiongying, Y., & Xiaoning, J. (1996). Bimetallic Thermally Actuated Micropump. Proceedings of International Mechnical Engineering Congross and Exposition (ASME 1996), 17–22.

Yasobant, S., & Rajkumar, P. (2014). Work-related musculoskeletal disorders among health care professionals: A cross-sectional assessment of risk factors in a tertiary hospital, India. *Indian Journal of Occupational and Environmental Medicine*, *18*(2), 75–81. doi:10.4103/0019-5278.146896 PMID:25568602

Yen, B. S., Wang, H.-M., Hou, M. C., Tcm, D., Huang, S.-C., & Chou, L.-C. (2010). The relationship between music processing and electrocardiogram (ECG) in vegetative state (VS). *Circuits and Systems (ISCAS), Proceedings of 2010 IEEE International Symposium on*. 10.1109/ISCAS.2010.5537211

Yoshimi, Y., Shinoda, K., Mishima, M., Nakao, K., & Munekane, K. (2004). Development of an artificial synapse using an electrochemical micropump. *Journal of Artificial Organs*, *7*(4), 210–215. doi:10.100710047-004-0269-5 PMID:15739055

Yueh, B., Shapiro, N., MacLean, C. H., & Shekelle, P. G. (2003). Screening and management of adult hearing loss in primary care: Scientific review. *Journal of the American Medical Association*, *289*(15), 1976–1985. doi:10.1001/jama.289.15.1976 PMID:12697801

Yu, J., Tan, J., & Wang, Y. (2010). Ultrasound speckle reduction by SUSAN-controlled anisotropic diffusion method. *Pattern Recognition*, *43*(9), 3083–3092. doi:10.1016/j.patcog.2010.04.006

Yun, K. S., Cho, I. J., Bu, J. U., Kim, C. J., & Yoon, E. (2002). A surface tension driven micropump for low voltage and low power operations. *Journal of MEMS.*, *11*(5), 454–461. doi:10.1109/JMEMS.2002.803286

Yusuf, K. K., Bulent, G., & Selda, G. (2005). Pure tone audiometery in children. *International Journal of Pediatric Otorhinolaryngology*, *69*(2), 209–214. doi:10.1016/j.ijporl.2004.08.018 PMID:15656954

Yu, Y., & Acton, S. (2002). Speckle reducing anisotropic diffusion. *IEEE Transactions on Image Processing*, *11*(11), 1260–1270. doi:10.1109/TIP.2002.804276 PMID:18249696

Zadeh, L. A. (1994). Soft computing and fuzzy logic. *IEEE Software*, *11*(6), 48–56. doi:10.1109/52.329401

Zaidi, A. M. A., Ahmed, M. J., & Bakibillah, A. (2017). *Feature extraction and characterization of cardiovascular arrhythmia and normal sinus rhythm from ECG signals using LabVIEW.* Paper presented at the Imaging, Vision & Pattern Recognition (icIVPR), 2017 IEEE International Conference on. 10.1109/ICIVPR.2017.7890871

Zanagnolo, V., Garbi, A., Achilarre, M. T., & Minig, L. (2017). Robot-assisted surgery in Gynecologic cancers. *Journal of Minimally Invasive Gynecology*, *24*(3), 379–396. doi:10.1016/j.jmig.2017.01.006 PMID:28104497

Zanen, P., Go, L. T., & Lammers, J. W. (1998). The efficacy of a low-dose, monodisperse parasympathicolytic aerosol compared with a standard aerosol from a metered-dose inhaler. *European Journal of Clinical Pharmacology*, *54*(1), 27–30. doi:10.1007002280050415 PMID:9591926

Zbilut, J. P., Thomasson, N., & Webber, C. L. (2002). Recurrence quantification analysis as a tool for nonlinear exploration of nonstationary cardiac signals. *Medical Engineering & Physics*, *24*(1), 53–60. doi:10.1016/S1350-4533(01)00112-6 PMID:11891140

Zeebregts, C. J., Heijmen, R. H., van den Dungen, J. J., & van Schilfgaarde, R. (2003). Non-suture methods of vascular anastomosis. *British Journal of Surgery*, *90*(3), 261–271. doi:10.1002/bjs.4063 PMID:12594661

Zhang, H. J., & Qiu, C. J. A. (2006). TiNiCu thin film micropump made by magnetron Co-sputtered method. *Materials Transactions*, *47*(3), 532–535. doi:10.2320/matertrans.47.532

Zhang, Y., Cheng, H. D., Tian, J., Huang, J., & Tang, X. (2010). Fractional subpixel diffusion and fuzzy logic approach for ultrasound speckle reduction. *Pattern Recognition*, *43*(8), 2962–2970. doi:10.1016/j.patcog.2010.02.014

Zhang, Y., Zhang, F., Shakhsheer, Y., Silver, J. D., Klinefelter, A., Nagaraju, M., ... Otis, B. P. (2013). A Batteryless 19μW MICS/ISM-Band Energy Harvesting Body Sensor Node SoC for ExG Applications. *IEEE Journal of Solid-State Circuits*, *48*(1), 199–213. doi:10.1109/JSSC.2012.2221217

Zhao, Z., Morstatter, F., Sharma, S., Alelyani, S., Anand, A., & Liu, H. (n.d.). *Advancing feature selection research – ASU feature selection repository.* Available online at http://featureselection.asu.edu/index.php

Zhou, F., Feng, J. F., & Shi, Q. Y. (2001). Texture feature based on local Fourier transform. *Proceedings - International Conference on Image Processing*, *2*, 610–613.

Zhou, Y., & Bai, J. (2007). Multiple abdominal organ segmentation: An atlas-based fuzzy connectedness approach. *IEEE Transactions on Information Technology in Biomedicine*, *11*(3), 348–352. doi:10.1109/TITB.2007.892695 PMID:17521085

Zhou, Z., Wu, S., Chang, K. J., Chen, W. R., Chen, Y. S., Kuo, W. H., ... Tsui, P. H. (2015). Classification of benign and malignant breast tumors in ultrasound images with posterior acoustic shadowing using half- contour features. *Journal of Medical and Biological Engineering*, *35*(2), 178–187. doi:10.100740846-015-0031-x PMID:25960706

Zhou, Z., Wu, W., Wu, S., Tsui, P. H., Lin, C. C., Zhang, L., & Wang, T. (2014). Semi-automatic breast ultrasound image segmentation based on mean shift and graph cuts. *Ultrasonic Imaging*, 1–21. PMID:24759696

Zimmermann, S., Frank, J. A., Liepmann, D., & Pisano, A. P. (2004). A planar micropump utilizing thermopneumatic actuation and in-plane flap valves. In *17th IEEE International Conference on Micro Electro Mechanical Systems (MEMS): Maastricht MEMS 2004 Technical Digest* (pp. 462–465). IEEE. 10.1109/MEMS.2004.1290622

Zou, J. X., Ye, Y. Z., Zhou, Y., & Yang, Y. (1997). A Novel Thermally Actuated Silicon Micropump. *Proceedings of International Symposium on Micromechatronics and Human Science.*

About the Contributors

Sandip Bag, Assistant Professor in the Department of Biomedical Engineering, JIS College of Engineering, Kalyani since 2005. Completed PhD, Post Graduation and Graduation from Jadavpur University, Kolkata. Published more than 26 nos of paper in national & international journal and proceedings and also presented papers in India and abroad. Received travel grant and research grant from DST & UGC respectively. Developed various laboratories such as Biomaterials & Biomedical Instrumentation laboratory in JIS College of Engineering, Kalyani.

Ranjit Barua is a M.Tech in Mechanical Engineering, also associate member of Institution of Engineers(India),and Chartered Engineer from Institution of Engineers(India). Currently Pursuing Ph.D from Centre for Healthcare Science & Technology at IIEST-Shibpur, Howrah. Research area is Additive manufacturing and Tissue Engineering.

Dinesh Bhatia pursued his PhD in Biomechanics and Rehabilitation Engineering from MNNIT, Allahabad, India in 2010 with Bachelor's (2002) and Master's degree (2004) in Biomedical Engineering from Mumbai University. He completed his MBA from IMT Ghaziabad in 2007. He is currently working as Associate Professor and Head, Department of Biomedical Engineering, North Eastern Hill University (NEHU), Shillong, Meghalaya, India since August 2013. Previously, he was employed as an Assistant Professor (Sr. Grade) at the Department of Biomedical Engineering, Deenbandhu Chhotu Ram University of Science and Technology, Murthal (Sonepat), Haryana (State Government University), India from July 2006 to July 2013. He was selected for the "Young Scientist Award (BOYSCAST)" in (2011-12) by Government of India to pursue research in osteoarthritis (OA) for one year at Adaptive Neural Systems Laboratory, Biomedical Engineering Department, Florida International University, Miami, Florida, USA. He is also the recipient of "INAE fellowship award" in 2011 by Indian National Academy of Engineering. He was selected as one of the twelve young Biomedical scientists by the ICMR, Govt. of India to pursue research fellowship (2014-15) in the field of sensory prosthetics at University of Glasgow, Scotland, UK. He has attended Biomechanics and human Gait training at Munich, Germany in March, 2017 and training of use of rTMS, EEG and EMG in disabled children in Ivanovo, Russia in September, 2017. He has several research papers in reputed journals, conference, seminars and symposia with teaching and research experience of more than thirteen (13) years. He is invited panel member of many professional bodies, editorial boards, committees, societies and forums. He is currently having several funded projects from Government of India on physically challenged, disabled and paralyzed persons. He authored a book titled "Medical Informatics" published (2015) by PHI and "Current aspects in Stroke Rehabilitation" (2016) by ABS Publishers. His research focuses on understanding muscle mechanics, joint kinematics and dynamics involved in performing locomotion and routine tasks and undermining it effects during an injury or disease. His interest areas are medical instrumentation, biomechanics and rehabilitation engineering, medical informatics, signal and image processing, marketing and international business.

Biswajeet Champaty is an Assistant Professor in the department of Biomedical Engineering at Ajeenkya D Y Patil Unversity, Pune since August 2016. He is a B.Tech in Biomedical Engineering from Biju Patnaik University of Technology Odisha and M.Tech in Biomedical Engineering from SRM University, Chennai. He holds a PhD in Biomedical Engineering from National Institute of Technology Rourkela, Odisha. He has a profound interest in research in the field of medical electronics and instrumentation with specialization in biosignal-based intelligent human-computer interface design for controlling assistive devices. He has extensive expertise in device development for biosignal acquisition, MATLAB based graphical user interface design for real-time signal processing and event monitoring, biosignal-based wireless control of rehabilitative devices and assistive robotics and applications of IoT in healthcare. He has published 4 research publications in referred journals, 23 international publications in various IEEE conferences and 11 book chapters of international repute. 7 of his research papers have received best international paper awards.

Pallab Datta completed his B Pharm from AISSMS College of Pharmacy, University of Pune, M Pharm in Pharmaceutics from NIPER Mohali and PhD from SMST, IIT Kharagpur, India. He has been recipient of DST Inspire Faculty Award from Govt. of India. His areas of interest are in biomaterials, biofabrication and drug delivery. He has around 20 publications and 3 extra mural projects.

J. Satya Eswari is currently working as an Assistant professor in Department of Biotechnology at National Institute of Technology (NIT)- Raipur, India. She did her M.Tech in Biotechnology and biochemical engineering from Indian Institute of Technology (IIT), Kharagpur and Ph.D. in chemical engineering from Indian Institute of Technology (IIT), Hyderabad. During her research career, she worked as a Woman Scientist for a Department of Science and Technology (DST) project at Indian Institute of Chemical Technology (IICT) Hyderabad. She has rigorously pursued her research in areas of bioinformatics and bioprocess and product development. She gained pioneering expertise in the application of mathematical and engineering tools in biotechnological processes. Her fields of specializations include bioinformatics, biotechnology, process modeling, evolutionary optimization and artificial intelligence. She has more than 20 publications in SCI/Scopus indexed journals and 27 proceedings in international and national conferences. Her research contributions have received wide global citations. She completed one DST woman scientist project (22 lakhs) and is currently handling two projects, a DST-Early career research project (43 lakhs) and a CCOST (Chhattisgarh Council of Science and Technology) project (4 lakhs). She has a teaching experience of more than 4 years along with a research experience of 3 years. She has conducted 2 short-term courses. She has delivered invited lectures in various institutes. She visited two countries for international conferences. She has guided more than 33 B.Tech and post-graduate students and is currently supervising two research scholars, two project fellows and six B.Tech students. She is an active participant in both academic and research activities. She is the convener of Departmental Academic Committee (DAC) and BITSA in-charge at National Institute of Technology (NIT) Raipur. She has reviewed various research articles in 11 international journals. She is a member of various societies.

Akash Handique, presently working as an Associate Professor in the Department of Radiodiagnosis, NEIGRIHMS Shillong. His prime area of interest is interventional radiology including neurointervention. He has 15 years work experience in the field of Radiodiagnosis and Medical Imaging and has published 30 scientific publications, presented guest lectures in more than 80 scientific meets and has received awards and honours in recognition of his work.

Geshwaree Huzooree was born in Mauritius. She received the M.Sc. Software Engineering Projects and Management degree with distinction from the University of Mauritius, Réduit, Mauritius in 2013, and B.Sc (Hons.) Computer Science and Engineering degree from the University of Mauritius in 2007. She is currently a full-time Lecturer at Charles Telfair Institute, affiliated with Curtin Business School in the department of IT. She was a Software Engineer for 7 years. Her area of interest is geared towards healthcare informatics.

Aditi Joshi is an undergraduate student in the department of Biomedical Engineering at A D Y Patil University, Pune, Maharashtra, India. Her research interests include Medical Electronics and Instrumentation, Human-Computer Interface, Bioinformatics, Prosthetic Organs, Biomaterial and Biomechanics.

Salman Siddique Khan is currently pursuing his B.Tech degree from the Department of Electronics and Communication Engineering, National Institute of Technology, Rourkela, India. His research interests include Signal and Image Processing, and Machine Learning.

Kavi Kumar Khedo is an Associate Professor at the Department of Digital Technologies at the University of Mauritius. He has a B.Eng (Hons) Computer Science and Engineering with First Class Honours and a PhD in Computer Science from the University of Mauritius. Dr Kavi Khedo was awarded UoM Research Excellence Award in 2010 and ICT Personality of the Year 2013. Dr Khedo has published more than 50 research papers on mobile computing, ubiquitous computing, health informatics and wireless sensor networks. Dr Khedo has published research papers in renowned journals and has presented his researches in reputed international conferences. He has also served on numerous editorial boards of distinguished international journals and on technical program committees of popular international conferences such as IEEE Sensors, WILEY International Journal on Communication Systems, International Journal of Sensor Networks, IEEE Africon 2013, IEEE ICIT 2013 and IEEE ICACCA 2017.

Sanjay Kotadiya is presently working as Technical Officer at Division of Physiology & Ergonomics, ICMR-National Institute of Occupational Health, Ahmedabad. He has more than 10 years of research experience in the application of noise, audiometry and occupational ergonomics.

Anushka Kumar is an undergraduate student in the Department of Mechatronics Engineering at A D Y Patil University, Pune, Maharashtra, India. Her research interests include Electronics and Instrumentation, Electro-Mechanical technologies and Automotive research.

Sunil Kumar is Scientist G and Former Director-in-Charge of ICMR-National Institute of Occupational Health, Ahmedabad. He is the recipient of the Shakuntala Amir Chand Prize for the year 1984 of ICMR for significant research contribution in the field of chemical radiation protection. He is the member of several committees on health at the national level. He is the recognized PhD. guide of three universities of India and 08 students have already been awarded PhD. under his guide ship. Dr. Kumar has about 100 original papers/review articles published in various national and International journals.

Naeem A. Mahoto received Master degree in Computer Engineering from Mehran University of Engineering and Technology, Pakistan and Ph.D in Information and System Engineering from Politecnico di Torino, Italy in 2013. He is currently working as Assistant Professor at Department of Software Engineering, Mehran UET Pakistan. His research interests are focused in the field of data mining and bioinformatics. His research activities are also devoted to summarization of web documents, sentiment analysis, data visualization and educational data mining. He is member of IEEE Computer society and Pakistan Engineering Council (PEC).

Joydeep Majumder is presently Scientist C (Ergonomics) at ICMR-National Institute of Occupational Health, Ahmedabad. He has more than 15 years of research experience in the application of ergonomics in industry, agriculture and office workplace. Earlier, he served as Assistant Research Officer (Scientific) at Min. of AYUSH, New Delhi for 3 years, and associated with Central Institute of Agricultural Engineering (ICAR), Bhopal as Human Physiologist for 6 years. He did his masters in Physiology and Ergonomics from Presidency College, University of Calcutta in 2002 and presently pursuing his PhD. in Life Science from Gujarat University, Ahmedabad. He joined NIOH in 2011 as Scientist B and for the last 6 years, he has been involved in research, teaching, training and client projects in the field of occupational ergonomics. He has published 30 papers in peer-reviewed International Journals, 10 co-authored/edited books and over 50 papers in in international and national conference proceedings.

Areej Fatemah Meghji is an Assistant Professor in the Department of Software Engineering at Mehran.U.E.T, Pakistan. She received her M.E from Mehran U.E.T., Pakistan and is presently pursuing her PhD working on Predictive Analysis of Big Data emerging from the sector of Higher Education. Her research interests include Knowledge Management, Data Mining, Natural Language Processing, Artificial Intelligence and Big Data Analytics.

Gajendra Kumar Mourya received his B.E. degree in Biomedical Engineering from Samrat Ashok Technological Institute (SATI) Vidisha, INDIA in 2007. He received his M.Tech degree in Biomedical Engineering from IIT-BHU Varanasi, INDIA in 2010. He is currently an Assistant Professor in the Department of Biomedical Engineering, School of Technology, North-Eastern Hill University (NEHU), Shillong. His research area is Medical Image Processing, Signal Processing and Bioinstrumentation.

Miss Shikshya Nayak is a B.Tech in Electrical and Electronics Engineering from the Department of Electrical Engineering & EEE, Veer Surendra Sai University of Technology, Burla, India.

Suraj Kumar Nayak received his B. Tech. in Electrical Engineering from Government College of Engineering Keonjhar, Odisha, India (formerly known as OSME Keonjhar) and M. Tech. in Biomedical Engineering from National Institute of Technology Rourkela, Odisha, India. Currently, he is pursuing his PhD degree in Biomedical Engineering from National Institute of Technology Rourkela, Odisha, India. His research interests include Biomedical Instrumentation, Biomedical Signal Processing, and Drug Delivery.

Kunal Pal pursued his graduation in Pharmacy from University of Delhi, New Delhi, India in the year 2002 followed by post-graduation in Biomedical Engineering from Jadavpur University, Kolkata, India in the year 2004. Later, he did his Ph.D. in Materials Science from Indian Institute of Technology, Kharagpur, India in the year 2006. Subsequently, he joined Ryerson University, Toronto, Canada as a post-doctoral fellow in the year 2007. During his tenure at Ryerson University, he served as Vice-Chair (Elect), HQPA, AFMNet Network of Excellence, Canada. He joined National Institute of Technology, Rourkela, India in the year 2009 as an Assistant Professor in Biomedical Engineering. He is currently the Professor-in-Charge of Medical Electronics and Instrumentation Laboratory in the Department of Biotechnology and Medical Engineering, National Institute of Technology, Rourkela, India. His major research interests revolve around Biomedical Signal Processing and Biomedical Equipment Design. He is also working in the fields of soft materials and controlled drug delivery. He has more than 150 publications in SCI cited journals of high repute, Book Chapters, and peer-reviewed conferences. He is a very well cited researcher having more than 2000 citations.

Karan Pande received his B. Engg. in Electrical Engineering from The Maharaja Sayajirao University of Baroda, Vadodara, Gujarat, India and M. Tech. in Biomedical Engineering from National Institute of Technology Rourkela, Odisha, India, he is currently working as a Research Associate in BIS Research, NOIDA, India. His research interests include Biomedical Instrumentation, Biomedical Signal Processing, Electrical and Electronics Engineering, Market Research and Consultation.

Sudip Paul is currently an Assistant Professor in the Department of Biomedical Engineering, School of Technology, North-Eastern Hill University (NEHU), Shillong, India since June 2012. He completed his B.Tech and M.Tech degree in Biomedical Engineering. Also he received his Ph.D degree from Indian Institute of Technology (Banaras Hindu University), Varanasi with specialization in Electrophysiology and brain signal analysis. He has also presented his research accomplishments in USA, Greece, France and South Africa. He has many credentials in his credit out of which his First Prize in Sushruta Innovation Award 2011 sponsored by Department of Science and Technology, Govt. of India and also he also organized many workshops and conferences out of which most significant are the 29th Annual meeting of the Society for Neurochemistry, India and IRBO/APRC Associate School 2017. He selected as Post Doc Fellow under Biotechnology Overseas Associateship for the Scientists working in North Eastern States of India: 2017-18 supported by Department of Biotechnology, Government of India. Dr. Sudip published more than 70 International journal and conference papers and also filled one patent. Recently he wrote a book on "Introduction to Rat Brain EEG Signal and its Significance" published by LAP LAMBERT Academic Publishing, Germany.

Ashirbad Pradhan obtained his B.Tech. (Hons.) in Biomedical Engineering from National Institute of Technology, Rourkela in 2016. He has currently joined the Masters program in Faculty of Kinesiology, University of New Brunswick. His areas of interest include myoelectric control, pattern recognition and prosthetic devices

Amit Roy Chowdhury is Professor of Department Aerospace Engineering and Applied Mechanics, IIEST Shibpur and Head of Centre for Healthcare Science and Technology, IIEST, Shibpur. He has obtained his B E from Bengal Engineering College Shibpur (now IIEST), M Tech from IIT Kharagpur and PhD from Jadavpur University, Kolkata. He has been a visiting scientist to State University of New York. He has been the Editor of the Indian Journal of Biomechanics.

Minerva Sarma is an undergraduate student in the department of Biomedical Engineering at A D Y Patil University, Pune, Maharashtra, India. Her research interests include Medical Electronics and Instrumentation, Human-Computer Interface, Prosthetic Organs.

Hiba Shah did Bachelors in Software Engineering from Mehran University of Engineering and Technology, currently doing masters in Software Engineering and working as a Teaching and Research Assistant in Department of Software Engineering, Mehran UET Pakistan.

Bikesh K. Singh received his PhD in 2015 from National Institute of Technology, Raipur (C.G) India. He is presently Assistant Professor and Head of the Department of Biomedical Engineering at National Institute of Technology, Raipur (C.G.) India. He received the Young Scientist Award from C.G. Council of Science and Technology, Raipur in 2010, Young Engineer Award from Institution of Engineers, India (IEI) in 2012 and Gowri Memorial Award from IETE India in 2016. He has published over 40 research papers in International Journals and Conference Proceedings. His research interests include biomedical image processing and analysis, biomedical signal processing and analysis, and soft computing.

Index

I

K

L

M

O

P

R

S

T

W

X

Z

www.ingramcontent.com/pod-product-compliance
Lightning Source LLC
LaVergne TN
LVHW060405300926
849162LV00006B/1344